YALE TEXTBOOK OF PUBLIC PSYCHIATRY

YALE TEXTBOOK OF PUBLIC PSYCHIATRY

EDITED BY

Selby C. Jacobs, MD
PROFESSOR EMERITUS OF PSYCHIATRY
AND PUBLIC HEALTH

Jeanne L. Steiner, DO
ASSOCIATE PROFESSOR OF PSYCHIATRY

EDITORIAL BOARD

Samuel A. Ball, PhD
PROFESSOR OF PSYCHIATRY

Robert M. Rohrbaugh, MD
PROFESSOR OF PSYCHIATRY

Larry Davidson, PhD
PROFESSOR OF PSYCHIATRY

Michael J. Sernyak, MD
PROFESSOR OF PSYCHIATRY

Joanne DeSanto Iennaco, PhD, APRN
ASSOCIATE PROFESSOR, SCHOOL OF NURSING

Thomas H. Styron, PhD
ASSOCIATE PROFESSOR OF PSYCHIATRY

Esperanza Díaz, MD
ASSOCIATE PROFESSOR OF PSYCHIATRY

Howard Zonana, MD
PROFESSOR OF PSYCHIATRY

Thomas J. McMahon, PhD
ASSOCIATE PROFESSOR OF PSYCHIATRY
AND CHILD STUDY CENTER
ASSOCIATE CLINICAL PROFESSOR
SCHOOL OF NURSING

YALE SCHOOL OF MEDICINE

OXFORD
UNIVERSITY PRESS

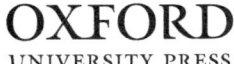

Oxford University Press is a department of the University of Oxford. It furthers
the University's objective of excellence in research, scholarship, and education
by publishing worldwide.Oxford is a registered trade mark of Oxford University
Press in the UK and certain other countries.

Published in the United States of America by Oxford University Press
198 Madison Avenue, New York, NY 10016, United States of America.

© Oxford University Press 2016

First Edition published in 2016

All rights reserved. No part of this publication may be reproduced, stored in
a retrieval system, or transmitted, in any form or by any means, without the
prior permission in writing of Oxford University Press, or as expressly permitted
by law, by license, or under terms agreed with the appropriate reproduction
rights organization. Inquiries concerning reproduction outside the scope of the
above should be sent to the Rights Department, Oxford University Press, at the
address above.

You must not circulate this work in any other form
and you must impose this same condition on any acquirer.

Library of Congress Cataloging-in-Publication Data
Yale textbook of public psychiatry/edited by Selby C. Jacobs and Jeanne L. Steiner.
  p. ; cm.
Textbook of public psychiatry
Includes bibliographical references and index.
ISBN 978-0-19-021467-8 (alk. paper)
I. Jacobs, Selby, 1939–, editor.   II. Steiner, Jeanne L., editor.   III. Title: Textbook of public psychiatry.
[DNLM: 1. Community Mental Health Services—United States.   2. Community Psychiatry—United States.   WM 30.6]
RC443
362.1968900973—dc23
2015020897

9 8 7 6 5 4 3 2 1

Printed by Sheridan, USA

This material is not intended to be, and should not be considered, a substitute for medical or other professional advice. Treatment for the conditions described in this material is highly dependent on the individual circumstances. And, while this material is designed to offer accurate information with respect to the subject matter covered and to be current as of the time it was written, research and knowledge about medical and health issues is constantly evolving and dose schedules for medications are being revised continually, with new side effects recognized and accounted for regularly. Readers must therefore always check the product information and clinical procedures with the most up-to-date published product information and data sheets provided by the manufacturers and the most recent codes of conduct and safety regulation. The publisher and the authors make no representations or warranties to readers, express or implied, as to the accuracy or completeness of this material. Without limiting the foregoing, the publisher and the authors make no representations or warranties as to the accuracy or efficacy of the drug dosages mentioned in the material. The authors and the publisher do not accept, and expressly disclaim, any responsibility for any liability, loss or risk that may be claimed or incurred as a consequence of the use and/or application of any of the contents of this material.

To people recovering from serious mental illnesses and substance use disorders and to those who serve them through clinical services, education, and research.

CONTENTS

Foreword ix
Preface xi
Acknowledgments xiii
Contributors xv

1. Introduction and Significance   1
   Selby C. Jacobs, Samuel A. Ball, Larry Davidson, Esperanza Díaz, Joanne DeSanto Iennaco, Thomas J. McMahon, Robert M. Rohrbaugh, Jeanne L. Steiner, Thomas H. Styron, Michael J. Sernyak, and Howard Zonana

PART I
THE SERVICE SYSTEM OF PUBLIC PSYCHIATRY

2. The Service System of Public Psychiatry   15
   Selby C. Jacobs, Andres Barkil-Oteo, Paul DiLeo, Patricia Rehmer, and Larry Davidson

3. Recovery and Recovery-Oriented Practice   33
   Larry Davidson, Janis Tondora, Maria J. O'Connell, Chyrell Bellamy, Jean-Francois Pelletier, Paul DiLeo, and Patricia Rehmer

4. Community Supports and Inclusion   49
   Thomas H. Styron, Janis L. Tondora, Rebecca A. Miller, Marcia G. Hunt, Laurie L. Harkness, Joy S. Kaufman, Morris D. Bell, and Allison N. Ponce

PART II
SYSTEM INTEGRATION CHALLENGES IN PUBLIC PSYCHIATRY

5. Integrated Health Care   63
   Aniyizhai Annamalai, Cenk Tek, Michael J. Sernyak, Robert Cole, and Jeanne L. Steiner

6. Substance Use Disorders and Systems of Care   81
   Donna LaPaglia, Brian Kiluk, Lisa Fucito, Jolomi Ikomi, Matthew Steinfeld, and Srinivas Muvvala

7. Public Health Concepts in Public Psychiatry   97
   Joanne DeSanto Iennaco, Jacob Kraemer Tebes, and Selby C. Jacobs

8. The Interplay Between Forensic Psychiatry and Public Psychiatry   115
   Reena Kapoor, Susan Parke, Charles C. Dike, Paul Amble, Nancy Anderson, and Howard Zonana

PART III
SERVICES AND CLINICAL COMPETENCIES OF PUBLIC PSYCHIATRY

9. Children, Adolescents, and Young Adults in the Publicly Funded System of Care   133
   Thomas J. McMahon, Nakia M. Hamlett, Christy L. Olezeski, Timothy C. Van Deusen, Natasha Harris, and Doreen J. Flanigan

10. Early Intervention and Prevention for Psychotic Disorders   155
    Jessica M. Pollard, Cenk Tek, Scott W. Woods, Thomas H. McGlashan, and Vinod H. Srihari

11. Hospital Services   171
    Charles C. Dike, Marc Hillbrand, Richard Ownbey, Daniel Papapietro, John L. Young, Srinivas Muvvala, and Selby C. Jacobs

12. Outpatient Behavioral Care Services   185
    Deborah Fisk, Joanne DeSanto Iennaco, Donna LaPaglia, and Aniyizhai Annamalai

13. Clinical Competence in Outreach and for Special Populations   197
    Anne Klee, Lynette Adams, Neil Beesley, Deborah Fisk, Marcia G. Hunt, Monica Kalacznik, Howard Steinberg, and Laurie Harkness

14. Cultural Competence and Public Psychiatry   211
    Esperanza Díaz, Michelle Silva, Elena F. Garcia-Aracena, Luis Añez, Manuel Paris, Andres Barkil-Oteo, Aniyizhai Annamalai, Miriam Delphin-Rittmon, and Selby Jacobs

15. Global Mental Health   223
    Carla Marienfeld, Andres Barkil-Oteo, Aniyizhai Annamalai, and Hussam Jefee-Bahloul

PART IV
SYSTEM DEVELOPMENT IN PUBLIC PSYCHIATRY

16. Education and Workforce Development in Public Psychiatry   235
Jeanne L. Steiner, Chyrell Bellamy, Michael A. Hoge, Joanne DeSanto Iennaco, Anne Klee, Allison N. Ponce, Robert M. Rohrbaugh, David A. Ross, Thomas H. Styron, and Selby C. Jacobs

17. Evidence-Based Public Psychiatry   249
Jack Tsai, Joanne DeSanto Iennaco, Julienne Giard, and Rani A. Hoff

18. Administrative Best Practices in Public Psychiatry   261
Andres Barkil-Oteo, Margaret Bailey, Robert Cole, Miriam Delphin-Rittmon, Susan Devine, Selby C. Jacobs, Jeanne L Steiner, Louis Trevisan, and Michael J. Sernyak

19. Conclusion and Future Challenges   273
Selby C. Jacobs, Samuel A. Ball, Larry Davidson, Esperanza Díaz, Joanne DeSanto Iennaco, Thomas J. McMahon, Robert M. Rohrbaugh, Jeanne L. Steiner, Thomas H. Styron, Michael J. Sernyak, and Howard Zonana

Index   287

FOREWORD

The emergence of this important textbook on public psychiatry signals a new era of transformative work in this area from a department with a long and distinguished history in the field. The Yale Department of Psychiatry was established by the Yale Medical School in 1930, under the leadership of Eugen Kahn, a protégé of the pioneer Emil Kraeplin. However, the Department emerged in its current form in 1948, as a result of a fundamental restructuring of its mission and organization under the leadership of Francis ("Fritz") Redlich, who was chair of the Department for 20 years. Dr. Redlich was a pioneer in public psychiatry whose research identified significant disparities in mental health treatments available to patients from upper socioeconomic groups compared with those available to poor patients in New Haven, as documented in his seminal book *Social Class and Mental Illness*. Through his personal example and through his leadership, Dr. Redlich demonstrated his commitment to the development of public psychiatry as an academic discipline with prominence in the Department equal to that of biological and psychological research. In 1957, Dr. Redlich began pioneering discussions with Abraham Ribicoff, then Governor of Connecticut, about the creation of a public psychiatry institute to address mental health disparities. After President Kennedy signed the Community Mental Health Center Act in 1963, Dr. Redlich implemented these plans with federal and state assistance. The Connecticut Mental Health Center (CMHC), opened in 1966, remains an exemplar of a public–academic partnership between the State of Connecticut Department of Mental Health and Addiction Services and Yale University. As we near the 50th anniversary of CMHC's founding, Dr. Redlich's vision of a public psychiatry institute fostering lively interdisciplinary faculty exchanges leading to improved outcomes for patients in the public sector has been fully realized. The programs at CMHC, including a clinical neuroscience unit to develop new biological treatments, have helped vulnerable and disadvantaged populations, with a special emphasis on those from ethnic and cultural minorities. The public psychiatry research portfolio at CMHC helped establish the evidence base for many public psychiatry clinical interventions and currently includes projects on ensuring patient's perspectives are included in service development and delivery, prevention of mental health disorders through school-based interventions, early interventions for patients with emerging psychotic symptoms, jail diversion for patients with mental illness in the justice system, and interventions for patients with addictions. A recent partnership between the CMHC and a local Federally Qualified Health Center provides an opportunity to explore integrated medical and psychiatric care and wellness for indigent people with serious mental illnesses and/or addictions.

Although the CMHC was founded to promote a public psychiatry mission, Yale faculty at the VA Connecticut Healthcare System (VACHS), Yale-New Haven Hospital (YNHH), and other affiliated sites in the Yale Department of Psychiatry have also made substantial contributions to the field. Over the past three decades, VA Connecticut has been a leader in pioneering and evaluating psychosocial rehabilitation programs, many of which have been disseminated widely within the national VA system. The Errera Community Care Center at VA Connecticut is widely viewed as a national model for the integration of recovery-oriented psychosocial rehabilitation into the continuum of mental health care. Treatment for many patients at the YNHH, a general, not-for-profit hospital, is reimbursed by Medicaid and Medicare. With the expansion of Medicaid eligibility in Connecticut under the Affordable Care Act, the YNHH is increasingly serving patients previously treated in public psychiatry settings. Evidence of the importance of the public psychiatry mission across all three institutions in the Yale Department of Psychiatry can be found in the contributions of 74 of our faculty members to this textbook.

Our public psychiatry faculty members provide outstanding training to students of the health professions. Medical students and psychiatric residents have opportunities to work on interdisciplinary teams caring for highly stigmatized, vulnerable patients, alongside nursing, psychology, and social work trainees. Community mental health workers, some of whom are also consumers of mental health care, provide an important recovery-oriented perspective to our trainees' education. Our faculty members have developed toolboxes to educate others in culturally sensitive mental health care. Exposing trainees from various disciplines to a public psychiatry perspective and to compelling state-of-the-art clinical care and research programs has inspired generations of our trainees to become involved in public psychiatry careers. Opportunities to gain additional specialized expertise are available through highly regarded advanced fellowships in public psychiatry and in psychosocial rehabilitation. The deep public–academic partnerships between the Yale Department of Psychiatry and the State of Connecticut at CMHC, and our Department and the federal government at VACHS, have been and continue to be mutually beneficial to each partner. The public partners have provided invaluable support, and, in return, the academic partner has advocated for the mission, educated large numbers of professionals who pursue careers within the public psychiatry system, and developed national model programs that provide the evidence base to meet contemporary challenges in public psychiatry. These widely disseminated programs illustrate our commitment to meet the challenge of the Yale Department of Psychiatry's mission statement to diminish the disability caused by mental illness. We commend this textbook to the next generation of professionals and leaders of public psychiatry.

Robert M. Rohrbaugh, MD
Professor and Deputy Chair for Education
and Career Development
Residency Program Director
Department of Psychiatry
Director, Office of International Medical Student
Education Yale University School of Medicine

John H. Krystal, MD
Robert L. McNeil, Jr. Professor of Translational
Research and Professor of Neurobiology
Chair, Department of Psychiatry
Yale University School of Medicine
Chief of Psychiatry, Yale-New Haven Hospital

PREFACE

This textbook is authored and edited by faculty members of the Yale Department of Psychiatry who practice, teach, and conduct clinical and evaluative research in public psychiatry. It is a comprehensive, integrated, and interdisciplinary introduction to public psychiatry for advanced professional students. As such, it is conceived in relation to the core, discipline-based educational programs of professional students. It is guided by unified educational aims, a shared teaching philosophy, and an integrated perspective (public psychiatry in relation to primary care, addiction medicine, public health, and forensic psychiatry) with regard to the service system and practices of public psychiatry. It emphasizes the competencies necessary for professional careers in public psychiatry.

Interdisciplinary professional education is a central tenet of the educational philosophy of this textbook. This education principle stems from a conviction that interdisciplinary team practice is the best organizational unit for providing services within a system of care to people with serious mental illnesses and substance use disorders. Essentially, the authors and editors believe that those who learn together—not only about the elements of care and the system, but also about their respective strengths, limitations, and professional aspirations—will practice better together. The net result is a stronger service unit that serves as a cornerstone of the workforce of public psychiatry. Although coming from an academic setting in a particular locality in the United States, the description of American public psychiatry in the textbook is generally applicable to other settings. All programs in public psychiatry serve a population of individuals with serious mental illnesses and substance use disorders. In every locality, federal policies and funding sources support and shape the service structures for this population. Professionals in public psychiatry, through meetings and publications, shape universal practices. Shared evidence-based practices unite practice in public psychiatry across the country. Despite variation from state to state and locality to locality, a basic foundation and knowledge base of public psychiatry prevails.

Although intended as a textbook for use in advanced, year-long internships or fellowships in public psychiatry, selected chapters can also serve as an introductory module for beginning professional students. For example, the first four chapters include an introduction to public psychiatry by providing definitions for terms such as serious mental illnesses and substance use disorders, a discussion of the service system of public psychiatry, an introduction to recovery concepts and practices, and a description of community supports and inclusion programs. Other chapters might be chosen for an introductory module given the educational aims of an introductory module.

This textbook is timely for a number of reasons. Health care reform under the Affordable Care Act considerably expands access to behavioral services for previously uninsured people. Medicaid is a vehicle for much of the expansion. Those gaining coverage under Medicaid will gravitate to community health centers and behavioral health centers for care. Meeting this new demand for service requires an expanded and well-trained workforce. Already, departments of psychiatry are anecdotally reporting an increase in applicants interested in public psychiatry. Many advanced fellowships in public psychiatry already exist, but more will be needed to provide essential interdisciplinary education while working with the target population within a public service system.

In a concluding chapter, this textbook suggests that academic centers of public psychiatry can play an essential role in moving the field forward. Academic divisions of public psychiatry that bring together veterans' services and state-funded services, for example, can make rich contributions to their home departments. Some departments of psychiatry already have such divisions, and others are contemplating it. In this regard, July 1 and September 28, 2016, mark, respectively, the 50th anniversary of the opening and the dedication of the Connecticut Mental Health Center in the Yale Department of Psychiatry, an illustration of an enduring, mutually beneficial partnership between the State of Connecticut and Yale University. In part, this textbook is a celebration of that anniversary.

As noted earlier, this textbook is intended primarily for advanced, professional students of public psychiatry. Certainly, psychiatric educators will also take an interest, not only those directly teaching public psychiatry but also other faculty members involved in departmental education, in order to appreciate how public psychiatry may fit into a broader curriculum. The textbook may also be of interest to public administrators who wish for an overview of the field. Finally, the textbook may be useful to people, such as individuals in recovery from serious mental illnesses and substance use disorders, and their families, who are seeking a greater understanding of treatment approaches and community supports available to them.

Although the editors and authors have done their utmost to provide a comprehensive introduction to current, public psychiatry, given the anticipated transitions in public psychiatry over the next several years, it is almost inevitable that the content of the textbook will become outdated. The authors and editors anticipate this possibility. Accordingly, the textbook will be updated regularly to reflect new developments. The authors and editors are pursuing academic careers in public psychiatry and will be informed of transitions that are occurring. In addition, they welcome feedback from readers of the textbook about omissions or needed updates.

The Editorial Board
March 31, 2015

ACKNOWLEDGMENTS

The Editors are grateful for support from the Connecticut Department of Mental Health and Addiction Services and the Department of Psychiatry of the Yale University School of Medicine. We thank Annette Forte and Nina Levine for their editorial assistance.

CONTRIBUTORS

All authors are faculty members within the Yale Department of Psychiatry, who hold academic appointments at the Yale School of Medicine, Yale School of Nursing, Yale Child Study Center and/or the Yale School of Public Health

Lynette Adams, PhD
Assistant Clinical Professor
Women Veterans Program Manager
VA Connecticut Healthcare System

Paul Amble, MD
Assistant Clinical Professor
Chief Consulting Forensic Psychiatrist
CT Department of Mental Health Service

Nancy Anderson, APRN
Lecturer
Director, Community Forensic Services
Connecticut Mental Health Center

Luis Añez-Nava, PsyD
Associate Professor
Director, Hispanic Clinic
Connecticut Mental Health Center
Director, CT Latino Behavioral Health System

Aniyizhai Annamalai, MD
Assistant Professor
Medical Director, Wellness Center
Connecticut Mental Health Center

Margaret Bailey, LCSW
Clinical Instructor
Director, Clinical Services
Connecticut Mental Health Center

Samuel A. Ball, PhD
Professor
Assistant Chair for Education and Career Development
President and Chief Executive Officer,
CASA Columbia

Andres Barkil-Oteo, MD, MSC
Assistant Professor
Medical Director, Acute Services
Connecticut Mental Health Center

Neil Beesley, LCSW
Lecturer
Chief, Social Work Service
VA Connecticut Healthcare System

Morris D. Bell, PhD, ABPP
Professor
Senior Research Career Scientist
Department of Veterans Affairs, Rehab R&D
Program Director, NIMH Research Fellowship in Functional Disability Interventions

Chyrell D. Bellamy, PhD, MSW
Assistant Professor
Director of Peer Services and Research
Yale Program for Recovery and Community Health

Robert Cole, MHSA
Lecturer
Chief Operating Officer, Connecticut Mental Health Center

Larry Davidson, PhD
Professor
Director, Yale Program for Recovery and Community Health

Miriam Delphin-Rittmon, PhD
Assistant Professor
Commissioner, CT Department of Mental Health and Addiction Services

Joanne DeSanto Iennaco, PhD, APRN
Associate Professor
Specialty Coordinator, Psychiatric-Mental
Health Nurse Practitioner Program
Yale School of Nursing

Susan Devine, APRN
Lecturer
Director, New Haven Office of Court Evaluations
Director, Risk Management
Connecticut Mental Health Center

Esperanza Díaz, MD
Associate Professor
Medical Director, Hispanic Clinic
Connecticut Mental Health Center
Medical Director, CT Latino Behavioral Health System
Associate Director,
Psychiatry Residency Program

Charles C. Dike, MD, MPH, FRCPsych
Assistant Professor
Associate Program Director,
Fellowship in Forensic Psychiatry
Deputy Medical Director, Department of
Mental Health and Addiction Services

Paul J. DiLeo, FACHE
Lecturer
Chief Operating Officer,
Department of Mental Health and Addiction Services

Deborah Fisk, PhD, LCSW
Assistant Clinical Professor
Team Director, Outpatient Services
Connecticut Mental Health Center

Doreen Flanigan, LCSW
Clinical Instructor
Clinician, West Haven Mental Health Clinic
Connecticut Mental Health Center

Lisa Fucito, PhD
Assistant Professor
Program Director, Tobacco Treatment
Smilow Cancer Hospital at Yale-New Haven

Elena F. Garcia-Aracena, MD
Clinical Instructor
Attending Psychiatrist, Hispanic Clinic
Connecticut Mental Health Center

Julienne Giard, LCSW
Lecturer
Director, Evidence-Based Practices
CT Department of Mental Health
and Addiction Services

Nakia M. Hamlett, PhD
Assistant Professor
Clinician, Young Adult Service
Connecticut Mental Health Center

Laurie L. Harkness, MSW, PhD
Clinical Professor
Director, Errera Community Care Center
VA Connecticut Healthcare System

Natasha Harris, APRN
Lecturer
Clinician, West Haven Mental Health Clinic and Young
Adult Service
Connecticut Mental Health Center

Marc Hillbrand, PhD
Assistant Clinical Professor
Former Chief of Psychology, Connecticut Valley Hospital

Rani A. Hoff, PhD, MPH
Professor
Associate Director, Robert Wood Johnson Clinical
Scholars Program
Director, Northeast Program Evaluation Center,
Office of Mental Health Operations,
Department of Veterans Affairs
Director, Evaluation Division, National Center for PTSD

Michael A. Hoge, PhD
Professor
Director, Yale Behavioral Health
Director, Clinical Training in Psychology

Marcia G. Hunt, PhD
Assistant Professor
Associate Director, Veteran Affairs Northeast Program
Evaluation Center
Office of Mental Health Operations, Veterans Health
Administration

Jolomi Ikomi, MD
Assistant Professor
Former Medical Director, Substance Abuse Treatment Unit
Connecticut Mental Health Center

Selby C. Jacobs, MD
Professor Emeritus
Attending Psychiatrist, Hispanic Clinic
Former Director, Connecticut Mental Health Center

Hussam Jefee-Bahloul, MD
Lecturer
Division of Substance Abuse

Monica Kalacznik, MD
Lecturer
Medical Director, Assertive Community
Treatment Team
Connecticut Mental Health Center

Reena Kapoor, MD
Assistant Professor
Associate Program Director,
Fellowship in Forensic Psychiatry
Attending Psychiatrist, Community Forensic Team
Connecticut Mental Health Center

Joy S. Kaufman, PhD
Associate Professor
Deputy Director for Operations,
Yale Consultation Center
Director, Evaluation Research,
Division of Prevention and Community Research

Brian Kiluk, PhD
Assistant Professor
Psychologist, Substance Abuse Treatment Unit
Connecticut Mental Health Center

Anne Klee, PhD
Assistant Professor
Director, Peer Services and Education and Training,
Errera Community Care Center
Director, Interprofessional Residency in Psychosocial
Rehabilitation and Recovery Services
VA Connecticut Healthcare System

John H. Krystal, MD
Robert L. McNeil, Jr. Professor of Translational Research
and Professor of Neurobiology
Chair, Department of Psychiatry
Chief of Psychiatry, Yale-New Haven Hospital

Donna LaPaglia, PsyD
Assistant Professor
Director, Substance Abuse Treatment Unit
Connecticut Mental Health Center

Carla Marienfeld, MD
Assistant Professor
Site Training Director, Yale Addiction
Psychiatry Fellowship
Director, Psychiatry Residency Global Mental
Health Program

Thomas H. McGlashan, MD
Professor Emeritus & Senior Research Scientist
Founder, PRIME Psychosis Prodrome
Research Clinic

Thomas J. McMahon, PhD
Associate Professor
Director, West Haven Mental Health Clinic and Young
Adult Service
Director of Clinical Research
Connecticut Mental Health Center

Rebecca A. Miller, PhD
Assistant Professor
Director, Peer Support
Connecticut Mental Health Center

Srinivas Muvvala, MD, MPH
Assistant Professor
Medical Director, Substance Abuse Treatment Unit
Connecticut Mental Health Center

Maria J. O'Connell, PhD
Associate Professor
Research & Evaluation Area Leader
Yale Program for Recovery and Community Health

Christy L. Olezeski, PhD
Assistant Professor
Clinician, Young Adult Service
Connecticut Mental Health Center

Richard Ownbey, MD
Assistant Clinical Professor
Director of Medical Education,
Connecticut Valley Hospital

Daniel Papapietro, PsyD
Assistant Clinical Professor
Chief of Psychotherapy Services,
Connecticut Valley Hospital

Manuel Paris, PsyD
Associate Professor
Deputy Director, Hispanic Services
Connecticut Mental Health System

Susan Parke, MD
Assistant Professor
Attending Psychiatrist, Community Forensic Service
Connecticut Mental Health Center

Jean Francois Pelletier, PhD
Assistant Clinical Professor
Psychologist, Yale Program for Recovery
and Community Health

Jessica M. Pollard, PhD
Assistant Professor
Director of Clinical Services,
Program for Specialized Treatment Early in
Psychosis [STEP]
Connecticut Mental Health Center

Allison N. Ponce, PhD
Associate Professor
Associate Director, Community Services
Network of Greater New Haven
Connecticut Mental Health Center

Patricia Rehmer, MSN
Lecturer
Former Commissioner, CT Department
of Mental Health and Addiction Services

Robert M. Rohrbaugh, MD
Professor and Deputy Chair for Education
and Career Development
Residency Program Director, Department of Psychiatry
Director, Office of International Medical Student
Education, School of Medicine

David Ross, MD, PhD
Assistant Professor
Associate Director, Psychiatry Residency Program

Michael J. Sernyak, MD
Professor
Chief Executive Officer, Connecticut
Mental Health Center
Deputy Chair, Clinical Affairs and Program Development,
Department of Psychiatry
Director, Division of Public Psychiatry

Michelle Silva, PsyD
Assistant Professor
Associate Director, CT Latino Behavioral Health System

Vinod H. Srihari, MD
Associate Professor
Director, Program for Specialized Treatment Early in
Psychosis [STEP]
Connecticut Mental Health Center
Associate Director, Psychiatry Residency Program

Howard Steinberg, PhD
Assistant Professor
Director, Psychosocial Residential Rehabilitation
Treatment Program
VA Connecticut Healthcare System

Jeanne L. Steiner, DO
Associate Professor
Medical Director, Connecticut Mental Health Center
Director, Yale Fellowship in Public Psychiatry

Matthew Steinfeld, PhD
Assistant Professor
Psychologist, Substance Abuse Treatment Unit
Connecticut Mental Health Center

Thomas H. Styron, PhD
Associate Professor
Director, Community Services Network of
Greater New Haven
Connecticut Mental Health Center

Jacob Kraemer Tebes, PhD
Professor
Director, Division of Prevention and Community
Research
Director, The Consultation Center
Chief Psychologist, Connecticut Mental Health Center
Director, NIDA T32 Postdoctoral Research Training
Program in Substance Abuse Prevention

Cenk Tek, MD
Associate Professor
Director, Psychosis Program
Connecticut Mental Health Center

Janis L. Tondora, PsyD
Assistant Professor
Systems Transformation Area Leader
Yale Program for Recovery and Community Health

Louis Trevisan, MD
Associate Professor
Associate Chief, Mental Health Service Line
VA Connecticut Healthcare System

Jack Tsai, PhD
Assistant Professor
Co-Director, Yale Division of Mental Health Services and Treatment Outcomes Research

Timothy C. VanDeusen, MD
Assistant Professor
Medical Director, West Haven Mental Health Clinic and Young Adult Service
Connecticut Mental Health Center

Scott W. Woods, MD
Professor
Chief, PRIME Psychosis Prodrome Research Clinic
Attending Psychiatrist, Connecticut Mental Health Center

John L. Young, MD, MTh
Clinical Professor

Howard Zonana, MD
Professor
Director, Law and Psychiatry Division
Director, Fellowship in Forensic Psychiatry

1.

INTRODUCTION AND SIGNIFICANCE

Selby C. Jacobs, Samuel A. Ball, Larry Davidson, Esperanza Díaz, Joanne DeSanto Iennaco, Thomas J. McMahon, Robert M. Rohrbaugh, Jeanne L. Steiner, Thomas H. Styron, Michael J. Sernyak, and Howard Zonana

---

EDUCATIONAL HIGHLIGHTS

- Public psychiatry encompasses special clinical competencies for practice in a complex system designed to serve the needs of people with serious mental illnesses (SMIs) and/or substance use disorders (SUDs).

- Public psychiatry is particularly important at this moment in history, as public sector practice is considerably expanded under the Affordable Care Act of 2010.

- Public psychiatry is a large sector of the field of psychiatry, one that makes an essential impact on the lives of people with SMIs and SUDs.

- The educational principles that guide this textbook derive from a commitment to an integrated system of care informed by public health.

- Important features of the service system include person-centered care, recovery orientation, interdisciplinary teams, community-based practice, cultural competence, integrated practice, population-based practice, evidence-based practice, and quality assurance, including peer and family satisfaction.

The educational principles of this textbook include the development of advanced interdisciplinary education (assuming basic clinical skills are already in place), integration of all aspects of practice, attention to a full range of services, and the cultivation of continuing self-education in a structure of supervised clinical placements, seminars, and faculty supervision.

INTRODUCTION

Mental health professionals who specialize in public psychiatry must master a body of knowledge and domain of practice. What is public psychiatry? Who does public psychiatry serve? Does practice require special skills? Is there a special system of services for public psychiatry? Are there special educational needs for people interested in entering public psychiatry? What is the special content, if any, of education in public psychiatry? Is a textbook needed at this point in time? What are the educational principles of this textbook? This introduction sets out to answer these questions and thereby previews the education in public psychiatry embodied in this book.

WHAT IS PUBLIC PSYCHIATRY?

Building on definitions offered by others,[1,2] this textbook uses the following definition of public psychiatry[3]: public psychiatry is that part of the practice of psychiatry that is (1) financed by the general funds of state departments of mental health or (2) by reimbursement income from entitlements such as Medicaid. For disabled, chronically ill individuals, Medicare also funds acute services, with eligibility determined by the Social Security Administration. In addition, the US Department of Housing and Urban Development supports residential services. Public psychiatry provides a safety net of services for low-income persons with serious mental illnesses (SMIs) and co-occurring or independent substance use disorders (SUD). The practice of public psychiatry incorporates evidence-based treatments, psychosocial rehabilitation, person-centered recovery plans of care, integration with primary care through medical homes, integration with substance use services, community supports such as housing and money management, and attention to social issues such as legal status, child protection, or homelessness. Public psychiatry is practiced in many settings. These include mental health and addiction agencies, community health centers, residential and nursing care facilities, psychosocial rehabilitation agencies, hospital-based primary care centers, and organizations offering forensic or public health programs. Practice typically occurs through interdisciplinary teams (IDTs). Also, given the multiplicity of settings and tasks, and also given the organizations such as community mental health centers or community health (primary care) centers where public psychiatry is practiced, system knowledge, management skills, and a community perspective are important for clinical success. Public psychiatry uses not only a clinical perspective while caring for the individual service user, but also a population perspective. It attends to public health data, epidemiologic studies, and health services research for the purpose of planning, evaluating, implementing, and managing services.

This definition of public psychiatry incorporates elements from major historical and policy developments since 1963, when Congress enacted the Community Mental Health Centers Act during the Kennedy Administration.[3] The definition is professional, medical, clinical, and administrative. It incorporates a broad clinical and public health perspective on psychiatric disorders and clinical services. Because public practice now takes place in both private and public locations, blurring the distinction between these two settings, this definition avoids the trap of defining public psychiatry in terms of the place or system where it is practiced.

Psychiatric services of the Veteran's Administration (VA) Healthcare System are not included in this definition, nor are they routinely incorporated into definitions of public psychiatry. The VA is sufficiently distinct as a national health service for veterans that it deserves separate consideration. The VA system deserves and, indeed, would require an entire textbook itself. Still, public psychiatry can learn much from many parallel programs in the VA system, such as outreach programs, rehabilitation programs, and services research. Indeed, some veterans move back and forth between the systems and differ in their preferences for public versus veteran services. This textbook takes advantage of the overlap between the systems and cites VA programs and examples in subsequent chapters. In the Yale Department of Psychiatry, faculty members at the Connecticut Mental Health Center and the West Haven Campus of the VA Connecticut Healthcare System collaborate in teaching and investigations and make up a departmental academic division of public psychiatry (see Chapter 19) devoted to education and research.

The chapters following this introduction amplify a description of the service system of public psychiatry; subsequent chapters address clinical competence, and additional chapters cover additional skills and themes that are important for successful practice in public psychiatry.

WHO IS SERVED BY PUBLIC PSYCHIATRY?

There is no simple answer to the question of who is served by public psychiatry. The short answer is that public psychiatry serves both children and adults who suffer from SMIs and/or addictions and who sometimes make up special populations, such as people with traumatic brain injury or problematic sexual behavior, that fall to state responsibility to provide care to, if not protect society from.

The term "serious mental illness" is often used to refer to the disorders of the core, target population served by public psychiatry. The term "serious mental illness" was coined to denote people with severe, recurrent, chronic, or persistent disabling mental illnesses and addictions.[4,5] It is used interchangeably in this text with "severe and persistent mental illness," a term that originated in studies done in the Yale Department of Psychiatry.[6] SMIs typically include schizophrenia spectrum disorders with residual symptoms; recurrent bipolar illness; chronic, relapsing depressive disorders; severe anxiety syndromes; and severe personality disorders, all with comorbidity and psychosocial disabilities. When substance abuse is added into the picture, which is often the case, SMI becomes even more challenging to treat. On the substance abuse side, severe addictions can be intractable and are often multiple, chronically relapsing, and disabling. Many of these chronic disorders are also associated with the risk of suicide and/or a risk of violence to others. As noted earlier, public psychiatry also cares for special populations, many of whom have severe and persistent illness as defined and for whom the state takes responsibility to provide care and to protect society in circumstances of high risk. In epidemiologic studies, which estimate a 26% prevalence of all psychiatric illnesses in the American population, about 6% of the total population have the most serious illnesses (see Chapter 7). Indeed, the population that public psychiatry serves is one of the most salient characteristics of public practice.

The root causes for psychiatric illnesses remain unknown. Although evidence-based treatments relieve symptoms, and recovery occurs in the community, cures are rarely achievable. Estimates of shortened life expectancy and years lost to disability from SMIs, known as *burden of disease*, place them among the top ten of all kinds of diseases (see Chapter 7). As the Mental Health Services Act of 1980 asserted, persons with SMIs served in the public sector are the most needy and vulnerable of all the people served by American psychiatry and medicine.

The pathway of a person with SMI or a SUD into public sector services varies by the nature of the illness, the course of illness over time, and access to care. Historically, examples have included young people with psychotic disorders who are no longer eligible for health insurance coverage under their parents and persons for whom the limited insurance benefits offered for treatment of psychiatric disorders have been exhausted. Also, many people become incapacitated and unemployed, thus making employer-based insurance inaccessible. How these various scenarios will change with current health reform efforts remains to be seen. Many people living in poverty are eligible for Medicaid and, once an illness is chronic, Medicare. These payers can serve as a pathway into the system. Finally, many people with SMIs or SUDs are identified primarily, at least at first, by a major social problem, whether it is homelessness, of which about 40% are considered seriously ill, or people transitioning out of prisons, of which about 80% are estimated to have SUDs.

In contrast to the rest of psychiatric practice, is there something distinct or different about those people with mental health and SUDs who are served by public psychiatry? Arguably, the answer is yes. The illnesses typically encountered in public practice are chronic and associated with disability. It is this combination of acute, often recurrent illness; chronic residual symptoms; comorbidity with various other psychiatric disorders, mental health disorders and addictions, and physical health problems; disabilities; the need for psychosocial rehabilitation and community supports; and aspirations for recovery as well as full citizenship that characterizes the typical person served in the public system. Furthermore, social problems of poverty, legal embroilments, and homelessness are commonplace and intermingle inextricably with the clinical picture. This clinical complexity is a hallmark of the population served.

The target population of people served by public psychiatry has varied over the years since inception of the modern era in 1963. This variation has been a function of ongoing budget crises and policy initiatives that invariably lead to discussions of exactly who is the target population. (See Chapter 2 for a brief discussion of the major periods of modern public psychiatry.) At first, during the 1970s, the definition of the target population emphasized those who resided in a particular community (the so-called *catchment* in the community mental health lexicon), especially those coming out of state hospitals.

Next, as the system seemed to be failing people with chronic conditions who were discharged from hospitals into the community, the definition of the target population swung to people with severe and persistent mental illness living in the community. During the same time in the 1980s, the target population slowly expanded as states began to use Medicaid to finance services. In these circumstances, the definition of the target population emphasized payer status and those eligible for Medicaid. Many of these people had SMIs or SUDs; however, many others who were single and poor were excluded. Services funded by state general funds targeted the latter group, but these resources shrank as states contended with budget problems.

Throughout the modern history of public psychiatry, populations have been identified as the special responsibility of the state, either as a last resort or to protect society. Although many special populations contained a number of people with SMIs or SUDs, the responsibility of public psychiatry for its core target population was often diluted. Despite these variations in target population definition, the central challenge for the public system of services is still to remain true to the core population of people with severe, persistent, and disabling behavioral disorders.

IS THERE A SYSTEM OF PUBLIC PSYCHIATRY?

Despite its apparent disorganization, there is indeed a public psychiatry service system. The current service system is a historical overlay of service and support components laid down over many years, in successive periods of development. The system for SUDs has distinct historical roots and is often orthogonal to mental health services, although many services for co-occurring disorders exist. The system also is stratified at federal, state, and local levels. The US Substance Abuse and Mental Health Services Administration (SAMHSA) and state departments of behavioral health define the purpose and function of the system through policies, demonstration projects, and the financing of services. County and local stratifications of management also contribute to the policies, services, supports, and financing of the system. The mission of serving people with SMIs and/or SUDs unites these parts of the system. Evaluation, treatment, case management, early intervention, outreach to people who are homeless, psychosocial rehabilitation including work and educational supports, other community supports such as housing, integrations with primary care, forensic consultation, peer-run programs, and prevention of behavioral disorders make up the current system of public psychiatry. A full spectrum of mental health and addiction professionals, community-based specialists, and program managers work through IDTs within this system. Federal, state, and local sources finance the services, community supports, and personnel that make up the system. On a local level, the system comprises a variety of organizations: community mental health centers, federally qualified community health (primary care) centers, general hospitals, emergency rooms, state-operated agencies, and private nonprofit agencies provide treatment, rehabilitation, and community supports. Each of these has particular policies, budgets, and a program of services and/or supports that they manage.

As a result of the broad array of services and supports, their disparate sources, and the historically piece-meal development of the current system (see Chapter 2), the service system of public psychiatry is complex, disjointed, and difficult to navigate. To understand it fully requires effort studying it and time working in it. Working on the most basic level of the system, the professional in public psychiatry marshals the multiple elements of the system into individual plans of care for people with SMI and/or addiction. This process is the strongest source of cohesion currently available for making the system work effectively for people who need care.

Chapter 2 fleshes out this starting definition of the service system of public psychiatry with a more detailed description, provides a brief history of its development as a strategy for understanding it, and amplifies a discussion of its financing. Subsequent chapters in this textbook elaborate on public health, substance abuse services, primary care, recovery and social inclusion, forensic services, and other parts of the system.

This definition of the system is universal and generic for the United States. However, below the federal level, considerable variation exists among state authorities for mental health and addiction services, not to mention state Medicaid programs. At the local, county, and city level, considerably more variation exists from place to place depending on state policies and local agency initiatives and development. The array of services available in each locale is a function of all of these levels. At a local level, a description of the system becomes particular and concrete. Still, the particulars of one place (such as New Haven, Connecticut, in the case of this textbook) illustrate usefully the outline of the system in many locations.

The bottom line for the service system is the array of clinical programs and community supports it provides for people with SMIs and/or SUDs, thereby enabling person-centered, individualized plans of care. A key value of this textbook is that it emphasizes that a system ought to incorporate as full a range of services and supports as possible. In this regard, several aspects of the system, including rehabilitative community support, public health, integrated health care, and services for co-occurring disorders and chronic addictions, deserve special emphasis because they have often been given short shrift if not ignored on the clinical side. Subsequent chapters will give full consideration to these parts of the system.

CLINICAL COMPETENCE IN PUBLIC PSYCHIATRY

Professionals in public psychiatry must acquire expertise in caring for people with SMIs and SUDs, the central target population. Psychopharmacologic and psychotherapeutic expertise and psychiatric consultation skills are cornerstones, but they must be supplemented by additional knowledge and skills in the areas of rehabilitation, accommodation, navigation, and the provision of in vivo supports in various life domains affected by these conditions.

Psychopathology for the professional in public psychiatry is more than knowledge of the disorders listed and defined in the *Diagnostic and Statistical Manual, Fifth Edition* (DSM 5)[6] In public psychiatry, the clinical picture is larger and all-encompassing. In the public sector, more so than in other domains of practice, psychiatric disorders defined by DSM5 are associated not only with morbidity caused by relapses, but also with mortality (suicide and premature death from a variety of causes) and impairment in functioning (disability or burden of disease). It is essential for the professional in public psychiatry to attend to all these aspects of illness and their interrelationships. Accordingly, this textbook addresses the entire course of illness, all of its outcomes, and the competencies needed to be effective in practice.

Furthermore, clinical competence in public psychiatry involves mastery of this complex clinical picture as part of an IDT of caregivers in different settings, not just in the hospital and clinic. These include residential settings, the street, rehab centers, legal offices, and homeless shelters. Not only must public psychiatry professionals learn to practice in all these settings, they must be savvy about the system in which they work in order to mobilize it for the people they care for. In contemporary public practice, a supported apartment or other residential setting, as opposed to a hospital, is often the platform for arranging care. These are the settings in which professionals practice without the "white coat" of the hospital setting. The key for making public services work for individuals with SMI and SUDs is the practicing professional in public psychiatry who works as part of, and often leads, an IDT that creates personal, comprehensive, coherent, recovery-oriented, and integrated plans of care in the community while using the hospital, emergency room, and other alternatives (such as respite care) for backup in the case of acute crises.

Furthermore, it is not sufficient for educators and practicing professionals in public psychiatry to assure themselves that their practice is competent. It is also necessary to measure key process and outcome indicators in the various domains of practice in order to document and then strive to improve the quality of care. Quality data, together with the cost of services, are two factors in an equation of value (with value equaling the ratio of quality over cost). Quality measures are useful not only for monitoring and improving outcomes, but also for reporting transparently about the quality of services. In each domain of practice covered in this textbook, such as treatments for SUDs, ambulatory treatment for major disorders, or assertive community treatment, the authors provide a discussion of key quality metrics in that area. A humble attitude of continually striving for improvement, in contrast to assertions of professionalism and even perfection, is the foundation for achieving quality care. Attention to quality metrics, along with independent learning, provides a building block for ongoing clinical competence in the future.

While maintaining a focus on person-centered clinical competence for the professional, the authors of this textbook also assume that many public psychiatry professionals will advance in their careers into positions of leadership. The content, integration, and comprehensiveness of the didactics in this textbook are a foundation not only for clinical competence but also for effective leadership in the field. The best leaders will need clinical competence; a comprehensive, integrated, interdisciplinary understanding of the field of public psychiatry; and well-honed management skills.

IS PUBLIC PSYCHIATRY A SUBSPECIALTY OF GENERAL PSYCHIATRY?

Predicated on the logic developed so far, it is important to recognize that public psychiatry is an important subspecialty of the general mental health professions. Advanced education in public psychiatry builds on general education in the mental health professions. In general education, the professional student learns interviewing, diagnosis, psychotherapies, psychopharmacology, consultation, and other aspects of practice in hospital, clinical, and community settings. Advanced education in public psychiatry builds on these foundational skills and addresses the knowledge and practice defined earlier.

At present, public psychiatry is not officially a subspecialty of psychiatry. In the past 20 years, however, several groups have made the case for such certified training.[1,3,7] There is a special body of knowledge to master and professional organizations to support such specialists, and the development of certified education programs would fill an existing need, improve educational quality, and offer a bridge to the future. Within the context of current health care reform and as a result of other factors shaping practice in public psychiatry, it is all the more important to have dedicated, specialized, and certified professionals in public psychiatry.

There is no doubt that public psychiatry makes important contributions to academic departments of psychiatry. In a previous volume, the authors considered the contributions to public psychiatry of academic programs at the Connecticut Mental Health Center of the Yale Department of Psychiatry[8] (see Chapter 19 for a more detailed discussion of this idea). The establishment of advanced qualifications in public psychiatry would enhance these academic pursuits. Also, advanced qualifications would support and consolidate a cadre of academic professionals who are needed to move the field of public psychiatry forward in teaching and research departments of psychiatry during a time of great change. Reflecting this need, the American Association of Community Psychiatrists began certification of advanced credentials in public psychiatry in 2015.

WHAT ARE THE EDUCATIONAL PRINCIPLES OF THIS TEXTBOOK?

The editors and authors have imbued this textbook with their shared beliefs and commitments to a comprehensive curriculum in public psychiatry. Shared educational principles and philosophy guide the content, and an education structure made up of multiple interrelated parts offers many platforms for educational experiences. This textbook contains the core didactics for teaching the care of people with SMIs and co-occurring or independent SUDs. In addition, the didactics are supplemented with selected, current citations in the literature, reflected in the bibliographies for each chapter.

The educational principles of this textbook derive from the authors' shared conviction in and commitment to a publicly funded system of service delivery. Optimal service delivery in the system of public psychiatry is characterized as a full range of services (1) provided by IDTs made up of professionals and specialists; (2) informed by an understanding, derived from public health, of the local community and its population; (3) based in the community; (4) person-centered; (5) recovery-oriented; (6) culturally competent; (7) integrated with primary care, addiction medicine, public health, and forensic psychiatry; (8) evidence-based; (9) competency-based (through training); and (10) driven by consumer and family satisfaction as part of quality improvement. The educational principles apply to the features of the service system defined and itemized earlier, and the organization of the textbook corresponds largely to the typology of the system and the educational principles presented earlier.

It is important to emphasize that the curriculum offered in this textbook is predicated on the assumption that the professional student already has accomplished basic clinical and professional education in interviewing, evaluation, diagnosis, formulation, treatment, and rehabilitation. Assuring this premise is a function of screening and selection of candidates for advanced education in public psychiatry. This principle does not exclude the possibility that selected chapters from the textbook can be used as an introductory module in public psychiatry for beginning professional students.

Second, this textbook is interdisciplinary in editing, authorship, content, consideration of roles, and teaching. It is not designed for just one professional group. The interdisciplinary character of the textbook reflects a conviction that practice in public psychiatry ought to be accomplished through IDTs. Psychiatrists, psychologists, nurses, social workers, rehabilitation therapists, and peer staff bring special skills to the task of caring for people with SMI and addictions. Working together effectively as a team is a professional skill in itself.

Also, the textbook teaches an integrated approach to the practice of public psychiatry. The text integrates the diverse parts of a complex public system with the complementary clinical, rehabilitative, and support tasks of care in the community. It integrates both public health and clinical perspectives. It addresses the integration of public psychiatry and primary care through medical homes, and it also emphasizes the challenge of integrating psychiatry and addiction medicine. The text strives for integration in order to (1) achieve a complete picture of psychiatric and SUDs in the community where they occur, (2) understand the continuum of practice from prevention and early intervention through treatment of acute illness and relapse prevention to finally easing the burden of disease while supporting recovery and citizenship, and (3) have an appreciation of how public psychiatry can help meet the challenges communities face, such as untreated illness, suicide, violence, addictions, and burden of disease.

Furthermore, this textbook emphasizes clinical competence in the educational program. In this textbook, clinical competence is fundamentally person-centered and focused on people with SMIs and SUDs in a variety of settings. Although the human encounter is essentially the same in all of psychiatric practice, the clinical relationship varies in a population of largely poor, culturally diverse people with limited educational opportunities and long-term disabilities. Beyond that, the setting of practice in public psychiatry is not just the short-term hospital, clinic, or emergency room but also the residential program, the street corner, the home, the homeless shelter, the laundromat, and the courthouse. Clinical competence includes not only up-to-date knowledge but also a commitment to continue to learn and to strive for the highest quality of service using transparently reported quality metrics. An educational program requires a curriculum that is designed to meet the various needs of people cared for in public practice, in the settings in which they are encountered, with the highest quality of care.

In addition, this textbook has universal application. Although rooted in a particular institution of an academic department of psychiatry in a particular city and state, the educational program embodied here prepares students for success in public psychiatry anywhere in the United States. Needless to say, the target population of people with SMIs and/or SUDs share common features regardless of setting. Also, the American service system, although varying from state to state and location to location, shares fundamental features. It is for these reasons that the educational content of the textbook is applicable in any setting, any system, and any educational program within the United States.

Finally, this textbook reflects an educational conviction that a system for public psychiatry ought to incorporate a full range of community-based services: acute and long-term clinical, rehabilitation, primary care, addiction, public health, and forensic services and community-based supports. Perhaps the rehabilitative, community support, and public health aspects of the system deserve special emphasis because they are sometimes given short shrift. Rehabilitative programs address disability, including psychological, social, and cognitive approaches. Community-based support focuses on increasing persons' access to housing, jobs, school, faith communities, and other naturally occurring community activities. Public health components of the system include programs for prevention of substance abuse, early intervention in the course of illness, programs to establish and maintain wellness, attention and amelioration of health disparities among subpopulations, and commitment to maintaining a population perspective in the development of the system and the allocation of resources.

As educators, the authors aim to kindle a flame of learning while beginning to fill gaps in existing knowledge. They aspire to spark a lifelong commitment to independent study through reading the literature and using independent judgment about new data. As a starting point, the bibliographies in each chapter offer an entry into the literature. Small seminars in the local fellowship program in public psychiatry are designed to encourage critical thinking and discussion. Students are encouraged to evaluate new evidence and to conduct independent research, with a goal of achieving up-to-date, evidence-based practice throughout a career in public psychiatry. In addition to small seminars, the optimal pedagogical structure includes personal and clinic-based supervision and the creation of a community of curious, science-oriented, public professionals, all of which support this aim. In Chapter 16, a discussion of discipline-based and interdisciplinary teaching of public psychiatry resumes with respect to the elements of education and the important issue of workforce development.

WHAT IS THE VISION FOR THIS TEXTBOOK?

The authors' vision is to contribute through scholarship and teaching to the best possible education in public psychiatry. Using this textbook, the editors' and authors' aim is to prepare advanced professional students as outstanding clinicians, as leaders, and, in some cases, as scholars. The goal is to equip them with up-to-date, clinical, person-centered knowledge and practice within a public service system. Given that the service system is broad, extensive, and complex, the authors believe that the most powerful force for the integration of services and supports is the well-educated, individual professional in public psychiatry. It is the professional clinician and leader—properly and well educated in caring for people with SMIs and/or SUDs; capable of advanced clinical practice in the public sector; knowledgeable in the value of residential and community supports; prepared for integrated health care, addiction medicine, public health, and forensic psychiatry; and expert in recovery—who connects the disparate parts of the system into a plan of care on behalf of and in collaboration with individuals living with SMIs and/or SUDs and their families. The quality of care derives from the incorporation of all these elements into a comprehensive, integrated, systemic, person-centered clinical process.

THE ORGANIZATION AND CONTENT OF THIS TEXTBOOK

This textbook can be seen as a summary of the didactics in a curriculum for public psychiatry. Each chapter, alone or in combination, supplemented by citations from the literature, might serve as a foundation reference for a seminar in a series that provides advanced, professional education in public psychiatry. Selected chapters can serve as the elements of a brief module in public psychiatry for beginning professional students (e.g., the Introduction, Systems, Public Health, Recovery, and the Conclusion).

The textbook has 19 chapters organized into four parts. Chapter 1 introduces the textbook, and Chapter 19 concludes it. The four parts in between are Part I "The Service System of Public Psychiatry, Part II "System Integration Challenges in Public Psychiatry, Part III "The Services and Clinical Competencies of Public Psychiatry," and Part IV "System Development in Public Psychiatry." When appropriate, the chapters offer brief histories of their topic. Most chapters consider quality metrics applicable to their domain, and most chapters cross-reference other chapters to emphasize overlapping and integrative themes. Some of the chapters use case examples to illustrate content. Each chapter includes an opening box summarizing the educational highlights of the chapter. Finally, each chapter has a selected bibliography to serve as an entry into the literature for the purposes of in-depth self-education.

Part I, "The Service System of Public Psychiatry," contains three chapters. The service system is a distinguishing feature of public psychiatry. Chapter 2 offers three perspectives on this complex service system: (1) historical and developmental, (2) descriptive and structural, and (3) economic. It reviews the status of the "de facto" system, the management of the system, the tendency for skewed system development, and system transformation. The chapter identifies the IDT as the fundamental unit of service in the system. The system is an essential constellation of resources and a context for practice in public psychiatry. Chapter 2 covers not only professional and scientific initiatives but also political and economic policies that shape the service system.

Chapter 3 on recovery begins with a brief history of the recovery movement in psychiatry. Recovery is now one of the basic assumptions of public psychiatry. This chapter covers three major implications of recovery: (1) the provision of person-centered care, (2) the development of peer-provided supports, and (3) involvement of peers in assessments of quality and health care outcomes. The "discovery" of recovery is one of the most important developments in public psychiatry in the past 50 years. The fundamental process of person-centered care planning creates a framework for integrating clinical care of symptoms, rehabilitation, and living in the community while responding to the goals and priorities of the person seeking help. It goes beyond symptom reduction to social inclusion and integration into society.

Chapter 4 covers the crucial importance of community supports for practice outside the walls of the hospital. It emphasizes the value of the social inclusion of people with SMIs and addictions in recovery. It covers residential services, supported employment, supported education, and the techniques of psychosocial rehabilitation. It considers the need for all professionals in public psychiatry to integrate clinical care, community supports, and psychosocial rehabilitation within a framework of person-centered care. It takes a "village" committed to community-based integrated care and social inclusion to establish an optimal system of services.

Part II, "System Integration Challenges," includes four chapters regarding four major integrative tasks currently facing the service system of public psychiatry: (1) integrated health care, (2) addiction medicine, (3) public health, and (4) forensic psychiatry. "Integration to the fourth power" is an expression that captures the exponential challenge ahead. Ultimately, the integration of plans of care for individuals seeking service is the most fundamental goal.

Chapter 5 addresses integrated health care and wellness as the latest expression of mainstreaming in public psychiatry, a concept originating in the health policy debates of 1993. Most of the shortened life expectancy of people with SMIs and addictions is related to chronic conditions such as diabetes mellitus, hypertension, cancer, and infectious diseases. This chapter considers the models, levels, and principles of integrated health care. It discusses medical homes, behavioral health homes, and the impetus given to integrated care by the Affordable Care Act (ACA).

Chapter 6 advocates for a greater integration of addiction medicine into public psychiatry and the leadership to carry this out. The chapter considers the service system of addiction medicine; the neurobiology and environmental factors in addiction; diagnosis, pharmacologic, and psychotherapeutic treatments; and dispositions for continuing care. It covers the evaluation and treatment of co-occurring disorders, and it argues for full equity of addiction services with mental health and primary care services. The ACA presents an opportunity to achieve better integration of addiction medicine into medicine and psychiatry, and public psychiatry may be instrumental in making this happen.

Chapter 7 argues that the incorporation of public health and population perspectives into public psychiatry is yet another key integrative task. The chapter provides definitions of key concepts in psychiatric public health. It illustrates how public health data on morbidity, mortality, and disability can inform psychiatric practice. Public health interventions, or prevention, when integrated into practice, offer an amplified spectrum of practices and facilitate adaptation to new models of practice-based population health. An ounce of prevention in public psychiatry has the potential to better balance the service system through enabling reallocation of finite resources to reaching as many people in need of services as possible.

Chapter 8 discusses how the interdigitation of forensic psychiatry and public psychiatry supports essential skills and competencies that need to be integrated into public practice. Many people with SMIs and SUDs have legal problems. Forensic psychiatry has grown, especially in the era of deinstitutionalization, as a large, independent subspecialty to address these issues. Forensic psychiatry provides expertise to the public professional regarding special forensic hospitals, oversight of forensic populations, forensic community services, risk assessment, and collaborations with court, probation, and parole officers.

Part III, "The Services and Clinical Competencies of Public Psychiatry," describes the services and competencies that are essential for public practice. The topics covered are (1) children, adolescent, and young adult services, (2) early intervention for psychosis, (3) hospital services,

(4) ambulatory services, (5) outreach services and services for special populations, (6) cultural competency, and (7) global mental health.

Chapter 9 reviews the public system for children, adolescents, and young adults, where a developmental perspective is essential for clinical practice and services. It covers a spectrum of special treatment considerations for these target populations. Youth who are transitioning out of the child system and into adult services, many of whom are already chronically ill and disabled, are particularly difficult to care for in the community. The chapter considers the challenges facing the child-focused system, including the long-standing need for better integration with the adult-focused system and the need for more manpower.

Chapter 10 presents early intervention programs for psychosis; these are probably the most important program developments in contemporary public psychiatry. These interventions, which distantly echo ideas about community-based crisis intervention that were part of the launch of community mental health in the 1960s, shift the focus of public practice from the end stages of persistent illness and disability to strategies for prevention of disability. Chapter 10 reviews the timing of interventions and first-episode services for the purpose reducing the duration of untreated psychosis. As evidence accumulates and the service system tools up, early intervention is potentially game-changing for the service system of public psychiatry.

Chapter 11 presents clinical services in hospitals. It covers acute care in emergency rooms and on inpatient units of general hospitals and long-term care in state hospitals, including forensic programs. It also reviews partial hospitalization. It elaborates on the IDT in the hospital setting, where team functions are codified in accreditation requirements, hospital departments, and procedures. Skill in working on an IDT is a core competency for professionals in public psychiatry, differentiates them from solo practitioners in psychiatry, and supports this fundamental unit for the delivery of services in the system. Finally, this chapter discusses the hospital as a microcosm in which system variables play out.

Chapter 12 reviews ambulatory services in both community mental health centers and federally qualified community health centers. It breaks down ambulatory services into walk-in, continuing care, transitional care in and out of hospitals, and specialty programs. A broad, truly bio-psychosocial, clinical consciousness underlies the clinical competencies considered in this chapter. Professionals in public psychiatry are the transducers of the system for a person seeking services. Through creative and professional plans of care, the professional in public psychiatry helps to pull the system of services together for the person with SMI and/or SUDs. It is the personal encounter and the cohesion, management, and adaptation of person-centered plans of care for individuals developed by the individual clinician that lies at the heart of practice in public psychiatry.

Chapter 13 presents special outreach services and services for special populations. These include homeless outreach; assertive community treatment; residential treatment programs; programs for those with traumatic brain injury; lesbian, gay, trans-sexual, and transgender services; veterans' services; and elderly services. When public professionals enter many of these domains, the white coat of the hospital usually is left behind and different rules of engagement and competencies are necessary. The chapter discusses clinical competencies in each of these domains.

Chapter 14 describes the cultural competence necessary for professionals in public psychiatry to engage effectively and sustain in treatment people of diverse backgrounds. Cultural competence figures prominently in strategies for reducing disparities in the treatment outcomes for people from cultural or ethnic minorities. The chapter reviews special evaluation modules and general education as fundamental strategies for preparing behavioral professionals to serve a wide range of populations. Person-centered care is a template for cultural competency. Cultural curiosity can be a lifelong pursuit that not only enhances practice but also can lead to considerable personal growth.

Chapter 15 introduces the burgeoning area of global mental health. Public psychiatry can be a pathway to global mental health and international practice. This chapter discusses the right to treatment and the need for psychiatry to have an international perspective. The challenge of meeting the needs of vulnerable populations such as refugees and recent immigrants brings home lessons learned in international practice. The development of telemedicine in low-resource settings may have applications in rural settings at home or for special populations. These examples suggest a useful, reciprocal relationship between global mental health and public psychiatry.

Part IV, "System Development in Public Psychiatry," has three chapters focusing on education and workforce development, evidence-based practice, and administrative best practices for the service system.

Chapter 16 discusses interdisciplinary teaching of professionals in public psychiatry with an eye to workforce development. It describes the elements of teaching programs in public psychiatry, both as part of core, discipline-based education and also in advanced fellowships, using the Yale Department of Psychiatry as an example. It emphasizes the value of interdisciplinary learning in advanced education programs, which are needed to address the inadequacies of core preparation. Only by attending to preparatory and continuing education in public psychiatry is it possible to adequately meet the field's future workforce needs.

Chapter 17 on evidence-based practice addresses another basic strategy for system development. New discoveries, the evaluation of services, and their translation into evidence-based practices move public psychiatry forward. This chapter emphasizes the need for training and fidelity monitoring and discusses challenges in implementation, as well as implementation strategies. It reviews the use of technology to achieve the goal of evidence-based practice. These topics are essential knowledge for scientist-professionals who aspire to evidence-based practice in the public system.

Chapter 18 considers administrative best practices in public psychiatry. The service system is only as good as its management at all levels, from the clinical team leader to the chief executive officer. This chapter is predicated on this axiom and describes how to get the best out of the system and those who work in it. Through a variety of measures within the context of recovery-oriented, person-centered care, and practice-based population health, creative and effective management provides ongoing stewardship for and development of the system. Acknowledging that "leadership is a relay race" current leaders must teach leadership to their junior colleagues, who in turn must develop and plan for their personal development as leaders.

Chapter 19 describes how the system of public psychiatry is in a state of flux. It discusses the major policies and variables that are driving development in the system, including insurance reform, new service delivery models, and variables reshaping practice. It suggests that public–academic partnerships can be powerful alliances for developing and sustaining the system. It also suggests that academic divisions of public psychiatry in departments of psychiatry are instrumental in achieving future development in the field.

THE SIGNIFICANCE OF PUBLIC PSYCHIATRY

Public psychiatry is the safety net of services for people with severe and persistent mental illnesses and SUDs. Ultimately, the significance of public psychiatry is found in the changed lives and hopeful futures of these people who are successfully supported as they recover in the public system. Take, for example, a young student whose life is disrupted by acute psychosis and who is successfully treated, receives cognitive training, and is supported by the psychoeducation of his or her family, thus paving the way for recovery rather than a lifetime of chronic illness. Or consider a single mother, threatened with the loss of her children unless her psychotic depression is treated. With successful treatment of her depression and delusions, and while attending a support group for young mothers, she is able to organize her daily life, establish a stable place to live, and care consistently for her children. Or consider a woman with an addiction who is precariously holding on to a job that her whole family depends on. With treatment, she can attend work regularly and productively. Although not all interventions in public psychiatry are fully successful, and there is much to learn and improve, these few examples illustrate the crucial value of public practice in the lives of those it serves.

It is possible and important to conceptualize the significance of public psychiatry not only for the individual, but also for the community. Recent tragic events involving gun violence and public health problems in American society dramatize the challenges to be addressed. Public psychiatry, among other professional disciplines, has a role to play in solving these challenges, and education in public psychiatry supports this role. Integration of knowledge and practice in public psychiatry is critical in addressing the challenges of isolated, young adults falling into psychosis or of suicide among young adults and military veterans. Public health strategies and the public system of care help to transform psychiatric practice so that it focuses more on prevention, when possible, and early intervention to address these problems.

Another perspective on the significance of public psychiatry is the enormous size of the enterprise. In 2009, about half of all mental health and substance abuse expenditures were in the arena of public psychiatry (combined cost to Medicaid, state agencies, Social Security Disability Insurance, and federal block grants; see Chapter 2, Figures 2.1 and 2.2). According to data from the Surgeon General's 1999 report on mental health, 2% of the American population received care that year in the public sector, out of the 15% of the population receiving mental health care.[9] Although larger in comparison with other professional groups, 40% of psychiatrists work full or part time in the public sector. Under the auspices of the ACA, the number of behavioral professionals and the entire enterprise will continue to grow because public psychiatry plays a key role in managing the vast increase in access to services through Medicaid for behavioral disorders.

SUMMARY

This textbook strives for excellent, comprehensive, integrated, advanced, professional education in public psychiatry. This chapter introduces the textbook by providing definitions of public psychiatry, the target population of people with SMIs and co-occurring or independent SUDs, and the service system. It discusses the special clinical competencies of public practice, and it reviews the educational principles that guide the book's various chapters while presenting the book's organization and content. The authors conclude that the present is a time of great significance for public psychiatry, given its critical role in the lives of people with serious, persistent behavioral disorders and disabilities; its size as part of the behavioral health care enterprise; and its expansion under health care reform.

REFERENCES

1. Brown DB, Goldman CR, Thompson KS, Cutler DL. Training psychiatrists for community psychiatric practice: guidelines for curriculum development. *Community Ment Health J*. 1993;29(3):271–283.
2. Ranz JM, Deakins SM, LeMelle SM, Rosenheck SD, Kellerman SL. Core elements of a public psychiatry fellowship. *Psychiatric Serv*. 2008;59(7):718–720.
3. Jacobs SC. The significance of public psychiatry and an overview. In *Inside Public Psychiatry*. Shelton, Connecticut: Peoples Medical Publishing House; 2011:1–19.
4. Schimar AP, Rothbard AB, Kanter R, Jung RS. An empirical literature review of definitions of severe and persistent mental illness. *Am J Psych*. 1990;147(12):1602–1608.
5. Staruss JS, Hafez H, Lieberman RP, et al. The course of psychiatric disorders, III: longitudinal principles. *Am J Psych*. 1985;142(3):289–296.
6. American Psychiatric Association. *Diagnostic and Statistical Manual of Mental Disorders*. 5th ed. Arlington, VA: American Psychiatric Association; 2013.
7. Yedidia MJ, Gillespie CC, Bernstein CA. A survey of psychiatric residency directors on current practices and preparation for public sector care. *Psychiatric Serv*. 2006;57(2):29–43.
8. Steiner JL, Anderson N, Belitsky R, et al. In: Jacobs SC, Griffith EEH, eds. *40 Years of Academic Public Psychiatry*. West Sussex, UK: Wiley; 2007: 159–174.
9. US Department of Health and Human Services. *A Report of the Surgeon General*. Rockville, MD: USDHHS, SAMHSA, CMS, NIH, NIMH; 1999.

PART I

THE SERVICE SYSTEM OF PUBLIC PSYCHIATRY

2.

THE SERVICE SYSTEM OF PUBLIC PSYCHIATRY

Selby C. Jacobs, Andres Barkil-Oteo, Paul DiLeo, Patricia Rehmer, and Larry Davidson

---

EDUCATIONAL HIGHLIGHTS

- Since 1963, five periods of development have shaped the system of public psychiatry: community mental health, community support systems, mainstreaming, transformation, and health care reform.

- The system includes a wide array of services and supports for people with serious mental illnesses (SMIs) and substance use disorders (SUDs), varying from state to state and locale to locale as a function of state policies and local stewardship. The broad system structure with multiple components is necessary to meet the large spectrum of individual needs of people served by the system.

- Economic and fiscal policies repeatedly have been instrumental in shaping the system of care, in some cases skewing the system toward particular modalities of treatment and care.

- The mission of serving people with SMIs and addictions unifies the system of public psychiatry.

- The "de facto" system of services for people with SMIs and addictions is fragmented and midstream, undergoing a process of transformation to recovery-oriented care and system policies in the face of a wide expansion of access to services, the emergence of new service delivery models, and changes in practice as a result of the Affordable Care Act.

- System knowledge is essential for successful practice in public psychiatry.

INTRODUCTION

This chapter sets out to answer three questions about the service system of public psychiatry. How did it develop over the modern era since 1963? What does it look like now? How is it financed? The chapter ends with a discussion of the present status of the system, the management of the system, and the need to advocate for certain components of the system.

In 2003, the US Presidential New Freedom Commission on Mental Health described the system of services for public psychiatry as a "patchwork relic" in a state of "shambles."[1] Since then, the system has continued to evolve as a result of a transformational agenda recommended by the New Freedom Commission and guided primarily by the Substance Abuse and Mental Health Services Administration (SAMHSA). As well, health care reform through enactment of the Affordable Care Act (ACA) in 2010 added impetus to system change. The primary challenge of this chapter is to describe this "de facto system,"[2] one characterized by disorganization and lack of internal coherence.

A central thesis of this chapter is the proposition that a distinguishing feature of public psychiatry is the service system in which practice takes place. The system is a constellation of resources that supports practice. It is essential for professionals in public psychiatry to understand the system and work as effectively as possible within it while also contributing to ongoing efforts to improve it. The cumulative knowledge of the service system, derived from clinical experience and applied in service of people with serious mental illnesses (SMIs) and substance use disorders (SUDs), is a defining characteristic of professionals in public psychiatry.

For learning purposes, this chapter utilizes three perspectives on the public system of care. One focuses on the history and evolution of policy over the past 50 years, since 1963, when Congress enacted the Community Mental Health Centers Act during the Kennedy administration. The second perspective describes the structure and components of the system. The third perspective is a review of the financing of public psychiatric services. Having already said that the system is disarticulated, is there a unifying concept for understanding the system? This textbook suggests that the mission of public psychiatry to serve people with SMIs and addictions is the overarching concept that holds the system together. Also, this mission is the criterion by which the system ultimately must be judged.

Chapter 1 served as an introduction to the service system by providing definitions of public psychiatry, the target population, and the system itself. This chapter builds on that introduction. Subsequent chapters included in Part I of the textbook expand on essential components of the system, such as recovery, community-based supports, and public health.

A BRIEF HISTORY OF THE SYSTEM OF PUBLIC PSYCHIATRY

Over the past 200 years, several important landmarks define major eras of development in the history of public psychiatry in the United States. Many of the service system elements created in each era remain as residual parts of the complex service system today. In 1813, during a time when many people with mental illnesses were imprisoned or confined in alms houses, the Quakers opened Friend's Hospital in Philadelphia. This institution was based on the belief that people with mental illnesses could lead "a moral, ordered existence if treated with kindness, dignity and respect." The opening of this hospital ushered in an era of "moral treatment" in American psychiatry, a concept imported from France and England. Following the advocacy efforts of Dorothea Dix, a retired school teacher who had experienced personal episodes of mental illness, the 19th century saw the widespread construction of both private and state hospitals, built largely in parallel. These state hospitals established the initial foundation of the early public mental health services system.[4] Across the country, many state hospitals, such as Connecticut Valley Hospital in Middletown, Connecticut, and some private hospitals, such as the Institute of Living in Hartford, Connecticut, remain in continuous operation to this day.

In 1913, Clifford Beers opened a clinic in New Haven, Connecticut, and launched a national mental hygiene movement that emphasized early intervention and ambulatory care for children and their families. Beers suffered from manic-depressive illness, spent 2 years in Connecticut Valley Hospital, and was convinced that an alternative to long-term hospital care was necessary. His aim was to avoid chronic illness and the social breakdown that resulted from institutionalization. Mental hygiene clinics are still found in the community today as part of the public system of care for children. The Clifford Beers Child Guidance Clinic in New Haven celebrated its 100th anniversary in 2013.

In 1963, President Kennedy proposed and Congress enacted the Community Mental Health Center Act, launching the modern era of public psychiatry. The modern era can be seen as a progressive dialectic in response to the challenges of developing community-based services and supports to cope with the deinstitutionalization of patients from state mental hospitals. The modern era breaks down into five main periods, with some overlap among them (see citation 3 for a more detailed discussion). Evolving policies on how best to serve people with SMIs and SUDs characterize each period and sow the seeds of the succeeding one, and the accumulation of these structures and services makes up the present "de facto" system of public services. No single period of modern public psychiatry "got it all right"; instead, an accumulation of services and community supports accrued during different phases of modern development accounts for the current system (see Table 2.1).

In the first period, the federally financed community mental health movement brought about the construction of 675 community mental health centers over approximately 20 years. One example is the Connecticut Mental Health Center (CMHC), which opened in 1966, in New Haven.[7] The community mental health movement considerably expanded community-based ambulatory care for people with SMIs. The federally initiated community mental health movement, which spawned community psychiatry as a special area of psychiatric practice, was predicated on public health concepts of social determinants of health status, early intervention, treatment in the community, and continuity of care.[4]

Roughly coincident with the Community Mental Health Center Act, Congress enacted Medicare and Medicaid in 1965. Both programs provided reimbursement for acute psychiatric services in general hospitals and freestanding psychiatric hospitals. Notably, Medicaid legislation, out of fear of cost-shifting to the federal government by states, excluded reimbursement to institutions for mental disorders (IMDs), which were defined as state-owned

Table 2.1 DEVELOPMENT OF MODERN PUBLIC PSYCHIATRY

MODERN PERIODS	FEATURES
Community mental health, 1963–82	Community-based services, public health and crisis intervention, large expansion of mental health professionals
Community support systems, 1982–93	Community-based services and supports for people with serious mental illnesses and addictions
Mainstreaming, 1993–2003	Striving for parity in insurance benefits for psychiatry and beginning integration into medicine
Transformation, 2003–2010	Recovery, focus on early stages of illness, and integration of mental health and substance abuse services
Health care reform, 2010–Present	Access, accountability, quality, new service delivery models, integrated heath care, health homes, and population-based practice

and -operated hospitals. The financial incentive provided by Medicaid reimbursement stimulated enormous growth in general hospital-based, acute psychiatric care that remains an essential part of the system today.

A second period of modern public psychiatry began during the Carter Administration with a Presidential Commission that laid the groundwork for community supports for people with SMIs and SUDs. In 1980, Congress, in the last year of the Carter Administration, enacted the Mental Health Systems Act. With the election of Ronald Reagan in 1980, the sweeping recommendations of the Carter Presidential Commission on Mental Health for expansion of the national community mental health system, as embodied in the Act, were rejected. Nevertheless, a policy focused on people with SMIs and many innovative ideas survived in a National Plan for the Chronically Mentally Ill, published by the National Institute of Mental Health.[5] Over the course of the ensuing decade, piecemeal policy and legislative initiatives took place on a federal level largely using Medicaid as a vehicle.[6] At the same time, under renewed federalism, states, through their departments of mental health, led local communities in developing community-based services, supports, and systems. A key resource that emerged in this period, one largely financed through the federal Department of Housing and Urban Development, as well as through local and state financing, was the development of community-based housing resources. This development was fundamental in making the transition from institutional to community care. In addition, emphasis was placed on system development through system-wide integration. During this time, replacing the earlier language of community mental health, "public psychiatry" emerged to characterize a system of services that included hospitals, clinics, rehabilitative services, community supports, and housing.

During this second period, Medicaid—as a result of a series of legislative victories—began to reimburse for medically necessary community-based services for people with SMIs and disabilities. These included clinic-based services, case management, psychosocial rehabilitation, and assertive community treatment (ACT). These services were provided together in local community mental health centers, many of which were products of the first period of community mental health development. Periodic state budget deficits during the 1980s induced states and private nonprofit community mental health centers to turn to Medicaid for reimbursement of mental health services, a process known as "medicaiding" services. By medicaiding, states became eligible for federal Medicaid matching reimbursement (FMAP). The logic was simple: if states could manage and control the volume of services they offered, they could reduce their expenditures by 50% or more. Using Medicaid, private nonprofit agencies established a revenue stream to support staff and administration. Medicaid Supplemental Security Income (SSI), by providing income supports for people living in poverty, and Medicaid acute and ambulatory health insurance, including reimbursement for community-based outreach and supports, laid the foundation for community living for large numbers of low-income individuals with SMIs. By 2001, the two main payers of public services were Medicaid and state departments of behavioral health services.[7] Medicaid was the single largest payer. The role of Medicaid financing was so central that some refer to this period as one of *Medicaid expansion*. Success in this arena was a harbinger of *mainstreaming*, the next period of modern public psychiatry.

This third period, which arose in 1993 out of the national debate on health insurance reform during the first Clinton Administration, aimed to mainstream mental health insurance and social benefits into existing federal entitlements, welfare, and health programs.[8,9] Mainstreaming in psychiatry provided an alternative to an expanded national system, originally stimulated by the community mental health movement, of special services for people with SMIs and SUDs. Mainstreaming echoed policy strategies that emerged from the community mental health debates of the early modern era. For example, during the health care debates of 1993, it became apparent that psychiatric services needed to integrate with medicine in order to achieve the benefits of universal health insurance and end discriminatory health insurance benefits for behavioral health disorders. A 1999 Surgeon General's report on mental health, which described the system, questioned its cohesion, pointed out delays in implementation of evidence-based practice, and called for a reorientation of care to the promotion of recovery, was a landmark appearing near the end of this period.

Mainstreaming and the growth of Medicaid as a payer introduced *payer status* into consideration as a determinant of access to services. The effects were complex. A Medicaid entitlement enabled access to managed Medicaid plans of service through private nonprofit providers. Given scarce resources, access to state-owned and -operated services was restricted to avoid duplicate financing. The problem was that many people, such as single adults with SMI, were not qualified to receive Medicaid. Using Medicare as an example, another problem arising from mainstreaming was disabled people on Medicare alone; these people had trouble accessing rehabilitative services because Medicare only covered acute care (see the later discussion on financing). Thus, payer status entered public practice as an important factor to consider when developing individualized plans of care.

The fourth period of modern public psychiatry embraced *transformation*. This was an outgrowth of mainstreaming, launched by a 2003 report of the New Freedom Commission on Mental Health during the Bush Administration.[1] Transformation shifted attention to the integration of mental health into primary care, the integration of mental health with substance abuse services, and the reorienting of services away from symptom reduction and rehabilitation of chronic disabilities to the promotion of recovery and social inclusion. All three of these goals remain prominent in today's agenda of the public mental health services system. The SAMHSA put $100 million into transformation grants to states, one of which was received by the Department of Mental Health and Addiction Services of Connecticut. Through these grants, the federal government provided initiative to state and local authorities to explore alternatives to a system that was considered to be in "shambles."

The recovery movement that the Surgeon General's report heralded and that figured prominently in the New Freedom Commission report historically developed as the vehicle for pursuing the rights and empowerment of people with mental illnesses and addictions. In the words of the 1999 Surgeon General's report, recovery is the notion that "a person with mental illness can recover even though the illness is not cured" and defined recovery as "a way of living a satisfying, hopeful, and contributing life even with the limitations caused by illness." The recovery movement was indigenous to psychiatry (e.g., addiction services with 12-step programs), but it was also part of a mainstream medical movement toward ownership and consumerism in general health and welfare policy. In this sense, it was yet another example of the mainstreaming of mental health care with the rest of medicine. One potentially influential policy outgrowth of the recovery movement was the development of the concept of a recovery-oriented system of care (ROSC), a concept initially launched in Connecticut in 2002 and then taken up and disseminated by the SAMHSA through its guidance for state systems. This idea of a managed system of complementary services and supports integrated through the vehicle of individualized, interdisciplinary recovery plans developed in collaboration with the person and his or her natural supports, is now the leading policy direction supported by the US government. As a step further down the road in pursuit of the full rights and empowerment of persons with SMIs and addictions, the promotion of social inclusion and full citizenship for what is increasingly being recognized as a marginalized population is now being proposed as a next iteration of the ROSC.[10]

The fifth and present period of public psychiatry opened in the first two decades of the 21st century. It grew out of the crowning achievement of mainstreaming: the federal enactment of parity for psychiatric insurance benefits. Central to these developments was the elimination of restrictive insurance benefits and prejudicial cost-cutting procedures in the management of mental health insurance and services. The enactment of health care reform in 2010 addressed the plight of uninsured persons through a mandate for universal insurance coverage, the establishment of community insurance ratings, and health insurance subsidies for people living in poverty. The ACA was a landmark achievement for increased access to mental health and substance abuse services [11]. Since then, most of the new policies and structures in health care stem from and support the objectives of access expansion, accountability in provision of care, integrated health care, population health, and quality of care. The implementation time table of health care reform is 9 years, and it is still playing out. The ACA provides a vehicle for accelerating the implementation of key components of recovery-oriented care through its focus on person-centered medical homes, consumer choice and peer services, and the deployment of *health navigators*, which many see as a primary role for peer staff in the future. (Further discussion of the ACA is presented in the final chapter, which considers directions for future service system development.)

On the heels of the ACA, Congress enacted and President Obama signed into law the Excellence in Mental Health Act of 2014. It is the single most important federal initiative specific to mental health since 1963, and it adds to the impetus for change in the current period of system development under the ACA. The Excellence Act provides for demonstration projects in eight states. It creates criteria developed by the federal Department of Health and Human Services for Certified Community Behavioral Health Clinics (CCBHCs), which will be certified by states. The Act requires that CCBHCs offer a specific set of services and that states develop a prospective payment system for reimbursement under their Medicaid plans. Reimbursement is essentially cost-based, which provides an enormous incentive for fiscally strapped agencies with revenue-driven budgets to comply with the requirements of the act. Within this framework, CCBHCs may become important vehicles—along with other new service delivery models (see Chapter 19)—for meeting the requirements for expanded access to mental health and addiction services created by the ACA.

When all the contemporary developments are said and done, it is conceivable that some people with SMIs and addictions will continue to fall through the cracks. Transitionally, probably 5–8% of the population will remain uninsured, mostly undocumented individuals and those moving on and off Medicaid or having difficulty navigating insurance exchanges. These individuals will need to be served through a publicly funded grant system. This is a critical role, one that state departments of mental health and addiction services will continue to play.

Going forward, the variety of factors discussed in this section will further shape public psychiatry, forging yet another version of the "de facto" system of services. Over the past generation, five major and interrelated themes have dominated policy and development: (1) mainstreaming of insurance benefits, (2) parity of insurance benefits, (3) the integration of mental health and primary care through medical homes and accountable care organizations, (4) the values of recovery and social inclusion of people with SMIs and addictions, and (5) improved access to care. These themes will continue to project into the future.

A DESCRIPTIVE OVERVIEW OF THE SERVICE SYSTEM

This chapter shifts now from a historical, evolutionary policy perspective on the system of public psychiatry to consider the question of what the de facto system looks like today. This section provides a description of the structures and components of services in the current system. According to the old anatomical dictum, "structure is destiny," the structure and components of the system determine how it functions and, ultimately, what the clinician can do within it.

At the outset, it is important to appreciate that there is no single, universal system of care for public psychiatry in the United States. As noted in Chapter 1, the system intends to be universal and generic only at the federal level. For example, Medicare, as a funder of care, operates at this level. At the state level, considerable variation exists among state authorities for mental health and addictions; how much is invested in the system also varies by state, not to mention the variation in state Medicaid and demonstration programs. Considerable variation also exists at the local, county, and city levels related to local agency development and decisions. The array of services available in each locale is a function of inputs from all these levels. More important than the particular description of services in this section is the conceptual framework employed here for thinking about the system.

To anchor the description of services in a concrete example, this section presents an overview of the system extant at the CMHC in the city of New Haven, Connecticut. The system described here has many basic similarities to all systems in all states and localities, and it has many unique features as well. One difference from many systems is that county government plays no role in Connecticut's mental health services system. Also, Connecticut, unlike many other states, separates adult and child services into two independent state agencies. Although a full range of adult and child services exists in Connecticut, this division of state agencies adds yet another wrinkle to the system. Finally, Connecticut expends more dollars per capita for behavioral health services than most other states, and it has invested more of its state dollars in recovery supports by decreasing overreliance on acute care.[12]

In the description that follows, it is interesting and useful to compare the service system for public psychiatry to the federally funded system for primary medical care. The state structures for mental health and addiction care make public psychiatry unique in comparison with primary care. Whereas states have departments of public health for general medical purposes, their role is generally limited to licensing, the collection of public health data, establishing prevention programs such as vaccinations, and generating statistical reports. It is the state departments of mental health and addiction services, engaged as they are in providing services, contracting for services, and stewarding the system, that make public psychiatry unique in comparison with primary care.

Finally, a major agenda of the ACA is the integration of primary care and public psychiatry through health homes and accountable care organizations. It will be helpful moving forward to have a basic idea of the system of community-based primary care to better appreciate that integration.

STRATIFICATION

In all states, the system of public psychiatry is stratified at the federal, state, and local levels. The stratifications are both independent and connected through policy and funding mechanisms.

FEDERAL LEVEL

At the federal level, the SAMHSA shapes national policy and innovates by means of service demonstration projects. An example of a demonstration project is the recent grants to local community mental health centers to create wellness centers to address the shortened life expectancy of people with SMIs. The SAMHSA is made up of three parts: the Center for Substance Abuse Prevention (CSAP), the Center for Substance Abuse Treatment (CSAT), and the Center for Mental Health Services (CMHS). Each focuses on its cognizant area. The SAMHSA corresponds to the Health Resources and Services Administration (HRSA) for primary care.

Another key federal agency is the Centers for Medicare and Medicaid Services (CMS). These centers administer Medicare and Medicaid policies. For Medicare, the federal agency operates reimbursement mechanisms. This task is relegated to the states for Medicaid, and there is great variation from state to state. These federal agencies finance the system of public psychiatry in each state. In Medicaid, states have considerable freedom to define policy and implement operations through their state plans written by their Medicaid agencies and reviewed by CMS. States can engage constructively with the federal agencies or try to thwart them.

STATE LEVEL

At the state level, most states have a department of mental health services and SUDs that either stands alone or is a division of an umbrella, superordinate human services agency. For example, Connecticut has an integrated Department of Mental Health and Addiction Services (DMHAS), which is a cabinet-level state agency.

Many states, due to budget stringency, have downsized their departments of mental health and switched state-funded programs to Medicaid. Some have closed their state hospitals and contracted for community-based services while maintaining some specialized programs, such as forensic services. In Connecticut, for example, the DMHAS manages one state-owned psychiatric hospital (reduced from five) and four community mental health centers. It also contracts with 17 private, nonprofit community mental health centers across the state to provide ambulatory care and community supports to people with SMIs and substance abuse disorders. With regard to special populations, DMHAS is responsible for both hospital- and community-based services for people aging out of child services (because of the split in state agencies mentioned earlier), people with traumatic brain injury (TBI), or people with sexual disorders. DMHAS also provides forensic psychiatry services that include a forensic institute with hospital beds, consultation to courts, evaluations of competency to stand trial, monitoring of individuals under not guilty by reason of insanity (NGRI) judicial decisions, jail diversion, and transitional services for people coming out of prison. Connecticut has been slow to "medicaid" services, and thus DMHAS remains a prominent player in public mental health policy and services.

All states have a state Medicaid agency; in Connecticut, this agency is the Department of Social Services. Within federal guidelines and according to a state plan approved by the CMS, these agencies administer Medicaid policies and benefits for people living in poverty, single mothers with children, and disabled people living in poverty. Some people are "dually eligible" by virtue of having a disability, qualifying for Medicare, and also being poor enough to qualify for Medicaid. Medicaid sets reimbursement rates and pays for services. Under the ACA, which expands Medicaid to uninsured populations, state Medicaid agencies play a growing role in the public psychiatry service system.

LOCAL LEVEL

Given the complex evolution of the system in response to various federal, state, scientific, professional, political, and economic forces, the best perspective on a system often is from the bottom up rather than top down. Each person with a SMI or SUD has different needs, and a spectrum of services is needed to meet those particular needs. Local agencies strive to make these two service spectrums converge. Community mental health services offered through local agencies correspond to the primary care services offered by federally qualified health centers (FQHCs).

At the local level of service, while service delivery has entered a period of major transition under the ACA (see Chapter 19), three models of service delivery have become well established in the past 25 years. They are (1) state-owned and -operated community mental health centers, which flourished in the first period of modern public psychiatry up until 1982; (2) the spectrum of private nonprofit mental health centers, which grew during the 1980s, stimulated by new sources of Medicaid reimbursement; and (3) mental health services in primary care FQHCs, which expanded considerably after enactment of cost-based reimbursement for FQHCs in 1989. Each corresponds roughly to the first three major periods of development in modern public psychiatry.

There are fundamental similarities in the missions of the three models, but there are differences as well. First, both state-owned and private, nonprofit behavioral agencies are tightly tied into the system of community supports, psychosocial rehabilitation, and outreach services. In general, community health centers are not, which limits their ability to provide comprehensive services to the most disabled parts of the population. Second, although the integration of primary care and behavioral health is a challenge for all three, community health centers have well-developed primary care as a foundation on which to build. Generally, the other two, not having in-house primary care services, face serious challenges in how and where to develop these services. Third, community health centers and private, nonprofit behavioral health centers can build and grow their budgets with revenue streams largely derived from Medicaid fees. For community health centers, Medicaid revenue is cost-based, which is a distinct advantage. For private, nonprofit community mental health centers, revenue is not cost-based, it makes up a smaller proportion of their total budget, and it often is supplemented with grants for services from state authorities. State-owned community mental health centers may collect fees for service on a sliding scale; however, their budgets come from state general funds and are usually independent of fees.

The governance of state-owned and -operated agencies is a state authority. By contrast, private, nonprofit community mental health centers and public community health centers have autonomous agency boards. Finally, depending on the health insurance benefit, each of the three serves somewhat different segments of the population of people with SMIs and addictions. Community health centers primarily serve those on Medicaid, with some exceptions. State-owned community mental health centers principally serve those on state assistance or without health insurance benefits. Private, nonprofit community mental health centers straddle these poles, given their hybrid budget structure.

A Description of Local Services

This section focuses down on the system, turning again to Connecticut to illustrate an array of services at the local level. In Connecticut, there are four state-owned, community mental health centers. One is the CMHC. Although the CMHC has some unique features, it shares in common with other state-owned and private nonprofit agencies the task of mounting an array of services to meet the needs of the surrounding population it serves. The CMHC, in addition to being state-owned, is also a major training institution for the Yale Medical School Department of Psychiatry. As such, it represents a public–academic partnership among the State of Connecticut, Department of Mental Health and Addiction Services, and Yale University.

The CMHC, as a continuously functioning community mental health center since 1966, illustrates a thoroughly developed, wide array of clinical services and supports ranging from the hospital to a network of community-based services and supports including peer support. As a state-owned and -operated facility not subject to shifts in funding sources (but still subject to recurrent periodic budget stringency), it has been able to maintain most essential services over the years. On each of the services, interdisciplinary teams (IDTs) of physicians, psychologists, nurses, social workers, rehabilitation therapists, and peer staff collaborate to offer comprehensive bio-psychosocial care. Subsequent chapters of the textbook provide expanded expositions of the services listed here. Those services in parentheses are operated by other institutions with which the CMHC maintains collaborative agreements:

- Acute and intermediate term hospitalization for adults
- (Acute hospitalization, adult and child, through the general hospital)

- (Long-term hospitalization in a state hospital)
- (Long-term care through local nursing homes)
- (Step-down partial hospitalization, intensive outpatient)
- Ambulatory outpatient care, both adult and child
- Early intervention in psychosis
- Addiction services
- Co-occurring mental health and substance abuse services
- Forensic psychiatry evaluations and consultations
- Community-based forensic, clinical services
- (Emergency services through the general hospital emergency department)
- Urgent care, crisis intervention including mobile crisis evaluations, and brief treatment
- Assertive community treatment
- Vocational rehabilitation
- Psychosocial rehabilitation
- Case management
- Community supports
- (Residential services, both child and adult), supported by clinical teams
- (Home-based services by visiting nurses)
- Outreach to people who are homeless
- Peer-delivered supports
- Integrated primary care through a Wellness Clinic
- Disaster readiness and critical incident stress management
- Services for special populations such as those with traumatic brain injury
- Young adult services
- Child ambulatory services (child guidance clinic)
- (Foster care services through the state agency)
- Consultation to nursing homes
- Home-based services for people leaving nursing homes

PREVENTION PROGRAMS

This spectrum of services grew during the modern era of public psychiatry as each period of development emphasized particular aspects of care. This broad array allows flexible, personalized planning of care for individuals and families. At the same time, program capacity is limited because balanced program development constrains resources in any particular area. It is incumbent on the local facility and its clinical teams to manage access and maintain movement to the extent possible through the system.

Compiling a list of services also serves as a vital step in a needs assessment process for local agencies. Each local agency has amassed a unique array of services over the years depending on how long it has been in operation and what inputs it receives from federal, state, and local sources. A list helps to identify gaps. It also reinforces an understanding of the broad array of services needed, and, combined with local community and population needs assessment processes, it plays an important role in the maintenance and development of the service system (see Chapter 18).

RESIDENTIAL RESOURCES

Among the broad array of services and supports needed to adequately serve a variety of people, residential supports (discussed more in Chapter 4) are particularly important in the public service system. They characterize the profound change seen in the system over the past 50 years as it deinstitutionalized the care of people with SMIs. Development of residential resources began in the 1980s for several reasons: they served as a low-cost alternative to hospitalization, as step-down placements for people coming out of hospitals, and as placements for people who were homeless. Although supported by clinical teams (although not a clinical service per se), residential supports are now an essential platform for community-based care.

Again taking the CMHC as an example, for years, the city-wide New Haven Continuum consortium, co-chaired by mental health professionals from the CMHC, conducts a census of persons who are homeless, assesses needs, and collaborates on annual grants for supportive housing from the federal Department of Housing and Urban Development. Federal Section 8 funding for low-income people supplements the supportive housing program. These federal sources supplement investments made by the State of Connecticut using general fund dollars in supportive housing.

In recent years, "housing first" programs provided evidence that initial or intensive clinical services sometimes were not needed to reduce readmissions or incarceration. It was discovered that stable housing arrangements could be achieved by persons with SMIs when they were offered their own apartment with on-site support.[13] The implications of housing first for the identity of the service system are profound because the essential problem addressed is the lack of adequate living arrangements for people coming out of hospitals and the social blight of homelessness, not symptoms of mental illness. Clinicians often viewed the task of finding a residential placement for patients as an adjunctive social variable in making a plan of care. The opposite proved true for many people with SMIs. Under this view, the hospital and clinic were no longer the center of the system. This perspective represents a seismic shift for the CMHC, which first applied for accreditation in 1984 under the hospital standards instead of behavioral standards of the Joint Commission on Accreditation of Healthcare Organizations.

As a final note, it is useful to consider both the historical development of the system and the levels of care as described in this section, given that increasing demand under the ACA may spur concern about rising costs. This could lead to a renewed sense of urgency about cost control, managed care, and utilization review. In this scenario, aggressive utilization review could once again become a tool for aligning the resources of the public psychiatry system without paying attention the needs of particular people with SMI and addictions, and it could potentially threaten a balanced spectrum of evidence-based services that has taken years to build.

THE INTERDISCIPLINARY TEAM

The IDT is the basic unit of organization for the service system of public psychiatry, although it is not unique to this field. Rather, it is found in most medical and behavioral practice, with the exception of the solo practitioner in a private office. In public psychiatry, the IDT may be unique in the amplitude of team professionals and specialists required to effectively navigate a complex system. In public psychiatry, the IDT is the essential unit of organization that encounters the person with SMIs and SUDs. The plan of care for each person draws on an array of services offered through the IDT to meet particular needs; the IDT and plan of care put the system in service of the individual seeking help.

The IDT is made up of physicians, nurses, psychologists, social workers, case managers, vocational specialists, and peer specialists. Commitment to the mission and practice principles, such as recovery and person-centered care, bind an IDT. Core competencies within each professional group may differentiate the members of the team. These differences are most often complementary and fit together in a package that enhances care for the service user. For example, physicians have biomedical skills; psychologists bring skills regarding psychological dynamics, personality assessment, and cognitive science; social workers are experts in understanding and working within the social welfare system, especially for support services; nurses have special skills in hospital, residential, and home care; case managers assist efforts to put benefits and resources in place; vocational specialists support adjustment to work; and peer specialists have special skills in navigating the care system; all work in collaboration with the service user.

Core competencies of team members may be redundant in several domains. Psychotherapy, which all of the professional groups learn, is an example. In this instance, finding ways to assign the work on the IDT may be more competitive than complementary. These potential conflicts are often sorted out by cost, as a result of what payers are willing to reimburse. In some cases, roles and responsibilities, such as risk assessment or civil commitment, are statutory; in this case, team members must respect statutory requirements. Algorithms for team decision-making, which acknowledge these issues and are discussed transparently by team members, are useful in working out relationships. These will vary by setting, from inpatient to outpatient and out on the street.

The ability to work on an IDT is a core competency for mental health and addiction professionals in public psychiatry, differentiates them from other professionals in psychiatry, and supports this fundamental unit for service delivery in the system.

FINANCING THE SYSTEM

This section provides a description of how the array of safety net services just described is financed, the third question posed in the introduction.

Even as policy initiatives have introduced new services and the system of public psychiatry has grown during the modern era, it has faced periodic political and economic headwinds and cutbacks. During the first wave of retrenchment from the community mental health center movement of the 1970s, an early director of the CMHC wrote about the "politico-economics" of the system.[14] Indeed, since then, and despite the stewardship of the system by SAMHSA and many state authorities, politico-economic pruning has redefined, truncated, and moth-eaten the system.

The final common pathway of politics and economics is the reimbursement mechanism and the services that are covered. Each financing mechanism insures or reimburses a particular and sometimes limited range of services, which in turn may open or restrict treatment options. The public service system, always faced with fiscal limitations, is very sensitive to the services covered by reimbursement. For community mental health centers, following sources of income to cover the costs of personnel and operations has substantially shaped the system; thus, it is useful to understand how services are financed. There is often a dialogue between political/economic agendas and professional and scientific policy initiatives. The 1980s presented a conspicuous example, as federal retrenchment from community mental health occurred while major policy initiatives were pursued piecemeal under Medicaid and implemented by the states.

A recent publication offered a view of the "economic anatomy" of American health care.[15] Because mental health care has recently achieved parity of insurance coverage in the United States and is progressively integrated into general medical care, this analysis is pertinent, and this section begins to develop an "economic anatomy" of the system of public psychiatry.

Through their analysis, Moses et al. identify four major factors driving the growth of the medical economy: price of particular services, costs for professional services, drug and device costs, and administrative costs. In other words, it is not aging, chronic diseases, particular health insurance initiatives, or a variety of other factors that are often cited. Sometimes, in conflict with each other, several additional forces catalyze this growth: (1) consolidation of health service delivery, (2) information technology, and (3) the rise of patients as consumers who choose the services they will use. Additional forces presently at play are (1) cost, (2) a focus on group or population health outcomes instead of individual outcomes, (3) the substitution of social and economic goals for goals related to the needs of individual patients, and (4) the pressure of demand for services resulting from expansion of insurance and access to care under the ACA. Note that none of these factors is essentially professional, medical, or based on research data, yet they have a powerful potential to shape, if not distort, the system of care. This picture of the general medical care system serves as background for a view of the economic anatomy of the system of public psychiatry. For example, in the later section "System Status, Management, Skew, and Transformation," there is an example of how the soaring cost of pharmaceuticals has dominated system economics without offering significant therapeutic advantage and to the exclusion of other evidence-based practices with proved efficacy in helping people with SMIs and addictions (e.g., cognitive behavioral psychotherapy, supported employment).

Virtually all the financing mechanisms discussed here have been operating throughout the modern era of public psychiatry. They have evolved considerably (e.g., mental health benefits under Medicaid). Also, in each period of the modern era, particular mechanisms prevailed and largely set the course of development for the system. During the community mental health center period, federal funding dominated in the construction and policies of community mental health centers. During the second period, at the beginning of the Reagan administration, Congress rescinded the Community Mental Health Systems Act, and federal money, repackaged as block grants to states, fell dramatically. State general fund dollars prevailed in picking up the slack at first, then Medicaid, jointly funded by the federal government and the states, grew as an essential payer for services. Over both these early periods, Medicare grew in importance for elderly and disabled people. Starting with mainstreaming in the 1990s, there has been a successful process of advocating for parity under Medicaid, Medicare, and, eventually, commercial health insurance under the ACA. Going forward, public benefits and commercial insurance policies will shape the system of care.

As in the case of describing a local service system, this description of financing draws on Connecticut as a concrete example. Whereas Medicare is universal, Medicaid policies vary from state to state according to state plans, and other state programs are locally determined.

MEDICAID

Medicaid, enacted in 1965, is a national health insurance program for families and individuals with low incomes and resources. It is a means-tested program that is jointly funded by federal and state governments. It is managed by state Medicaid agencies in concert with policies negotiated with and approved by the federal CMS. On the state level, Medicaid agencies become counterparts to state departments of mental health and addiction services. Medicaid covers a wide range of acute care and, notably, many long-term care, outreach, and community-based services for people with SMIs. In addition, Medicaid covers nursing home care, which is commonly used for discharge from the hospital to avoid long-term hospital costs. States control the level of reimbursement under Medicaid, which, depending on the state, at times is so low (even below costs) as to discourage participation by individual professional practitioners. Even in states that have increased levels of reimbursement equal to those of Medicare (such as Connecticut), professional participation remains low, not only because of the marginal reimbursement rates but also perhaps because of the special challenges of the patient population served in the public sector (see the Kaiser Commission report for a general discussion of mental health care financing and Medicaid).[16]

CHIPS

The State Children's Health Insurance Program (CHIP) is a health insurance program for children in families with incomes that are modest but too high to qualify for Medicaid. It is administered by the federal Department of Health and Human Services through state Medicaid agencies.

MEDICARE

Medicare, enacted in 1965, is a national health and social insurance program administered by the US government through its CMS. Medicare guarantees access to health care for Americans aged 65 and older. Younger people with disabilities and special populations such as people with end-stage renal disease or amyotrophic lateral sclerosis are also eligible for Medicare. Medicare Part A covers hospital costs. Medicare Part B covers ambulatory costs. Medicare Part D covers drug costs under managed pharmacy benefits. Medicare's health benefits cover acute care. With the exception of the special populations just mentioned, these benefits do not include long-term or rehabilitative services. For the Medicare beneficiary, the latter services are difficult to access unless a person is dually eligible (see next) or the service is underwritten through a state budget.

Dual Eligibility

Dually eligible people are those Medicare Part A and B recipients who qualify for a Medicare Savings Program (MSP) or for Medicaid benefits. Many qualify for Qualified Medicare Beneficiary (QMB) benefits, which cover Medicare Part A and B premiums and Medicare deductibles, co-insurance, and co-payments, paid for by Medicaid. This arrangement provides full health care coverage. Essentially, the dually eligible population is both disabled and poor.

Many people with SMIs and addictions who are living in poverty are dually eligible and are provided access to a full range of acute and long-term care services covered by both Medicare and Medicaid. This population is very costly to serve. Dually eligible people with mental illness accounted for 16% of the Medicare population in 2007 and for 27% of Medicare spending. Fifteen percent of Medicare enrollees were dually eligible and accounted for 39% of Medicaid spending.

STATE GENERAL FUNDS

Each state annually appropriates money into budgets for human services, including mental health and addictions. Administered by free-standing state departments of mental health and addiction services or as departments under human services, these state funds cover a range of services and supports, including hospital care, ambulatory care, rehabilitation, residential supports, and services for special populations. In some cases, the services are provided through state-owned and -operated agencies such as hospitals or mental health centers. In other cases, the state offers grants or contracts for a service. Generally, states build their general fund programs in a way to supplement or complement those services reimbursed by Medicare or Medicaid in order to fill gaps and provide a full spectrum of services in each state.

LOW-INCOME ADULT MEDICAID PROGRAMS

Low-income adult Medicaid programs, formerly known as state administered general assistance (SAGA), provide a social safety net for people who are very poor and do not qualify for other types of public assistance. These programs provide both income and health benefits. Many states have eliminated these programs recently; however, 30 states still offer them to people who are poor, do not have minor children, are not elderly, and are not disabled enough to qualify for disability income. Although variation exists among the 30 states that offer general assistance programs, most recipients qualify for health coverage, generally through Medicaid.

Figures 2.1 and 2.2 summarize the components of public funding for services and place them in the context of overall funding for psychiatric services for both mental health and substance abuse services using SAMHSA data from 2012, the latest year for which data are available.[16]

Public funding combining Medicaid, Medicare, other federal funding (which includes block grants from the SAMHSA to states), and state and local funding is the largest source of financing for both mental health and substance abuse services. It accounts for 60% for mental health services and 68% for substance abuse services. Medicaid is the

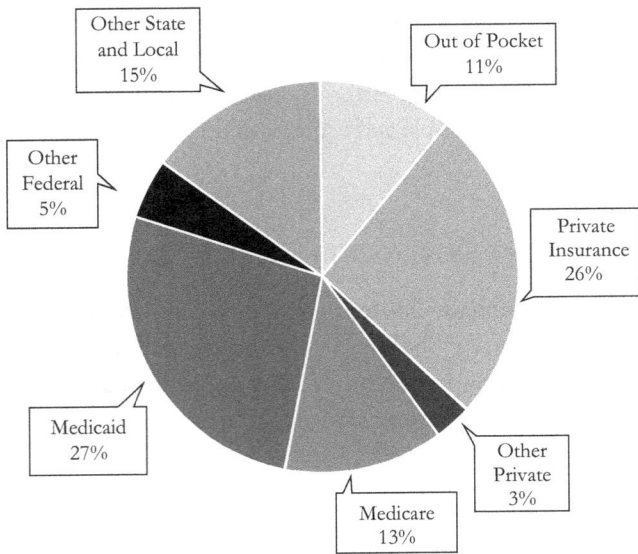

Figure 2.1 Mental health expenditures by payer: 2009 (by millions of dollars)

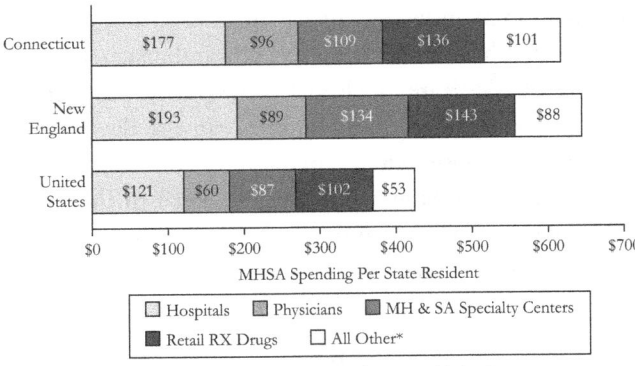

* Includes Other Professionals, Nursing Home and Home Health Services.

Figure 2.3 Mental health and substance abuse services spending per person by region and service, 2005

single largest payer for mental health public services, and state and local sources are the largest funders for substance abuse services. If you combine Medicaid and CHIPs, which is sometimes placed under the state and local category depending on where it is managed, Medicaid is even more prominent. When data are available for 2014 and the years following, they will undoubtedly show Medicaid's expanding role due to new enrollment under the ACA. Medicaid's prominence explains why state Medicaid agencies, in contrast to cognizant state departments of mental health and addictions, have a growing and perhaps dominant voice in setting policies regarding who is covered and what services are covered in public psychiatry. In addition, there is much variation among states regarding how much is invested in public psychiatry (see Figure 2.3).[18]

New England invests more than the national average in services. In contrast, many states in the Southwest and South invest less than New England, which brings down the national average and raises questions—given scarce state funding on average—about whether funding of the mental health and addiction services is adequate.

PUBLIC BENEFITS FOR SOCIAL WELFARE AND COMMUNITY SUPPORTS

SOCIAL SECURITY DISABILITY INSURANCE (SSDI)

SSDI is a federally administered program that provides aid to people who are unable to achieve gainful employment due to a permanent disabling condition. The Social Security tax finances SSDI. People must have worked in gainful employment and paid Social Security taxes long enough to achieve sufficient work credits to qualify. The Social Security Administration adjudicates the existence of disability and eligibility for the benefit. Many people with SMIs fell ill after sufficient work history to qualify for SSDI, which provides income for them to live in the community.

SUPPLEMENTAL SECURITY INCOME

SSI is a federal income supplement program funded by general tax revenues (not Social Security taxes). It provides cash to pay for basic needs such as food, clothing, and shelter to disabled adults and children who have limited income and resources. Individuals who are aged 65 or older, without disabilities, and who meet the financial limits are eligible. Individuals who have worked long enough may also

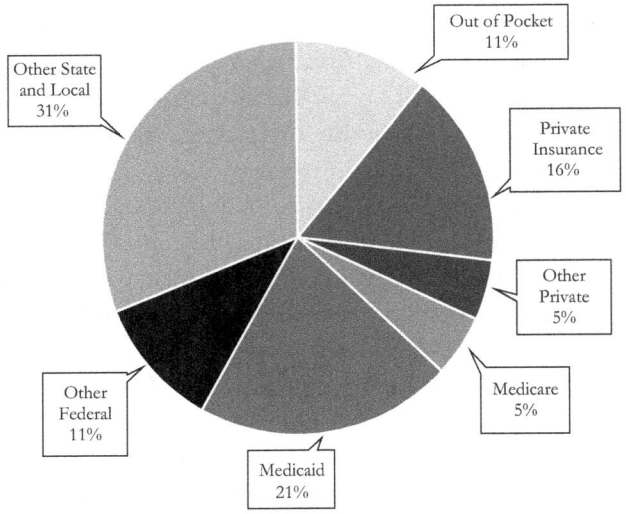

Figure 2.2 Substance abuse expenditures by payer: 2009 (by millions of dollars)

be eligible for SSDI or Social Security retirement benefits. Many people with SMIs are eligible for this welfare benefit.

HOUSING AND URBAN DEVELOPMENT (HUD) SUPPORTIVE HOUSING GRANTS

HUD offers grants through an annual competitive bidding process for new construction, acquisition, rehabilitation, or leasing of buildings to provide transitional or permanent housing, as well as supports to homeless individuals and families. HUD also offers grants to fund a portion of annual operating costs and grants for technical purposes. Many people with SMIs who are homeless are eligible for these benefits and establish residences, with community supports, via the process.

SECTION 8 RENTAL HOUSING ASSISTANCE

Section 8, managed by HUD in conjunction with state Medicaid and public housing agencies (PHA), authorizes the payment of rental housing assistance to private landlords on behalf of low-income households. It operates through several programs, the largest of which, the Housing Choice Voucher program, pays a large portion of the rents and utilities of eligible households. Housing subsidies are paid directly by the PHA to landlords on behalf of the participating family.

CONNECTICUT HOUSING ASSISTANCE FUND PROGRAM

The Housing Assistance Fund Program is a state-funded program that provides for monthly housing subsidies to persons with a SMI on a temporary basis while an individual or family is on a waiting list for a permanent state or federal subsidy.

CONNECTICUT PERMANENT SUPPORTIVE HOUSING

Using state general fund dollars, Connecticut has created more than 2,000 units of Supportive Housing through the establishment of the Interagency Committee on Supportive Housing to address the needs of the homeless population in the state. Connecticut Supportive Housing combines affordable housing, most often through a rental subsidy, with intensive yet flexible supports for people with SMIs.

All these health and social welfare benefits, either singly or in combination, enable people with SMIs and SUDs to live in the community, outside of hospitals and nursing homes, as they utilize treatment and pursue recovery. The public psychiatry professional with a working knowledge of these benefits can plan efficiently and effectively for the care of the individuals they serve. Also, when the mental health professional is asked to support an application for a benefit or disability, it is useful to have a working understanding of the system.

COST SHIFTING

Given both the federal and state sources of financing for the public system of psychiatry, at times of budget stringency, federal or state authorities may try to shift costs from one to the other. Cost shifting plays out through Medicaid in particular. It was the concern about cost shifting that motivated the federal rule against reimbursement for IMDs when Medicaid was enacted in 1965. Another example is the "medicaiding" of services, which began in the 1980s. States faced with severe budget problems during this decade limited their general fund expenditures (in which they paid 100% of the costs) by shifting to Medicaid (in which they paid 50% or less). Medicaid became a major source of support for services for people with SMIs. Yet another example of cost shifting may be developing, this one involving the risk of retrenchment in state general fund dollars when Medicaid is fully instituted as the payer of services for previously uninsured people with SMIs and addictions. As a corollary, the federal government may retrench on block grants for the same reason. The risk for the service system is that a net loss of resources may occur, and the people needing services may be lost in the shuffle. It is important to monitor this process to minimize this risk, through provisions for maintenance of effort by states in federal/state Medicaid agreements. For example, the expansion of access under Medicaid as part of the ACA is financed largely by the federal government in the first few years after 2014. As the state share rises in the future, it is likely that cost-sharing maneuvering between the states and the federal government will intensify. At this point, mental health advocates must pay attention.

This look at the "economic anatomy" of public psychiatry reveals a collage of multiple sources of funding and reimbursement mechanisms for health and welfare services. This hodge-podge is the financial foundation of the fragmented, de facto system of public psychiatry. No single level of government or agency is in charge of striving for a coherent whole. This "patchwork relic," supported by a multiplicity of sources, has motivated the call for a new federal agency charged with coordinating policy for services to people with SMIs and addictions.[12]

SYSTEM STATUS, MANAGEMENT, SKEW, AND TRANSFORMATION

Who is in charge of the system? What are strategies for managing the system? What is the current status of the system? How can the system be shaped to better serve people with SMIs and addictions? Are there distortions in the system? The next few sections set out to address these questions.

Obviously, no single person takes responsibility for the whole services system. In the large, complex, and stratified system that exists, a variety of people take responsibility. Two essential ideas are worth emphasizing when addressing this question. First, at the lowest level, it is the professional in public psychiatry, working as part of an IDT and through individualized plans of care, who takes charge of the system on behalf of a person seeking care for a SMI or addiction. Second, the service user as the ultimate consumer of services, through governance structures, consumer choice of where to obtain care, involvement in quality control, and consumer satisfaction data, plays an essential and growing role as custodian and shaper of the system.

SYSTEM MANAGEMENT AND UTILIZATION

During the 1980s, the community system expanded the administrative and clinical leadership of local mental health authorities who were responsible for the management of the system in order to assure proper use of the multiple levels of care. Then, first in the private sector and eventually in public psychiatry, payers hired managed care companies or administrative service organizations to manage utilization, improve efficiency, and reduce costs. Although savings could conceivably be applied to service expansion or development, in most cases, the savings went toward administrative costs or profit. In response to the challenges posed by this new type of utilization review, the American Association of Community Psychiatrists developed the LOCUS tool for determining level of care as part of a utilization review.[19]

LOCUS brought clinical assessments and clinical rationales back into the process of determining the proper level of care. LOCUS uses quantifiable ratings on six dimensions of risk management, functional status, co-morbidity, recovery environment, treatment/recovery history, and engagement to place a person in one of six levels of care. The levels of care are, starting from the lowest, recovery/health management, low-intensity community services, high-intensity community services, medically monitored nonresidential, medically monitored residential, and medically managed residential services (i.e., hospitalization). The local array of services enumerated earlier fits into these categories in obvious ways.

SYSTEM STATUS

The primary purpose of this chapter is descriptive, not analytic or judgmental. Indeed, there is no single, universal service system on which to render judgment. Each locale and situation is different, state by state and locality by locality. Nevertheless, a brief discussion of the current state of the public system provides perspective on how well it is doing.

As noted earlier, two recent national reports on the public psychiatry service system rendered judgments on it that give pause. One was the 1999 Surgeon General's report, which referred to the system as "fragmented" and "de facto." It noted that the public system had little logic or coherence and was instead an accumulation of developments formed over the years. In 2003, the New Freedom Commission described the system as a "patchwork relic," "in shambles," and failing to meet the needs of recovering people with SMIs and addictions. No fundamental system change has occurred since these reports.

Adding insult to injury, the economic recession of 2009 and ensuing years led to deep budget cuts for services for people with SMIs and addictions. The National Association of State Mental Health Program Directors (NASMHPD) estimates that states cut public services by $4.35 billion from 2009 to 2012.[20] That is $81 million per state on average, although wide variation exists among the states with some, like Connecticut, cutting less and others more. Also, 4,417 state psychiatric hospital beds, 9% of capacity, have been eliminated. Many of the remaining beds are filled by patients under court order for evaluation or other forensic purposes. In addition, the American Hospital Association estimates that the number of acute beds for psychiatry in general hospitals has fallen by 32.5%. The number of general hospitals with psychiatric units has declined from more than 1,500 in 1995 to fewer than 300 in 2010. Forty percent of people with SMI and 60% of people with any psychiatric disorder go without treatment. The new asylums are nursing homes, emergency departments, jails, and homeless shelters,[21] although the exact causes of this are still uncertain.[22] These budget cuts for services have occurred despite the knowledge that psychiatric disorders account for a substantial burden of disease in American society (see Chapter 3) and that mortality rates from psychiatric disorders are high from suicide and untreated chronic medical conditions (see Chapter 3). It will take time to simply restore services lost to recent budget cuts and address this disarray in services. In the meantime, much of the management of behavioral health services is fundamentally the management of scarcity.

Two mental health policy experts concluded that, over the past 50 years (1950–2001), there has been improvement in the well-being of people with mental illnesses and that the population served was "better but not well."[8] Yet the system of services and the substantial—yet insufficient—investment in behavioral health care, along with deficient scientific models for prevention, diagnosis, and treatment,[22] has not delivered reasonably expected reductions in morbidity, mortality, and disability from mental and addictive disorders.[23]

The ACA and the Excellence in Mental Health Acts are the latest major health policy initiatives that will further shape the service system of public psychiatry. The "de facto" system under the ACA will feature a prominent role for new service delivery models (see Chapter 19). For example, the major source of treatment for depression may become the community health center.[26] On the other hand, community mental health centers probably will continue to play a key role in caring for the most severely, persistently ill and disabled. Connecticut, for instance, stimulated substantially by the Excellence Act, is developing a model of behavioral health homes (a medical home with emphasis on a broader agenda for behavioral services) to offer persons with more SMIs more choices in care, with many of them being able to receive their primary care within traditional mental health settings. Interestingly, it is easy to see the potential for competition between primarily primary medical care agencies and primarily behavioral health care agencies. If so, the role of consumer satisfaction and consumer choice will become a big variable in determining the locus of care. On a state level, both departments of mental health and addictions, which have the requisite expertise in public psychiatry, and state Medicaid agencies will continue to share important fiscal and policy decisions regarding the system of public psychiatry.

Given the disorganized, uneven, and chronically insufficient resources of the service system for public psychiatry, the challenge for the practicing, public-sector professional is to know the system, take advantage of its strengths, try to compensate for its weaknesses, and advocate for adequate and wisely managed resources. It is essential to use knowledge of the service system to respond to people seeking services and help them access the system in whatever way is possible and right for them. In addition, given the "disarray" in the service system, it is a challenge for professional service managers to sustain a broad spectrum of services to provide the range of options, including all evidence-based practices, needed by individuals at different points in the trajectory of serious and persistent mental illnesses or addictions. Finally, mental health professionals should advocate for resources allocated to effective practices and for patients' freedom of choice by offering all evidence-based options, including psychosocial ones, in a balanced array of services. These professional responsibilities are part of an ongoing obligation to establish a social priority for the least well off in the circumstances of mainstreaming and health care reform.

SERVICE SYSTEM SKEW

Throughout the modern history of the service system of public psychiatry, sometimes single-minded, telescopic policies or commercial zeal have skewed the system. Given finite resources, professionals in public psychiatry need to be vigilant and able to correct for such system distortions, which create an illusion of progress and can constrict practice.

For example, in the earliest stages of the modern era, emphasis on development of community-based services and early intervention was associated with relative neglect of chronically ill people deinstitutionalized out of the hospital and into the community. In the 1980s, single-minded devotion to creating community-based services for people with SMIs and addictions was associated with inattention to early intervention and hospital services. This eventually led to a relative neglect of early stages of illness and shortages of acute, intermediate, and long-term hospital services. The emergence of Medicaid as a prominent payer during the 1980s and '90s led to increased access to public services for people on Medicaid; although this is desirable, it also attenuated the focus of the public system on some needy people with SMIs and SUDs who were not on Medicaid.

Currently, despite a nagging shortage of hospital beds, there is improved overall balance in the system. Still, there is a "pharmacologic bias," apparent in three prominent, interrelated problems persistent in the treatment of SMIs: excessive reliance on a limited number of antipsychotic medications at the expense of other effective treatments[27], nonadherence to evidence-based practices, and the crucial problem of access to care for people who need it. Whereas medically ill patients in the United States receive the recommended care about half the time, the corresponding rate for people with SMIs is no more than 1 in 4.[34] Rather than be consoled by the general inadequacy of medical treatment in the United States, the field of public psychiatry needs to ask itself, "Why is this happening? And can we do better?"

Large comparative effectiveness trials (like CATIE) discredited the widely held belief created by incomplete data from pharmaceutical companies that newer, often more expensive atypical antipsychotic medications are more effective than older, less expensive ones.[25] Yet, the only consistently superior medication is clozapine, and, ironically, it is widely underprescribed. Two reasons often cited for this are the frequent blood draws required to avoid the risk of agranulocytosis and general side effects like weight gain, constipation, and sedation. Other countries with similar compulsory lab schedules have higher prescription rates, and clozapine's side effects are not much different from the side effects of the polypharmacy regimens that result when patients are not prescribed clozapine.

Over the past 15 years, psychotropic medication use in general and polypharmacy in particular have increased, with little indication of concurrent changes in patients' illness severity, comorbidity, or outcomes as measured by burden of disease, mortality, or prevalence of disorders.[24] Psychiatrists continue to prescribe some atypical antipsychotic drugs despite their higher cost—some of them with increased risk for causing metabolic syndrome and diabetes—and with no demonstrated superior efficacy. To make things worse, fewer than 13% of patients taking atypical antipsychotic drugs are screened for glucose imbalances and dyslipidemia, and only 3% receive follow-up laboratory tests. This has serious consequences for patients because iatrogenetically induced metabolic syndrome is one of the four main risk factors identified as a cause of early mortality in persons with schizophrenia treated with antipsychotic medications. Typical antipsychotic drugs have their side effects as well, particularly the risk for tardive dyskinesia; however, recent reports found no differences in the extrapyramidal side effect rates between conventional and atypical antipsychotic drugs. To make things worse, people on atypical antipsychotic medications are less likely to be prescribed adjunctive anticholinergic medication despite equivalence in terms of extrapyramidal side effects.

Some evidence-based approaches (see Chapter 17) to SMI, such as cognitive behavioral therapy (CBT) groups for psychotic symptoms, supported employment, family psychoeducation, and supportive housing programs are underutilized. The schizophrenia Patient Outcomes Research Team (PORT) study, for example, found that, in the late 1990s, patients were receiving only 10–46% of the approved treatment interventions for schizophrenia; later studies confirmed these results. Constraints on mental health funding from Medicaid and state general funds, coupled with increased spending on new and expensive medications, are responsible for this shortage in the delivery of effective treatments because they led to reduced funding for other evidence-based services such as housing, vocational training, and case management programs.[25] Such situations not only limit the basic right of choice for service users, but also increase the cost of services by concentrating treatment in a few interventions of limited effectiveness. For example, 80% of the money spent on antipsychotics is allocated to only three medications (although this situation may change, given that two out of the three medications are in the process of becoming available in generic forms). Still, there is no guarantee that the savings in cost will be used to provide other, more effective treatments.

In an era of person-centered practice (see Chapter 3), personal choice should be highly valued, and the right to be offered all evidence-based interventions, both pharmacological and psychosocial, must be assured. Behavioral professionals must serve as guides in selecting high-value options for each individual based on the evidence, clinical expertise, and patient values. Given finite resources, in order to support such practice, it is important to strive for balance when choosing from an evidence-based array of services to meet the entire needs spectrum of individuals with SMIs and SUDs. Furthermore, it is important for behavioral professionals, who take note of skew in the system, to use this understanding to advocate for constructive change, consistent with the core mission of improving care for people with SMIs and addictions. Optimally, professionals in public psychiatry need to steward the system: to be not only creative clinicians who shape their practice wisely, but also mangers, advocates, and agents of change.

SYSTEM TRANSFORMATION

Given the challenges facing the service system of public psychiatry, what can be done to improve and expand it, to transform it as the New Freedom Commission called for, with an eye on the original target population of vulnerable people with SMIs and SUDs? This chapter begins a discussion of system transformation. The final chapter picks it up and addresses the full spectrum of factors now active in shaping the public system of services. These include policies regarding insurance reform, new service delivery models including integrated health care, and new models of practice, accountability, and quality assurance (see Chapter 19).

Optimal transformation depends on engaging the whole service system from top to bottom. It requires both clinical and population perspectives (see Chapters 3 and 18). Most behavioral professionals are deeply trained in a clinical perspective that places the needs of a particular person above everything else. The challenge for a system manager is to develop a community and population perspective and integrate it with the clinical one. Using a population perspective, system managers must take an overview of the system, maintain a balanced spectrum of services, and implement innovative practices as they are developed and proved.

Translating into practice those innovative services supported by evidence is essential for transformation. (Subsequent chapters of this textbook discuss evidence-based practices in several domains of practice; Chapter 17 more generally discusses evidence in public psychiatry.) Scientific discovery from clinical trials and services research is only part of the process. The challenge is to shorten the estimated 17 years between discovery of evidence-based practices and implementation in the field. This goal requires not only an eye to new, evidence-based practices as they develop, but also training clinicians in new interventions and using creativity in finding new resources or reallocating existing resources where the demand does not justify current levels of service. The objective is a range of services that meets the needs of a variety of individuals with SMIs and addictions.

Thus, coincident with innovation in services is the need for workforce development and training (see Chapter 16 on education). For innovative practice to take hold and figure in person-centered care, frontline clinicians must be part of the equation. Effective leadership at all levels of the system—from chief executive officers, to agency policy directors and medical directors, down to the clinical team leaders—is essential. Advanced training in public psychiatry, including preparation for leadership and management, supports this task.

Also, it is important to note that consumer empowerment and consumerism play an increasingly important role in system transformation and the allocation of services (see Chapter 3). Data on cost and quality of services, collected, managed, and publicly accessible in real time, will provide a foundation for documenting consumer satisfaction and supporting consumer choice. Contemporary information management resources make this possible. In addition, system leaders must incorporate service users and family members into every level of governance and operational roles in the system.

SUMMARY

System knowledge, acquired through special training, differentiates professionals in public psychiatry from their counterparts in general psychiatry. The "system" as described in this chapter figures prominently in teaching programs for professional students of public psychiatry. Learning about the system occurs not only in didactic seminars, but also in placements in various parts of the system, in supervision, and, on a daily basis, in working out comprehensive plans of care with individuals served by the system. The central thesis of this chapter is that the system—knowing it, working in it, using it, managing it, developing it, and sustaining it—is one of the most important features of public psychiatry that distinguishes it from the rest of psychiatry.

System knowledge, together with understanding of the special needs of the key target population of people with SMIs and addictions, is the foundation for effective practice in public psychiatry. Working within an IDT, professionals in public psychiatry, drawing on an integrated view of care and a thorough knowledge of the strengths and weaknesses of the service system in which they work, are lynchpins in creating comprehensive, coherent, integrated plans of care in collaboration with persons in recovery that will enable them to access and navigate the system of services. For the purpose of making accessible as many necessary services as possible, knowledge of the system is essential. A transition in practice is under way that will lead from procrustean programs of service that are offered practically to everyone to person-centered care, in which elements of service are mobilized into individualized plans of care.

Using three perspectives—an evolutionary, historical approach to development; a descriptive, structural approach; and a sketch of the economic anatomy of the system of public psychiatry—this chapter offers an introduction to the system of public psychiatry. The chapter describes how not only scientific and professional principles have guided the evolution of the system but also, inevitably, how political and economic forces have shaped it as well. The net result is a de facto system with multiple sources of funding that has little coherence or logic. Focusing on the recovery of people with SMIs and addictions as a value helps to also maintain focus on the needs of this key target population as other political, economic, scientific, and professional forces shape the system going forward. The bottom line is that the system must be monitored to keep an eye on the array of services offered to assure they are reasonably comprehensive, balanced, and evidence-based in order to meet the needs of people with SMIs and addictions—the essential target population of public psychiatry.

As mental health professionals work in the domain of public psychiatry and serve those seeking help, they learn about and operate in the service system, where they weave together plans of care to meet the needs of individuals.

This chapter is intended to help the advanced professional student get started. From state to state, county to county, and city to city, the system differs, and professionals must develop their own understanding of their particular locale. It is the individualized, person-centered plan of care, developed through an interdisciplinary clinical team that provides a roadmap of care within each system. It is also a key professional task, while serving individuals, to try to compensate for deficiencies in the system. Outside the clinic, there is also an opportunity to advocate for missing services. The system faces many challenges over the next few years, including managing increased access, maintaining a focus on people with SMIs and addictions, implementing integrated health care, integrating a population perspective into practice, and maintaining a full spectrum of acute and long-term clinical, rehabilitative, and mental health services and supports.

Although it is possible to describe the service system of public psychiatry and characterize its status, it is important to appreciate that the system is not static. Indeed, it constantly evolves as new evidence, new policy initiatives, new professional standards, and new political and social events occur. Looking at the system as dynamic, the final chapter of the textbook discusses the multiple factors shaping the system of public psychiatry at present.

REFERENCES

1. President's New Freedom Commission Report. *Achieving the Promise: Transforming Mental Health Care in America.* Rockville, MD: President's New Freedom Commission on Mental Health; 2003.
2. Department of Health and Human Services. *A Report of the Surgeon General.* Rockville, MD: USDHHS, SAMHSA, CMS, NIH, NIMH; 1999.
3. Jacobs S. *Inside Public Psychiatry.* Shelton, CT: PMPH Press; 2011.
4. Foley HA, Sharfstein SS. *Madness and Government: Who Cares for the Mentally Ill.* Washington, DC: American Psychiatric Press; 1983.
5. Goldman H, Morrissey J, Ridgeley M, Frank R, Newman S, Kennedy C. Lessons from the program on chronic mental illness. *Health Aff.* 1992;11:51–68.
6. Grob G, Goldman H. *The Dilemma of Federal Mental Health Policy: Reform or Incremental Change.* New Brunswick, NJ: Rutgers University Press; 2007.
7. Mark TL, Levit KR, Buck JA, Coffey RM, Vandivort-Warren R. Mental health treatment expeditures trends, 1986–2003. *Psychiatr Serv.* 2007;58(8):1041–1048.
8. Frank R, Glied S. *Better But Not Well: Mental Health Policy in the United States since 1950.* Baltimore, MD: Johns Hopkins University Press; 2006.
9. Glied S, Frank R. Trends in the well-being of the mentally ill. *Health Aff.* 2009;28:639–648.
10. Davidson L, Tondora J, O'Connell MJ, Kirk T, Rockholz P, Evans AC. Creating a recovery-oriented system of behavioral health care: moving from concept to reality. *Psychiatr Rehab J.* 2007;31(1):23–31.
11. Mechanic D. Seizing opportunites under the Affordable Care Act for transforming the mental and behavioral health system. *Health Aff.* 2012;31:376–382.
12. Kirk T, Di Leo P, Rehmer P, Moy S. Case and care management can improve outcomes while reducing costs and service demand. *Psychiatr Serv.* 2013;64(5):491–493.
13. Stefancic A, Tsemberis S. Housing first for long-term shelter dwellers with psychiatric disabilities in a suburban county: a four-year study of housing access and retention. *J Prim Prev.* 2007;28(3–4):265–279.
14. Astrachan B. The pragmatics of health care delivery. *Conn Med.* 1974;37:1774–1779.
15. Moses H, Matheson D, Dorsey E, Benjamin P, Sadoff D, Yashimura S. The anatomy of health care in the United States. *JAMA.* 2013;310(18):1947–1964.
16. Kaiser Comission on Medicare and the Unisured. *Mental Health Financing in the United States: A Primer.* 2011. https://kaiserfamilyfoundation.files.wordpress.com/2013/01/8182.pdf. Accessed 10/22/15.
17. Substance Abuse and Mental Health Services Administration, National Expenditures for Mental Health Services and Substance Abuse Treatment, 1966-2009, HHS Publication No. SMA 13-4740, Rockville, Maryland, SAMHSA, 2013.
18. Substance Abuse and Mental Health Services Administration, State Level Spending on Mental Health Services and Substance Abuse Treatment, 1997-2005, Rockville, Maryland, Center for Mental Health Services and Center for Substance Abuse Treatment, SAMHSA, 2012.
19. Sowers W, Benacci R. *LOCUS, Training Manual: Levels of Care Utilization System for Psychiatric and Addiction Services Adult Version 2000.* http://www.ct.gov/dmhas/lib/dmhas/publications/CSPlocustrainingmanual.pdf. Published 2000. Accessed January 3, 2015.
20. Glover RW, Miller JE, Sadowski SR. Proceedings on the State Budget Crisis and the Behavioral Health Treatment Gap. Paper presented at: National Association of State Mental Health Program Directors meeting; March 22, 2014; Washington, DC.
21. Szabo L. The cost of not caring. *USA Today.* May 12, 2012. http://www.usatoday.com/story/news/nation/2014/05/12/mental-health-system-crisis/7746535/. Accessed 8-24-15
22. Prinz S. Does trans-institutionalization explain explain the over-representation of people with serious mental illness in the criminal justice system? *Comm Ment Health J.* 2011;47:716–722.
23. Insel T. Translating scientific opportunity into public health impact: a strategic plan for research on mental illness. *Arch Gen Psychiatry.* 2009;66:128–139.
24. Lieberman JA, Stroup TS, McEvoy JP, et al. Effectiveness of antipsychotic drugs in patients with chronic schizophrenia. *N Engl J Med.* 2005;353(12):1209–1223.
25. Wang P, Ulbricht C, Schoenbaum M. Improving mental health treatments through comparative effectiveness research. *Health Aff.* 2009;28(3):783–791.
26. Barkil-Oteo A. Collaborative care for depression in primary care: how psychiatry could "troubleshoot" current treatments and practices. *Yale J Biol Med.* 2013;86(2):139–146.
27. Kreyenbuhl J, Buchanan RW, Faith B, Dickerson FB, Dixon LB. The Schizophrenia Patient Outcomes Research Team 8. (PORT): updated treatment recommendations. 2009. *Schizophr Bull.* 2010;36:94–103.

3.

RECOVERY AND RECOVERY-ORIENTED PRACTICE

Larry Davidson, Janis Tondora, Maria J. O'Connell, Chyrell Bellamy,
Jean-Francois Pelletier, Paul DiLeo, and Patricia Rehmer

> ### EDUCATIONAL HIGHLIGHTS
>
> The central theme of this chapter is how recognition of the fact that many people recover from behavioral health conditions, and many others find ways to live self-determined and meaningful lives in the face of prolonged behavioral health conditions, has changed and will continue to change public psychiatric practice. Key points include:
>
> - Serious mental illnesses are not necessarily life-long or permanently disabling conditions, which has been accepted as conventional wisdom since the era of institutionalization.
>
> - People have figured out how to live full and meaningful lives in the community despite mental illnesses and/or addictions. Treatment has played a limited role in their efforts to reclaim their lives and has been most effective when it builds on the foundation of a positive identity and sense of belonging.
>
> - Recovery-oriented practice reverses the traditional order of "recover first and return to the community after"; instead, it establishes a meaningful life first and, within that context, uses treatment as a tool to further the person's recovery.
>
> - Peer-delivered services can play effective and important roles in assisting people to create and sustain meaningful lives of their choice.
>
> - In the future, behavioral health services will be assessed based on the degree to which they enable people to live the lives they have reason to value.

INTRODUCTION

As noted in Chapter 2, calls began as early as 1999, in the US Surgeon General's *Report on Mental Health*, for all mental health services to become more consumer-oriented and to promote recovery. By the 2003 US Presidential New Freedom Commission, a new definition of recovery—in contrast to the traditional medical notion of recovery that requires eliminating or overcoming an illness—was being heralded as "the process in which people are able to live, work, learn, and participate fully in their communities."[1] Since that time, the transformation to a recovery orientation and to recovery-oriented systems of care[2] has become the overarching policy direction for publicly funded behavioral health services across the United States and abroad.[3,4] How did this happen? Where did the concept of recovery as different from cure come from? And what implications does this concept have for transforming public psychiatric practice? These are the questions we take up in this chapter.

We begin with a brief historical introduction to the concept of "being in recovery" or "personal recovery" (as differentiated from "recovering from" or "clinical recovery"[5,6]), and then we turn to its implications for practice. We will discuss some of these implications as they relate to offering person-centered care, implementing peer support, and using new tools to assess care quality and outcomes. Although these categories do not exhaust the many components of recovery-oriented practice, they do cover a majority of the territory that students, trainees, and new practitioners will likely encounter in their early days in public psychiatry service settings. Resources are included at the end of the chapter for readers who are interested in delving into any of these topics in more depth or detail.

As noted in the introductory chapter, being "recovery-oriented" is the fifth characteristic that we envision as embodied in optimal service delivery in public psychiatry. Here, we suggest that recovery-oriented practice cannot stand alone but instead requires the following nine characteristics of optimal service delivery as well: it is (1) provided largely by interdisciplinary teams of professionals and specialists; (2) informed by an understanding of the assets and resources of the local community and the values, preferences, experiences, and needs of the population served; (3) systemic (offered within a ROSC); (4) person-centered; (5) culturally competent; (6) community-based; (7) evidence-based; (8) competency-based (through training); and (9) driven by service user and family involvement as part of both quality improvement and all other levels of system, agency, and program operations.

A BRIEF INTRODUCTION TO RECOVERY

Where did this new meaning for the term "recovery" come from in relation to mental illness and addiction, and how did it come to exert such influence on public policy in the United States? We should not infer from the use of the term in federal policy documents (such as the Surgeon General's and New Freedom Commission reports) that it was introduced or promoted initially by policy-makers themselves. Rather, the call for services to be reoriented to the promotion of recovery came about gradually, in response to increasingly visible and effective lobbying efforts by the mental health consumer/survivor movement, which began to coalesce in the United States in the 1970s, and by the new recovery advocacy movement in addictions, which began in the 1990s.[7]

Mental health consumer/survivors (also called ex-patients, ex-inmates, "mad" people, and, most recently, service users) are people who describe themselves as having a history of receiving (or using) mental health services in the past and who, based on those (often harmful) experiences, have taken up an advocacy role to change the nature of the services offered and the ways in which such services are provided. Although there have been such ex-patient advocates throughout the history of mental health care—most notably perhaps Dorothea Dix and Clifford Beers—it was not until the 1970s that a political movement made up of large numbers of such individuals began to gain traction. Beginning at the grassroots level in urban areas on the West and East Coasts, by the time the Carter Commission on Mental Health got under way, there was an increasing number of mutual support/self-help groups made up of articulate and effective mental health consumers across the country. These consumer leaders were included in the initiation and development of the Community Support Program (CSP) at the National Institute of Mental Health, which was the primary accomplishment of the Carter Administration's efforts to improve mental health care. Two key components of the CSP model were that persons with serious mental illnesses (SMIs) would have access to mutual support/self-help groups in their local community and, perhaps more importantly, that consumer and family advocates would have "a seat at the table" in the development and governance of the community-based systems of care that were to be developed to serve them within each geographic catchment area.

As noted in Chapter 1, the Reagan Administration cut all new funding that had been allocated to develop such systems of care, but a foundation for the Recovery Movement had been established nonetheless. By the 1980s, increasing numbers of persons with histories of involuntary confinement and other negative experiences with mental health care were joining the consumer/survivor movement, developing mutual support programs, and becoming outspoken role models for others. It was within this context that Patricia Deegan (a mental health consumer advocate who had gone on to receive a doctorate in clinical psychology) and William Anthony (a long-time leader in psychiatric rehabilitation who directed the Center for Psychiatric Rehabilitation at Boston University) first began to talk and write about a new meaning for the term "recovery."

Deegan's 1988 paper, "Recovery: The Lived Experience of Rehabilitation," was perhaps the first to make the distinction between having recovered from a mental illness and being in an ongoing process of recovering. In what became a highly influential passage, she wrote that "Recovery refers to the lived or real life experience of people as they accept and overcome the challenge of the disability . . . they experience themselves as recovering a new sense of self and of purpose within and beyond the limits of the disability."[8] Soon thereafter, Anthony offered his own influential definition of recovery:

A deeply personal, unique process of changing one's attitudes, values, feelings, goals, skills, and roles. It is a way of living a satisfying, hopeful, and contributing life even with limitations caused by the illness. Recovery involves the development of new meaning and purpose in one's life as one grows beyond the catastrophic effects of mental illness.[9]

Anthony went on to declare this new meaning of recovery as the "guiding vision of the mental health service system in the 1990s," referring to the 1990s as "the decade of recovery."

No doubt, this new vision of recovery appealed to large numbers of persons who had been diagnosed with SMIs not only because of the combination of Deegan's eloquence and Anthony's hopefulness, but also because of their own real-life experiences. At around the same time, an emerging body of longitudinal research was showing that outcomes for SMIs were much less predetermined, much more diverse than had previously been thought. Despite the lack of funding for community-based care and the myriad other difficulties encountered during deinstitutionalization, studies beginning in the late 1960s were showing that, outside of hospital settings, many persons with SMIs were experiencing significant improvements in their conditions over time.

Ground-breaking studies by Strauss and Carpenter[10–12] and Harding and colleagues[13–15] in the United States, along with work by colleagues abroad,[16] were consistently disproving the long-held, mainstream view (attributed to Kraepelin, 1904[17]) that schizophrenia was a life-long illness that inevitably led to progressive deterioration. Rather, they were finding that up to 67% of their samples experienced significant improvements over time, with many recovering fully from the disorder. Among those who did not recover fully, there was a range of functioning found both across and within individuals.[18] In other words, some people improved in some areas (e.g., social functioning) while not others (e.g., symptoms), and the remaining 33% of the sample fell at many different points along a broad continuum of outcomes from progressive deterioration to clinical stability.

By the 1980s, these data led to a reconceptualization of outcome in schizophrenia and other SMIs, from one of a chronic course leading to inevitable decline to one of heterogeneity in both course and outcome.[19] In brief, a body of scientific evidence not only allowed for but actively supported an emerging vision of recovery as a process by which people led self-determined and meaningful lives either in the absence or in the ongoing presence of an SMI. Full recovery is possible, but even for those who do not recover fully, who are not cured, it is still possible to "be in recovery," to derive a sense of "personal recovery" in living one's life despite or in the face of the lingering effects of illness. What remained to be determined was how such a reconceptualization of SMI, and an analogous redefinition of recovery in addiction, would change practice.

A BRIEF INTRODUCTION TO RECOVERY-ORIENTED PRACTICE

As this vision of recovery took hold, mental health advocates joined forces with other disability rights advocates to develop and lobby for the 1990 passage of the Americans with Disabilities Act (ADA). Passage of the ADA may be considered a watershed event in ushering in the recovery movement because inclusion of mental illnesses and addictions as disabilities under the purview of the ADA reframes much of the legal and cultural context in which behavioral health practitioners now practice. If an SMI is a disability, then a person with an SMI, under the ADA, retains all of the rights and associated responsibilities of community membership as do other citizens. He or she is to be afforded access to a life in the community of his or her choice, as are other citizens, and, should accommodations be required to afford such access, they are to be provided (as long as they are considered "reasonable").

By "reasonable accommodations," the ADA refers to such things as wheelchairs, wheelchair ramps, and handrails in bathrooms that are provided so that persons with mobility impairments will be able to access public spaces as much as possible like everyone else. Although we are still in the learning phase as to what psychiatric accommodations may end up looking like, adoption of a disability model of mental illness and addiction has allowed advocates to insist that people not be cured of their mental illnesses or substance use first before rejoining community life as full, contributing members. Adoption of this model has dramatic and far-reaching implications for how behavioral health care needs to change to support people in rejoining their communities even while they may remain disabled by a mental illness or addiction.

One way to think about the nature of this change is to consider much long-stay hospital practice has changed over time in most places. People were admitted to the hospital because they were sick, they received treatment in the hospital that would make them better, and then they were discharged to the community when they were well. In the hospital, people adopted the "sick role," which would absolve them of any responsibilities but also of any sense of personal agency or autonomy. Under this form of practice, in the hospital, other people make decisions for you and do things to you because you are in no condition to do so for yourself. Although the adoption of the sick or patient role may be appropriate to acute illnesses and acute care, doing so undermines long-term recovery by ignoring those internal resources the person needs to do battle with illness or, even worse, leading to their atrophy (along with brain cells). Yet, as many critics have pointed out, this hospital framework followed people with mental illness or addictions out of long-stay institutions into the community during deinstitutionalization and has, according to recovery proponents, permeated community-based services since. We still operate largely with a "be cured or recover first and then take your life back afterward" perspective, even though we no longer practice primarily in hospitals. Changing this perspective has been a major focus of the recovery movement.

We should acknowledge at this point that there is a tremendous amount of diversity to be found under the rather broad tent of recovery when it comes to discerning its implications for practice. Advocates who identify as "ex-inmates," "survivors," or "mad" typically view the mental health system as beyond repair and also view the diagnosis of "mental illness" to be other than an illness per se (e.g., mental illness as the effects of distress or trauma). Similarly, there are differing views in the addiction treatment field, with some advocates arguing for a narrow standard of complete abstinence as required by the 12-step fellowship and therefore showing little interest in transforming behavioral health care, preferring to argue for self-help options for persons experiencing difficulties in their lives. Other advocates have entered into partnerships with behavioral health practitioners and system leaders to develop new practices that could be considered recovery-oriented and for which an evidence base could then be established. The next two sections of this chapter will focus on describing a few of those developments, along with presenting data that have been collected thus far relative to each practice.

By way of introduction, though, it might be useful first to list the principles for recovery-oriented care that resulted from a consensus development conference convened by the Substance Abuse and Mental Health Services Administration (SAMHSA) in 2010.[20] These principles were offered to guide service system development for persons with either mental health and/or substance use conditions, in response to growing recognition of the high prevalence of co-occurring disorders and the need to integrate mental health and addictions services under one conceptual framework that will allow for integration at the person, program, and system levels.[21] The definition developed by SAMHSA to span mental health and addiction states that recovery is "A process of change through which individuals improve their health and wellness, live a self-directed life, and strive to reach their full potential."[2] Based on this definition, the following ten principles were established to guide the development of recovery-oriented practices:

- Recovery emerges from hope;
- Recovery is person-driven;
- Recovery occurs via many pathways;
- Recovery is holistic;
- Recovery is supported by peers and allies;
- Recovery is supported through relationship and social networks;
- Recovery is culturally based and influenced;
- Recovery is supported by addressing trauma;
- Recovery involves individual, family, and community strengths and responsibility; and
- Recovery is based on respect.

These principles suggest that, for persons with mental illnesses and/or addictions, they, their families, and their communities are responsible for the person's recovery. The role of the practitioner is perhaps best framed as that of an expert consultant who has information, skills, education, treatments, and other interventions to offer in support of the person's and family's own efforts at recovery. Each party, including the broader community, possesses strengths and resources that can be identified and built on in the recovery process, which can evolve in many different ways for different people. People are supported in their recovery when they are respected and treated with dignity as whole human beings who are more than just their diagnosis or illness; when they are offered hope; and when their cultural identity, values, affiliations, and preferences are honored. Many persons with mental health and/or substance use disorders (SUDs) have histories of trauma, and, if left unaddressed, this history can impede recovery efforts. Finally, a main avenue for promoting recovery is through the person's relationships with others, including but not limited to family. These relationships need to offer the person a sense of being accepted and cared for as a worthwhile, unique individual who is, or has the potential to be, valued as a contributing member of society. In contrast to the hospital or detox/rehab-based model of "recover first and have a life second," the model for recovery-oriented practice is "accept me as a whole person with a unique and important story first, and then we can work together on finding and traveling together down those pathways that are most conducive to my recovery."

Implicit in this last sentence, a substantive shift in our conceptualization of mental health and addiction care occurs when we move from the perspective of the practitioner and what treatments or other interventions he or she has to offer his or her clients or patients to the perspective of the person receiving or using the care and what he or she needs from others in order to pursue his or her own recovery. In the case of the new recovery advocacy movement in addictions, this has involved moving from an acute care model of disconnected episodes of practitioner-driven treatments to a "recovery management" model that supports the person's own long-term efforts to pursue, enter into, and sustain recovery among a community of supportive family and peers.[22] As with mental health care, services and supports for persons in active addiction seek to help the person establish a solid sense of community membership as a foundation for pursuing recovery in the community, rather than focusing primarily on detoxification and the reduction of substance use and cravings, often in institutional settings. Treatment is reconceptualized as a tool for the person to use in his or her everyday and ongoing life as opposed to something to be completed following an acute episode. This shift is made operationally in the provision of person-centered care, to which we turn next.

Prior to doing so, though, it is important to point out a common misunderstanding of the terms "recovery," "recovery-oriented practice," and "psychiatric rehabilitation." The field of psychiatric rehabilitation predated the advent of the recovery movement and refers primarily to what psychiatric rehabilitation practitioners do in their practice, including skills training, remediation of functional deficits, and provision of community-based supports (see Chapter 4). Recovery, as pointed out by Deegan, refers to what a person with a mental illness (or addiction) is doing to manage his or her condition and to live the fullest and most meaningful life possible. It refers to the real-life or lived experiences of the person with the condition. Recovery-oriented practice refers to what behavioral health and other practitioners do to support people and their loved ones in their own efforts at recovery. Recovery-oriented practice may therefore include a number of psychiatric rehabilitative interventions, as well as other interventions that are clinical or supportive in nature, as long as they are offered in a respectful, collaborative manner as part of a person-driven recovery plan.

PERSON-CENTERED CARE

Although the origins of person-centered care are to be found in the seminal work of Carl Rogers[23] and the Independent Living Movement of persons with physical disabilities beginning in the early 1970s, the case for all of medicine, including psychiatry, to shift to this paradigm was made more recently in a 2001 Institute of Medicine (IOM) report entitled *Crossing the Quality Chasm: A New Health System for the 21st Century*. This report argued that the active involvement of patients in their own care and the tailoring of that care to meet their own individual needs were necessary measures for improving the safety, quality, and outcomes of all health care.[24] This belief also permeates the design of the Affordable Care Act (ACA) passed in 2010 and currently under implementation across the United States.

As part of the ACA, practitioners are encouraged not only to offer person-centered care, but also to integrate all the services a person receives by ensuring that each person is provided with a person-centered health "home." A key mechanism for coordinating care, especially for persons with multiple or complex conditions, is through development of a person-centered care plan, which we have defined previously as "involving a collaborative process between the person and his or her service providers and supporters that results in development and implementation of an action plan that will assist the person in achieving his or her unique, personal goals."[25]

Within the context of behavioral health specifically, we suggest that, for the plan to be considered "person-centered," it needs to "(1) be oriented toward promoting recovery rather than only minimizing illness; (2) be based on the person's own goals and aspirations; (3) articulate the person's own role and the role of others, both paid and natural supports, in assisting the person to achieve his or her own goals; (4) focus and build on the person's capacities, strengths, and interests; (5) emphasize the use of natural community settings rather than segregated program settings; and (6) allow for uncertainty, setbacks, and disagreements as inevitable steps on the path to greater self-determination."[25]

In previous publications, we identified the following five guiding principles for ensuring that recovery-oriented care is provided in a person-centered fashion.[26,27]

1. Person-centered care identifies and builds on people's own strengths and the resources and opportunities that exist in their community.

Person-centered care focuses on the restoration or continued support of the person living a meaningful and gratifying life in the community of his or her choice. Disease, disability, and various forms of dysfunction are not ignored but are viewed instead as potential obstacles to the life the person wishes to lead. For this reason, practitioners first need to get to know the person and what he or she is trying to do in life because this provides the context for treatment and other interventions. What the person is trying to do, where he or she is trying to do these things, what strengths and resources the person brings to these pursuits, and who else will support him or her in doing so are all important dimensions to consider in the planning and provision of recovery-oriented care.

2. Person-centered care focuses on equipping and empowering people to play an active role in the self-management of their conditions.

Person-centered care is based on the premise that people are the primary agents in their own lives and will make their own decisions as to how they will (or will not) take care of themselves on an everyday basis. This remains true even in the lives of those who have been demoralized by an SMI and/or addiction and the discrimination associated with these conditions. For such individuals, an early step in person-centered care may be to help them view themselves as agents in their own lives who can learn how to exercise self-care. In this way, the focus in person-centered care shifts from what the practitioner needs to do to treat and manage the illness to what the individual needs to know and know how to do in order to take good care of him- or herself given the conditions that he or she has.

3. The planning and provision of person-centered care are collaborative processes in which persons and their natural supports are encouraged and enabled to play active, substantive roles.

In parallel to the active role people play in their own self-care, person-centered care involves people playing an active role in collaborating with their practitioners in all decision-making processes. These include not only making decisions about specific treatments, perhaps using shared decision-making tools, but also decisions about who will be involved in care planning discussions and about the life goals on which the care to be provided is based. For individuals who prefer to have others involved in their decision-making based on cultural or other preferences, practitioners are to honor these preferences because it would not be very "person-centered" to insist that people make their own decisions when their preference is to defer to the wisdom of family or elders.[28]

4. Person-centered care recognizes the "dignity of risk" and the "right to fail" that most people with most mental illnesses retain most of the time.

Person-centered care is also based on the premise that, in the absence of serious, imminent risk or grave disability, adults with mental illnesses and/or addictions retain the right to self-determination. This means that these adults, unless assigned conservators or guardians by a judge, retain the right to live the lives of their choosing. Acknowledging this right in person-centered care requires not only "allowing" people to set their own goals and make their own decisions (and therefore their own mistakes), but also actively encouraging them to do so. This does not absolve practitioners from their societal obligation to protect the person and community from harm, but it does limit that obligation to circumstances in which there is clear and compelling evidence of such a risk. In this respect, person-centered care is offered within a framework of competent risk assessment and management, balanced by recognition of the fact that most persons with most mental illnesses pose no more of a risk to self or the community most of the time than most persons without mental illnesses do.[29] The same cannot be said, however, for persons with addictions. Here, the argument is made that people are more likely to use and sustain pathways to recovery that they find more consistent with their own values, preferences, and cultural identity and affiliations.

5. The provision of person-centered care is based on a person-centered care plan that the person and his or her supports have played integral roles in creating in partnership with his or her health care practitioners.

As noted earlier, the provision of person-centered care is based on a person-centered care plan. A person-centered care plan is a plan for how the person will be enabled to live a life he or she has reason to value,[30] and it includes the services and supports he or she may need in order to do so, including those treatments required for reducing or overcoming symptoms and other barriers posed by mental illness or addiction. Because the plan also is oriented toward promoting self-care, it includes the action steps the person will need to take on his or her own behalf, as well as those tasks family and friends have agreed to take on in support of the plan. Finally, it is important that the person and his or her natural supporters play as significant a role in collaborating with practitioners in developing the plan as they are expected to play in implementing the plan.

In addition to these guiding principles, a number of characteristics of person-centered care planning have been articulated and serve as the basis for a fidelity tool.[31] These characteristics pertain to details of the planning process, care plan document, and process of implementation and documentation to ensure that the process of developing and using the plan embodies the principles just described and illustrates how these principles translate concretely into actual practice.[27] Key characteristics include conducting a strength-based assessment, eliciting and assisting people to articulate their own life goals, involving the person and his or her natural supports in the scheduling and conduct of the planning meeting, offering the person a copy of his or her plan, identifying a range of professional and community-based supports and alternative interventions to support the person's recovery from which he or she may make meaningful choices, identifying the steps the person and his or her natural supports will take in pursuit of the person's goals, and using person-first language—and avoiding professional jargon—in documenting the plan and progress made (or not made) in implementing the plan.

In terms of the accumulating evidence base supporting this approach to care, a recent review paints a consistent picture of positive effects resulting from enabling persons to take on active roles in and to make decisions about their own care.[32] First, offering people choices in their care enhances their initial engagement and the likelihood that they will stay in care long enough to derive benefit from it.[33-39] Second, once engaged, persons offered person-centered care are more likely to adhere to prescribed medications,[40-44] with both quantitative and qualitative studies showing an inverse relationship between perceived coercion and adherence.[45,46]

Finally, reductions in symptoms and improvements in functioning have been found in both psychiatric and medical conditions as a result of emphasizing autonomy and affording people more choices.[47-52] Rates of rehospitalization and use of costly emergency and acute care services have been reduced,[33,53-55] while improvements in other domains include patient satisfaction,[49,56-60] residential stability,[50,53,54] cost-effectiveness,[61] rates of job placement, length of job tenure and satisfaction with earnings,[62-64] and quality of life.[64-66]

PEER SUPPORT

Peer support has become perhaps the most visible and rapidly growing outgrowth of the mental health consumer/survivor and new recovery advocacy movements to date. In its contemporary form, hiring people who have experienced their own mental illness and/or addiction and who have recovered or are "in" recovery to provide support to others began in the late 1980s in the United States. Early efforts were a somewhat natural extension of the growth of self-help/mutual support groups around the country, as practitioners became aware of these community groups and their members and began to realize that some of the benefits of these relationships could be brought into the behavioral health system. One strategy for doing so was to invite people who were doing well to come back and mentor others who were not as far along in their own recoveries. Initially, these positions were created as volunteer opportunities, but, by the early 1990s, they had become paid positions in which persons in recovery were beginning to play a variety of roles, from case management assistants and residential staff to the new role of recovery educator.

What has happened since then has been nothing short of extraordinary. The number of peer support staff in the United States practicing both inside and outside of the formal behavioral health system currently numbers in the tens of thousands. The Veterans Administration alone has already employed more than 1,000 peer staff in its hospitals and medical centers. More than 30 states have used waivers to secure Medicaid reimbursement for peer-delivered services, an international peer support network has been formed (with a listserv topping 3,000), and more than 3,000 practitioners of peer support have had input into a first set of US practice guidelines for their rapidly emerging profession (with an ethics statement and set of competencies soon to follow), with similar advances occurring in other countries (e.g., Canada, Scotland). And although mental health practitioners may have initially opened the doors of the system to invite peers in, it has been the peers who have generated the energy, excitement, and effects that are coming to be associated with this relatively new form of service delivery.

We refer to peer support as "relatively new" because it actually has a much longer and more distinguished lineage in psychiatry than most readers might realize. In fact, one of the first references found to hiring former patients to help care for current patients appears in Pinel's 1801 *Treatise on Insanity* (English translation, 1806). Pinel describes the "simple" yet central strategy employed by Jean Baptiste Pussin, governor of the Bicetre Hospital in Paris when he arrived there to be Chief Physician in the 1790s: "His servants were generally chosen from among the convalescents."[67] Pinel knew this prior to his arrival at the Bicetre because he had sent Pussin a letter asking him to describe his strategies for managing the hospital and what he had found helpful in caring for his patients. In what is most likely the first documentation of this practice, Pussin replied in his letter that: "As much as possible, all servants are chosen from the category of mental patients."[68] Once at the Bicetre, Pinel came to see the transformative effect this practice had on the hospital first-hand and soon came to describe Pussin's management practices as "moral treatment."[69]

In the history of psychiatry, there are other examples of rediscoveries of the power of peer support, such as Harry Stack Sullivan's practice of hiring his own recovered patients to staff his inpatient unit for young men experiencing psychosis in Baltimore in the 1920s. One certainly could argue that a key therapeutic agent in the therapeutic community model that dominated inpatient psychiatry in the 1950s and '60s was the role of recovering patients, even though in this case they were not paid for their work because their participation in the therapeutic milieu was considered part of their own treatment. The addiction field has been stimulated and populated by various mutual support approaches throughout its history, with the most prominent contemporary example being Alcoholics Anonymous and other 12-step derivatives. Similarly, one can look outside of psychiatry to many other branches of medicine to see the role that recovered or recovering peers can play in supporting people who are struggling, with a prominent example currently being the growing population of cancer survivors, many of whom now choose to run peer support groups or outreach to persons newly diagnosed. The point of mentioning these earlier and concurrent forms of peer support is simply to establish that the idea of having a person in recovery from a health condition play a useful role in supporting others with the same or similar condition is well-accepted in the general community. Even though this also may have been true in previous decades in psychiatry as well, when peer support was first reintroduced into mental health settings in the 1990s it was considered by many to be an irresponsible, unethical, and potentially harmful practice.

We note the reception that peer support initially received in the mental health system because the form of discrimination it represents continues to challenge and undermine the effectiveness of peer support being offered in many settings across the country. The most formidable obstacles to the successful hiring and deployment of peer staff in mental health organizations are not the conditions from which people are recovering, but rather the cultures of the agencies themselves and the discriminatory attitudes and behaviors of (some) non-peer staff. Underlying this form of discrimination is the deeply held belief that once a person has a mental illness or addiction, he or she will have it for the remainder of his or her life and will be permanently compromised in his or her ability to function as a result. The very presence of peer support staff in mental health settings challenges this long-standing, entrenched belief. And it was, in part, for this reason (i.e., to challenge and disprove such beliefs) that peer staff were initially introduced.[70]

Since their introduction, though, peer staff have quickly shown that there are many more benefits to their employment than the transformative effects they have on organizational culture. Early studies were primarily feasibility studies, showing that it was in fact possible to train and hire persons in recovery with histories of SMIs or addictions to provide behavioral health services. In most of these studies, however, the peers had been hired to provide conventional services, such as functioning as case management assistants or residential staff. In these roles, peer staff were found to function equally as well as non-peer staff, with no differences found in outcomes or other variables.[71]

The only positive difference for peer staff functioning in conventional roles was found in one study of outreach and engagement to persons who would have been eligible for mandated outpatient treatment in a state that did not yet have outpatient commitment. To be eligible, participants had to have an SMI, have shown a positive response to acute care during a previous hospitalization, have a pattern of refusing outpatient services once discharged, and have a history of violence or be at risk for violence. Participants were randomly assigned to either an outreach team that had hired peer staff or an outreach team that had not hired peer staff. Participants who were assigned to peer outreach staff became engaged in treatment more quickly and reported having a better relationship with staff than those assigned to non-peer staff. In this particular study, no adverse events were reported for participants in either study condition over the 2-year duration of the project.[72]

Although some proponents of peer support found these overall results disappointing, it soon became evident that many people hired into peer staff roles were not in fact trained or hired to provide peer support per se. They were hired to function as case managers, as residential or employment support staff, or as generic aides, with little emphasis (if any) on using their own life experiences of illness and recovery to inform their work. In fact, some peer staff report being told that they could not disclose any information about their own recovery to their clients because this would violate professional "boundaries." Such misunderstandings of the role of peer staff in providing peer support unfortunately continue to permeate the field.[73]

More recent studies have begun to focus on the unique strengths and contributions that peer staff can bring to the provision of peer support—in contrast to conventional behavioral health services—and have begun to produce consistently positive findings. In the role of peer supporter, people with histories of SMIs and/or addictions use their personal experiences of illness and recovery—along with relevant training and supervision—to facilitate, guide, and mentor another person's recovery journey by instilling hope, role modeling recovery, and supporting people in their own efforts to reclaim meaningful and self-determined lives in the communities of their choice.[74] The numerous ways in which peers perform these functions as a rapidly growing part of the behavioral health workforce are further described in Chapter 4 on community supports.

The most robust and tangible research finding thus far related to the deployment of peer support staff in this uniquely "peer" capacity has been reductions in the rate and length of stay of costly readmissions for persons with SMIs and/or addictions leaving hospitals. Evaluations of programs in New York and Tennessee, for example, demonstrated reductions of 72% and 73% in rate of rehospitalization and days spent in hospital, respectively.[75] Our own study in Connecticut found a 42% reduction in readmissions and 48% reduction in days spent in hospital by persons with histories of multiple readmissions who were offered peer mentors.[76] A 2013 review commissioned by the National Health Service in England, entitled "Peer Support in Mental Health Care: Is It Good Value for the Money?" calculated that, on average, every British pound (£) spent on peer support resulted in a savings of £4.75 due to reductions in hospital use.[77]

Finally, peer support has been shown to increase hope, empowerment, well-being, and quality of life and reduce substance use and depression among persons with mental illnesses and/or SUDs with histories of multiple hospitalizations and criminal justice involvement.[74,78,79] Peer support has also been shown to increase the involvement of persons with mental illnesses and/or addictions in their own care. A recent study conducted within the VA system, for example, found that veterans who were randomly assigned to care teams that included peer specialists became significantly more active and interested in taking care of themselves.[80]

As health care reform efforts focus on improving the quality of care and on promoting self-management, especially among persons with long-term conditions, there will likely be heightened interest in building on this ability peers have to motivate persons with mental illnesses and/or addictions and teach them self-care skills as members of interdisciplinary health home teams. Peers may also be particularly well suited to function as health navigators, and several studies are currently examining the various physical and behavioral health outcomes of peers functioning in this way as wellness coaches. Preliminary findings suggest that the use of peers may enhance the timely access of persons with mental illnesses to primary care and specialty medical services and may improve their physical and behavioral health, thus addressing their current disparity in life span while at the same time potentially reducing their overall Medicaid costs.[74,78,81]

Recent developments in peer-delivered supports have been somewhat different in the addiction field. Here, there is a long history of substance use services being provided by persons who have their own personal history of recovery from addiction, and Alcoholics Anonymous and its many 12-step derivatives have long been seen as important mutual support complements to professionally provided treatment. In this case, new advances have been made in training and deploying peers—which here means persons in recovery from an addiction—to offer an array of what are described as "recovery support services."[2,82]

The primary aims of recovery support services are to assist persons with SUDs to (1) establish and maintain environments supportive of recovery; (2) remove personal and environmental obstacles to recovery; (3) enhance linkage to, identification with, and participation in local communities of recovery, and (4) increase the hope, inspiration, motivation, confidence, efficacy, social connections, and skills needed to initiate and sustain the difficult and prolonged work of recovery. These services are far more likely to be delivered in the person's natural environment than in clinical settings and, nested within the person's social network, often involve a larger cluster of family and community relationships.

In contrast to the acute care model, the recovery management model emphasizes a sustained continuum of pre-recovery (and pre-treatment), recovery initiation, and recovery maintenance supports. Recovery management models also include sustained recovery monitoring (including recovery checkups), stage-appropriate recovery education, active linkage to indigenous communities of recovery, and early reintervention.[83–85] Finally, recovery support services may be provided by paid or volunteer staff and may be delivered by treatment agencies, local community providers (church, school, labor union), or grassroots and peer-run recovery advocacy or recovery support organizations.[82]

Examples of recovery support services include assertive outreach and engagement, case management (adapted from mental health), recovery coaching or mentoring (provided by peers), and other strategies and interventions that assist people in gaining the resources and skills needed to initiate and sustain recovery, such as transportation, child care, sober housing, social support, and community-based supports to enable people to return to school, obtain and maintain employment, and parent effectively. Although in the past such supports might have been considered to enable continued substance use (i.e., keep people from "hitting bottom"), in the new recovery advocacy movement they are seen as enabling engagement in care and ensuring that people make effective and sustained use of the treatment resources available. Initial research confirms these functions, as well as suggests that the use of recovery support services can reduce acute care costs, increase "connect-to-care" rates following detox and residential treatment, and enhance the effectiveness of treatments in reducing substance use and maintaining abstinence over time.[82,86] This use of peer-delivered interventions—as well as many other aspects of the growing peer support profession—appear to offer fruitful directions for innovation and future research.

ASSESSING QUALITY AND OUTCOMES

In terms of new evaluation tools, governments need to rely on evidence and accurate measurements to justify the allocation of public funds for the development and implementation of new approaches regardless of their appealing, innovative, or progressive nature or outlook. Systematic measurement of impact has thus been highlighted as a means of improving the evidence base and legitimacy of recovery as a recognized best practice.[87] In terms of what is meant by recovery and how to measure it, though, two broad perspectives have generated quite different kinds of data. The first perspective focuses on the dimensions of clinical recovery measured objectively through outcome studies and expressed as approximations to cure. When clinical recovery is understood as an outcome, it can be assessed by an observer with a focus on symptom reduction and the effectiveness of treatments administered by behavioral health services. The other perspective of "personal recovery," in contrast, takes the form of subjective and self-evaluated accounts of how an individual has learned to accommodate living with an illness.[88] As discussed previously, the personal recovery perspective is commonly understood as a process, one that can best be judged by the individual service user, with or without involving symptom reduction or referring to the actions of mental health services.[6]

Clinical recovery and personal recovery are different, and Bellack[89] has referred to scientific versus consumer models of recovery to distinguish between these perspectives. These perspectives are not necessarily mutually exclusive, but they do come from very different backgrounds, with the consumer model being associated with the consumer/survivor movement much more than with the scientific or clinical communities. A plethora of measures already exist to assess clinical recovery from an observer point of view and in terms of specific symptom reductions. These will not be discussed here. Instead, we wish to highlight the importance of person-identified and person-rated outcomes and how new tools have been systematically and rigorously developed to reliably assess personal recovery and the recovery orientation of services. These methods and tool are recognized as being no less scientific than measures of clinical recovery. In that respect, we are grateful to draw on the work done by the Australian Mental Health Outcomes and Classification Network.

In 2010, Burgess, Pirkins, Coombs, and Rosen proposed a systematic review of existing recovery measures. Their identification of potential instruments drew on a search of Medline and PsycInfo that explicitly considered instruments designed to either measure individuals' recovery or instruments designed to assess the recovery orientation of services. Their search yielded 33 instruments, of which 22 were designed to measure individuals' recovery, and 11 were designed to assess the recovery orientation of services (or providers). The researchers were looking for scientifically scrutinized instruments with sound psychometric properties (e.g., internal consistency, validity, reliability). They further applied exclusion criteria to assess whether given instruments might be candidates for measuring recovery in Australian public-sector mental health services from a consumer perspective, including being acceptable to consumers. Assessing these 33 instruments against these supplementary criteria resulted in eight instruments (seven emanating from the United Sates): four for individuals' recovery (Table 3.1) and four for recovery orientation of services (Table 3.2). A more recent review that focused only on measures of personal recovery by Sklar and colleagues[90] assessed the psychometric properties, ease of administration, and degree of service user involvement in the development of each of these measures. The interested reader is referred to this review for details.

It is useful to note that the degree of service user involvement is considered especially crucial in assessing both personal recovery and the recovery orientation of services, programs, and agencies. Personal recovery, as we have defined it, is subjective in nature and thus based in the service user's own perspective. For this reason, service

Table 3.1 INSTRUMENTS FOR MEASURING INDIVIDUALS' RECOVERY

INSTRUMENT	AREAS OF ASSESSMENT	NUMBER OF ITEMS	RESPONSE FORMAT	REFERENCE
Recovery Assessment Scale (RAS)	5 domains: • Personal confidence and hope • Willingness to ask for help • Goal and success orientation • Reliance on others • No domination by symptoms	Original version: • 41 items Short version: • 24 items	Both versions: • 5-point Likert Scale • Provider interview • Consumer self-report	Corrigan, Giffort, Rashid, Leary, & Okeke, 1999[93]
Illness Management and Recovery (IMR) Scales	Does not purport to measure cohesive domains but instead to assess a variety of aspects of illness management and recovery	Both client and clinician versions: • 15 items	Both versions: • 5-point Likert scale	Mueser, Gingerich, Salyers, McGuire, Reyes, & Cunningham, 2004[94]
Stages of Recovery Instrument (STORI)	Five stages of recovery: • Moratorium • Awareness • Preparation • Rebuilding • Growth	• 50 items	• 6-point Likert scale • Consumer self-report	Andresen, Caputi, & Oades, 2006[95]
Recovery Process Inventory (RPI)	Six domains: • Anguish • Connectedness to others • Confidence/purpose • Others care/help • Living situation • Hopeful/cares for self	• 22 items	• 5-point Likert scale • Provider interview	Jerrell, Cousins, & Roberts, 2006[96]

Adapted from Burgess, Pirkins, Coombs, & Rosen, 2010.[92]

users have the only direct access to the body of lived experience and expertise needed to conceptualize and measure this domain. As a result, they must be represented in any attempt to assess personal recovery, not only as participants (obviously) but also as members of the research team as well.

As for measuring recovery orientation, some of the tools just described have already been incorporated into practice and program evaluation efforts, with the Recovery Self-Assessment, for example, having been used by more than 40 states and a dozen other countries to determine the recovery-orientation of existing or newly developed programs. Their use in more rigorous research, however, is just beginning and will likely increase significantly over the next decade. A key challenge facing all stakeholders—from practitioners, agency directors, and system leaders to clients, families, and researchers—is that, thus far, recovery has been implemented more in rhetoric than in actual practice. Perhaps it is for this reason that so many different tools have been developed to assess the recovery orientation of services even before we have established a consensus on what recovery-oriented care looks like in actual practice. In the development of an evidence-base for recovery-oriented practice, it will be important to ensure that what is being evaluated for its effectiveness is recovery-oriented in more than name alone. And, as has been implied in this chapter, the people who will be in the best position to determine this will be those using the services being offered, along with their loved ones. For this reason, recovery proponents argue—if not insist—that service users also be members of research teams that evaluate recovery-oriented practices. This is currently a central focus of the growing movement in "service user-involved" research.[91]

SUMMARY

As one example of the challenge in determining the nature of recovery-oriented practice, readers of this volume will undoubtedly hear practitioners use some recovery-oriented language in their clinical sites. Unfortunately, referring to someone as "a person with schizophrenia" or even "a person in recovery," as opposed to "a schizophrenic," is not all there is to adopting a recovery orientation. A basic sense of respect for the person is certainly important and provides an essential foundation for any other changes to be made in professional

Table 3.2 INSTRUMENT FOR MEASURING RECOVERY ORIENTATION OF SERVICES

INSTRUMENT	AREAS OF ASSESSMENT	NUMBER OF ITEMS	RESPONSE FORMAT	REFERENCE
Recovery Oriented Systems Indicators Measure (ROSI)	Consumer Self-Report Survey: • Person-centered decision-making and choice • Invalidated personhood • Self-care and wellness • Basic life resources • Meaningful activities and roles • Peer advocacy • Staff treatment and knowledge • Access Administrative Data Profile: • Peer support • Choice • Staffing ratios • System culture and orientation • Consumer inclusion in governance • Coercion	Adult Consumer Self-Report Survey: • 41 items Administrative Data Profile: • 23 items	Combination of response formats: • Closed-ended questions • Likert scales • Open-ended questions	Dumont, Ridgway, Onken, Dornan, & Ralph, 2005[97]
Recovery Self-Assessment (RSA)	Five domains: • Life goals • Involvement • Diversity of treatment options • Choice • Individually-tailored services	Four versions of the same survey designed to elicit the views of consumers, family members and care, providers and agency directors Each version: • 36 items	Each version: • 5-point Likert scale	O'Connell, Tondora, Croog, Evans, & Davidson, 2005[98]
Recovery-Oriented Practices Index (ROPI)	Eight domains: • Meeting basic needs • Comprehensive services • Customization and choice • Consumer involvement/participation • Network supports/community integration • Strengths-based approach • Client source of control/self-determination • Recovery focus	• 20 items	• 5-point Likert scale • Interviews with consumers, family members or carers, service managers and service providers • Document review	Mancini & Finnerty, 2005[99]
Recovery Promotion Fidelity Scale (RPFS)	Five domains: • Collaboration • Participation and acceptance • Self-determination and peer support • Quality improvement • Development	• 12 items	• 5-point Likert scale (with some items attracting bonus points) • Survey which draws on the views of consumers, service managers/administrators, providers and family members or carers	Armstrong & Steffen, 2009[100]

Adapted from Burgess, Pirkins, Coombs, & Rosen, 2010.[92]

practice. But our field has espoused such respect for personhood and even the need for our practice to be "person-centered" at least since the time of Pinel—if not, some would argue, all the way back to Hippocrates. Now we are being challenged once again to find ways to embody these principles in ways that are hopeful, strength-based, culturally relevant, and based on the democratic values of self-determination and social inclusion. We anticipate that the coming generation of practitioners will see a plethora of innovative and idealistic efforts to establish multiple new pathways to recovery both inside and outside of the formal behavioral health system. We invite you, the reader, to join in.

REFERENCES

1. President's New Freedom Commission on Mental Health. *Achieving the Promise: Transforming Mental Health Care in America*. Rockville, MD: President's New Freedom Commission on Mental Health; 2003.
2. SAMHSA. *Recovery-Oriented Systems of Care (ROSC) Resource Guide*. Rockville, MD: Department of Health and Human Services; 2011a.
3. Slade M, Amering M, Oades L. Recovery: an international perspective. *Epidemiol Psichiatr Soc*. 2008;17(2):128–137.
4. Slade M, Leamy M, Bacon F, et al. International differences in understanding recovery: systematic review. *Epidemiol Psichiatr Soc*. 2012;21(4):353–364.
5. Davidson L, Roe D. Recovery from versus recovery in serious mental illness: one strategy for lessening confusion plaguing recovery. *J Ment Health*. 2007;16(4):459–470.
6. Slade M. Measuring recovery in mental health services. *Isr J Psychiatry Relat Sci*. 2010;47(3):206–212.
7. White W. *Let's Go Make Some History: Chronicles of the New Addiction Recovery Advocacy Movement*. Washington, DC: Johnson Institute and Faces and Voices of Recovery; 2006.
8. Deegan P. Recovery: the lived experience of rehabilitation. *Psychiatr Rehabil J*. 1988;11(4):11–19.
9. Anthony WA. Recovery from mental illness: the guiding vision of the mental health service system in the 1990s. *Psychiatr Rehabil J*. 1993;16(4); 11–23.
10. Strauss JS, Carpenter WT. The prediction of outcome in schizophrenia, I: characteristics of outcome. *Arch Gen Psychiatry*. 1972;27(6):739–746.
11. Strauss JS, Carpenter WT. The prediction of outcome in schizophrenia, II: relationships between predictor and outcome variables. *Arch Gen Psychiatry*. 1974;31(1):37–42.
12. Strauss JS, Carpenter WT. Prediction of outcome in schizophrenia, III: Five-year outcome and its predictors. *Arch Gen Psychiatry*. 1977;34(2):159–163.
13. Harding CM, Brooks GW, Ashikaga T, Strauss JS, Breier A. The Vermont longitudinal study of persons with severe mental illness, I: methodology, study sample, and overall status 32 years later. *Am J Psychiatry*. 1987a;144(6):718–726.
14. Harding CM, Brooks GW, Ashikaga T, Strauss JS, Breier A. The Vermont longitudinal study of persons with severe mental illness, II: long-term outcome of subjects who retrospectively met DSM-III criteria for schizophrenia. *Am J Psychiatry*. 1987b;144(6):727–735.
15. Harding CM, Zubin J, Strauss JS. Chronicity in schizophrenia: fact, partial fact, or artifact? *Hosp Community Psychiatry*. 1987;38(5):477–486.
16. Ciompi L. The natural history of schizophrenia in the long-term. *Br J Psychiatry*. 1980;136:413–420.
17. Kraepelin E. *Clin Psychiatry*. New York: Macmillan; 1904.
18. Davidson L, McGlashan TH. The varied outcomes of schizophrenia. *The Can J Psychiatry/La Revue canadienne de psychiatrie*. 1997;42(1):34–43.
19. Carpenter WT, Kirkpatrick B. The heterogeneity of the long-term course of schizophrenia. *Schizophr Bull*. 1988;14(4):645–652.
20. SAMHSA. *Consensus Definition of Recovery in Behavioral Health*. Washington, DC: Department of Health and Human Services. http://blog.samhsa.gov/2011/12/22/samhsa%E2%80%99s-definition-and-guiding-principles-of-recovery. Published 2011. Accessed February 1, 2015.
21. Davidson L, White W. The concept of recovery as an organizing principle for integrating mental health and addiction services. *J Behav Health Serv Res*. 2007;34(2):109–120.
22. Kelley JF, White W. *Addiction Recovery Management: Theory, Research, and Practice*. New York: Humana; 2011.
23. Rogers CR. *On Becoming a Person*. New York: Houghton Mifflin; 1961.
24. Institute of Medicine. *Crossing the Quality Chasm: A New Health System for the 21st Century*. Washington, DC: Institute of Medicine; 2001.
25. Tondora J, Miller R, Davidson L. The top ten concerns redux: Implementing person-centered care (in Spanish). In: *Sociedad Iberoamericana de Informacion Cientifica*. May 1, 2010.
26. Davidson L, Tondora J, Miller R, O'Connell M. Person-centered care. In: Corrigan P, ed. *A New Orientation to Adherence and Self-Determination for People With Mental Illness*. Washington, DC: American Psychological Association. In press.
27. Tondora J, Miller R, Slade M, Davidson L. *Partnering for Recovery in Mental Health: A Practical Guide to Person-centered Planning*. London: Wiley Blackwell; 2014.
28. Tondora J, O'Connell M, Dinzeo T, et al. A clinical trial of peer-based culturally responsive person-centered care for psychosis for African Americans and Latinos. *Clin Trials*. 2010;7(4):368–379.
29. Institute of Medicine. *Improving the Quality of Health Care for Mental and Substance Use Conditions*. Washington, DC: Institute of Medicine; 2006.
30. Sen, A. *Development as Freedom*. New York: Anchor Books; 1999.
31. Tondora, J, Miller, R. *Person-Centered Care Planning Questionnaire*. New Haven, CT: Yale Program for Recovery and Community Health; 2000.
32. Davidson L, Roe D, Stern E, Zisman-Ilani Y, O'Connell M, Corrigan P. If I choose it, am I more likely to use it? The role of choice in medication and service use. *Int J Pers Cent Med*. 2012;2(3):577–592.
33. Alakeson V. *The Contribution of Self-Direction to Improving the Quality of Mental Health Services*. Rockville, MD: US Department of Health and Human Services; 2007.
34. Calsyn RJ, Morse GA, Yonker RD, Winter JP, Pierce KJ, Taylor MJ. Client choice of treatment and client outcomes. *J Community Psychol*. 2003;31(4):339–348.
35. Calsyn RJ, Winter JP, Morse GA. Do consumers who have a choice of treatment have better outcomes? *Community Ment Health J*. 2000;36(2):149–160.
36. Hamann J, Langer B, Winkler V, et al. Shared decision making for in-patients with schizophrenia. *Acta Psychiatr Scandinav*. 2006;114(4):265–273.
37. Rokke PD, Tomhave JA, Jocic Z. The role of client choice and target selection in self-management therapy for depression in older adults. *Psychol Aging*. 1999;14(1):155–169.
38. Ryan RM, Plant RW, O'Malley S. Initial motivations for alcohol treatment: relations with patient characteristics, treatment involvement and dropout. *Addict Behav*. 1995;20(3):279–297.
39. Stefancic A, Tsemberis S. Housing First for long-term shelter dwellers with psychiatric disabilities in a suburban county: a four-year study of housing access and retention. *Am J Public Health*. 2007;28(3–4):265–279.
40. Day JC, Bentall RP, Roberts C, Randall F, Rogers A, Cattell D, et al. Attitudes toward antipsychotic medication: the impact of clinical variables and relationships with health professionals. *Arch Gen Psychiatry*. 2005;62(7):717–724.
41. Laugharne R, Priebe S. Trust, choice and power in mental health: a literature review. *Soc Psychiatry Psychiatr Epidemiol*. 2006;41(11):843–852.
42. Ludman E, Katon W, Bush T, et al. Behavioral factors associated with symptom outcomes in a primary care-based depression prevention intervention trial. *Psychol Med*. 2003;33(6); 1061–1070.
43. Wilder CM, Elbogen EB, Moser LL, Swanson JW, Swartz MS. Medication preferences and adherence among individuals with severe mental illness and psychiatric advance directives. *Psychiatr Serv*. 2010;61(4):380–385.
44. Williams GC, Rodin GC, Ryan RM, Grolnick WS, Deci EL. Autonomous regulation and long-term medication adherence in adult outpatients. *Health Psychol*. 1998;17(3):269–276.
45. Kaltiala-Heino R, Laippala P, Salokangas RKR. Impact of coercion on treatment outcome. *Int J Law Psychiatry*. 1997;20(3):311–322.

46. Roe D, Goldblatt H, Baloush-Klienman V, Swarbrick P, Davidson L. Why and how do people with a serious mental illness decide to stop taking their medication: exploring the subjective process of making and activating a choice. *Psychiatr Rehabil J.* 2009;33(1):38–46.
47. Greenfield S, Kaplan S, Ware JE. Expanding patient involvement in care: effects on patient outcomes. *Ann Intern Med.* 1985;102(4):520–528.
48. Greenwood RM, Schaefer-McDaniel NJ, Winkel G, Tsemberis SJ. Decreasing psychiatric symptoms by increasing choice in services for adults with histories of homelessness. *Am J Community Psychol.* 2005;36(3/4):223–238.
49. Langer E, Rodin J. The effects of choice and enhanced personal responsibility for the aged: a field experiment in an institutional setting. *J Pers Soc Psychol.* 1976;34(2):191–198.
50. Srebnik D, Livingston J, Gordon L, King D. Housing choice and community success for individuals with serious and persistent mental illness. *Community Ment Health J.* 1995;31(2):139–152.
51. Stewart M, Brown JB, Donner A, et al. The impact of patient-centered care on outcomes. *J Fam Pract.* 2000;49(9):796–804.
52. Williams GC, McGregor HA, Zeldman A, Freedman ZR, Deci EL. Testing a self-determination theory process model for promoting glycemic control through diabetes self-management. *Health Psychol.* 2004;23(1):58.
53. Chipperfield S, Aubry T. The supportive housing program in Winnipeg. *Psychiatr Rehabil J.* 1990;13(4):91–94.
54. Gulcur L, Stefancic A, Shinn M, Tsemberis S, Fischer S. Housing, hospitalization, and cost outcomes for homeless individuals with psychiatric disabilities participating in continuum of care and housing first programmes. *J Community Appl Soc Psychol.* 2003;13(2):171–186.
55. Loh A, Leonhart R, Wills CE, Simon D, Härter M. The impact of patient participation on adherence and clinical outcome in primary care of depression. *Patient Educ Couns.* 2007;65(1):69–78.
56. Carlson BL, Foster L, Dale S, Brown R. Effect of cash and counseling on personal care and well-being. *Health Serv Res.* 2007;42(1):467–487.
57. Gattellari M, Butow PN, Tattersall MN. Sharing decisions in cancer care. *Soc Sci Med.* 2001;52(12):1865–1878.
58. Ullman R, Hill JW, Scheye EC, Spoeri, RK. Satisfaction and choice: a view from the plans. *Health Aff.* 1997;16(3):209–217.
59. Loh A, Simon D, Wills CE, Kriston L, Niebling W, Härter M. The effects of a shared decision making in primary care of depression: a cluster-randomized control trial. *Patient Educ Couns.* 2007;67(3):324–332.
60. Malm U, Ivarsson BB, Allebeck PP, Falloon IH. Integrated care in schizophrenia: a 2-year randomized controlled study of two community-based treatment programs. *Acta Psychiatr Scandinav.* 2003;107(6):415–423.
61. O'Connell MJ, Kasprow W, Rosenheck R. Direct placement versus multistage models of supported housing in a population of veterans who are homeless. *Psychol Serv.* 2009;6(3):190–201.
62. Becker GR, Drake RE, Farabaugh A, Bond GR. Job preferences among people with severe psychiatric disorders in supported employment programs. *Psychiatr Serv.* 1996;47(11):1223–1226.
63. Drake RE, Becker DR, Clark RE, Mueser KT. Research on the individual placement and support model of supported employment. *Psychiatr Q.* 1999;70(4):289–301.
64. Wehmeyer M, Schwartz M. Self-determination and positive adult outcomes: a follow-up study of youth with mental retardation or learning disabilities. *Except Child.* 1997;63(2):245–255.
65. O'Connell M, Rosenheck R, Kasprow W, Frisman L. An examination of fulfilled housing preferences and quality of life among homeless persons with mental illness and/or substance use disorders. *J Behav Health Serv Res.* 2006;33(3):354–365.
66. Swanson JW, Swartz MS, Elbogen EB, Wagner HR, Burns BJ. Effects of involuntary outpatient commitment on subjective quality of life in persons with severe mental illness. *Behav Sci Law.* 2003;21(4):473–491.
67. Pinel P. A treatise on insanity. In: Davis DD, trans. Sheffield, UK: W. Todd; 1806.
68. Weiner DB. The apprenticeship of Philippe Pinel: A new document, "Observations of Citizen Pussin on the insane." *Am J Psychiatry.* 1979;36(9):1128–1134.
69. Davidson L, Rakfeldt J, Strauss JS. *The Roots of the Recovery Movement in Psychiatry: Lessons Learned.* London: Wiley-Blackwell; 2010.
70. Davidson L, Weingarten R, Steiner J, Stayner D, Hoge M. Integrating prosumers into clinical settings. In: Mowbray CT, Moxley DP, Jasper CA, Howell LL, eds. *Consumers as Providers in Psychiatric Rehabilitation.* Columbia, MD: International Association for Psychosocial Rehabilitation Services; 1997:437–455.
71. Davidson L, Chinman M, Sells D, Rowe M. Peer support among adults with serious mental illness: a report from the field. *Schizophr Bull.* 2006;32(3):443–450.
72. Sells D, Davidson L, Jewell C, Falzer P, Rowe M. The treatment relationship in peer-based and regular case management services for clients with severe mental illness. *Psychiatr Serv.* 2006;57(8):1179–1184.
73. Davidson L. Peer support: coming of age or miles to go before we sleep? *J Behav Health Serv Res.* 2013;96–99. doi: 10.1007/s11414-013-9379-2.
74. Davidson L, Bellamy C, Guy K, Miller R. Peer support among persons with severe mental illnesses: a review of evidence and experience. *World Psychiatry.* 2012;11(2):123–128.
75. New York Association for Psychiatric Rehabilitation Services. *New York State Peer Services Fact Sheet.* Albany: New York Association for Psychiatric Rehabilitation Services; 2012. http://www.policyresearchinc.org/fcnhome/SiteAssets/SCN2012/Session11_PS_FactSheet.pdf. Accessed February 1, 2013.
76. Sledge WH, Lawless M, Sells D, Wieland M, O'Connell M, Davidson L. Effectiveness of peer support in reducing readmissions among people with multiple psychiatric hospitalizations. *Psychiatr Serv.* 2011;62(5):541–544.
77. Trachtenberg M, Parsonage M, Shepard G, Boardman J. *Peer Support in Mental Health Care: Is it Good Value for the Money?* London: Centre for Mental Health; 2013.
78. Chinman M, George P, Doughtery RH, et al. Peer support services for individuals with serious mental illnesses: assessing the evidence. *Psychiatr Serv.* 2014;65(4):429–441.
79. Repper J, Carter T. A review of the literature on peer support in mental health services. *J Ment Health.* 2011;20(4):392–411.
80. Chinman M, Oberman RS, Hanusa BH, et al. A cluster randomized trial of adding peer specialists to intensive case management teams in the Veterans Health Administration. *J Behav Health Serv Res.* 2013;42(1):109–121.
81. Druss BG, Zhao L, von Esenwein SA, et al. The Health and Recovery Peer (HARP) program: a peer-led intervention to improve medical self-management for persons with serious mental illness. *Schizophr Res.* 2010;118(1):264–270.
82. Davidson L, White W, Sells D, Schmutte T, O'Connell M, Bellamy C, et al. Enabling or engaging? The role of recovery support services in addiction recovery. *Alcohol Treat Q.* 2010;28(4):391–416.
83. Dennis ML, Scott CK, Funk R. An experimental evaluation of recovery management checkups (RMC) for people with chronic substance use disorders. *Eval Program Plann.* 2003;26(3):339–352.
84. White W, Boyle M, Loveland D. Recovery management: transcending the limitations of addiction treatment. *Behav Health Management.* 2003;23(3):38–44.
85. Kelley JF, White W. *Addiction Recovery Management: Theory, Research, and Practice.* New York: Humana; 2011.

86. Kirk TA, DiLeo P, Rehmer P, Moy S, Davidson L. Case and care management can improve outcomes while reducing costs and service demand. *Psychiatr Serv.* 2013;64(5):491–493.
87. Gilburt H, Slade M, Bird V, Oduola S, Craig T. Promoting recovery-oriented practice in mental health services: a quasi-experimental mixed-methods study. *BMC Psychiatry.* 2013;13:167. doi:10.1186/1471-244X-13-167.
88. Roberts G, Wolfson P. The rediscovery of recovery: open to all. *Adv Psychiatr Treat.* 2004;10(1):37–49.
89. Bellack, A. Scientific and consumer models of recovery in schizophrenia: concordance, contrasts, and implications. *Schizophr Bull.* 2006;32(3):432–442.
90. Sklar M, Groessl EJ, O'Connell MJ, Davidson L, Aarons GA. Instruments for measuring mental health recovery: a systematic review. *Clin Psychol Rev.* 2013;33(8):1082–1095. doi: 10.1016/j.cpr.2013.08.002.
91. Wallcraft J, Amering M, Schrank B, eds. *Handbook of Service User Involvement in Mental Health Research.* London: Wiley; 2009.
92. Burgess P, Pirkis J, Coombs T, Rosen A. Review of recovery measures. Australian Mental Health Outcomes and Classification Network: "Sharing Information to Improve Outcomes": February, 2010. http://www.recoverydevon.co.uk/download/Review_of_Recovery_Measures.pdf accessed 8/27/2015.
93. Corrigan P, Giffort D, Rashid F, Leary M, Okeke I. Recovery as a psychological construct. *Community Ment Health J.* 1999;35(3):231–239.
94. Mueser K, Gingerich S, Salyers M, McGuire A, Reyes R, Cunningham H. *The Illness Management and Recovery (IMR) Scales (Client and Clinician Versions).* Concord: New Hampshire-Dartmouth Psychiatric Research Center; 2004.
95. Andresen R, Caputi P, Oades L. Stages of recovery instrument: development of a measure of recovery from serious mental illness. *Austral New Zeal J Psychiatry.* 2006;40(11–12):972–980.
96. Jerrell J, Cousins V, Roberts K. Psychometrics of the Recovery Process Inventory. *J Behav Health Serv Res.* 2006;33(4):464–473.
97. Dumont J, Ridgeway P, Onken S, Dornan D, Ralph R. *Mental Health Recovery: What Helps and What Hinders?* A National Research Project for the Development of Recovery Facilitating System Performance Indicators. Phase II Technical Report: Development of the Recovery Oriented System Indicators (ROSI) Measures to Advance Mental Health System Transformation. Alexandria, VA: National Technical Assistance Center for State Mental Health Planning; 2005.
98. O'Connell M, Tondora J, Croog G, Evans A, Davidson L. From rhetoric to routine: Assessing perceptions of recovery-oriented practices in a state mental health and addiction system. *Psychiatr Rehabil J.* 2005;28(4):378–386.
99. Mancini A, Finnerty M. *Recovery-oriented Practices Index.* New York: New York State Office of Mental Health; 2005.
100. Armstrong N, Steffen J. The Recovery Promotion Fidelity Scale: assessing the organizational promotion of recovery. *Community Ment Health J.* 2009;45(3):163–170. doi: 10.1007/s10597-008-9176-1.

4.

COMMUNITY SUPPORTS AND INCLUSION

*Thomas H. Styron, Janis L. Tondora, Rebecca A. Miller, Marcia G. Hunt,
Laurie L. Harkness, Joy S. Kaufman, Morris D. Bell, and Allison N. Ponce*

INTRODUCTION

The move away from living in institutions to a life in the community for people with serious mental illnesses (SMI) and co-occurring disorders characterizes mental health care in the United States in the last half of the twentieth century. Before this period, much of treatment and rehabilitation for individuals with SMI and co-occurring disorders took place during long-term hospital stays and was provided—to the extent it was provided at all—within those walls. Since the 1960s, and in the past two decades in particular, a variety of community supports and strategies for inclusion have emerged to assist individuals with SMI and co-occurring disorders in developing and sustaining lives not in the hospital but in the community (see Chapter 3 for a broader historical context).

The crucial importance of community supports and related strategies for community inclusion for individuals with SMI and co-occurring disorders served as a focal point of the president's 2003 New Freedom Commission.[1] In 2004, the Substance Abuse and Mental Health Services Administration (SAMHSA) assembled a panel of consumers, families, and professionals who agreed that "recovery is a journey of healing and transformation enabling a person with a mental health problem to live a meaningful life in a community of his or her choice while striving to achieve his or her full potential."[2] Subsequently, the SAMHSA[3] delineated four major dimensions that support a life in recovery: *Health*—overcoming or managing one's disease(s) as well as living in a physically and emotionally healthy way; *Home*—a stable and safe place to live; *Purpose*—meaningful daily activities, such as work, school, creative endeavors; and *Community*—relationships and social networks that provide support, friendship, love and hope. This chapter provides an overview of evidence-based supports and strategies for community inclusion. These include housing, employment, education, peer support, and psychosocial rehabilitation (PSR). Professionals in public psychiatry are encouraged to understand and employ these in their efforts to assist individuals with SMI and co-occurring disorders establish and maintain meaningful lives in communities of their choice.

HOUSING

In the wake of deinstitutionalization, supported housing was developed to provide opportunities for people with psychiatric disabilities to live in the community rather than in hospitals, jail, or on the streets.[4] Although many people with SMI and co-occurring disorders live self-sufficiently and independently in their communities of choice *without* supported housing, for others, housing supports are central to recovery. Multiple factors may lead to the desire or need for supported living arrangements. Poverty is a significant factor because low income affects most people who live with SMI and co-occurring disorders,[5] and the modest income that many people in recovery receive creates significant problems in obtaining suitable housing,[6] including increased risk for repeated or chronic homelessness.[7] Personal choice is another important element in determining the best living situation for someone, although these preferences are sometimes at odds with the desires of clinicians and family members, with people sometimes preferring to live alone and supporters sometimes suggesting congregate options like group homes.[8]

A range of housing and residential options are available for individuals with SMI and co-occurring disorders, both for those who experience homelessness and those with housing. These can be in congregate or scattered-site locations and can vary in type from custodial care settings to permanent supportive housing arrangements.

Congregate living situations are those in which several people who have mental illness reside together in one location. These settings may include the structure of a group home or nursing home, or they might be apartment buildings where case management is provided to residents who maintain their own leases and units.

Scattered-site living arrangements are those in which people live in apartments located throughout the community, and these sites are not specifically identified as units for people with disabilities. This model is employed as a means of promoting community inclusion and to increase opportunities for interaction with people outside of the mental health system. Those living in scattered-site locations may still take advantage of services such as clinical care and case management, which are generally based off-site. Tsemberis and colleagues[9] summarize several studies that indicate both advantages and disadvantages for congregate and scattered-site models, and they note the need for further research in this area.

In addition to the distinction between congregate and scattered-site models, which represent *approaches* to housing programs, there are several *types* of residential and housing options that exist within these approaches. These generally include custodial or residential care, housing continuum or housing array, and permanent supportive housing. These options vary in terms of the level of support offered to residents, the amount of independence exercised, and the permanency of the arrangement.

Custodial or *residential care settings* are those in which individuals receive a significant level of support from caregiver staff. These programs are often called "rest homes" or board-and-care facilities. These settings, which usually operate as for-profit businesses, are not generally designed to teach people independent living skills or facilitate rehabilitation and thus often serve as long-term placements.

Housing continuum and *housing array* programs are usually transitional in nature and vary in terms of how much support is offered to residents. An assumption in these models is that rehabilitation can occur in the residential setting. Traditional housing continuum models, which originated in the era of deinstitutionalization,[8] generally employ a stepwise approach: as a person moves toward higher levels of independence, he or she will move to successively less supportive settings, with the ultimate goal of helping a person achieve independent housing. In contrast to the continuum model, the *housing array* model is more flexible and does not prescribe any particular order in which residents should access different levels of care or require that they transition at any particular juncture. Both continuum and array programs usually require engagement in clinical services and sobriety, and they range in intensity from group homes offering around-the-clock staffing to apartment programs that are staffed for portions of the day and allow residents to experience more opportunity to develop independent living skills.

Permanent supportive housing (PSH) is an evidence-based practice[10] that provides permanent housing to individuals with SMI and co-occurring disorders and offers treatment and other supportive services that are individually tailored and may be intensive. According to Tsemberis and colleagues,[9] the goal of PSH is "to improve social integration and quality of life of people with psychiatric disabilities, to reduce the problems people have in achieving stable housing, and to increase the potential for successful recovery from psychiatric disability." The housing is affordable or subsidized and can be either congregate or scattered-site. Individuals in PSH have a lease or sublease in their own names and enjoy the full rights of tenancy. Their leases have no requirements that are not expected of tenants who do not have SMI and co-occurring disorders (such as sobriety), and they cannot lose housing for failure to participate in services. Tenants are offered a range of flexible services that may vary in intensity over time, based on the individual's needs and preferences.

An extensive literature base summarized by the SAMHSA[11] demonstrates that PSH is effective for individuals with SMI and co-occurring disorders. One particularly well-cited study conducted in conjunction with the Corporation for Supportive Housing demonstrated reductions in shelter use, number of hospitalizations, and length of hospitalizations and incarcerations among nearly 5,000 homeless individuals with SMI and co-occurring disorders.[12]

Professionals in public psychiatry can play an important role in supporting individuals in residential settings and PSH. Tsemberis and colleagues discuss the role of psychiatrists in housing and describe the importance of a team-based approach, with care given to clear communication and a consistent definition of responsibilities among team members. Flexible psychiatric outreach and engagement and creative treatment strategies to connect with individuals in the community are recommended. There is also an important role for professionals in public psychiatry as consultants and liaisons to supportive housing staff and other providers.

SUPPORTED EMPLOYMENT AND SUPPORTED EDUCATION

The vast majority of persons with SMI and co-occurring disorders are still unable to claim the valued roles of "employee" or "student" as a core of what they do and who they are. Historically, public mental health systems have tended to divorce the meanings of work and education for people with SMI and co-occurring disorders from the various meanings that work and education have for the general public.[13] For many years, this perspective perpetuated models of care in which participation in work or school was viewed primarily as something that came *after* an individual had successfully completed treatment and achieved clinical stability. This view neglects the fact that meaningful jobs and education are not the reward at the end of the recovery journey but more often the reason a person takes the first step toward wellness.

SUPPORTED EMPLOYMENT

Traditional models of vocational rehabilitation (VR), such as sheltered or protracted "train-and-place" approaches, have been harshly criticized as being (1) disrespectful of the preferences and potential of those accessing VR services, (2) inaccessible to the majority of people with SMI and co-occurring disorders, (3) poorly integrated with clinical services, and (4) unreasonable in the compliance expectations placed on those accessing VR services.[14] Individuals with SMI and co-occurring disorders served in such models could literally spend years, if not decades, "getting ready to work" without ever actually spending a single day in a "real job."[15] For these reasons and more, pre-vocational and transitional approaches began to fall by the wayside in the early 1990s as public mental health systems began to adopt promising alternative rehabilitation interventions, collectively referred to as "supported employment" (SE).

Unlike other vocational approaches, SE programs do not "screen" people for work readiness, but help all who say they want to work; they do not provide pre-vocational or intermediate work experiences, and they actively facilitate rapid job acquisition and often send staff to accompany individuals on interviews and job sites.[16] SE stresses on-the-job training through individualized vocational support plans in recognition of the fact that work behavior is best learned in its natural setting. SE, recognized as an evidenced-based practice for more than a decade by the SAMHSA provides support, instruction, and supervision that are initially intensive then decrease as the individual achieves greater independence. However, the model does not assume that all people will achieve full, autonomous functioning over time. In recognition of this, supports are continuous and are tailored based on individual need. This feature helps to avoid the all-too-frequent situation wherein initial services are withdrawn according to arbitrary time parameters thus leaving insufficient supports to promote job retention in the competitive employment arena.[17]

One specific SE approach, the Individual Placement and Support (IPS) model developed at the New Hampshire–Dartmouth Psychiatric Research Center, has been able to effectively embrace and implement the multiple principles of SE in furthering the community work tenure of people with SMI and co-occurring disorders.[18,19] In addition to the SE principles just described, a core fidelity feature within the IPS model is the integration of vocational and clinical services in one comprehensive interdisciplinary team.

Although IPS emerged in community mental health centers less than 25 years ago, the empirical foundation for the efficacy of the model has been well established. IPS is three times more effective than other vocational approaches in helping people with SMI and co-occurring disorders to work competitively.[20] Similar positive effects have been consistent for nonvocational outcomes as well, such as improved self-esteem, enhanced quality of life, and reduced symptoms.[21] The model has been found effective for numerous populations for which it has been tried, including people with many different diagnoses, educational levels, and prior work histories.[22] Finally, IPS is an excellent investment because studies have demonstrated a significant reduction in community mental health treatment costs for people receiving SE largely due to associated decreases in psychiatric hospitalization days and emergency room usage.[23]

LEARNING-BASED RECOVERY OF COGNITIVE AND WORK CAPACITY

Cognitive impairments are a common feature of SMI and co-occurring disorders and are more closely related to functional disability than clinical symptoms. Moreover, they are often present before the onset of illness and persist in the absence of other clinical manifestations of illness. These impairments often occur in multiple domains including attention, verbal memory, visual memory, processing speed, and executive function.[24] They are likely to be most impaired in schizophrenia and related psychotic disorders, but cognitive impairments are also reported in bipolar disorder, depression, and post-traumatic stress disorder. These impairments may be rate-limiting factors in the recovery of lost function due to psychiatric illness[25] and, for that reason, have become targets for pharmacological and behavioral interventions. Although no psychopharmacological agents have yet demonstrated cognition-enhancing effects, there is growing evidence that cognitive training that takes advantage of the brain's neuroplastic capacity for experienced-based changes may be effective in improving neurocognitive performance. When combined with activating rehabilitation programs, these improvements may lead to significant functional improvements.[26]

For example, recently, a series of studies found that computer-based cognitive remediation that provided exercises that trained attention, memory, and executive function in both verbal and visual domains could improve neurocognitive performance and lead to significant improvements in work performance over time. Moreover, these studies demonstrated that when cognitive remediation was combined with SE services, participants were more likely to achieve competitive employment and to work more hours and earn more money over a two-year period than those who received SE without cognitive remediation.[27,28] Cognitive remediation was found to be most beneficial for those participants who had poor community function at baseline.[29] Thus, it appears that cognitive remediation, when combined with rehabilitation programs, may be especially beneficial to those who need it most—people in recovery less able to do well in the community.

These encouraging findings suggest that systematic learning approaches founded on growing neuroscience understanding of brain plasticity may have broad applications for psychiatric rehabilitation and recovery. Computer-based cognitive training methods are evolving rapidly and becoming more sophisticated, targeted, and user-friendly. They provide the person with greater autonomy and choice because the person being trained may have the option of using these programs at home or in the clinic, and the programs may be shaped to the person's interests and needs. The focus of such training is on positive change and self-improvement, with the cognitive training specialist serving as facilitator and guide. The adaptive nature of computer-based training ensures that the tasks provide the optimum amount of challenge (neither too easy nor too hard) so that the person experiences earned success. These successes may increase motivation and self-confidence as well as improve cognitive performance. These successes may then make it more likely that the person will get the most out of the opportunities provided by SE and other PSR and recovery programs.

SUPPORTED EDUCATION

SMI and co-occurring disorders often emerge in late adolescence or early adulthood and interrupt the attainment of typical educational milestones (e.g., a high school diploma or completion of postsecondary academic or technical training programs). Even in systems of care where evidence-based SE is more widely available, the absence of these educational milestones may limit people to entry-level, low-pay, or part-time positions that relegate them to a life of poverty and dependence on state and federal entitlement programs. In a recovery-oriented system of care, "employment services" should, therefore, be conceptualized broadly to include supported education (SEd) as a critical element of meaningful career development.

SEd, designated as a promising practice by the SAMHSA,[30] is a recovery-oriented practice that was developed to assist individuals with mental illness who want to start or return to school to complete their educational goals.[31] Although SEd is generally geared for postsecondary education, it has also assisted people in getting their General Education Diploma (GED) to help them apply to college or vocational technical school. A comprehensive program of SEd should include methods to strengthen basic educational competencies, immersion in a normalizing educational environment such as a college campus, access to recreational and cultural resources, opportunities for career planning, and professional support for navigating academic environments and negotiating necessary accommodations and peer support from other SEd students.[32] SEd also places a strong emphasis on the need for systems-level change and the widespread offering of awareness building to decrease stigma and increase support for students living with SMI and co-occurring disorders. Successful SEd projects therefore involve collaborative work and the sharing of resources among multiple stakeholders, including students, instructors, family members, tutors, classmates, SEd alumni, and mental health providers.

Research has demonstrated numerous benefits from involvement in SEd programs including decreased hospitalization[33] and increased educational attainment, competitive employment, self-esteem, and personal empowerment.[34,35] More recently, pilot projects combining the interventions of SE and SEd have shown highly promising results, with nearly half of those completing the intervention working in the skilled occupation of their choice at the conclusion of the study.[36]

Service users participating in SE and SEd echo these diverse benefits when describing how participation in work and school helps them achieve a sense of "normalcy" despite the influences of the illness. This phenomenological process is poignantly illustrated in the following statement made by an individual living with a serious psychiatric disorder:

> It lessens the stigma for me, my own personal stigma and how I feel about myself having schizophrenia. I feel more of a normal person. I feel more of a capable person, that I'm just as good as anybody else.[37]

In summary, many individuals identify the pursuit of employment and higher education as a critical ingredients in their personal growth, recovery, and sense of community belonging. The valued roles of "employee" or "student" are particularly crucial for people living with SMI and co-occurring disorders because they afford them the opportunity to define themselves as something other than "mental patients"[38,39] in a service system and society that has traditionally focused on pathology rather than competency.

PEER SUPPORT

As discussed in Chapter 3, the discipline of peer support is a growing area of service provision within public psychiatry and a key element of recovery-oriented care. Emerging from the addictions field and the consumer-survivor movement,[40] peer support has a growing evidence base, national recognition, and a burgeoning labor force last estimated at 10,000–15,000 in the United States.[41] Peer support can play a central role in strategies that promote community inclusion for individuals with SMI and co-occurring disorders.[42] This section offers brief highlights of this important area of practice; see Chapter 3 for a more detailed discussion.

Peer support involves persons in recovery from mental illness working in roles to support others in their recovery journeys and is defined by Mead as "a system of giving and receiving help founded on key principles of respect, shared responsibility, and mutual agreement of what is helpful."[43] Peer support staff share their own experience of mental illness and/or addiction to provide support, hope, and education, and they serve as role models. As a service delivery model, peer support dates back to the early 1990s, but historical roots extend to France in the late 18th century, with other examples across the centuries.[44] Titles of people in this role may include *peer support specialist, recovery coach, recovery support specialist, peer mentor, peer coach*, and others.[45]

Peers provide a wide range of supports in a variety of settings including individual support, groups, education, case management, advocacy, employment support, skill development, support around developing recovery plans, and facilitating specific curricula such as *Wellness Recovery Action Plan*,[46] a commonly peer-provided evidence-based self-directed wellness tool. Peers often act as a bridge to clinical providers, educating people about what to expect from clinicians and alleviating common fears and misconceptions, particularly early in treatment.[47] A recent article also identifies peers as potential consultants to public psychiatry professionals in training, acting as advisors to clinical work.[48] Johnson and colleagues[49] found significant positive impacts on recovery and quality of life for those working as peer support specialists, a finding illustrated by this quote from a provider: "getting back to work as a peer provider makes me feel good; makes me understand I can do [recovery]".[50] A range of certification processes exist in 37 states as of 2012.[51] Many states reimburse for peer-provided services through the Medicaid Rehab Option,[52] and the practice is growing within the Veterans Health Administration as well.[53] A national professional organization, the International Association of Peer Supporters (inaops.org), emerged in 2004, with practice standards for the discipline currently in development. Nevertheless, many challenges within peer support as a discipline persist, including the risk of being co-opted by—and the challenge of retaining one's "peerness" in the face of—more traditional mental health systems and how to create truly mutual relationships in the context of the medical model.[54] Peer staff also encounter discrimination in the workplace and may also encounter fears among clinical staff that the peer will "decompensate," thus becoming a burden rather than an asset to treatment teams,[55] despite research evidence to the contrary.

The evidence in support of peer programming is increasingly robust and promising. Evidence shows that peer support increases empowerment, helps reach people difficult to engage,[56] and inspires hope.[57] In a recent overview of peer support, Chinman and colleagues[58] considered the evidence strength "moderate" and identified improvements in the following six outcomes: reduced inpatient use, improved relationship with providers, better engagement with care, higher levels of empowerment, higher levels of activation, and higher levels of hopefulness for recovery.

One of the unique qualities of peer support is "conditional regard" and the ability to "call someone out" based on the legitimacy granted by a shared experience, illustrated by the quote here:

> I had been sitting back letting other folks call the shots, and then complaining when things got messed up. A Peer Specialist at the advocacy center called me out on it. I realized that I had gotten comfortable letting other folks make decisions for me, and I know now that I gotta take charge of my own recovery.[59]

As an essential part of an interdisciplinary team, peer support adds a unique resource for people with mental illness and for promoting recovery. As well as serving as role models for clients, peers are living examples of recovery and remind providers of its possibility, thus acting as advocates and assisting in decreasing discrimination. Peer support can be especially helpful in working with those who are harder to engage into care and who are mistrustful of the mental health system. A key point for professionals in public psychiatry is acknowledging that peer support team members are staff just like other staff, but can offer their unique perspective to the work and can provide invaluable insights around care.

PSYCHOSOCIAL REHABILITATION: PUTTING THE PIECES TOGETHER

Successful strategies for community inclusion depend, in a large part, on the identification, coordination, and integration of any and all community supports, be they housing, employment, education, peer, social supports, and/or life skills based on an individual's particular needs. PSR is an approach that can bring all these pieces together. PSR has been conceptualized in many ways but is defined generally as a process or approach that utilizes a broad variety of techniques, many of them evidence-based, to help an individual reach his or her highest potential or highest individual community functioning.[60-62] In addition to supported housing, employment, education, and peer supports, as discussed previously, core PSR practices include Assertive Community Treatment (ACT) (see Chapters 13 and 17), Medication Management (see Chapters 12 and 17), Family Psychoeducation (see Chapters 10 and 17) and, as will be discussed later, interdisciplinary case management, training to improve life skills, fostering of natural social supports, and clubhouses.

INTERDISCIPLINARY CASE MANAGEMENT

Case management is a key component in assisting people with SMI and co-occurring disorders to succeed in community-based living.[63,64] Case management services for adults with SMI and co-occurring disorders provide care and/or care coordination for needs including physical health, mental health, housing, employment, social roles, and community integration goals. In so doing, case management addresses each of the SAMHSA's four dimensions for recovery: health, home, purpose, and community. Interdisciplinary case management is a team-based service that utilizes the skills and discipline-specific expertise of team members to provide a holistic approach to providing and/or coordinating care.[65,66] Interdisciplinary case management is often central to—if not essential in—determining a comprehensive and holistic person-centered care plan. To help ensure a person-centered approach, many teams use an organizing tool such as "SNAP" to be sure to include a person's *strengths, needs, abilities,* and *preferences* in the care planning process.[67]

LIFE SKILLS TRAINING

Life skills training is another core PSR technique, and it may include Illness Management and Recovery (IMR) or similar evidence-based programs of self-management, such as money management[68] and social skills training.[69] IMR is a curriculum developed to help people with SMI and co-occurring disorders understand recovery, set goals for moving forward, gain greater understanding of mental illness and its treatment, develop medication support regimens and relapse prevention plans, learn coping skills for symptom management, and improve social support. Whereas IMR is a multifaceted approach drawing on several evidence-based practices including Cognitive Behavioral Therapy (CBT), money management and social skills training target a specific area of need.

FOSTERING NATURAL SUPPORTS

Fostering natural supports can include helping with the development of new relationships, the strengthening of current relationships, family reunification, and, ultimately, expanding roles within communities or groups with shared interests or values such as the arts community, faith community, and 12-step programs. Natural supports are best characterized as "naturally occurring, [largely] bi-directional and mutual relationships."[70] Like most PSR techniques, fostering natural supports necessitates *in vivo* work, so that context and group norms, among other variables, can be understood and the care team can best assist the person in building or strengthening social connections and supports.

CLUBHOUSES

Clubhouses are one of the best known models within PSR. The first clubhouse, which established the model, was Fountain House, located in New York City and established in 1948 by people who had previously formed a self-help group after their discharge from a nearby state hospital.[71] The clubhouse model is a member-driven therapeutic community in which members have specific rights and responsibilities, including self-governance, through which the model promotes hope and empowerment.[72] Clubhouse International, the accrediting body for clubhouses, considers a clubhouse to be a "local community center" with a focus on employment for members, either as a paid worker in the community or as a volunteer in the clubhouse working in various aspects of the program. Clubhouses often offer housing support, case management, supported education, and advocacy. Limited staff are hired by clubhouses. The Clubhouse International website notes that there are 341 clubhouses in 32 countries as of March 2014.[73]

THE IDENTIFICATION, IMPLEMENTATION, AND COORDINATION OF COMMUNITY SUPPORTS

One way to illustrate the identification, implementation, and coordination of community supports on an individualized basis and the PSR process more broadly is through a brief case vignette. Meet Mr. Harry Harcourt (whose name and other identifying information have been changed to protect confidentiality):

Mr. Harcourt is a 49-year-old white man, currently without housing, who has a diagnosis of bipolar disorder and a substance use disorder. He served in the military from the age of 18–26 and receives a small veteran's disability benefit. After the military, he worked in construction and later worked as a tool and die maker, but he hasn't worked steadily for around 15 years. He has a brother and an aunt living nearby with whom he is not in touch. He identifies as heterosexual, has never been married, and has no children. Mr. Harcourt has had several encounters with the police in the past when he drinks. He has multiple medical problems including diabetes, obesity, and congestive heart failure.

Mr. Harcourt has sporadically accessed mental health care through a community mental health center and, at times, a VA hospital. His physical health care has largely been through the VA. He usually sees an outpatient psychiatrist for medication management but has needed inpatient care during both manic and depressed episodes several times in the past.

Within a recovery paradigm, the approach to helping Mr. Harcourt includes understanding his strengths, needs, abilities, and preferences (SNAP) so that his care is both holistic and person-centered. This is a first step for professionals in public psychiatry working as a team to develop a wrap-around care plan.

Strengths: Mr. Harcourt honorably served in the military and has a small pension income and access to VA health care due to his veteran status. He has valuable work skills (carpentry, tool and die) and a high school education. Mr. Harcourt also has relatives who live near him and who may be a source of support.

Needs: Mr. Harcourt's needs from a health provider's point of view are his mental and physical health care, followed by his lack of safe and affordable housing. Mr. Harcourt indicates that working, addressing legal problems, and improving his relationship with his family are his primary needs.

Abilities: Mr. Harcourt is a strong self-advocate. He is able to voice his needs easily and will advise providers when his needs are not being met. This is sometimes viewed by providers as being disruptive or "noncompliant."

Preferences: Like many people, Mr. Harcourt is not able to easily articulate treatment preferences without assistance in determining which services in his care system are under his control. With assistance from his team, he indicates he prefers not to come to a mental health center for treatment and would like the opportunity to work with a peer who he feels may better understand his struggles.

After completing the SNAP assessment, the care team and Mr. Harcourt are able to develop a holistic view of his current situation, priorities, and needs. They decide that interdisciplinary case management using an ACT model will allow Mr. Harcourt to be served in the community and would be the best approach given his complex needs. Within this model, a number of steps and approaches are identified and recommended to Mr. Harcourt. These include:

1. IMR skill building, including an emphasis on continuing medication management and the introduction of peer supports to address Mr. Harcourt's mental health and substance use.
2. A case manager who is designated to support Mr. Harcourt during initial meetings with his lawyer in order to address his legal issues.

3. A referral to supported housing. Although housing is not a stated priority for Mr. Harcourt, he agrees that stable housing would ultimately be to his benefit, considering his employment needs and primary health issues.
4. Supported employment. Mr. Harcourt is connected with the SE specialist on his interdisciplinary care team, and, after an assessment, they immediately pursue a competitive employment placement with supports.
5. Therapy. Mr. Harcourt and his care team agree that, among other things, therapy will focus on helping him rebuild relationships with his aunt and brother, and the team will provide assistance in reaching out to them.
6. Finally, although Mr. Harcourt is ambivalent about giving up alcohol and making social connections, Mr. Harcourt and his care team identify community resources such as Alcoholics Anonymous and a local Clubhouse with a wide variety of available daily activities for him to consider. Through discussions with his care team and the use of motivational interviewing, Mr. Harcourt realizes that sobriety and use of these community supports can have a positive impact on achieving many of his goals, including those related to legal issues, employment, and family relationships.

With all of these supports in place, Mr. Harcourt is able to make slow and steady progress in achieving his goals.

ENSURING QUALITY IMPROVEMENT

The Health Resources and Services Administration[74] defines quality improvement (QI) as consisting of "systematic and continuous actions that lead to measurable improvement in health care services and the health status of targeted populations." A review of QI data for agencies that provide supports for individuals receiving publicly funded community-based psychiatric services can help professionals in public psychiatry understand both the impact of the services for their clients and also clients' perceptions of the care provided.

Although many community-based providers are required by their funders to collect and report client and services data, many of these agencies do not utilize these data to understand the impact of their services or to improve the quality of care provided. As a requirement of the Federal Community Mental Health Services Block Grant program,[75] states must report data on a myriad of outcomes including employment/education, stability in housing, social connectedness, access to care, client perceptions of care, and criminal justice involvement. With the goal of helping providers utilize collected data, some localities have implemented a network of care approach, which, along with other services and supports, provides core support to help build the capacity of community providers to employ a QI process.[76]

In an effort to promote transparency and service development, some states post on the Web a "dashboard" or summary of outcomes for each program they fund.[77] These reports provide information for both consumers and providers that can be helpful in determining the most appropriate service fit and promote QI: for example, given the consensus in the consumer literature that services are beneficial when they facilitate recovery.[78]

Consumer perspectives of care are an essential outcome to consider. For professionals in public psychiatry who work from a recovery orientation, the review of consumer satisfaction data provides an opportunity to understand if a community provider shares this orientation and, if not, there is an opportunity to address this discrepancy.

RECOMMENDATIONS FOR THE PROMOTION OF COMMUNITY INCLUSION

Community inclusion should be the shared commitment of all providers in public sector mental health. In addition, the creation of a wide spectrum of community-based care resources introduces a challenge with regard to its integration with other treatments. The following paragraphs detail recommendations for professionals in public psychiatry to maximize their contributions in an evolving recovery-based system of care for persons with SMI and co-occurring disorders.

In clinical practice and organizational leadership, professionals in public psychiatry should actively encourage and support all people in exploring and pursuing resources and opportunities that lead to socially valued community roles. Housing, employment, education, and social life are, for all people, usually the foundation for such roles.

Psychiatric expertise and treatment, including pharmacological management, need to be reframed so that they are squarely focused on outcomes that are most important to the individual. For example, employment- or school-related goals may call for modifications to medication schedules to promote maximum energy and cognitive functioning at certain times during the day. The care team may also need to discuss with the person how symptoms and side effects impact work or school performance and to brainstorm personal management strategies.

Professionals in public psychiatry should be mindful of referral procedures that preclude certain people from accessing supported housing, employment, education, and other resources. In some systems, people are still screened for "readiness" in one or more of these areas and are unable to access services unless they are deemed to be functioning at a high enough level. In general, readiness screening has no place in a recovery-oriented system of care, and professionals in public psychiatry can advocate for a science-based "zero reject policy" that does not exclude people based on symptomatology, substance use, or unwillingness to participate in community supports.

Along these same lines, many people served by the community mental health system often have substantial fears and doubts regarding their ability to pursue meaningful lives in the community and valued social roles after having heard the message for years that they "are not ready" and being repeatedly asked "what if you relapse?" Professionals in public psychiatry can play a critical role in addressing these fears by consistently sending the message that participation in their community of choice through supported housing, work, education, or other opportunities is fundamental for mental health and wellness.[79]

As team leaders and policy-makers, all professionals in public psychiatry can embrace the emerging best practice of person-centered recovery planning (PCRP) as a powerful tool in helping people to return to or continue in valued social roles. Person-centered planning models support individuals with SMI and co-occurring disorders to discover (or rediscover) themselves as healthy persons with a history, a future, and with strengths and interests beyond their clinical deficits or functional impairments. As such, PCRP is highly complementary to strategies for community inclusion, and professionals in public psychiatry are encouraged to develop their knowledge and competencies in this area.

Finally, individuals with SMI and co-occurring disorders continue to be the target of damaging and unremitting myths and assumptions that contribute to their exclusion from the community. The media is fraught with images of violence committed by people with psychiatric disabilities, despite the fact that there is limited empirical support for such a sensationalized caricature.[80] Leading professionals in public psychiatry are uniquely positioned to confront these myths and assumptions and communicate accurate facts within and beyond the community mental health system.

SUMMARY

Public psychiatry has undergone a revolution over the past 50 years as the care of people with SMI and co-occurring disorders moved from the hospital to the community. Nowhere is this change more evident than in the emergence of community supports and the goal of community inclusion in contemporary practice. This chapter has reviewed the evidence for essential community supports such as housing, SE, SEd, and peer support. Also, it has highlighted the multiple practices of community-based PSR. Supporting individuals with SMI and co-occurring disorders in the community raises the challenge of achieving true community inclusion through an integration of treatment and other essential support based on person-centered care within recovery-oriented systems. A case vignette highlighted this challenge through the lens of one individual's set of circumstances, needs, and desires. Finally, the chapter discussed the importance of metrics for evaluating community supports and inclusion as a way of achieving continuous quality improvement.

REFERENCES

1. New Freedom Commission on Mental Health. *Achieving the Promise: Transforming Mental Health Care in America. Final Report.* DHHS Pub. No. SMA-03-3832. Rockville, MD: Department of Health and Human Services; 2003.
2. Substance Abuse and Mental Health Services Administration. National Consensus Statement on Mental Health Recovery. http://www.cibhs.org/sites/main/files/file-attachments/10_fundamental_components_of_recovery.pdf. 2006. Accessed date: 9/4/15.
3. Substance Abuse and Mental Health Services Administration. SAMHSA announces a working definition of recovery. 2011b. http://www.samhsa.gov/newsroom/press-announcements/201112220800. Accessed date: 9/4/15.
4. McQuistion HL, Sowers W, Ranz JM, Feldman JM (Eds). The role of psychiatry in permanent supported housing. *Handbook of Community Psychiatry*. New York: Springer; 2012:349–368.
5. Draine J. Role of social disadvantage in crime, joblessness, and homelessness among persons with serious mental illness. *Psychiatric Serv.* 2002;53(5):565–573. doi:10.1176/appi.ps.53.5.565.
6. Levstek DA, Bond GR. Housing cost, quality, and satisfaction among formerly homeless persons with serious mental illness in two cities. *Innovat Res.* 1993;2(3):1–8.
7. McQuistion HL, Sowers W, Ranz JM, Feldman JM (Eds). Homelessness and behavioral health in the new century. *Handbook of Community Psychiatry*. New York: Springer; 2012:407–422.
8. Corrigan, PW. *Principles and Practice of Psychiatric Rehabilitation: An Empirical Approach*. New York: Guilford; 2008.
9. Tsemberis S, Henwood B, Yu Vl, Whoriskey Al, & Stephanic, A. The role of psychiatry in permanent supported housing. In McQuiston HL, Sowers WE, Ranz JM, Feldman JM (Eds.). *Handbook of Community Psychiatry*. New York: Springer; 2012:349–368.
10. Substance Abuse and Mental Health Services Administration. *Permanent Supportive Housing: Building Your Program*. HHS Pub. No. SMA-10-4509. Rockville, MD: Center for Mental Health Services, Substance Abuse and Mental Health Services Administration; 2010a.

11. Substance Abuse and Mental Health Services Administration. *Permanent Supportive Housing: The Evidence*. HHS Pub. No. SMA-10-4509. Rockville, MD: Center for Mental Health Services, Substance Abuse and Mental Health Services Administration; 2010b.
12. Culhane DP, Metraux S, Hadley T. Public service reductions associated with placement of homeless persons with severe mental illness in supportive housing. *Hous Policy Debate*. 2002;13(1):107–163. doi:10.1080/10511482.2002.9521437.
13. Bonnie RJ, Monahan J. Mental disorders, work, and choice. In: *Mental Disorder, Work Disability, and the Law*. Chicago: University of Chicago Press; 1997:105–130.
14. Drake RE, Becker DR, Xie H, Anthony WA. Barriers in the brokered model of supported employment for people with psychiatric disabilities. *J Vocat Rehabil*. 1995;5:141–149.
15. Fabian E. The example of consumers with serious mental health disorders. *Rehabil Counsel Bull*. 1999;41(4):302–316.
16. Bond GR. Implementing supported employment as an evidence-based best practice. *Psychiatr Serv*. 2001;52(3):313–322.
17. Cook J. Research-based principles of vocational rehabilitation for psychiatric disability. *Int Assoc Psychosoc Rehab Serv*. 1999;4(1):6–7.
18. Drake RE. A brief history of the individual placement and support model. *Psychiatr Rehabil J*. 1998;22(1):3–7. doi:10.1037/h0095273.
19. Drake RE. A Randomized clinical trial of supported employment for inner-city patients with severe mental disorders. *Arch Gen Psychiatry*. 1999;56(7):627–633. doi:10.1001/archpsyc.56.7.627.
20. Bond GR, Drake RE. An update on randomized controlled trials of evidence-based supported employment. *Psychiatr Rehabil J*. 2008;31(4):280–290. doi:10.2975/31.4.2008.280.290.
21. Drake RE, Bond GR, Becker DR. *Individual Placement and Support: An Evidence-Based Approach to Supported Employment*. Oxford: Oxford University Press; 2012.
22. Campbell K, Bond GR, Drake RE. Who benefits from supported employment: a meta-analytic study. *Schizophr Bull*. 2011;37(2):370–380. doi:10.1093/schbul/sbp066.
23. Burns T, Catty J, White S, et al. The impact of supported employment and working on clinical and social functioning: results of an international study of individual placement and support. *Schizophr Bull*. 2009;35(5):949–958. doi:10.1093/schbul/sbn024.
24. Wexler BE, Nicholls SS, Bell MD. Instability of cognitive processing systems in schizophrenia. *Schizophr Res*. 2004;71(2–3):513–514.
25. Green M. What are the functional consequences of neurocognitive deficits in schizophrenia. *Am J Psychiatry*. 1996;153(3):321–330.
26. Wykes T, Huddy V, Cellard C, Mcgurk SR, Czobor, P. A meta-analysis of cognitive remediation for schizophrenia: methodology and effect sizes. *Am J Psychiatry*. 2011;168(5):472–485. doi:10.1176/appi.ajp.2010.10060855.
27. Bell MD, Bryson GJ, Greig TC, Fiszdon JM, Wexler BE. Neurocognitive enhancement therapy with work therapy: productivity outcomes at 6- and 12-month follow-ups. *J Rehabil Res Dev*. 2005;42(6):829. doi:10.1682/JRRD.2005.03.0061.
28. Bell MD, Zito W, Greig T, Wexler BE. Neurocognitive enhancement therapy with vocational services: work outcomes at two-year follow-up. *Schizophr Res*. 2008;105(1–3):18–29. doi:10.1016/j.schres.2008.06.026.
29. Bell MD, Choi K, Dyer C, Wexler BE. Benefits of cognitive remediation and supported employment for schizophrenia patients with poor community functioning. *Psychiatr Serv*. 2014;65(4):469. doi:10.1176/appi.ps.201200505.
30. Substance Abuse and Mental Health Services Administration. *Supported Education: How to Use the KITs*. HHS Pub. No. SMA-11-4654. Rockville, MD: Center for Mental Health Services, Substance Abuse and Mental Health Services Administration; 2011b.
31. Mowbray CT, Collins ME, Bellamy CD, Megivern DA, Bybee D, Szilvagyi S. Supported education for adults with psychiatric disabilities: an innovation for social work and psychosocial rehabilitation practice. *Social Work*. 2005;50(1):7–20. doi:10.1093/sw/50.1.7.
32. Bellamy CD, Root K, Mowbray CT, Szilvagyi S. *The Supported Education Program Implementation Manual*. Unpublished manuscript. Ann Arbor, MI: Supported Education Community Action Group; 2004.
33. Unger KV, Anthony WA, Rogers ES. A supported education program for young adults with long-term mental illnesses. *Hosp Community Psychiatry*. 1991;42:838–842.
34. Cook JA, Solomon, ML. The Community Scholar Program: an outcome study of supported education for students with severe mental illness. *Psychosoc Rehab J*. 1993;17(1):83–97. doi:10.1037/h0095623.
35. Mowbray CT, Collins M, Bybee D. Supported education for individuals with psychiatric disabilities: long-term outcomes from an experimental study. *Social Work Res*. 1999;23(2):89–100. doi:10.1093/swr/23.2.89.
36. Rudnick A, Gover M. Combining supported education with supported employment. *Psychiatr Serv*. 2009;60(12):1690–1690. doi:10.1176/appi.ps.60.12.1690.
37. Krupa T. *Work Recovery in Schizophrenia*. Unpublished manuscript, Department of Human Development and Applied Psychology, University of Toronto; 2000.
38. Arns P, Linney J. Work, self, and life satisfaction for people with severe and persistent mental disorders. *Psychosoc Rehab J*. 1993;17(2):63–69.
39. Bailey J. I'm just an ordinary person. *Psychiatric Rehab J*. 1998;22(1):8–10.
40. Chamberlin J. Speaking for ourselves: an overview of the ex-psychiatric inmates movement. *Psychiatric Rehab J*. 1984;8(2):56–64.
41. Goldstrom ID, Campbell J, Rogers JA, et al. National estimates for mental health mutual support groups, self-help organizations, and consumer-operated services. *Adm Policy Ment Health*. 2006;33(1):92–103. doi:10.1007/s10488-005-0019-x.
42. Davidson L, Bellamy C, Guy K, Miller R. Peer support among persons with severe mental illness: a review of evidence and experience. *World Psychiatry*. 2012;11(2):123–128.
43. Mead S. Defining peer support. 2003. http://chrysm-associates.co.uk/images/SMeadDefiningPeerSupport.pdf. P. 135. Accessed date: August 28th, 2015.
44. Davidson L, Bellamy C, Guy K, Miller R. Peer support among persons with severe mental illness: a review of evidence and experience. *World Psychiatry*. 2012;11(2):123–128.
45. International Association of Peer Supporters. Peer Support Definition. 2014. http://inaops.org/definition-peer-specialist/. Accessed date: August 28th, 2015.
46. Copeland ME. *Wellness Recovery Action Plan: A System for Monitoring, Reducing and Eliminating Uncomfortable or Dangerous Physical Symptoms and Emotional Feelings*. West Dummerston, VT: Peach Press; 2002.
47. Davidson L, Bellamy C, Guy K, Miller R. Peer support among persons with severe mental illness: a review of evidence and experience. *World Psychiatry*. 2012;11(2):123–128.
48. Agrawal S, Edwards M. Personal accounts: upside down: the consumer as advisor to a psychiatrist. *Psychiatr Serv*. 2013;64(4):301–302. doi:10.1176/appi.ps.640413.
49. Johnson G, Magee C, Maru M, Furlong-Norman K, Rogers, ES, Thompson, K. Personal and societal benefits of providing peer support: a survey of peer support specialists. *Psychiatr Serv*. 2014;65(5):678–680.
50. Davidson L, Rowe M, O'Connell M, Lawless MS. *A Practical Guide to Recovery-Oriented Practice: Tools for Transforming Mental Health Care*. Oxford University Press: New York; 2008: 95.
51. Kaufman L, Brooks W, Steinley-Bumgarner, M., Stevens-Manser, S. *Peer Specialist Training and Certification Programs: A National*

Overview. University of Texas at Austin Center for Social Work Research; 2012. http://www.dbsalliance.org/pdfs/training/peer-specialist-training-and-certification-programs-a-national-overview UT 2013.pdf. Accessed date: August 28, 2015.
52. US Department of Health & Human Services, Center for Medicare and Medicaid Services; SMDL 07-11;2007. Downloads.cms.gov/cmsgov/archived-downloads/SMDL/downloads/smd081507A.pdf. Accessed date: August 28, 2015.
53. Resnick SG, Rosenheck RA. Integrating peer-provided services: a quasi-experimental study of recovery orientation, confidence, and empowerment. *Psychiatr Serv*. 2008;59(11):1307–1314. doi:10.1176/appi.ps.59.11.1307.
54. Braiterman K. Peer support in CMHC's is an oxymoron, peer support pioneer says. http://www.madinamerica.com/2012/07/peer-support-in-cmhcs-is-an-oxymoron-peer-support-pioneer-says/ 2008. Updated July 19, 2012. Accessed date: August 28, 2015.
55. Davidson L, Bellamy C, Guy K, Miller R. Peer support among persons with severe mental illness: a review of evidence and experience. *World Psychiatry*. 2012;11(2):123–128.
56. Sells D, Black R, Davidson L, Rowe M. Beyond generic support: incidence and impact of invalidation in peer services for clients with severe mental illness. *Psychiatr Serv*. 2008;59(11):1322–1327. doi:10.1176/appi.ps.59.11.1322.
57. Sledge W, Lawless M, Sells D, Wieland M, O'Connell M, Davidson L. Effectiveness of peer support in reducing readmissions among people with multiple psychiatric hospitalizations. *Psychiatr Serv*. 2011;62:541–544.
58. Chinman M, George P, Dougherty RH, et al. Peer support services for individuals with serious mental illnesses: assessing the evidence. *Psychiatr Serv*. 2014;65(4):429. doi:10.1176/appi.ps.201300244.
59. Tondora J, Miller R, Slade M, Davidson L. *Planning for Recovery in Mental Health: A Practical Guide to Person-Centered Planning*. London: Wiley-Blackwell; 2014.
60. Anthony WA, Cohen MR, Farkas MD, Gagne C. *Psychiatric Rehabilitation*. 2nd ed. Boston, MA: Center for Psychiatric Rehabilitation, Boston University, Sargent College of Allied Health Professions; 2002.
61. Bachrach LL. Psychosocial rehabilitation and psychiatry in the care of long-term patients. *Am J Psychiatry*. 1992;149:1455–1463.
62. World Health Organization. Psychosocial Rehabilitation: A Consensus Statement. http://www.who.int/iris/handle/10665/60630. Issued 2006. Accessed date: January 25, 2014.
63. Horvitz-Lennon M, Kilbourne AM, Pincus HA. From silos to bridges: meeting the general health care needs of adults with severe mental illness. *Health Aff*. 2006;25(3):659–669.
64. Mueser KT. The illness management and recovery program: rationale, development, and preliminary findings. *Schizophr Bull*. 2006;32(Suppl 1):S32–S43. doi:10.1093/schbul/sbl022.
65. Jessup RL. Interdisciplinary versus multidisciplinary care teams: do we understand the difference? *Austral Health Rev*. 2007;31(3):330.
66. Rapp CA, Goscha, RJ. The principles of effective case management of mental health services. *Psychiatr Rehabil J*. 2004;27(4):319–333. doi:10.2975/27.2004.319.333.
67. CARF International. 2014 Behavioral Health Program Descriptions. www.carf.org/programdescriptions/bh/. Accessed date: January 25, 2014.
68. Marson DC. Financial capacity in persons with schizophrenia and serious mental illness: clinical and research ethics aspects. *Schizophr Bull*. 2005;32(1):81–91.
69. Kopelowicz A. Recent advances in social skills training for schizophrenia. *Schizophrenia Bulletin*. 2006;32(Suppl1):S12–S23.
70. Davidson L, Chinman M, Sells D, Rowe M. Peer support among adults with serious mental illness: a report from the field. *Schizophr Bull*. 2005;32(3):443–450. doi:10.1093/schbul/sbj043.
71. Macias C, Jackson R, Schroeder C, Wang Q. What is a clubhouse? Report on the ICCD 1996 survey of USA clubhouses. *Community Ment Health J*. 1999;35:181–190.
72. Jacobs HE, DeMello C. The clubhouse model and employment following brain injury. *J Vocat Rehabil*. 1996;7:169–179.
73. Clubhouse International. Mission. http://www.iccd.org/mission.html. Accessed January 25, 2014.
74. Health Resources and Service Administration. Quality improvement. 2011. http://www.hrsa.gov/quality/toolbox/methodology/qualityimprovemement/ Accessed date: March 24, 2014.
75. Substance Abuse and Mental Health Services Administration. National outcome measures (NOMS). http://www.samhsa.gov/co-occurring/topics/data/nom.aspx, Accessed date: March 27, 2015.
76. Kaufman, JS, Crusto, CA, Quan, M, Ross, E, Friedman, SR, O'Rielly, K, Call, S. Utilizing program evaluation as a strategy to promote community change: Evaluation of a comprehensive community-based family violence initiative. *Journal of Community Psychology*, 2006;38(3-4):191–200.
77. Department of Mental Health and Addiction Services. EQMI-Provider Quality Reports Info. 2014. http://www.ct.gov/dmhas/cwp/view.asp?a=2900&q=489554. Accessed date: March 20, 2015.
78. Torrey WC, Wyzik P. The recovery vision as a service improvement guide for community mental health center providers. *Psychiatr Rehabil J*. 2010;36(2):209–217.
79. Marrone J, Golowka E. If work makes people with mental illness sick, what do unemployment, poverty, and social isolation cause? *Psychiatr Rehabil J*. 1999;23(2):187–193.
80. Monahan J. Mental disorder and violent behavior: perceptions and evidence. *Am Psychol*. 1992;47(4):511–521.

PART II

SYSTEM INTEGRATION CHALLENGES IN PUBLIC PSYCHIATRY

5.

INTEGRATED HEALTH CARE

Aniyizhai Annamalai, Cenk Tek, Michael J. Sernyak, Robert Cole, and Jeanne L. Steiner

---

EDUCATIONAL HIGHLIGHTS

- Integrated medical and behavioral health services are imperative for improving the morbidity and mortality of seriously mentally ill people.

- Health care models integrating primary care into behavioral health show early promise for improving health outcomes in this population.

- The Center for Integrated Health Solutions funded by the Substance Abuse and Mental Health Services Administration and the Health Resources and Services Administration promotes integrated care and provides training to community health organizations.

- The Affordable Care Act creates options for providing health homes for those with chronic conditions; although these homes have traditionally been based at primary care centers, there is now opportunity for community mental health centers to serve as medical homes.

- Psychiatrists and other mental health professionals can be at the forefront of integrated health care in the era of health care reform.

INTRODUCTION

People with serious mental illness (SMI) frequently have comorbid general medical conditions, and this largely accounts for the shortened life expectancies of those with SMI compared with the general population.[1] In addition to patient and provider factors, health care system factors contribute significantly to the poor quality of medical care. For example, patients receiving care at community mental health centers have problems with access to care and receive a lower quality of primary care than does the general population.[2] Traditionally, general medical care is segregated from mental health care. Medical and behavioral health systems are not colocated, often do not share information, and have separate funding streams.[3]

These challenges are faced by community mental health centers where the majority of SMI population is seen. A survey of leaders at these mental health centers indicated that even though more than two-thirds reported protocols to screen for common medical conditions, only half could provide treatment and referral sources, and only a third could provide medical services on site. Barriers to medical care include insufficient physical infrastructure on site, reimbursement issues, and lack of referral sources.[4]

Among integrated care models, those in which mental health providers are brought into medical settings have been well-studied. More recently, models in which medical providers are brought into behavioral health settings are being implemented. Interventions designed to improve medical care in persons with mental illness have shown improved linkage with primary care, better quality of primary care, and some improvement in medical outcomes.[5]

In this chapter, the authors review the need for integrated care among those with SMI and commonly encountered medical comorbidities, describe different models of integrated care and required competencies for an integrated practice setting, and then outline the concepts and structure of a medical home. The authors then use a case example to illustrate clinical and administrative challenges in implementing an integrated clinic.

MEDICAL CARE FOR PEOPLE WITH SERIOUS MENTAL ILLNESS

HISTORY OF MEDICAL SERVICES IN COMMUNITY MENTAL HEALTH CENTERS

By the 1990s and early 2000s, momentum grew for the development of national policies and initiatives regarding integrated care within the public sector. There was clear evidence that individuals with serious mental illness were not utilizing the health care system effectively, often using emergency rooms rather than outpatient settings to meet their medical needs.[6] One study conducted at Yale demonstrated that patients enrolled at the Connecticut Mental Health Center experienced lower access to medical care than did the general population, as well as lower quality of care in four essential domains: care provided at first contact, ongoing care, comprehensiveness of care, and coordination of care.[2]

The Bazelon Center published a report in 2004 outlining "How to Integrate Physical and Mental Health Care for People with Serious Mental Disorders," one of the first publications to address new models of integrated care within the context of a recovery-oriented mental health system.[7]

The Medical Director Council of the National Association of State Mental Health Program Directors (NASMHPD) published a comprehensive blueprint for integrated care within state mental health authorities.[8] Under the auspices of the National Council for Community Behavioral Healthcare, which published its own reports in 2006, the leaders of these entities provided a template for mechanisms to improve health care outcomes for individuals who receive services in the public sector.[9]

MEDICAL NEED

An analysis of 10,084 patients at public mental health facilities showed high rates of obesity and metabolic syndrome in patients with schizophrenia, bipolar disorder, and other SMI.[10] Rates of obesity (body mass index [BMI] ≥ 30) and hypertension (blood pressure [BP] ≥ 130/85) were greater than 50%. Elevated glucose levels (fasting ≥ 100) were seen in 33% patients. An abnormal lipid profile was seen in more than half of patients. Among those with metabolic syndrome, 60% were not receiving treatment. Among those being treated, more than 50% continued to have high levels of BP, cholesterol, and blood sugar. Similarly, baseline data from the Clinical Antipsychotic Trials of Intervention Effectiveness (CATIE) study showed that more than 40% of patients had metabolic syndrome.[11] In this sample, the 10-year risk for coronary heart disease for patients with schizophrenia was significantly increased compared to a control population.[12] Treatment rates for these metabolic disorders are low in the SMI population.[13] In addition to metabolic syndrome and cardiovascular risk, people with SMI are also at higher risk for other chronic conditions such as hypothyroidism,[14] chronic obstructive pulmonary disease,[14,15] hepatitis C, HIV,[14,16] obstetrical problems, and dental issues.[16]

BARRIERS IN MEDICAL CARE OF PEOPLE WITH SMI

The etiology of increased medical comorbidity in people is manifold and related to provider factors, patient factors, treatment variables, and issues with access to quality primary care.

Healthcare Providers

Traditionally, psychiatrists have distanced themselves from physical health evaluations. In a 1978 survey of practicing psychiatrists, none was found to perform physical examinations in their outpatient practice. Those in inpatient practice delegated the hospital admission physical examination to others.[17] Medical diagnoses were missed in more than 50% of patients in a 1989 study done in a state mental health facility.[18] In later years, even with the advent of newer psychotropic medications that cause or exacerbate chronic medical conditions, psychiatrists did not focus on preventive health screening or physical health.[19]

In more recent years, it has been reassuring to note that psychiatric providers do have an increased awareness of the risks of psychotropic treatment regimens and the need to tailor treatment based on metabolic risk factors.[20] However, it is unclear if this knowledge and awareness translates into the greater involvement of psychiatrists in physical health care. Primary care physicians may not be comfortable caring for the medical needs of people with SMI due to a perceived need for specialized care.[21] And, with competing demands on their time, primary care physicians may not have the resources to address the special needs of severely impaired, mentally ill patients.

Patient Factors

Patients with SMI have cognitive impairments across several neurocognitive domains limiting their adaptive and social functioning.[22] This affects their ability to adapt to the fast-paced environments found in a typical medical clinic and to communicate effectively with health care providers. Noisy and crowded waiting areas were cited as one of the barriers in accessing primary care by people with SMI.[21] Poor understanding of physical illness, inability to navigate complex health care systems, lack of motivation to follow through on treatment, and fear and mistrust of providers who are not familiar to them can all contribute to patients with SMI not engaging in primary care.

Symptoms of psychiatric illness such as paranoia and severe depression or anxiety also influence patient behaviors. Patients also may not have adequate social and economic resources to adhere to healthy lifestyles. Furthermore, adverse life experiences significantly impact physical as well as mental health.[23]

Adverse Effects of Pharmacologic Treatment

Patients with SMI are usually on treatments that include psychopharmacologic agents. In the past two decades, there has been a tremendous increase in use of second-generation antipsychotics.[24] Many of these contribute significantly to obesity and metabolic syndrome, although there are variations in the magnitude of risk among different agents.[25] This leads to an increased cardiovascular risk, especially with those agents associated with greater changes in weight.[26]

Access to Medical Care

Access to primary care is a significant barrier in the medical care of people with SMI and contributes to poor outcomes.[4,27] The mental health sector is the only site of health care for the majority of people with SMI. However, the treatment model in mental health settings has mostly been centered on treatment of psychiatric disorders. Organizational supports that facilitate coordinated medical and psychiatric care are infrequent. Funding streams for mental health care are often separate from those for medical care. As a result, the cost benefits of preventive care and improved medical outcomes accrue outside the mental health system. Hence, the financial incentive for medical screening and treatment within mental health settings is not compelling.

Information exchange between mental health and primary care providers is limited by restrictive policies and overzealous adaptation of the Health and Insurance Portability and Accountability Act (HIPAA) of 1996.

THE ROLE OF BEHAVIORAL HEALTH CARE PROVIDERS

All mental health professionals can and should play a role in the prevention and treatment of disease. The role of psychiatrists, especially in the public sector, may be changing with health care reforms and the push toward integrated care.[28] Many continuing medical education programs at scientific meetings now provide content intended to enhance the primary care skills of psychiatrists. Some innovative educational curricula are being developed in psychiatry residency programs to address this need.[29] In their role of promoting health for their patients, at a minimum, psychiatrists must minimize the deleterious effect of the medications they prescribe and conduct appropriate screenings for chronic medical conditions, especially those affected by psychotropic medications. Addressing medication side effects early in treatment is crucial in preventing long-term morbidity. Psychiatrists are trained to be experts in behavior change and can be in the forefront of preventive counseling in lifestyle issues, treatment adherence, and self-management of chronic conditions. Psychiatrists, who train in basic medicine as well as behavioral health, are uniquely qualified to be leaders in integrated health settings. Finally, psychiatrists may need to provide some treatment of medical conditions for those mentally ill patients who are unable to access care or unwilling to receive care in primary care settings. This last role is probably the most debated at this time.

All mental health professionals should also play a role in promoting health and wellness. Wellness goes beyond disease management and refers to a holistic approach to health. The focus is on active patient participation in a lifestyle that promotes physical, social, spiritual, intellectual, financial, occupational, environmental, and emotional well-being.[30] Part of enhancing wellness is engaging in illness prevention activities such as healthy eating, maintaining physical activity, and avoiding harmful practices such as tobacco use. The Center for Integrated Health Solutions (CIHS) at the Substance Abuse and Mental Health Services Administration (SAMHSA) provides a guide to a number of wellness strategies.[31]

Counseling on wellness strategies for a healthier lifestyle can be provided by nonphysician professionals such as nurses, social workers, mental health workers, and case managers. A growing number of people with a diagnosis of mental illness have become providers of psychiatric rehabilitation in the last few decades (see Chapters 3 and 4 for a more extensive discussion on the role of peer support in mental health care); these specialists are more recently integrating health and wellness into the concept of recovery.[30] Peer support among those with SMI is known to increase satisfaction in various life domains and the ability to effect changes among participants.[32] Peers can help deal with the challenges of maintaining healthy lifestyle activities such as increasing physical exercise or eliminating tobacco use. Peers can also help bridge the gap between patients and physicians by providing education on treatment and facilitating appointments and referrals.

A public health approach to improving the medical care of those with SMI includes primary prevention by modifying risk factors for chronic illness, secondary prevention by screening for medical conditions, and tertiary prevention by providing treatment for existing chronic medical conditions to reduce disability. A multidisciplinary team-based approach is required to achieve these goals. A brief review of selected medical conditions follows in the next section.

CHRONIC MEDICAL CONDITIONS

Obesity and Metabolic Syndrome

SMI patients who typically utilize community mental health services are likely to suffer from two or three times higher rates of obesity than the general population.[10] This is partly related to socioeconomic reasons but mostly due to the weight-producing effects of psychiatric medications that are commonly used in this population. Given that obesity is at epidemic proportions in the general population, SMI patients are likely to be overweight when they initially receive services. When they are started on medications (mainly antipsychotics), they rapidly gain weight, which first leads to an increase in a constellation of risk factors commonly referred to as *metabolic syndrome*. Metabolic syndrome eventually leads to a multitude of diseases, mainly diabetes and cardiovascular disease.[33,34]

Metabolic syndrome denotes an increase in risk factors for diabetes and cardiovascular disease. It is not a disease in itself and does not have a treatment. On the other hand, components of the metabolic syndrome, such as obesity, hypertension, high cholesterol, and impaired glucose tolerance, require treatment to prevent the loss of health-related quality of life, excess morbidity, and early mortality observed in SMI populations.

Psychiatrists can play a major role in management of obesity. As with any medical illness, primary prevention is key. Metabolic syndrome almost always follows obesity; thus, prevention of obesity, if at all possible, will have significant health benefits decades later. Primary prevention of obesity in community mental health starts with medication selection. Practitioners must be keenly aware of the weight increase liability of different psychiatric medications and attempt to use the least weight-producing medications. Regardless, some patients will gain weight on the first medication that they are prescribed. Rapid weight gain is a perfectly good reason to switch medications, and available data show that medication switch to medications with lower weight liability produces metabolic benefits.[35]

The second leg of prevention is utilization of lifestyle interventions that are shown to be effective in the treatment of obesity as well as its prevention.[36] Lifestyle interventions are based on nutritionally informed cognitive behavioral therapy (CBT) principles that can be provided with minimal educational burden and relative ease. Clinicians at community mental health centers who are already familiar with the cognitive behavioral component of these interventions can perform this therapy. The authors suggest using lifestyle interventions early in the process, before overweight turns into obesity. Simple changes such as weekly self-monitoring on relatively inexpensive bathroom scales; reduction or elimination of calorie-dense foods from the diet, such as sugared beverages and candy bars; increased everyday activity, such as switching to stairs instead of elevators or increasing the amount and speed of walking; stimulus reduction, such as changing shopping habits and eliminating high-calorie foodstuff from the household environment; and stress management techniques can be effective. These strategies, as well as learning to recognize nonhunger emotional eating, go a long way in reducing weight in a consistent and steady manner. These and other suggestions are components of manualized lifestyle interventions and can be readily accessed for free on the Internet.[37] Small improvements in body weight have been shown to provide disproportionately large health benefits.[38]

For patients for whom metabolic syndrome has already set in, lifestyle interventions and a medication switch to lower weight-liability agents need to be supplemented with medical treatment for high BP and high cholesterol. These patients need to be monitored regularly for the early detection of diabetes. The antidiabetic medication metformin has not only been shown to delay development of diabetes for patients with metabolic syndrome, but also to provide modest weight loss regardless of SMI or antipsychotic use status.[39] The authors suggest using metformin early on, when signs of impaired glucose tolerance are discovered through regular monitoring, even if diabetes diagnosis is not present.

Pharmacotherapy for obesity is a burgeoning field, and new medications are developed and approved every day. Unfortunately, many of these medications are centrally acting, with psychiatric side effects. Currently, the data on using obesity medications in SMI populations are very limited, and familiarity with the medications and caution is required. Some psychotropic medications commonly prescribed by psychiatrists are approved as weight loss medications; examples are topiramate, the use of which may be limited by neurocognitive side effects, and naltrexone/bupropion, for which evidence of safety and efficacy in SMI is limited.

Finally, for very obese patients or obese patients with medical problems, bariatric surgery provides intensive weight loss and significant benefits, including remission of diabetes. Evidence for bariatric surgery is good in SMI patients with affective disorders[40]; however, there is extremely limited evidence for schizophrenia spectrum patients. Patient selection is key due to intensive and critical compliance requirements both pre- and post-bariatric surgery. Regardless, bariatric surgery can be utilized with eligible SMI patients in the context of close collaboration between surgical and mental health providers.

Tobacco Dependence

More than 50% of adults with SMI are tobacco smokers.[31,41,42] Smoking is a known risk factor for cardiovascular disease, lung cancer, chronic obstructive pulmonary disease, and reduced life expectancy.[43] Smoking also plays a causal role in multiple other health conditions, such as other malignancies, bone disease, reproductive disorders, gastric ulcers, and periodontal disease. Smoking cessation dramatically reduces morbidity and mortality,[44] and mortality benefits can be seen as early as 1 year after quitting. In the SMI population, smoking adds to the already high burden of medical morbidity. In addition to cardiovascular disease, the prevalence of pulmonary diseases such as asthma, chronic obstructive pulmonary disease, and obstructive sleep apnea (OSA) is high in patients with SMI.[15,45–47] These conditions are aggravated by smoking and independently contribute to physical morbidity and mortality. OSA is also a significant risk factor for cardiovascular disease.

People with SMI have lower rates of success with smoking cessation.[41] Smoking cessation can be harder for people with SMI due to the mood altering effects of nicotine, higher levels of stress, social factors such as poor education, lower motivation due to psychiatric symptoms or cognitive defects, and poor access to resources for help quitting.[48] Pharmacological therapies licensed in the United States are varenicline, bupropion, and nicotine replacement therapy (NRT). In the general population, varenicline has shown superior efficacy to bupropion and single NRT and equivalent efficacy to combination NRT.[49] Most studies of smoking in people with SMI show good tolerability and efficacy of all three agents. Psychosocial interventions are often combined with pharmacological treatment, and these include supportive group therapy, cognitive behavioral approaches, social skills training, and contingency monetary reinforcement.

Relapse rates were found to be high after abstinence following smoking cessation therapy.[50] More recent studies have found maintenance treatment for up to 1 year to be effective in reducing relapse rates with bupropion, NRT,[51] and varenicline in combination with CBT[52] in the SMI population.

The role of psychiatrists and other mental health professionals in smoking cessation ranges from advocating for smoke-free mental health facilities, education on the risks of smoking and benefits of cessation, providing both behavioral and pharmacologic treatment, and referral to appropriate community resources. Weight loss and smoking cessation are the cornerstones for prevention and management of many of the illnesses mentioned here. (See Chapter 6 for a further review of tobacco dependence in people with SMI, recommended assessment and treatment modalities, and available community resources for smoking cessation.)

Infectious Diseases

Adults with SMI are more likely than their counterparts without SMI to engage in risky behaviors associated with sexually transmitted diseases.[53] These behaviors are correlated with factors related to psychiatric illness, substance use, cognitive capacity, and social relationships. People with SMI have a high prevalence of HIV,[54] as well as other infectious diseases such as chronic hepatitis and tuberculosis.[55] Data on the prevalence of syphilis in SMI are limited, but it is known to coexist in patients infected with HIV, and the prevalence may be high due to high numbers of people with SMI and comorbid HIV.

The Centers for Disease Control provides guidelines on testing for these and other infectious diseases. Screening for tuberculosis is recommended for those with a close contact with tuberculosis; a person with a immunosuppressive disease such as HIV; and those who live in homeless shelters, jails, or nursing homes. Testing for syphilis should be routinely performed in pregnant persons, those who engage in sexually risky behaviors, and in at-risk groups such as men who have sex with men. HIV screening is recommended for patients in all health care settings, and in high-risk patients it is recommended annually. Screening for hepatitis C is recommended for those at risk, such as injection drug users, those infected with HIV, and as a one-time test for those born between 1945 and 1965. Routine screening for hepatitis B is not recommended, although vaccination is recommended for those with HIV or with sexual risk factors.

Mental health providers can reduce disease transmission in the SMI population by a combination of education on safe sex practices, treatment of substance use including injection drug use, robust infection control programs at mental health facilities, the facilitation of screening, and the provision of immunization for vaccine-preventable diseases.

Cancers

Cancer is among the top five leading causes of death in patients with SMI.[1] An 11-year prospective study showed cancer as the second leading cause of mortality, especially lung cancer for men and breast cancer for women.[56] A recent large study also found lung cancer death rates much higher in patients with schizophrenia and overall cancer rates high in middle-aged persons with schizophrenia compared to the rest of the population.[57] This is, at least in part, attributable to disparities in cancer screening in mentally ill patients due to multiple barriers.[58] A higher prevalence of risk behaviors such as tobacco smoking in the SMI population is also likely to contribute to higher rates of cancers.

Educating consumers of mental health services and facilitating their access to appropriate preventive services can help reduce disparities in screening. Cancer screening guidelines are published by the US Preventive Services Task Force (USPSTF) and other professional societies. The USPSTF guidelines, as well as those of some other organizations, are available free to the general public.[59] It is to be noted that guidelines are evidence-based and thus change when new evidence emerges on the long-term benefits and risks of screening, as well as the cost effectiveness of testing. For example, previously, there was no routine screening recommended for lung cancer detection. Now, the USPSTF recommends annual helical computerized tomography scanning for those with a 30-pack year smoking history and who either are current smokers or have quit less than 15 years ago. It also often happens that different professional societies disagree on recommendations. For instance, controversy is still raging over USPSTF recommendations in 2009 to start mammography at a later age of 50 years and at a lesser frequency of biennial. The USPSTF recommends against prostate specific antigen-based screening for prostate cancer whereas the American Urologic Society continues to recommend shared decision-making between providers and patients on the utility of screening with prostate specific antigen for men aged 55–69.[60] Hence, it is useful for psychiatrists and other mental health professionals to keep abreast of major developments in cancer screening and, to the extent possible, be aware of current guidelines.

Reproductive Health

A complete discussion of clinical issues related to women's health—specifically, contraception, pregnancy, and postpartum care—in patients with mental illness is beyond the scope of this chapter. Readers are referred to a review of services and recommendations for women with schizophrenia who are of childbearing age.[61] Although this review focuses on schizophrenia, the recommendations are applicable to all women with mental illness. The major recommendations are to (1) engage all women of childbearing age in discussions of sex, sexually transmitted disease, and contraception; (2) carefully monitor patients during all stages of pregnancy within an appropriate level of care; (3) adjust psychotropic agents as indicated; and (4) address substance use issues early in the preconception period so that adequate treatment can be initiated to prevent use during pregnancy.

DELIVERY OF INTEGRATED CARE

MODELS OF INTEGRATED CARE

As discussed earlier, there is increasing awareness of clinical integration across services, and this has become a focus for several policy initiatives. The Institute of Medicine, in its proposed strategy to improve quality of care for people with mental illness, gave importance to greater clinical integration among different service providers.[62] The Agency for Healthcare Research and Quality (AHRQ) reviews different models of integrated care across both primary care and specialty settings.[63] The President's New Freedom Commission for Mental Health advocates for improved detection of mental health issues in primary care.[64]

A Bazelon Center report in 2004 examined four approaches that still remain salient[7]: (1) the embedding of primary care providers within public mental health programs, (2) unified programs that offer mental health and physical health care through one administrative entity, (3) initiatives to improve collaboration between independent office-based primary care and public mental health, and (4) colocation of behavioral health providers in primary care offices. The role of the consumer was highlighted, with a recommendation for providers to provide education and support so that individuals could take an active role in managing their health.

The Medical Director Council of NASMHPD developed a "Four Quadrant Model" (Table 5.1) of service need, a population-based tool that has become the conceptual framework for many subsequent initiatives. The quadrants and populations are described as follows[9]:

I. Low to moderate risk/complexity for both behavioral and physical health issues
II. High behavioral health risk/complexity and low to moderate physical health risk/complexity
III. Low to moderate behavioral health risk/complexity and high physical health risk/complexity
IV. High risk and complexity in regard to both behavioral and physical health

Quadrants II and IV include individuals generally served within community mental health centers whose physical health needs have been challenging to address. Aspects of the chronic care model (see later discussion) are incorporated in these blueprints for integrated care, with an emphasis placed on creating comprehensive programs that provide education, care coordination, and self-management tools in order to enhance outcomes. Individuals in quadrants I and III are best served in the primary care setting.

Behavioral Health in Primary Care

Early models of integrated care, in which mental health providers are brought into medical settings, have been tested for depression, anxiety, and substance use disorders (SUDs). Most of these interventions have shown an improvement in symptom severity, treatment response, and remission, with the most robust results seen with depression treatment.[63,65] A 2012 Cochrane review showed that, in addition to depression and anxiety outcomes, there is some evidence of improvement in mental health quality of life although less so for physical quality of life.[66] However, there is promise for improvement in physical health indicators, as shown in some intervention studies.[67] Many of these models utilized a depression care manager who was supervised by a psychiatrist and provided education, care management, and brief psychotherapy and facilitated additional consultation by the

Table 5.1 FOUR QUADRANT MODEL OF CLINICAL INTEGRATION

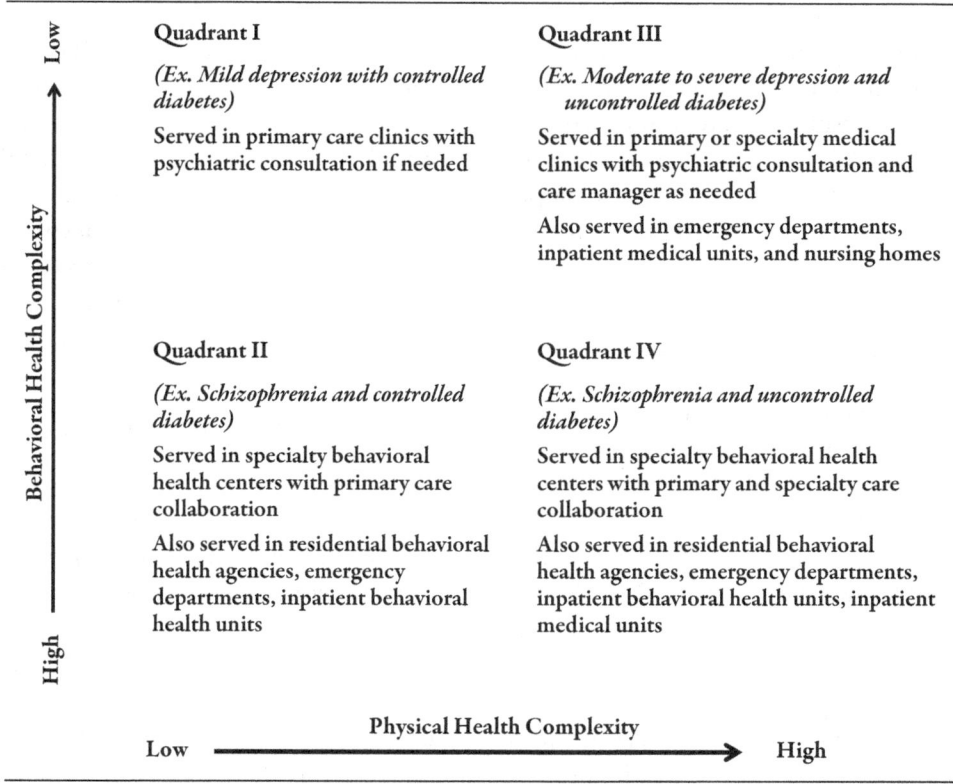

Adapted from National Council for Community Behavioral Health Care.[9]

psychiatrist to the primary care physician for medication management.

The Improving Mood Promoting Access to Collaborative Treatment (IMPACT) model is one such example of collaborative care across multiple primary care practices.[68] Patients requiring care beyond psychiatric consultation were referred to short- or long-term behavioral health specialty treatment. Hence, the elements of this collaborative model are (1) systematic psychiatric assessment; (2) a nonphysician care manager to perform longitudinal symptom monitoring, treatment interventions, and care coordination; and (3) specialist-provided stepped-care recommendations.[69] The TEAMcare model employing primary care provider consultants and nurse educators along with psychiatric consultants ensured improvement in medical disease targets.[67] Examples of this collaborative care model are Depression Improvement Across Minnesota, Offering a New Direction (DIAMOND); the Mental Health Integration Program in Washington state; and large national health care organizations like Kaiser Permanente.

Skills required of psychiatrists and other mental health professionals who work in these settings are flexibility, adaptability, ability to work in a team, availability for consultations outside of structured times, ability to appreciate cultural differences in primary and behavioral health care environments, and an interest in public health. Mental health providers in these settings usually provide both informal and direct consultation, education of primary care providers, and leadership within the collaborative care team. Traditionally, training programs have focused on collaborative and direct consultative care in inpatient settings. Many of the learned skills are applicable to outpatient practice also, and there is increasing recognition that outpatient mental health care is an important part of consultative training.

Primary Care in Mental Health

The approach of integrating primary care in mental health settings is less well studied. However, some experimental models have shown promise. These models spanned a continuum of approaches with intermediate to high levels of involvement by primary care providers and regular contact between medical and mental health staff. They showed improvement in quality of medical care and some evidence of improvement in health outcomes.[5,63] Care management was specifically tested as an approach in the Primary Care Access, Referral, and Evaluation (PCARE) trial. Care managers provided communication and advocacy with medical providers, health education, and support in overcoming system-level fragmentation and barriers to primary medical care. Those people with SMI who had a care manager were more likely to have received preventive services and treatment, and have an established primary care provider.[70]

The SAMHSA has a Primary and Behavioral Health Care Integration (PBHCI) grants program that supports the integration of primary care services into behavioral health treatment for adults with SMI. SAMHSA developed the PBHCI program to support the coordination and integration of primary care services into publicly funded, community-based behavioral health settings with goals of improved access to primary care, improved prevention and early identification of physical illness, and increased availability of integrated care. More than 100 grantees have been funded so far in regions across the United States. Program characteristics of each grantee organization and specifics of service integration vary considerably.[71] Early reports from evaluation of grantee programs show improved access to care within organizations that provide colocated care and demonstrate frequent communication between providers. There is also some indication that health outcomes, such as diabetes and BP control, improved in patients served in these integrated programs, although there was no reduction in the rates of obesity and tobacco use, which are markers of preventive care.[72]

Funding these integrated programs is challenging, especially outside of an existing program such as the PBHCI. Many programs have been initiated by community mental health agencies, and they have partnered with local federally qualified health centers (FQHC). The FQHCs are able to bill for primary care services at the prospective payment systems rates. Some mental health systems have also taken steps to attain FQHC status because of the funding advantages it offers for an integrated health system. A notable example is the Cherokee Health System in Tennessee. Some behavioral health organizations have set up their own primary care clinics outside of a grant program in response to medical need, but financial sustainability is an ongoing issue in these settings.

LEVELS OF INTEGRATION

Integration of care can occur across a spectrum from minimal collaboration between off-site practices to a completely merged primary and behavioral health practice.[73] Here, we present an overview of the levels:

1. *Coordinated care.* Practices are at different sites, but there is sharing of information either periodically or driven by specific clinical care issues.
2. *Colocated care.* Practices are in the same site, but funding is separate, records are usually separate,

treatment plans may be shared, and there is better communication between providers at the two practices.
3. *Integrated care.* Practices share the same space, providers communicate consistently at all levels, there is team-based resolution of systems issues, one treatment plan, a blended culture of practices, and there may be shared resources and integrated funding (Table 5.2).

PRINCIPLES OF INTEGRATED CARE

Successful integration involves screening for co-occurring conditions, determining the need for treatment of those conditions, implementing mechanisms for on-site treatment or outside referral, arranging for effective linkages between providers to coordinate care, and providing organizational support for collaboration.[27]

The Center for Advancing Integrated Mental Health Solutions at the University of Washington, a forerunner of the collaborative approach, lists the following core principles in integrating primary care and behavioral health[74]:

1. *Patient-centered care.* Team-based care; effective collaboration between primary care and behavioral health providers.
2. *Population-based care.* Patients tracked in a registry so that outcomes can be measured for groups or populations.
3. *Measurement-based treatment to target.* Measurable treatment goals and outcomes defined and tracked for each patient; treatments are actively changed until clinical goals are reached.
4. *Evidence-based care.* Treatments used are evidence-based.
5. *Accountable care.* Providers are accountable and reimbursed for quality of care, clinical outcomes, and patient satisfaction, not just the volume of care provided.

Regardless of the site of integration, the team-based approach is emphasized in an integrated model. A team of behavioral health and primary care professionals with a shared vision and values should be developed. Once formed, there should be continual assessment of the functioning and goals of the team. Care delivered should be patient-centered and evidence-based, with patient outcomes measured and monitored continually.[75] The SAMHSA-HRSA center for integrated health solutions (CIHS) recently developed a set of core competencies relevant to working in diverse settings and integrating primary care into behavioral health. They are also a resource for educators as they develop training programs on integrated care.[76] The competencies are arranged into the following major categories within the context of an integrated health care team:

1. Interpersonal communication
2. Collaboration and teamwork
3. Screening and assessment
4. Care planning and care coordination
5. Intervention
6. Cultural competence and adaptation
7. Systems-oriented practice
8. Practice-based learning
9. Quality improvement informatics

Table 5.2 CORE DESCRIPTIONS OF SIX LEVELS OF INTEGRATION BETWEEN PRIMARY CARE AND BEHAVIORAL HEALTH PRACTICES

INTEGRATION LEVEL	DESCRIPTION
Coordinated care (separate facilities)	
Minimal collaboration	Communication occurs rarely and is driven by provider need
Basic collaboration at a distance	Providers view each other as resources and communicate periodically for specific patient needs
Colocated care (same facility)	
Basic collaboration on-site	Separate systems. More regular communication and more reliable referral process due to proximity. Treatment team is ill-defined.
Close collaboration onsite with some system integration	Some sharing of systems. In-person communication as needed and coordinated plans for difficult patients. Better sense of an integrated treatment team.
Integrated care (shared space)	
Close collaboration approaching an integrated practice	Frequent communication. Collaboration with desire to be a single care team. Regular team meetings to overcome barriers and in-depth understanding of roles and culture
Full collaboration in a transformed/merged integrated practice	Most systemic barriers are resolved. Collaboration driven by shared concept of single treatment team. Blended roles and cultures.

Adapted from Substance Abuse and Mental Health Services Administration-Health Resources and Services Administration Center for Integrated Health Solutions.[73]

PATIENT-CENTERED MEDICAL HOME

CHRONIC CARE MODEL

The chronic care model serves as the foundation for the patient-centered medical home (PCMH) structure and concept. This model grew out of an awareness that primary care practice tends to be organized around acute care but must shift to a continuing care model. This model incorporates six elements for improving the quality of care for chronic illness[77,78]:

1. Providing self-management skills to patients and their families
2. Redesigning care delivery systems
3. Linking patients to community resources for support in illness management
4. Providing decision support to clinicians
5. Using computerized clinical information tools to support adherence with treatment protocols and monitoring health indicators
6. Aligning the health care organization's structures and values to support chronic care

COMPONENTS OF A MEDICAL HOME

A PCMH is a team-based model of care led by a primary care provider who provides continuous and coordinated care throughout a patient's lifetime to maximize health outcomes. The core principles include a personal physician for each patient, a physician-led practice team with responsibility for ongoing care across the patient's life span, and care coordination across health systems and aligned payment methods. Family physician and pediatric groups initially proposed the characteristics of a PCMH.[79] The health homes do not need to provide a full array of services themselves but must ensure availability of those services and coordinate care. The team at the medical home provides care that is patient- and family-centered, comprehensive, continuous, accessible, and culturally competent. The concept of the medical home model is intended to improve health care by transforming how primary care is organized and delivered. A successful medical home requires a collaborative relationship between primary care providers and specialists, including psychiatrists.

The Agency for Healthcare Research (AHRQ) defines the components of a medical home.[80] The National Committee for Quality Assurance (NCQA) uses this model to list the standards required for a health care center to qualify as a medical home.[81] Some of the core components are:

1. *Comprehensive care.* The care team is responsible for meeting the large majority of physical and mental health care needs including preventive, acute, and chronic care. The care team includes a physician provider, nurse, and health educator, among others.
2. *Coordinated care.* The team coordinates care across other elements such as specialty care, home health care, hospital-based care, and community supports.
3. *Patient-centered.* The team partners with patients and their families to develop a self-care plan and provide tools to manage their care. Patients needing additional care may be identified for proactive management.
4. *Accessibility.* The medical home is responsive to patient need and delivers culturally and linguistically appropriate services within convenient hours and options for after-hours care.
5. *Quality and safety.* The medical home is committed to using evidence-based care, performance measurement, population health management, and patient satisfaction.

The medical home is conceptually aligned with integrated care. However, a primary care-based medical home may not be the best treatment setting for people with SMI, especially given that, for many of them, the only connection with the health care system is at community mental health centers. There is recognition of the need for a strong focus on integrating behavioral health care management into the PCMH.[82-84] The National Council for Behavioral Health recommends that community mental health centers be defined as medical homes for the SMI population. In a related development, the SAMHSA-HRSA center for integrated health solutions released guidelines on core clinical features of behavioral health homes (BHHs) for people with substance use and mental health conditions.[85] The application of core principles of PCMH and the chronic care model and the structural frameworks to achieve this in BHHs are outlined in this document. Care management is an integral component of a BHH and combines the principles of health homes in an integrated health delivery system.

AFFORDABLE CARE ACT AND BEHAVIORAL HEALTH HOMES

The Affordable Care Act (ACA), passed in 2010, creates options for state Medicaid programs to provide health homes for those with chronic medical and mental health conditions. There is a financial incentive for states as there is federal assistance for health home-related services. The ACA requires many of the services just discussed—comprehensive care plan for each patient, person-centered and evidence-based care, preventive services, linkages to community resources, care management, and care coordination. States are instructed to address mental health and SUDs regardless of which chronic condition is selected as the primary focus. Individuals eligible for health home services must have either a serious and persistent mental health condition or two chronic conditions (or one condition with risk of developing another). Due to this strong emphasis on mental health in the Medicaid health home, there is opportunity for behavioral health organizations to become health homes for the SMI population. The PCMH is the model for the Medicaid health home.

States are authorized to develop prospective payment mechanisms for health home services, and the payment is for a team and not an individual provider. The Centers for Medicaid and Medicare Services (CMS) provide incentives for states to implement health homes. Each state has flexibility in designing the payment structure. Initiatives that are under way to develop BHHs within community mental health centers in Connecticut are described next.

Behavioral Health Home Initiative in Connecticut

Connecticut's Department of Mental Health and Addiction Services (DMHAS) has taken a strategic proactive approach to the development of BHHs for the Medicaid population with serious mental illnesses and co-occurring SUDs. In anticipation of a Medicaid State Plan Amendment (SPA) requesting federal funding for BHH services, $10 million in new state funding has been budgeted and a comprehensive planning process undertaken to build capacity among private nonprofit as well as state-operated community mental health centers to provide the comprehensive care management, care coordination, and other services identified in Section 2703 of the ACA.[86] Each community mental health center will serve as the BHH for eligible Medicaid enrollees in their designated catchment areas. To set the stage for the rollout of this initiative, the DMHAS has engaged the leadership of the community mental health centers in a series of collaborative planning and technical assistance discussions about the service delivery model, outcome goals, quality measures, eligibility, enrollment, staffing, billing, provider standards, data collection and management, and ongoing learning supports for BHH staff.

The goals of Connecticut's BHH initiative are:

1. Improve quality by reducing unnecessary hospital admissions and readmissions
2. Reduce substance use
3. Improve transitions of care
4. Increase the proportion of individuals with mental illness who receive preventive care
5. Improve chronic care delivery for individuals with SMI
6. Increase person centeredness and satisfaction with care delivery
7. Increase connection to recovery support services

DMHAS plans to utilize data from the Medicaid Management Information System (MMIS) and the services of an Administrative Services Organization (ASO) to improve coordination across the care continuum through use of a universal care plan and data sharing among BHH providers. The ASO will build and oversee an interoperable data system to support the provider network, oversee provider credentialing, provide training and technical assistance, support an ongoing "learning collaborative," enroll and track service recipients, analyze and report on data collected, and support the building and processing of Medicaid claims for BHH services.

The fiscal model includes the following elements:

1. Services will be billed on a statewide per member per month rate.
2. Services will be billable if one or more BHH services are provided during the month.
3. All claims must be substantiated by appropriate clinical documentation in each individual's service record.
4. CMS-approved Random Moment Time Studies will be conducted.
5. Providers will be paid by DMHAS with prospective quarterly contract distributions.
6. Funding from DMHAS will be based on expected enrollment at each community mental health center, based on Medicaid claims data from 2013 at the outset, as well as on a multidisciplinary staffing model that includes licensed clinicians as well as peer recovery specialists.

As of this writing, the plan is to negotiate staffing and funding with each community mental health center, allocate the dollars through the state's administrative processes, and bring the BHH staff on board at each location such that the capacity to provide services, track data, and generate the Medicaid claims is in place when the Medicaid state plan amendment is approved.

AN ILLUSTRATION OF INTEGRATED CARE AT THE CONNECTICUT MENTAL HEALTH CENTER

This section describes an example of an integrated care clinic serving the primary care needs of patients at a mental health center. It illustrates the clinical, administrative, and financial structures of this model along with the challenges of developing and sustaining such a clinic.

STRUCTURAL COMPONENTS

The Wellness Center (WC) at the Connecticut Mental Health Center (the CMHC) is a project formed in partnership between the CMHC and the Cornell Scott-Hill Health Center (CS-HHC), an FQHC. The WC is one of the projects funded by the PBHCI program of SAMHSA. The CMHC is the community mental health center serving the greater New Haven area, and it is operated as a collaboration between the Yale Department of Psychiatry and Connecticut's DMHAS. Approximately 5,000 patients with psychotic, affective, anxiety, and SUDs are seen every year. Services include outpatient care, inpatient care, walk-in services, and community rehabilitation services such as supported housing, supported employment, assertive community treatment, and jail diversion. Almost 70% of patients served are minority populations, and 36% of CMHC patients are uninsured. Prior to the recent SAMHSA funding, on-site medical services were provided by the medical evaluation unit that cared mostly for inpatients and for urgent consultative medical needs of outpatients.

The CS-HHC is a federally qualified community health center serving the New Haven population from 18 locations and provides comprehensive primary and preventive care. Services include medical, dental, laboratory, nutrition, nursing, pharmacy, and behavioral health programs and programs for special populations such as homeless people and those with AIDS. The CS-HHC has a community-controlled board of directors. Approximately 79% of the population served by the center belongs to a minority group, and 24% are uninsured.

The WC located at CMHC is a clinic that provides on-site primary care services to the CMHC patient population. It is a colocated model of integrated care. The staff at the WC include (1) a nurse practitioner who provides medical care, educates patients on health care and chronic disease management, and refers patients to specialty services as appropriate; (2) a nurse care manager who conducts intake assessments, assists in developing individualized wellness plans, provides health education, and coordinates with behavioral health providers and off-site specialty providers; (3) a medical assistant who supports the clinical activities of the medical provider and nurse care manager; and (4) three peer health navigators who assist patients to enroll in primary care services, engage patients in self-care and healthy lifestyles, help patients with health literacy, provide practical assistance to keep medical appointments, and assist patients in navigating health services in the community. One of the navigators is bilingual in English and Spanish. A sign language interpreter employed by CMHC is also available for patients with hearing disability. In addition to staff described here, several other key clinical and administrative personnel in both organizations are responsible for overseeing daily clinical operations, and they meet regularly to solve systems based issues. The medical director is a physician dually trained in internal medicine and psychiatry who oversees clinical activities at the WC and serves as a liaison between the primary care team and the mental health professionals.

CLINIC WORKFLOW

Patients are referred to the clinic by the outpatient behavioral health providers or they self-refer. Behavioral health providers routinely screen for health indicators such as engagement with a primary care provider, medical history, tobacco and other substance use history, fasting blood sugar or HbA1c, fasting lipid profile, BMI, and BP. When patients have medical needs that require specialty services, they are referred to community or hospital-based clinics that partner with CS-HHC. Patients can utilize pharmacy services on the main campus of CS-HHC, if needed. The CS-HHC maintains electronic medical records and CMHC maintains paper charts, but it is transitioning to electronic records as of this writing. For every patient seen at the clinic, consent is obtained for sharing medical information. The nurse care manager facilitates the transmittal of information from clinic visits to behavioral health providers immediately after each visit. The peer health navigators identify high-risk patients and assist with collaborative treatment planning for those patients. Direct communication between the behavioral health providers and primary care staff occurs based on need and allows for warm hand-offs when necessary. Patients are tracked in a registry that allows for population-based management as well as individualized health plans.

WELLNESS INITIATIVES

In addition to primary care services, the integrated program provides many health promotion services. The goals of these programs are to prevent development of medical conditions by risk modification and to effectively manage existing chronic conditions. These programs have targeted common conditions seen in the SMI population such as tobacco use and obesity that contribute to increased morbidity and mortality.

In addition to providing integrated care and wellness promotion activities for patients at the WC, the center has also begun a population-based program with a goal of improving the physical health of everyone in the center—both patients and staff. Based on the concept of primary prevention, this program attempts to provide multiple opportunities for all members of the CMHC community to live healthier lives. Activities such as smoking cessation programs and periodic health fairs have been well received. Recent activities have focused on providing opportunities to increase movement in daily life through the installation of showers and lockers, an exercise room with 24-hour access, and attaining a bicycle-friendly business designation; to improve the quality of food available through the colocation of a farmers' market, a complete redesign of the inpatient and outpatient food services emphasizing local fresh food, guest chef demonstrations, and community gardening; and to reduce stress through free yoga and meditation sessions.

The CMHC has also been a smoke-free facility since 2008. Smoking cessation aids are offered free of cost to patients. Psychiatrists are required to address smoking cessation and document smoking status in their clinical reviews.

Challenges in an Integrated Clinic

Financial Sustainability

From the outset, a key strategic goal of the CMHC's integrated clinic has been its long-term viability and sustainability. Addressing this goal requires a multifaceted approach to the separate but linked components of the initiative. There is no single funding stream or reimbursement mechanism currently in place to support all the pieces of this collaborative endeavor. That said, the core clinical service provided by the on-site FQHC-operated primary clinic is the most straightforwardly sustainable component as long as the volume of clinic visits continues to be near or at capacity, the no-show rates remain at no more than 30%, and the payer mix remains heavily Medicaid and Medicaid/Medicare eligible. In other words, assuming a reasonably favorable payer mix and sufficient volume, the FQHC's rate of reimbursement is sufficient to support the direct service time of a practitioner teamed with a medical assistant. However, it is questionable whether the revenue will support clinic staffing beyond these two positions, which means that other funding sources will be needed to continue paying for clerical/receptionist support, a full-time licensed practical nurse (LPN)/coordinator, and three peer health navigators. In the case of CMHC's clinic, the decision was made from the outset to provide the clerical/receptionist support on an in-kind basis. Thus, it would not be unreasonable to expect this to continue after the SAMHSA grant support is gone. Unfortunately, under current Medicaid guidelines, most of what the LPN does is not reimbursable. The same is true for the peer health navigators. But with the upcoming rollout of the BHH initiative in Connecticut, there may very well be an opportunity to keep these positions funded, albeit somewhat realigned to address the broader goals of the BHH. Given the critical importance of the primary care/behavioral health integration, it will be a very high priority for CMHC's leadership to identify resources (either new or reallocated) to continue to support as much of the staffing as possible.

Any strategic sustainability effort must also focus on aspects of the endeavor that extend outside the walls of the colocated primary care clinic. Most notably, it will be incumbent on leadership and the clinical and support staff at all levels within the CMHC to keep care coordination and the integration of health, wellness, and medical care issues into behavioral health service delivery at the forefront of clinical practice. This will require substantive and visible support from executive leadership, ongoing use of pertinent data, continuous training and technical assistance, and focused supervision in clinical rounds, as well as on an individual basis. Such efforts will be an enormous undertaking. Fortunately, the BHH rollout will inject critical resources and provide further impetus for organization-wide integration efforts well in advance of the end of the SAMHSA PBHCI grant.

Clinical Barriers

In addition to these administrative and financial issues, there are challenges in implementing effective clinical services. The clinic currently serves the primary care needs of a large volume of patients, but optimal care coordination is still a challenging goal to accomplish. The clinic's LPN has a multitude of clinical and administrative tasks that leave less time for direct care coordination. Also, as in many integrated health settings, staff turnover rates are high. This is partly due to multitalented staff leaving for better opportunities and partly due to the cultural challenges of working within an integrated setting. Another area of challenge is in the collection of data that track patient outcomes in real time. A web-based registry, which is an important tool for population-based chronic disease management, has not been readily available, and other less useful databases have had to suffice.

The biggest challenge is true clinical integration. Currently, there is frequent communication between the medical and behavioral health teams; however, treatment plans are still separate and unique to the teams. Communication is usually based on need and not routinely part of all patient encounters. Separate medical records make a truly shared care plan all the more challenging. Although the primary care staff are flexible in their approach, it is still an ongoing task to educate them on the special needs of the SMI population. A fast-paced environment, in part driven by the financial and clinical need to serve large numbers of patients, limits the amount of extra time that providers can spend in patient education.

Psychiatrists and other mental health professionals have also expressed a desire for better communication with the primary care team. Although the current model, with its on-site primary care provider, is perceived as being extremely useful, immediate and effective communication is still a challenge with a single part-time mid-level primary care provider. Mental health professionals also face some difficulty adapting to the primary care culture and incorporating screening and referrals for medical conditions as a routine part of their practice. Also, the process of referral was considered cumbersome and an additional burden by mental health clinicians in the initial phases. This, however, was much less of a barrier than at many other sites because CMHC leadership and staff have been long aware of the medical needs of SMI patients. Another clinical challenge is coordinating specialist referrals because these are off-site. Although the health navigators assist with reminders and transportation, it is still a challenge to maintain a high level of adherence. Also, mental health providers do not have direct communication with specialists, and any exchange of clinical information takes place mainly through the primary care provider.

Although the wellness clinic has placed significant emphasis on wellness initiatives, participation by patients in these activities still remains less than desired. At the end of the first year of clinic operations, there were no significant improvements in rates of smoking cessation and weight loss. This is consistent with the experience of other PBHCI grantees. Many creative methods of engaging patients are continually being developed.

THE CMHC AS A MEDICAL HOME

The wellness center is in the middle of the spectrum of integrated care, with colocation and coordination of services, but it is not a completely integrated practice. There are many challenges in building a fully integrated practice: (1) financial, in the form of a need for integrated funding, a single billing structure, and long-term sustainability; (2) administrative, in the form of a need for a common registration process and sharing and allocation of resources throughout the entire practice; (3) data sharing, in the form of a need for an integrated system for sharing medical information; (4) integrated treatment plans, in the form of a need to implement one evidence-based practice treatment plan across different disciplines; and (5) unified culture, in the form of a need to blend organizational roles and cultures among disciplines.

Within a colocated model, there must be regular communication between providers that is not driven simply by clinical need, but by a desire for improved sharing of clinical information between both sets of providers, a shared treatment plan, a system in which there is a seamless response to all health care needs, and a blended work culture.

For the wellness center to be transformed into a fully operational medical home, it will need to continue to develop along several lines. Team-based care will need to be refined, including more frequent use of single plans of care, and coordination with outside entities must be streamlined. More challenging will be the adoption of shared electronic health records that can be accessed easily and that have the capacity to provide meaningful data to patients and providers to maximize population-based initiatives.[87] The upcoming rollout of the BHH initiative in Connecticut will hopefully help surmount some, if not all, of these challenges.

FUTURE CHALLENGES

The challenge in integrated care and any PCMH is for a health care organization to achieve the triple aim of improved population health care, improved health outcomes, and reduced costs. The literature on integrated care is still in its infancy, and the evidence for improved health care access and outcomes for people with SMI is still emerging. Also, financial reimbursement models have to be continually redesigned before integrated care is sustainable in the long term.

ESSENTIAL QUALITY METRICS

In populations with chronic illness, outcomes improve with the use of care models that integrate clinical information, evidence-based treatments, and proactive management of care. Health registries can be an effective way of managing illness and measuring outcomes. Integrated care delivery operates on the principle that access to a unified and integrated source of care will result in improved health. Measuring outcomes in service delivery as well as health status in the target population is necessary to identify actionable targets. Population-based measurement and management of chronic health conditions are important for identifying determinants of health and wellness. Given the importance of continuous assessment of quality of care in an integrated practice, the SAMHSA calls for development of data registries to track primary care and behavioral health outcomes of participants in the PBHCI program. However, web-based registries to track health outcomes in real time are not yet widely available, and this remains an area under development. Health homes also need to follow these evaluation metrics, and the CMS requires states to collect and report information on health home services delivery.

SUMMARY

Integrated health care delivery systems are critical for the SMI population, given their poor health outcomes and increased mortality. There are multiple reasons for poor health in this population, including poor access to quality care. Although many models for improving behavioral health in primary care settings have been tested, there are fewer evidence-based delivery systems to improve the physical health of the SMI population. Emerging evidence for different models of integration shows promise for improving health outcomes for people with SMI. With the implementation of ACA, in many states, Medicaid health homes that incorporate the principles of a PCMH are becoming a viable financial option. BHHs stimulated by the SAMHSA may emerge as a key service delivery model for state behavioral authorities and community behavioral health centers. Many national organizations and federal agencies are facilitating the shift to an integrated and chronic care management system of health care delivery. Psychiatrists and other mental health professionals can be at the forefront of this change. They can be leaders in integrated care, both by providing high-quality clinical care and by designing service delivery systems in the era of health care reform.

REFERENCES

1. Colton CW, Manderscheid RW. Congruencies in increased mortality rates, years of potential life lost, and causes of death among public mental health clients in eight states. *Prev Chron Dis.* 2006;3(2):A42.
2. Levinson Miller C, Druss BG, Dombrowski EA, Rosenheck RA. Barriers to primary medical care among patients at a community mental health center. *Psychiatr Serv.* 2003;54(8):1158–1160.
3. Druss BG. Improving medical care for persons with serious mental illness: challenges and solutions. *J Clin Psychiatry.* 2007;68(Suppl 4):40–44.
4. Druss BG, Marcus SC, Campbell J, et al. Medical services for clients in community mental health centers: results from a national survey. *Psychiatr Serv.* 2008;59(8):917–920.
5. Druss BG, von Esenwein SA. Improving general medical care for persons with mental and addictive disorders: systematic review. *Gen Hosp Psychiatry.* 2006;28(2):145–153.
6. Berren MR, Santiago JM, Zent MR, Carbone CP. Health care utilization by persons with severe and persistent mental illness. *Psychiatr Serv.* 1999;50(4):559–561.
7. Koyanagi C. *Get It Together: How to Integrate Physical and Mental Health Care for People with Serious Mental Disorders.* Washington, DC: Bazelon Center for Mental Health Law; 2004.
8. Parks J, Pollack D, Bartels S, Mauer B. *Integrating Behavioral Health and Primary Care Services: Opportunities and Challenges for State Mental Health Authorities.* Alexandria VA: National Association of State Mental Health Program Directors; 2005.
9. Mauer B. *Behavioral Health/Primary Care Integration: The Four Quadrant Model and Evidence-Based Practices.* Rockville, MD: National Council for Community Behavioral Healthcare; 2006.
10. Correll CU, Druss BG, Lombardo I, et al. Findings of a US national cardiometabolic screening program among 10,084 psychiatric outpatients. *Psychiatr Serv.* 2010;61(9):892–898.
11. McEvoy JP, Meyer JM, Goff DC, et al. Prevalence of the metabolic syndrome in patients with schizophrenia: baseline results from the Clinical Antipsychotic Trials of Intervention Effectiveness (CATIE) schizophrenia trial and comparison with national estimates from NHANES III. *Schizophr Res.* 2005;80(1):19–32.
12. Goff DC, Sullivan LM, McEvoy JP, et al. A comparison of ten-year cardiac risk estimates in schizophrenia patients from the CATIE study and matched controls. *Schizophr Res.* 2005;80(1):45–53.
13. Nasrallah HA, Meyer JM, Goff DC, et al. Low rates of treatment for hypertension, dyslipidemia and diabetes in schizophrenia: data from the CATIE schizophrenia trial sample at baseline. *Schizophr Res.* 2006;86(1–3):15–22.
14. Carney CP, Jones L, Woolson RF. Medical comorbidity in women and men with schizophrenia: a population-based controlled study. *J Gen Intern Med.* 2006;21(11):1133–1137.
15. Himelhoch S, Lehman A, Kreyenbuhl J, Daumit G, Brown C, Dixon L. Prevalence of chronic obstructive pulmonary disease among those with serious mental illness. *Am J Psychiatry.* 2004;161(12):2317–2319.
16. Leucht S, Burkard T, Henderson J, Maj M, Sartorius N. Physical illness and schizophrenia: a review of the literature. *Acta Neurol Scand.* 2007;116(5):317–333.
17. Patterson CW. Psychiatrists and physical examinations: a survey. *Am J Psychiatry.* 1978;135(8):967–968.
18. Koran LM, Sox HC Jr., Marton KI, et al. Medical evaluation of psychiatric patients. I. Results in a state mental health system. *Arch Gen Psychiatry.* 1989;46(8):733–740.
19. Carney CP, Yates WR, Goerdt CJ, Doebbeling BN. Psychiatrists' and internists' knowledge and attitudes about delivery of clinical preventive medical services. *Psychiatr Serv.* 1998;49(12):1594–1600.
20. Newcomer JW, Nasrallah HA, Loebel AD. The Atypical Antipsychotic Therapy and Metabolic Issues National Survey: practice patterns and knowledge of psychiatrists. *J Clin Psychopharmacol.* 2004;24(5 Suppl 1): S1–S6.

21. Lester H, Tritter JQ, Sorohan H. Patients' and health professionals' views on primary care for people with serious mental illness: focus group study. *BMJ*. 2005;330(7500):1122.
22. Bowie CR, Harvey PD. Cognition in schizophrenia: impairments, determinants, and functional importance. *Psychiatr Clin North Am*. 2005;28(3):613–633.
23. Druss B, Walker, ER. *Mental Disorders and Medical Comorbidity: Research Synthesis Report*. Princeton, NJ: Robert Wood Johnson Foundation; 2011.
24. Verdoux H, Tournier M, Begaud B. Antipsychotic prescribing trends: a review of pharmaco-epidemiological studies. *Acta Neurol Scand*. 2010;121(1):4–10.
25. Meyer JM, Davis VG, Goff DC, et al. Change in metabolic syndrome parameters with antipsychotic treatment in the CATIE schizophrenia trial: prospective data from phase 1. *Schizophr Res*. 2008;101(1–3):273–286.
26. Ratliff JC, Palmese LB, Reutenauer EL, Srihari VH, Tek C. Obese schizophrenia spectrum patients have significantly higher 10-year general cardiovascular risk and vascular ages than obese individuals without severe mental illness. *Psychosomatics*. 2013;54(1):67–73.
27. Horvitz-Lennon M, Kilbourne AM, Pincus HA. From silos to bridges: meeting the general health care needs of adults with severe mental illnesses. *Health Aff (Millwood)*. 2006;25(3):659–669.
28. Raney L. Integrated care: the evolving role of psychiatry in the era of health care reform. *Psychiatr Serv*. 2013;64(11):1076–1078.
29. Annamalai A, Rohrbaugh RM, Sernyak MJ. Status of general medicine training and education in psychiatry residency. *Acad Psychiatry*. 2014;38(4):473–475.
30. Swarbrick MA. Integrated care: wellness-oriented peer approaches: a key ingredient for integrated care. *Psychiatr Serv*. 2013;64(8):723–726.
31. SAMHSA-HRSA Center for Integrated Health Solutions. *Wellness Strategies*. http://www.integration.samhsa.gov/health-wellness/wellness-strategies. Accessed January 11, 2015.
32. Davidson L, Bellamy C, Guy K, Miller R. Peer support among persons with severe mental illnesses: a review of evidence and experience. *World Psychiatry*. 2012;11(2):123–128.
33. De Hert M, Cohen D, Bobes J, et al. Physical illness in patients with severe mental disorders. II. Barriers to care, monitoring and treatment guidelines, plus recommendations at the system and individual level. *World Psychiatry*. 2011;10(2):138–151.
34. Druss BG, Zhao L, Von Esenwein S, Morrato EH, Marcus SC. Understanding excess mortality in persons with mental illness: 17-year follow up of a nationally representative US survey. *Med Care*. 2011;49(6):599–604.
35. Stroup TS, McEvoy JP, Ring KD, et al. A randomized trial examining the effectiveness of switching from olanzapine, quetiapine, or risperidone to aripiprazole to reduce metabolic risk: comparison of antipsychotics for metabolic problems (CAMP). *Am J Psychiatry*. 2011;168(9):947–956.
36. Daumit GL, Dickerson FB, Wang NY, et al. A behavioral weight-loss intervention in persons with serious mental illness. *N Engl J Med*. 2013;368(17):1594–1602.
37. Tek C. *Simplified Intervention to Modify Physical Activity, Lifestyle, and Eating Behavior*. Simple Program. http://www.simpleprogram.org. Accessed January 11, 2015.
38. Knowler WC, Barrett-Connor E, Fowler SE, et al. Reduction in the incidence of type 2 diabetes with lifestyle intervention or metformin. *N Engl J Med*. 2002;346(6):393–403.
39. Jarskog LF, Hamer RM, Catellier DJ, et al. Metformin for weight loss and metabolic control in overweight outpatients with schizophrenia and schizoaffective disorder. *Am J Psychiatry*. 2013;170(9):1032–1040.
40. Ahmed AT, Warton EM, Schaefer CA, Shen L, McIntyre RS. The effect of bariatric surgery on psychiatric course among patients with bipolar disorder. *Bipolar Disord*. 2013;15(7):753–763.
41. McClave AK, McKnight-Eily LR, Davis SP, Dube SR. Smoking characteristics of adults with selected lifetime mental illnesses: results from the 2007 National Health Interview Survey. *Amer J Pub Health*. 2010;100(12):2464–2472.
42. Centers for Disease Control. *Smoking Among Adults With Mental Illness*. 2013. http://www.cdc.gov/features/vitalsigns/smokingandmentalillness/. Accessed January 11, 2015.
43. Centers for Disease Control and Prevention (CDC). Smoking-attributable mortality, years of potential life lost, and productivity losses—United States, 2000-2004. *MMWR*. 2008;57(45):1226–1228.
44. Vollset SE, Tverdal A, Gjessing HK. Smoking and deaths between 40 and 70 years of age in women and men. *Ann Intern Med*. 2006;144(6):381–389.
45. Jones DR, Macias C, Barreira PJ, Fisher WH, Hargreaves WA, Harding CM. Prevalence, severity, and co-occurrence of chronic physical health problems of persons with serious mental illness. *Psychiatr Serv*. 2004;55(11):1250–1257.
46. Annamalai A, Palmese LB, Chwastiak LA, Srihari VH, Tek C. High rates of obstructive sleep apnea symptoms among patients with schizophrenia. *Psychosomatics*. 2015;56(1):59–66.
47. Winkelman JW. Schizophrenia, obesity, and obstructive sleep apnea. *J Clin Psychiatry*. 2001;62(1):8–11.
48. Ziedonis D, Hitsman B, Beckham JC, et al. Tobacco use and cessation in psychiatric disorders: National Institute of Mental Health report. *Nicotine Tob Res*. 2008;10(12):1691–1715.
49. Cahill K, Stevens S, Perera R, Lancaster T. Pharmacological interventions for smoking cessation: an overview and network meta-analysis. *Cochrane Database Syst Rev*. 2013;5:CD009329.
50. Tsoi DT, Porwal M, Webster AC. Interventions for smoking cessation and reduction in individuals with schizophrenia. *Cochrane Database Syst Rev*. 2013;2:CD007253.
51. Cather C, Dyer MA, Burrell HA, Hoeppner B, Goff DC, Evins AE. An open trial of relapse prevention therapy for smokers with schizophrenia. *J Dual Diagn*. 2013;9(1):87–93.
52. Evins AE, Cather C, Pratt SA, et al. Maintenance treatment with varenicline for smoking cessation in patients with schizophrenia and bipolar disorder: a randomized clinical trial. *JAMA*. 2014;311(2):145–154.
53. Coverdale JH, Turbott SH. Risk behaviors for sexually transmitted infections among men with mental disorders. *Psychiatr Serv*. 2000;51(2):234–238.
54. Meade CS, Sikkema KJ. HIV risk behavior among adults with severe mental illness: a systematic review. *Clin Psychol Rev*. 2005;25(4):433–457.
55. Pirl WF, Greer JA, Weissgarber C, Liverant G, Safren SA. Screening for infectious diseases among patients in a state psychiatric hospital. *Psychiatr Serv*. 2005;56(12):1614–1616.
56. Tran E, Rouillon F, Loze JY, et al. Cancer mortality in patients with schizophrenia: an 11-year prospective cohort study. *Cancer*. 2009;15(15):3555–3562.
57. Kredentser MS, Martens PJ, Chochinov HM, Prior HJ. Cause and rate of death in people with schizophrenia across the lifespan: a population-based study in Manitoba, Canada. *J Clin Psychiatry*. 2014;75(2):154–161.
58. Aggarwal A, Pandurangi A, Smith W. Disparities in breast and cervical cancer screening in women with mental illness: a systematic literature review. *Am J Prev Med*. 2013;44(4):392–398.
59. US Preventive Services Task Force. *Recommendations for Primary Care Practice*. 2013. http://www.uspreventiveservicestaskforce.org/Page/Name/recommendations. Accessed January 11, 2015.
60. American Urological Association. Detection of prostate cancer. http://www.auanet.org/education/guidelines/prostatecancer-detection.cfm. Accessed January 11, 2015.
61. Seeman MV. Clinical interventions for women with schizophrenia: pregnancy. *Acta Neurol Scand*. 2013;127(1):12–22.

62. Institute of Medicine. *Improving the Quality of Health Care for Mental and Substance-Use Conditions: Quality Chasm Series.* Washington, DC: National Academies Press; 2005.
63. Butler M, Kane RL, McAlpine D, et al. *Integration of Mental Health/Substance Abuse and Primary Care.* Rockville, MD: Agency For Healthcare Quality and Research; 2008.
64. President's New Freedom Commission on Mental Health. *Achieving the Promise: Transforming Mental Health Care in America.* Rockville, MD: Author; 2003.
65. Woltmann E, Grogan-Kaylor A, Perron B, Georges H, Kilbourne AM, Bauer MS. Comparative effectiveness of collaborative chronic care models for mental health conditions across primary, specialty, and behavioral health care settings: systematic review and meta-analysis. *Am J Psychiatry.* 2012;169(8):790–804.
66. Archer J, Bower P, Gilbody S, et al. Collaborative care for depression and anxiety problems. *Cochrane Database Syst Rev.* 2012;10: CD006525.
67. Katon WJ, Lin EH, Von Korff M, et al. Collaborative care for patients with depression and chronic illnesses. *N Engl J Med.* 2010;363(27):2611–2620.
68. Unutzer J, Katon W, Callahan CM, et al. Collaborative care management of late-life depression in the primary care setting: a randomized controlled trial. *JAMA.* 2002;288(22):2836–2845.
69. Huffman JC, Niazi SK, Rundell JR, Sharpe M, Katon WJ. Essential articles on collaborative care models for the treatment of psychiatric disorders in medical settings: a publication by the Academy of Psychosomatic Medicine Research and Evidence-Based Practice Committee. *Psychosomatics.* 2014;55(2):109–122.
70. Druss BG, von Esenwein SA, Compton MT, Rask KJ, Zhao L, Parker RM. A randomized trial of medical care management for community mental health settings: the Primary Care Access, Referral, and Evaluation (PCARE) study. *Am J Psychiatry.* 2010;167(2):151–159.
71. Scharf DM, Eberhart NK, Schmidt N, et al. Integrating primary care into community behavioral health settings: programs and early implementation experiences. *Psychiatr Serv.* 2013;64(7):660–665.
72. Scharf D, Eberhart NK, Hackbarth NS, et al. *Evaluation of the SAMHSA Primary and Behavioral Health Care Integration (PBHCI) Grant Program: Final Report.* Washington, DC: US Department of Health and Human Services; 2013.
73. SAMHSA-HRSA Center for Integrated Health Solutions. *Standard Framework for Levels of Integrated Healthcare.* http://www.integration.samhsa.gov/resource/standard-framework-for-levels-of-integrated-healthcare. Accessed January 11, 2015.
74. Advancing Integrated Mental Health Solutions (AIMS) Center. *Principles of Collaborative Care.* http://aims.uw.edu/collaborative-care/principles-collaborative-care. Accessed January 11, 2015.
75. Lardieri M, Lasky GB, Raney L. *Essential Elements of Effective Integrated Primary Care and Behavioral Health Teams.* Washington, DC: SAMHSA-HRSA, Center for Integrated Health Solutions; 2014.
76. Hoge M, Morris JA, Laraia M, Pomerantz A, Farley T. *Core Competencies for Integrated Behavioral Health and Primary Care.* Washington, DC: SAMHSA-HRSA, Center for Integrated Health Solutions; 2014.
77. Wagner EH. Chronic disease management: what will it take to improve care for chronic illness? *Eff Clin Pract.* 1998;1(1):2–4.
78. Bodenheimer T, Wagner EH, Grumbach K. Improving primary care for patients with chronic illness: the chronic care model, Part 2. *JAMA.* 2002;288(15):1909–1914.
79. American Academy of Family Physicians (AAoP), Americal College of Physicians, American Osteopathic Association. *Joint Principles of the Patient-Centered Medical Home.* Washington, DC: Patient-Centered Primary Care Collaborative; 2007.
80. Agency for Healthcare Research and Quality. *Defining the PCMH.* http://www.pcmh.ahrq.gov/page/defining-pcmh. Accessed January 11, 2015.
81. National Center for Quality Assurance. *Patient-Centered Medical Home Recognition.* http://www.ncqa.org/Programs/Recognition/Practices/PatientCenteredMedicalHomePCMH.aspx. Accessed January 11, 2015.
82. Croghan T, Brown JD. *Integrating Mental Health Treatment into the Patient Centered Medical Home.* Rockville, MD: Agency for Healthcare Research and Quality; 2010.
83. Amiel JM, Pincus HA. The medical home model: new opportunities for psychiatric services in the United States. *Curr Opin Psychiatry.* 2011;24(6):562–568.
84. Alakeson V, Frank RG, Katz RE. Specialty care medical homes for people with severe, persistent mental disorders. *Health Aff (Millwood).* 2010;29(5):867–873.
85. Alexander L, Druss BG. *Behavioral Health Homes for People with Mental Health and Substance Use Conditions: The Core Clinical Features.* Washington, DC: SAMHSA-HRSA Center for Integrated Health Solutions; 2012.
86. State of Connecticut Department of Mental Health and Addiction Services. *Behavioral Health Homes.* 2014. http://www.ct.gov/dmhas/bhh. Accessed January 11, 2015.
87. Nutting PA, Miller WL, Crabtree BF, Jaen CR, Stewart EE, Stange KC. Initial lessons from the first national demonstration project on practice transformation to a patient-centered medical home. *Ann Fam Med.* 2009;7(3):254–260.

6.

SUBSTANCE USE DISORDERS AND SYSTEMS OF CARE

Donna LaPaglia, Brian Kiluk, Lisa Fucito, Jolomi Ikomi, Matthew Steinfeld, and Srinivas Muvvala

---

EDUCATIONAL HIGHLIGHTS

- Recovery from substance use disorders (SUDs) is possible and is defined by individual progress.
- There is no single best approach to recovery from SUDs; however, it must happen in the context of a person's life.
- Addictions research shows promising interventions for the treatment of SUDs, and public psychiatry can help with the difficult task of system adoption.
- Public systems must make an "organizational diagnosis" to determine system strengths and weaknesses. Public systems need to make structural, policy, staff/training, and resource shifts to better care for the people they serve.

INTRODUCTION

People who seek treatment for their substance use disorders (SUDs) in public psychiatry settings tend to present with complex medical and psychiatric comorbidities. As a result, treatment engagement and adherence may be challenging due to the chronic nature of these issues and the hurdles in navigating what are frequently complicated systems of care. When people do present for treatment, the public professional is faced with the often difficult diagnostic task of formulating a clinical picture from fragmented information and from often murky clinical presentations complicated by numerous chronic health, psychiatric, and substance issues.

Although clinical formulation and treatment planning with this population is among the most challenging tasks for the public-sector professional, the authors suggest that the diagnosis and treatment of substance-using individuals occurs most efficiently in the context of interdisciplinary teams and can no longer occur in specialty addiction programs alone. The authors advocate for the development of dually competent public service professionals through an integrated approach to the treatment of mental illness and addiction that includes (1) an understanding of the neurobiology of addiction and genetic factors, (2) an understanding of the environmental and comorbid factors of addiction, (3) strong assessment and diagnostic skills, (4) the ability to assess and manage intoxication and withdrawal, (5) knowledge of local resources and their designated level of care, (6) knowledge of pharmacologic interventions for all substances including nicotine, (7) knowledge and skill in behavioral interventions for addictions, (8) an a priori understanding of systemic challenges and the ability to successfully navigate them, and (9) the need for participation in the research and implementation of new treatments. Systems of care benefit when high-quality research science and high-quality clinical practice inform and support each other and, in so doing, improve the care for the most chronically ill and vulnerable individuals served.

In this chapter, it is essential to carry forth the theme espoused by the textbook: that an essential role of the public professional is practicing without the "white coat." The authors contend that nowhere is it more important to practice this way than when working with addictions and traversing the gap between traditional therapeutic methods and the gathering of human data through the collection of urine, breath, and blood. The authors wholeheartedly agree that the public psychiatry professional must be comfortable and fluid in his or her approach and must, above all else, believe that therapeutic encounters happen beyond the clinic walls. In this way, the public psychiatry professional is poised to lead interdisciplinary professional teams in the practice of state-of-the-art care.

A final theme of the chapter highlights the importance of leadership training for the public psychiatry professional. Given that many public psychiatry fellows advance into leadership positions, it is essential that fellows develop an advanced reflective capacity and prepare themselves for the difficult and emotionally stirring work of leading teams in this effort. Curriculums need to expand to teach leadership theory that not only addresses knowledge of local, state, and federal systems; management skills; and the concept of community as treatment, but that also places value on fellows recognizing personal bias and attitudes and in developing a leadership identity. These curricula are delivered through the use of reflective writing, in class reflection exercises, and in peer interaction through the use of leadership cases. Public psychiatry can no longer afford to thrust trainees into leadership positions and hope for the best; rather, the field needs to create space for the intentional practice of leadership within a complex system (see Chapter 18).

A BRIEF INTRODUCTION TO THE CURRENT SYSTEM OF CARE

The 19th century saw the development of separate, publicly funded service systems in mental health and substance abuse, each with distinct care ideologies impacting service delivery. Unfortunately, most public behavioral health systems continue to operate with separate arms for treating mental health and SUDs. What happens for people with co-occurring mental health and SUDs? Recent reports from the Substance Abuse and Mental Health Services Administration (SAMSHA) indicate that, although there is a high prevalence of people with co-occurring disorders (COD) in treatment settings, only 7% of this population receives treatment for both disorders.[1,2] With increasing evidence supporting the effectiveness of integrated treatments for persons with COD,[3-5] professionals in public psychiatry must consider the factors that continue to impede optimal integration of care in public behavioral settings.

The most common factors accounting for this practice gap include issues at the systems, programmatic, and workforce level. The large-scale structural impediments include federal and state regulations around contracted services and funding streams.[6] Differing care ideologies, specifically around the treatment philosophy of mental health programs versus specialty substance abuse programs, also account for difficulty in implementing an integrated treatment approach.[7] The lack of trained and credentialed staff to carry out integrated treatment interventions,[8] along with shifting staff patterns due to high rates of staff turnover,[9] also impede successful programmatic implementation.

At the public policy level, discussions are focused on ways to increase knowledge of addictions in professional mental health programs around the nation. The relative inattention to this issue stands in stark contrast to data on the high frequency with which people with addictions present to the mental health system. The consequences of this imbalance lead to underdiagnosis of SUDs or treatment by an untrained practitioner.[8] Both practices are unacceptable, at the educational and at the individual practitioner level.

A BRIEF HISTORY OF ADDICTION MEDICINE IN AMERICA

To develop a working knowledge of how to treat SUDs, it is necessary to understand the historical development of the current system. The mid 1700s saw the emergence of a public awareness of the damaging effects of alcohol and intoxication. The first classification of intoxication as an addictive disease requiring proper medical care was helped by the observations of physician Benjamin Rush. His early recordings of behavioral symptoms associated with drunkenness led to his writing of "Inquiry into the Effects of Ardent Spirits on the Human Mind and Body," the first treatise on alcoholism. This work led to the "addiction disease" concept, which is defined by biologic predisposition, drug toxicity, pharmacologic tolerance, disease progression, craving, loss of volitional control of intake, and the pathophysiologic consequences of sustained alcohol and opiate ingestion[10] and leads to the designation of the disease *alcholismus chronicus*.[11]

In 1830, the field of addiction medicine emerged as a specialty, looking beyond the consequences of the addiction and focusing on the organic basis of "alcoholic behavior." Inebriety became a central organizing principle and helped to define a movement of distinct treatment approaches based on the type of inebriety—alcohol, opiate, or cocaine. Several other important advances occurred during this time, among them the formation of the American Association for the Cure of Inebriety (AACI),[12] texts on the nature of addiction and treatment methods, and the development of terms describing the mental health consequences induced by prolonged alcohol use. Carl Wernicke and Sergei Korsakoff both wrote about psychosis—Wernicke wrote about a psychotic state brought on by prolonged alcohol use, and Korsakoff described an alcohol-induced psychosis that included hallucinations, memory impairment, and confusion.

Following this period in which work on the topic proliferated, the early 1900s saw the collapse of addiction treatment programs in the wake of the Great Depression and the beginning of prohibition laws. Patients suffering from addictive disorders were sent to the back wards of state psychiatric hospitals instead of to addiction treatment centers. This period also saw the offshoot creation of private hospitals designed to care for wealthy patients suffering from addictive disorders.

In addition to the loss of addiction-specific programming, the passing of the 18th Amendment transferred responsibility for chronic alcoholism from physicians to the legal system. The Harrison Act (1914) took this idea one step further and threatened to punish physicians with loss of license or jail if they failed to steer patients toward rapid detox and abstinence.[13] To make matters worse, in 1919, the American Medical Association (AMA) opposed the practice of ambulatory treatments for narcotic maintenance. It was not until Charles Terry and Mildred Pellens wrote *The Opium Problem* (1928),[14] which provided the strongest argument in favor of maintenance treatment options for patients suffering from opiate addiction, that the AMA reconsidered its position.[14]

In addition to medication-assisted treatments, the field of addiction medicine made room for developing therapeutic approaches called *fellowship models*. Alcoholics Anonymous (AA) was one such program, founded in 1935 by Bill Wilson and Dr. Bob Smith. AA opened its doors to all those suffering from alcoholism regardless of socioeconomic status, gender, age, or race. The only requirement of the participant was "an honest desire to stop drinking."[15]

From roughly 1940 to 1960, the AA fellowship strengthened its advocacy for specialized medical treatment for their peers, which included medical detoxification and aftercare services necessary for continued support. Also helping to propel a rebirth of addiction-specific services was a mid-twentieth-century reform that removed people with addictions from the penal system and reinstated their care with the medical community.

Other pivotal treatment services emerged during this time and still exist today: peer-run residential therapeutic communities, methadone maintenance programs, and outpatient abstinence-based programs. One of the first outpatient alcoholism clinics opened in Connecticut in 1968, as a freestanding satellite clinic of the Connecticut Mental Health Center, with a mission to treat addiction disorders in an ambulatory care setting.

In the 1970s, local, state, and federal systems partnered to improve communication, pool resources, and expand the scope and quality of the addiction service system. In addition, the National Institute on Alcohol Abuse and Alcoholism (NIAAA) and the National Institute on Drug Abuse (NIDA) were founded with a research mission that continues today: to understand and develop treatments to reduce the staggering social costs of addiction.

THE SERVICE SYSTEM OF ADDICTION MEDICINE

As this brief history suggests, the service system of addiction medicine is largely orthogonal to the mental health system; however, it is important to note the distinct and structural elements of addiction medicine in comparison to the system of mental health services presented in Chapter 2. Levels of care within addiction services include detoxification (ambulatory, inpatient), inpatient, residential (therapeutic communities, wilderness/holistic recovery programs), partial hospital (PHP), intensive outpatient (IOP), outpatient including opioid agonist maintenance programs, self-help groups (AA, NA, etc.), and sober housing (Oxford Houses, Recovery Houses). The interface between the addiction services listed here and mental health services remains limited and continues to present navigational challenges for both staff and patients.

A similarly challenging interface exists between addiction and medicine, specifically in primary care where individuals with addiction frequently present with health issues. These health-related encounters offer health care professionals the opportunity to intervene in the cycle of addiction. However, despite regular access to patients with addiction, a service gap exists: medical staff are poorly educated in addictive disorders, staff often holds negative attitudes toward patients with addictions,[16] and there is a lack of insurance coverage for the provision of addiction services (which is not seen with mental health or health-related issues).

The burgeoning field of addiction medicine is making strides toward closing the gap between medicine and addiction. In 2007, addiction medicine established its own independent board, the American Board of Addiction Medicine (ABAM), to ensure quality training and certification for physicians in the diagnosis and treatment of addictive disorders. A model of integration and inclusion, the ABAM board includes eight specialties covering all aspects of addictions: emergency medicine, family medicine, internal medicine, obstetrics and gynecology, pediatrics, preventive medicine, psychiatry, and surgery. With increased priority given to addictions in organized medicine, it appears that the discipline of addiction medicine is poised to help manage the increased need for medically integrated addiction services under the Affordable Care Act (ACA).

THE NEUROBIOLOGY OF ADDICTION

Following this account of the historical evolution of addiction medicine, we now turn to understanding addictions at the individual and biological level. Drug addiction can be defined as compulsive seeking and use of drugs despite severe negative consequences.[17] This is brought about by various long-lasting changes induced in certain regions of an individual's brain that makes them susceptible to compulsively seek and use the drug, to lose control of this use despite negative consequences, to have a negative emotional state in the absence of the drug, and to have cravings and urges to use the drug for prolonged periods despite abstinence.[18,19]

Multiple brain systems have been connected with the development of addictive disorders. These include the dopaminergic, cannabinoid, opioid, GABAergic, serotonergic, cholinergic, glutamatergic, and neuromodulatory (via neuropeptide Y) systems. Various regions of the brain have been identified in which changes at the molecular and cellular level influence and mediate addictive behaviors. Out of these, the most studied is the mesolimbic dopaminergic system consisting of the dopamine neurons in the ventral tegmental area of the midbrain, which innervate the nucleus accumbens of the striatum and many forebrain regions including the hippocampus, amygdala, and prefrontal cortex.[17-19]

GENETIC FACTORS

Various genetic and environmental factors are believed to account for the individual variability found in becoming susceptible to drug addiction.[18,19] Genetic factors can either be directly responsible for the development of addictive disorders or the development of personality traits leading to potential addictive behaviors.[20] For example, a well-documented example of genetic variations that may lead to the expression of addictive disorders in individuals is the ALDH 2 gene variant, which is implicated in the production of an inactive aldehyde dehydrogenase enzyme. Individuals with a homozygous ALDH 2 gene are less likely to develop alcohol use disorders due to the occurrence of an alcohol–disulfiram-like reaction resulting from acetaldehyde accumulation.[21]

Genetic factors are also related to the expression of personality traits in individuals more likely to develop drug and alcohol use disorders. Some individuals act more impulsively than others and in an unplanned manner to satisfy a desire. DRD4 (dopamine receptor D4), DAT (dopamine transporter), TPH1 (tryptophan hydroxylase 1), SERT (serotonin transporter), MAOA (monoamine oxidase A), COMT (catechol-O-methyl transferase), and $GABRA_1$, $GAGRA_6$, $GABRB_1$ (GABA receptors) are all gene variants associated with this personality trait.[20]

Individuals who demonstrate excessive risk-taking behaviors do so when they undertake an act with uncertain or inherent negative consequences with little contingency planning; such people are associated with gene variants like DRD3 and DRD4.[20]

Additionally, a person's low stress responsivity can predispose him or her to express addictive disorders. Response to stress is modulated by the hypothalamic-pituitary-adrenal axis and can be affected by gene variants like OPRM1 (mu opioid receptor) and COMT.[20]

Transcriptional and Epigenetic Mechanisms of Addiction

Although there is individual variability in the risk of developing addictive disorder due to heritability, studies also have shown that individuals with lower genetic loading for addiction can develop an addictive disorder with exposure to sufficiently high doses of drugs for a prolonged period of time. Drug-induced adaptations can be seen as "molecular or cellular memory" wherein nerve cells undergo changes due to prolonged exposure to drugs and respond differently to the same and/or different drugs and various other stimuli.[18,19] Multiple mechanisms have been shown to change the transcriptional potential of genes. Proteins that bind to regulatory regions of genes, like ΔFOSB and cyclic AMP-responsive element-binding protein (CREB), have been shown to mediate the long-term effects of drug abuse on the brain.[18,19] More recently, epigenetic mechanisms have been shown to alter gene expression without directly changing the DNA sequence. Epigenetic mechanisms change the accessibility of genes by controlling the packaging of DNA within the cell nucleus.[18,19] Various brain regions, such as the hippocampus, amygdala, and prefrontal cortex, are affected by these changes; this results in abnormalities in the traditional memory circuits and leads to clinical outcomes like drug cravings and relapse. Addicts can remain at risk for relapse to drug use despite prolonged abstinence, thus suggesting that drugs can induce lasting changes in the brain.[18,19] Thus, our improved understanding of the biology of addiction challenges the age-old assumptions about addiction being a "moral problem" or a "weakness."

ENVIRONMENTAL FACTORS

The development of addictive disorders may also be the result of environmental factors, which may be familial or nonfamilial. Environmental factors influence the addictive behaviors in interaction with the individual's genetic composition. Availability of drugs and alcohol at home or within a community or society, age of first use, peer influence, a history of trauma, and other societal factors like lack of structure and increased antisocial behavior, may all contribute to the development of addictive behaviors.

COMORBID FACTORS

The prevalence of all psychiatric disorders is higher in substance-abusing patients than in the general populations. Furthermore, 50–60% of patients with an addictive disorder also have a coexisting psychiatric diagnosis. This may be either a primary psychiatric disorder occurring independently of the addictive disorder or a substance-induced psychiatric disorder. Mood disorders, anxiety disorders, psychotic disorders, antisocial personality disorder, and attention deficit hyperactivity disorder are the most common psychiatric problems seen among patients with SUDs. For these reasons, integrated care of both the substance use and the psychiatric disorder should be the standard approach in such cases.

ASSESSMENT, DIAGNOSIS, AND TREATMENT OF SUDS

Best practice in the treatment of SUDs starts with a thorough biopsychosocial assessment.[22] Box 6.1 includes key factors to include in the diagnostic interview with the goal of producing a comprehensive, person-centered care plan and treatment disposition.

Box 6.1 THE DIAGNOSTIC INTERVIEW

Motivation for change: Assess patient's current motivation/readiness for treatment and for changing his or her substance use behavior. Treatment approaches that address motivation may be useful (e.g., Motivational Enhancement Therapy, Contingency Management, etc.).

Psychiatric comorbidity: Assess whether there are comorbid psychiatric and/or personality disorders along with a SUD. Consider a treatment approach that addresses the multiple conditions (e.g., combination of pharmacotherapy and psychotherapy).

Medical: Assess for direct toxic effects of the substance on the body (such as alcohol on the liver) or effects due to procedures associated with drug use (needle sharing among heroin users leading to hepatitis C, HIV, etc.).

Social history: Assess for level of academic achievement, extent of social support, quality of relationships, employment, stability of living arrangements, and current or past legal issues.

Family history: Assess for SUDs across family systems; use genograms to depict patterns of use across biological and/or environmental family systems.

Trauma history: Assess if substance abuse began or increased following a period of abuse or a traumatic event, and assess the presence of symptoms indicating post-traumatic stress disorder (PTSD). If so, consider an approach that addresses both conditions simultaneously (e.g., Seeking Safety). Consider patient's strengths and resilience in surviving the trauma.

Cultural context: Assess the cultural context of the substance-using behaviors. Consider whether substance use is part of or violates a patient's cultural, spiritual, or religious values and practices. Consider enlisting members of the patient's faith community.

Substance use history: Assess patient's history of substance use beyond "drug of choice" including the range of psychoactive substances; assess the amount and frequency of use and period of longest "clean time." Consider what resources the patient utilized during periods of abstinence.

Coping skills: Assess if the patient has a limited repertoire of coping strategies. A treatment approach that incorporates skills training for avoiding substance use may be useful (e.g., Cognitive-Behavioral Therapy [CBT], 12-Step Facilitation, etc.).

Table 6.1 INTOXICATION AND WITHDRAWAL EFFECTS OF COMMON PSYCHOACTIVE SUBSTANCES

PSYCHOACTIVE SUBSTANCE	INTOXICATION	WITHDRAWAL
Alcohol	Supportive management. Hydrate, parenteral high dose thiamine (protective against Wernicke's encephalopathy), folic acid, prevent aspiration; manage hypothermia, hypoglycemia and metabolic derangement.	Benzodiazepines are the treatment of choice. Can be given as fixed dose and tapered or by symptom triggered approach with use of CIWAr protocol. Other drugs, which have been used for detoxification, are carbamazepine, valproic acid, propranolol, phenothiazines, gabapentin, and barbiturates, none of which has shown superior efficacy over benzodiazepines.
Opiates	Naloxone (IM/SC) administration, intubation and ventilation may be required. Due to short half-life of naloxone, continuous monitoring of respiratory rate is required and recurrent naloxone administration might be needed.	Detoxification 1. Non opiate detox: Symptomatic treatment with clonidine, ibuprofen, benzodiazepines, anti-diarrheal medications. 2. Opiate detox: methadone or buprenorphine initiation and taper.
Sedatives/ hypnotics	Supportive management. Flumazenil maybe used, but with caution, due to precipitation of benzodiazepine withdrawal.	Benzodiazepine taper is the treatment of choice. For ease and smoothness of detoxification, longer acting benzodiazepines like diazepam and clonazepam are preferred to shorter acting such as alprazolam. Anticonvulsants have also been used for benzodiazepine detoxification, but benzodiazepines remain the main stay of treatment.

MANAGEMENT OF INTOXICATION AND WITHDRAWAL

It is essential to be able to assess the signs and symptoms of intoxication and withdrawal and to be able to provide the necessary treatment interventions to prevent the potentially lethal consequences that accompany them. Table 6.1 outlines the management of intoxication and withdrawal for alcohol, opiates, and sedatives/hypnotics.[23] Medications are not required to manage intoxication or withdrawal from other classes of substances unless there are acute psychiatric symptoms or complicating medical problems.

DISPOSITION AND PLACEMENT

An appropriate level of care needs to be determined to formulate a treatment plan and to initiate appropriate psychopharmacological and psychotherapeutic interventions. These treatment recommendations are best made within the context of an interdisciplinary team with input from various providers creating the most comprehensive disposition/plan. The two parts to this process involve decision-making about the level of care or treatment (e.g., inpatient vs. outpatient vs. residential, etc.) and conducting a safe hand-off to the next provider. Factors for consideration are patients' goals (total abstinence vs. reduction), safety (is the patient at risk to self or others?), level of impairment (is the patient able to carry out regular activities of daily living or are they gravely disabled as a result of chronic substance use?), and amount of substance use (heavy, daily ingestion of a substances is best treated at a higher level of care with the availability of medical services).

Inpatient psychiatric care is required for patients at risk to self or others or for those who are considerably disabled to the point where they are unable to take care of themselves. Medically supervised detoxification in an inpatient setting is required for patients using considerable amounts of alcohol, benzodiazepines, or opiates and for patients for whom prior withdrawals evidenced conditions like delirium tremens or seizures. Residential treatment may be indicated if there is chronic daily use, severe medical comorbidity, lack of stable housing, lack of supportive social networks, high-risk surroundings, long history of addiction, or poor treatment adherence.

The length of stay varies greatly among treatment programs, with some lasting as long as a year. For patients who may benefit from a greater number of clinical contacts than weekly outpatient treatments, partial hospital programs and intensive outpatient programs are available. Partial hospital programs run every day for a total of 20 or more hours, and the clinical programming is highly structured. This level of care is a step down from 24-hour care.

Intensive outpatient programs involve 3 or more days per week for 3 or more hours per day with a varied length of treatment, generally between 6 and 12 weeks. Patients who benefit from this level of care are those with a high risk of relapse. They require more structure and need more intensive counseling. They may have minimal support networks within the community, and some of the focus should be on connecting the patient to supportive clinicians and networks of care within the community prior to being stepped down to a lower level of care. All other clients who are usually motivated with some history of treatment adherence, a binge pattern of SUD, or some community supports (family, engaged in 12-step program, case management) can generally be treated in less frequent forms of outpatient care.

PHARMACOLOGIC INTERVENTIONS

Pharmacological intervention for SUDs, heavily influenced by disposition and patient placement, can be effective in helping patients achieve abstinence and/or experience symptom reduction. The treatment of a comorbid mental illness is vital in this pursuit, as research has shown that doing so will result in more favorable outcomes as well as improved treatment adherence. Moreover, relapse rates are reduced when comorbid symptoms such as depression, anxiety, and insomnia are addressed. Detoxification alone is not necessarily adequate to promote abstinence or maintain decreased drug use and recovery.

Appropriate pharmacologic and psychotherapeutic treatment options must be discussed with patients and put into effect. Treatment of opiate use disorders with agonist medications like methadone or buprenorphine have been shown to be highly effective. Prolonged treatment with the optimum daily dosage of these medications is more effective than short-term tapers or detoxification treatments. Agonist maintenance treatment has been shown to be particularly effective in reducing craving, decreasing illicit opiate use and opiate overdoses, improving treatment adherence, and decreasing HIV risk and criminal behaviors in this population.[24] Opiate antagonists like naltrexone have also been used for maintenance treatment of opiate use disorders. Oral naltrexone is shown to be less efficacious due to poor compliance and retention rates. Extended-release naltrexone (depot) injection when combined with psychosocial interventions has been shown to improve the adherence and retention rates thereby improving the efficacy in preventing relapse on opiates.[25]

The US Food and Drug Administration (FDA) has approved disulfiram, naltrexone (oral and XR formulation), and acamprosate for the maintenance treatment of alcohol use disorders. When prescribing disulfiram, patients should be extensively counseled about disulfiram–alcohol reactions, and they must avoid all products that contain alcohol. Oral naltrexone is most efficacious in reducing heavy drinking days. Both Acamprosate and Naltrexone have been shown to prevent relapse to drinking.[26] Topiramate, an anticonvulsant, has been shown to have efficacy in treatment of alcohol use disorders, and, although it is not FDA approved, NIAA clinical guidelines have encouraged the use of this medication.[26]

Other non-FDA approved medications for the treatment of alcohol use disorders, which have shown some efficacy, are gabapentin, ondansetron, baclofen, and varenicline.[26–30] FDA-approved medications for tobacco use disorders are nicotine replacement, varenicline, and bupropion.[31] Despite extensive clinical research, there still remains no approved maintenance medication for the treatment of stimulants (cocaine, amphetamines, methamphetamines), cannabis, hallucinogens, and inhalants.

DIAGNOSIS, ASSESSMENT, AND TREATMENT OF CIGARETTE SMOKING

Cigarette smoking is frequently overlooked when performing substance abuse assessments and neglected in the course of treating SUDs. Yet cigarette smoking is the leading preventable cause of morbidity and mortality in the United States.[32,33] An estimated one-third of adults with mental illness smoke cigarettes compared to less than one-fifth of adults without mental illness.[32–34] Among individuals with SUDs, smoking prevalence exceeds 70%.[33] Smokers with psychiatric disorders are less likely to initiate and maintain smoking abstinence,[32,33] which contributes to the high premature mortality rates in this population.[32,34] For these reasons, there is an urgent need for primary and mental health providers to screen mentally ill patients for tobacco use and provide cessation assistance.[32,33,35]

The Tobacco Use and Dependence Clinical Practice Guidelines outline a treatment model with five major components (i.e., the 5A's; see Table 6.2).[33] Clinicians are advised to assess tobacco use for every patient, to encourage those who use tobacco to quit, to assess interest in quitting, to assist by providing counseling and pharmacotherapy, and to arrange follow-up to promote abstinence. Patients who receive this model of support are more likely to initiate and maintain abstinence compared to patients whose quit attempts are not supported.[33] In typical clinical practice, only the first two steps are implemented or the first two along with a referral for treatment (i.e., telephone quit-line or tobacco treatment specialist). Evidence-based treatment, however, dictates active clinician involvement through repeated assessments of tobacco use and the ongoing provision of counseling and pharmacotherapy.

Evidence-based behavioral and pharmacological interventions are effective for smokers with psychiatric disorders.[33] Moreover, there is little evidence that smoking cessation interferes with recovery from other SUDs.[33] In fact, a meta-analysis of smoking cessation interventions provided to patients in current addiction treatment or recovery

Table 6.2 THE 5 A'S MODEL FOR TREATING TOBACCO USE AND DEPENDENCE[1]

Ask about tobacco use	Identify and document tobacco use status for every patient at every visit.
Advise to quit	Provide clear, strong, and personalized advice to every tobacco user to quit.
Assess willingness to make a quit attempt	Determine if the tobacco user is willing to make a quit attempt at this time.

Assist in quit attempt	For the patient willing to make a quit attempt, provide assistance.
	• Recommend evidence-based medications and explain how they increase quitting success and reduce withdrawal symptoms.
	• Help patient develop a quit plan using the STAR algorithm (Set a quit date ideally within 2 weeks, Tell others and request support, Anticipate challenges, Remove tobacco products from the environment)
	• Provide information about smoking and successful quitting and practical counseling (problem solving/skills training) focused on recognizing, avoiding, and coping with triggers to use and
	• Offer intratreatment social support (encouragement about patient and quitting, communicate caring and concern)
	• Provide supplementary materials (e.g., self-help information) and encourage the use of additional resources (e.g., state quitlines, online resources such as www.smokefree.gov)
	For patients unwilling to quit, initiate motivational interventions to increase the likelihood of future quit attempts; encourage patient to consider reduction as a starting point.
	• Motivational interviewing/motivational enhancement therapy
	• Use the "five Rs"
	  • Discuss:
	    • Reasons to quit that are personally relevant
	    • Risks of continued smoking
	    • Rewards for quitting
	    • Roadblocks to successful quitting
	    • Repeat counseling at subsequent clinic visits
	Recommend smoking reduction and use of nicotine replacement therapies.

Arrange follow-up	For patients willing to make a quit attempt, arrange follow-up contacts to prevent relapse. For patients unwilling to quit at this time, repeat assessment of tobacco use and advice to quit at subsequent visits.

Adapted from Tobacco Use Clinical Practice Guidelines[33] and Fiore and Baker.[35]

Box 6.2 SMOKING CESSATION IN A MAN WITH ALCOHOL DEPENDENCE AND DEPRESSION

"Roger" is a middle-aged male with a history of alcohol dependence and depression. He presents for outpatient substance abuse treatment following inpatient treatment. He reports smoking a pack of cigarettes per day but states that he is unwilling to quit smoking at this time largely due to concerns that he will not be able to manage his other problems without smoking. He has chronic pain and peripheral arterial disease (PAD) that contributes to his distress. The patient states that pain is a trigger for both depression and alcohol use. How would you address smoking with this patient?

We would advise the use of motivational interviewing techniques or the "5A's"; see Table 6.2) with this patient at each visit to help move him toward smoking behavior change. In particular, it would be important to help the patient understand the cycle of smoking, PAD, pain, and alcohol use/depression. In his case, smoking cessation would have a major impact on his chronic medical condition, would reduce his pain, and, consequently, reduce his relapse risk for both Axis I disorders. By the same token, the clinician should also focus on building the patient's coping skills so that he feels better equipped to handle other problems without smoking. If the patient is willing to consider smoking reduction as an initial option, he should be encouraged to do so and provided with nicotine replacement therapy following the standard dose schedule (i.e., usually up to 3 months).[35] If the patient becomes willing to make a quit, the clinician should follow the "Assist" and "Arrange" steps outlined in Table 6.2. We would also recommend combination nicotine replacement therapy for this patient (i.e., nicotine patch plus a short-acting form of nicotine replacement) because it is effective for smokers with high nicotine dependence levels and depressive symptoms and safe for smokers with a history of alcohol.[35]

showed that smoking interventions were associated with a 25% increased likelihood of long-term abstinence from alcohol and illicit drugs.[36] Clinicians may also wish to provide smoking cessation treatment when SUD symptoms are not severe (see Box 6.2).[33]

PSYCHOTHERAPEUTIC INTERVENTIONS

The SAMHSA lists 69 different evidenced-based interventions for the treatment of SUDs on their National Registry of Evidenced-based Programs and Practices (NREPP; www.nrepp.samhsa.gov).[37] Some interventions have been found effective for treating a range of populations (e.g., ages, gender, races/ethnicities), substances (e.g., alcohol, drugs, tobacco), and settings (e.g., inpatient, outpatient, residential, etc.), whereas others are targeted to a specific population. Here, we review some of the behavioral therapies with the most empirical support for the treatment of primary substance use and for co-occurring mental health and substance use (in alphabetical order), including a brief description of their underlying theory, key strategies for facilitating change in behavior, and typical delivery format, as well as references to treatment manuals and further informational resources.

Behavioral Couples Therapy (BCT) for alcohol and drug use disorders is an approach that combines cognitive-behavioral methods for the treatment of substance use and BCT for distressed relationships.[37-39] It is grounded in the assumption that substance use is maintained in part by interactions between the substance user and partner and is changed most effectively by teaching both partners coping skills and improving the couple's interactions. Key strategies include development of a daily sobriety contract, completion of a decisional balance related to substance use, functional analysis to identify patterns and key triggers to substance use, teaching coping skills to the substance user and partner, and enhancement of positive exchanges between the partners. Typical course of treatment is 12–24 sessions (90 minutes each) on an outpatient basis, with both partners present for all sessions.

Cognitive-Behavioral Therapy (CBT) for substance abuse is based on social learning theory, such that alcohol and drug use are deemed learned behaviors (i.e., through modeling; operant and classical conditioning).[40-42] Providers help individuals recognize, avoid, and cope with triggers for alcohol/drug use by performing a functional analysis for identifying the patterns of substance use with respect to the triggers, thoughts/feelings, behaviors, and positive and negative consequences; coping skills training; and practice of coping skills outside of sessions through specified assignments. A typical format is generally 12–16 weeks and can be individual or group-based.

The *Community Reinforcement Approach* (CRA) and the *Community Reinforcement Approach And Family Training* (CRAFT) in treating substance abuse are based on principles of operant conditioning, with an underlying philosophy that in order to overcome substance use, a person's life must be rearranged so that abstinence is more rewarding than continued substance use.[43,44] Key strategies involve functional analysis of substance use, sobriety sampling, CRA treatment plan with happiness scale, behavioral skills training, job skills training, social and recreational counseling, relapse prevention, relationship counseling, and the inclusion of concerned family members to change the home environment to reward behaviors that promote sobriety and withhold rewards when drug/alcohol use occurs. The typical format for CRAFT is generally 12–24 weeks of individual treatment (with the addition of significant others).[45]

Contingency Management (CM) is an approach to treating substance abuse based on principles of behavioral modification, particularly operant conditioning, such that behaviors are reinforced by their consequences.[46-49] Key strategies involve the identification of a specific behavior to change (e.g., drug/alcohol use, treatment attendance, etc.), use of objective methods to verify desired behavior (e.g., urine testing), and providing incentives whenever the desired behavior has occurred (e.g., vouchers or cash, on-site prizes, clinic privileges, etc.). A typical format has a client monitored 2–3 times per week for 12–24 weeks.

Mindful-Based Relapse Prevention (MBRP) is an approach to treating substance abuse that integrates mindfulness practices and cognitive-behavioral relapse prevention; a mind–body approach for recognizing innate healing abilities coupled with awareness of triggers; and the teaching of coping skills.[50,51] Key strategies involve guided meditation, recognizing thoughts and emotions in relation to triggers, integrating mindfulness practices in daily routine, learning an awareness and acceptance of cravings/urges, and practicing skills in high-risk situations. Typical format is generally group-based for 8 weeks, with 2-hour sessions.

Motivational Interviewing (MI)/*Motivational Enhancement Therapy* (MET) is an approach to treating substance abuse that is grounded in humanistic psychology and that employs an empathic, client-centered, nonjudgmental although directive style of interacting with people to assist individuals to move toward change.[52,53] Key strategies involve using open-ended questions, affirmations, reflections, summaries, and importance/confidence rulers; learning decisional balance; rolling with resistance; expressing empathy; developing discrepancy; and supporting self-efficacy. Typical format is a brief intervention (fewer than eight sessions) and is commonly deployed in individual or group settings.

Twelve-Step Facilitation (TSF) is an approach to treating substance abuse that assumes that addiction is a progressive disease of mind, body, and spirit for which the only effective remedy is abstinence from all mood-altering substances (i.e., the disease model).[54] Key strategies involve encouraging attendance and engagement in AA/Narcotics Anonymous (NA) meetings; providing education about the 12 steps; giving feedback on negative consequences from substance use to facilitate acceptance of the problem; education on the process of denial; examination of "stinking thinking"; and identification of "people, places, things" as triggers to substance use. The typical format is 12 sessions of individual-based treatment and includes encouragement for the patient to attend 12-step meetings, undertake "sponsorship" from an individual with more "clean time" that the person seeking treatment, and undertake "step-work."

Supported employment and supported education can be integrated into standard treatment settings or be included as one of many "wraparound services"; these efforts seek to improve individual functioning and facilitate job acquisition.[55-57] Key strategies include (1) providing information about the job market, about the skills and experience necessary to obtain work, and about the benefits and stressors inherent in each job; (2) helping the client develop a realistic understanding of his or her vocational skill set; (3) teaching problem solving and coping skills; (4) helping the client to develop motivation for job seeking; and (5) aiding the client in obtaining the proper entitlements, educational services (GED), certificates, or skills training necessary to pursue employment (case management).[58]

FAMILY-FOCUSED APPROACHES

There are several approaches with significant research support for treating adolescent substance use by including family members in the intervention. These interventions can be relatively brief (e.g., 8–12 sessions) or more extensive (20+ sessions) depending on the severity of the problem and are generally flexible so that they can be adapted to a broad range of service settings (e.g., mental health clinics, drug abuse treatment programs, etc.) and treatment modalities (e.g., outpatient intervention, continuing care service to residential treatment, etc.). Some examples of family-focused approaches include *Family Behavior Therapy* (FBT),[59, 60] *Brief Strategic Family Therapy* (BSFT), and *Multidimensional Family Therapy* (MDFT), to name a few.

APPROACHES FOR CO-OCCURRING DISORDER

Integrated Dual Disorders Treatment (IDDT)[61] is a treatment model based on the integration of treatment services for individuals with co-occurring SUDs and mental illness. Treatment is provided in a single facility, by the same team, with no time limit or number of sessions attached to the care. Key elements include stage-wise interventions, motivational interventions, substance abuse counseling (relapse prevention), supported employment, and outreach. *Seeking Safety*[62] is a present-focused treatment for individuals with a history of trauma and substance abuse. It includes 25 topics that are evenly divided among cognitive, behavioral, and interpersonal domains, with each addressing a safe coping skill relevant to both PTSD and substance abuse. The treatment can be provided in individual or group format, with male and female clients, and in a variety of settings (e.g., outpatient, inpatient, residential). *Dialectical Behavior Therapy* (DBT) is a well-established treatment for individuals with severe psychosocial disorders (including suicidality) and has been adapted for those with co-occurring substance abuse.[63] DBT is a cognitive-behavioral treatment approach combined with acceptance-based strategies, with an emphasis on dialectical processes. It is a comprehensive program typically conducted in outpatient settings and includes four treatment modalities: individual therapy, group skills training, telephone consultation, and therapy for the therapist.

TREATMENT SELECTION

Although there is now ample evidence showing the efficacy of a range of treatments in their ability to increase treatment retention and to reduce the harmful effects of substance abuse, the question of how to know which validated intervention will have optimal effect for a given patient is one of the ongoing challenges faced by clinicians providing community-based mental health care in the course of their daily practice.

The most substantive research to date attempting to match patient characteristics with a psychotherapeutic modality best suited to treat their symptomatic presentations has underscored the real complexity involved in choosing an evidence-based therapy to treat addictive disorders[64,65]; the successful selection of treatment modality is as much an art as it is a science. Adding to the complexity of treatment selection is the fact that SUDs (along with certain paraphilias) are the only disorders in the *Diagnostic and Statistical Manual of Mental Disorders* (DSM 5) that are, generally speaking, illegal. This requires the clinician to decide whether a patient is disclosing the totality of his use history and to consider the extent to which real and perceived legal consequences stemming from such disclosure may lead to underreporting the severity of his addiction. Gathering collateral information through family members and significant others, as well as through urine toxicology analysis and an assessment of blood alcohol content, are vital in having a clear diagnostic picture with which to choose an appropriate level of care.

FUTURE OF ADDICTION RESEARCH

Despite the strong empirical evidence supporting the therapies described herein for the treatment of addictions, their overall effect is relatively modest. For instance, reviews of treatments for alcohol use (including more than 8,000 people) have indicated that only about one-third of alcohol-dependent individuals remained abstinent during the initial 12-month period following treatment.[66] Although this is a comparatively positive outcome, it suggests that a large percentage of individuals do not respond to treatment. Thus, the future of addiction research may be viewed with a goal of maximizing treatment effects so that they are applicable to the broader population. To maximize treatment effects, we must first understand how they work and for whom and under what conditions they work best. This has been a high priority in the field of addiction research for the past decade and will likely continue as new approaches, such as those described in this section, are integrated into future research designs.

RESEARCH-ENHANCING TREATMENT OUTCOMES

Although randomized controlled trials can demonstrate that a specific treatment led to or caused change in a given outcome variable (e.g., decreased substance use), showing that a treatment causes change does not in itself explain how this change occurred.[67] The "how" is explained through the identification of the specific "mechanisms of behavior change," which are the processes or events that are responsible for the change (i.e., the reasons that change occurred or how change came about).[68,69] Therefore, to improve treatment outcomes for larger percentages of individuals seeking treatment, the specific mechanisms need to be identified so that future treatments can be adapted for certain individuals based on a better understanding of how and for whom that treatment works.

Emerging research has seen the incorporation of neuroscience into the study of how addiction treatments may work, with neuroimaging being one such approach that has tremendous promise for furthering our understanding of addictions. Neuroimaging methodology includes structural brain imaging using magnetic resonance imaging (MRI) to measure the volume and shape of specific brain regions, positron emission tomography (PET) for measuring brain activation and metabolic activity, and functional MRI (fMRI) for measuring brain activity during experimental manipulation of specific cognitive processes.[70,71] These tools have been used to examine both predictors of relapse to alcohol or drugs, as well as changes in the underlying neural circuitry following treatment—valuable information that can be used to design more effective behavioral and pharmacological treatments.[72] For instance, incorporating fMRI can be useful for identifying specific neural mechanisms of treatments for addiction, which can then shed light on new targets to enhance and individualize addiction treatments, as well as move toward potential biomarkers of treatment response.

Along the lines of individualizing addiction treatment, information on gene expression or proteins has become more prevalent in treatment research studies, with a goal of someday using genetic information to tailor decisions about which pharmacologic treatment (and potentially which psychotherapeutic treatment) or what dose of a medication is most appropriate for a given individual.[73] There are several examples of early successes with this approach in other areas of medicine, such as tests of genetic variation used clinically to predict response to medications for breast cancer[74] or to guide clinical decisions regarding the use of antipsychotics.[75]

Although, in the aggregate, the corpus of addiction research is still in its infancy, studies have supported the premise that genetic differences may predict treatment outcomes from pharmacologic[76] and psychosocial treatments.[77] Moreover, future research that integrates genomic and neuroimaging methods may lead to a greater understanding of the links among genetic variation, brain-based phenotypes, and treatment outcome, which may in turn lead to significant improvements in treatment outcomes.[73]

Technology-based interventions provide another fruitful area for future addiction research as the rapid growth of technology and the omnipresent use of the Internet and mobile devices offer a potential way to reach patients who have traditionally been resistant to engage in traditional treatment settings. Several technology-based interventions have been developed based on existing evidenced-based treatments, such as CBT, CRA, MET and other brief interventions, and CM.[78-84]

Of note, several of these technology-based interventions are being implemented in public-sector programs. Such novel ways of delivering evidenced-based treatments may be particularly beneficial for the future of addiction treatment because the implementation of the ACA is likely to result in larger numbers of individuals attempting to access treatment, which may overwhelm the current resources available.

Thus, the future of addiction research will likely focus on attempting to develop a better understanding of how our current evidenced-based treatments work, providing them across a range of service platforms, and, in so doing, offering these treatments to larger populations of individuals and incorporating new methods into public-sector programs to increase access for diverse populations.

MEASURING TREATMENT OUTCOMES AT LOCAL, STATE, AND FEDERAL LEVELS

For decades, addiction treatment services have operated without knowing—beyond anecdotal evidence—whether the treatments provided were effective and, if so, in what ways. Under the pressure of health care reform, managed care companies began to force programs and providers to justify clinical decision-making, collect treatment outcomes, and survey consumers regarding satisfaction. In an era of increased program accountability, local, state, and federal agencies now require programs to collect data in order to maintain funding.

With an increasing emphasis on treatment efficacy and outcomes, state departments, like the Department of Mental Health and Addiction Services (DMHAS) in Connecticut, are designing elaborate real-time data collection systems that record program statistics like admissions, discharges, client demographics, insurance information, and drug of choice. These data are used to inform programming decisions on the state level and to petition federal agencies for resources and support when needed.

At the national level, the National Survey of Substance Abuse Treatment Services (N-SSATS) gathers program data by level of care and compares states on a series of treatment outcomes. This annual survey goes out to program directors, and the data are published online and in a comprehensive book of provider information. These types of comparative data are used to spark discussion about national trends and for program and policy development.

PROGRAM STANDARDS

Local addiction treatment services can seek accreditation in an effort to increase patient safety and improve patient outcomes. Program accreditation ensures that standards of patient care are met and that deficits or gaps in treatment are identified and addressed. Examples of health care accreditation bodies include the Joint Commission on Hospital Accreditation (JCAHO), the Commission on Accreditation of Rehabilitation Facilities (CARF), and the Council on Accreditation for Children and Family Services (COA). With program accreditation as the gold standard, the 2006 N-SSATS reported that less than 50% of the nation's addiction treatment facilities were accredited.[85]

Accredited and publicly funded programs in an era of staffing shortages, scarce resources, and the increasing cost of medications experience pressure to continually improve services. The Network for the Improvement of Addiction Treatment (NIATX), a national collaborative endeavor for programs to share resources, advocates for improving care through the use of *short-cycle process improvements*, a technique borrowed from the field of engineering. Trying small changes in short study cycles helps achieve relatively cost-free, quick-change practice improvements. The approach allows health care professionals to continually test and revise procedures in an effort to improve operations. The approach also helps build team moral, increases employee satisfaction, and enhances patient care.

FUTURE CHALLENGES

The passage of the Mental Health Parity and Addiction Equity Act in 2008 achieved equality among all medical benefits for behavioral health disorders including depression, anxiety, psychotic spectrum illnesses, and SUDs. Additionally, "the passage of the ACA in 2010 has the potential to profoundly affect the integration of the delivery of mental health and addiction care."[86]

In line with Mental Health Parity and the ACA, SAMHSA published the Treatment Improvement Protocol 42, which puts forth a "vision of fully integrated treatment."[87] Despite the compelling evidence base supporting integrated treatment for patients with comorbid addiction and other mental illnesses, care is still fragmented and in short supply. "In the United States, treatment for most mental illnesses is provided by psychiatrists or primary care physicians. In contrast, care for addiction is provided almost exclusively at specialty treatment centers by individuals of various disciplines, often with little input from physicians."[88]

Traditional mental health and addiction treatments have not adequately addressed these co-occurring disorders due to multiple challenges with training, program structure, and other systemic disconnects. Minkoff (1989) was one of the first to propose an integrated model of addiction treatment.[89] He set forth the design for treating co-occurring addiction and psychosis on an inpatient unit. His approach sought to help psychiatric clinicians by introducing them to 12-step philosophy while familiarizing addiction clinicians with the use of psychiatric medications. This dual training approach seeks to develop competencies in both mental health and addiction service professionals, but there is still a long way to go toward systems integration between mental health and addictions.

IMPLICATIONS FOR TRAINING

The authors contend that best practice in public psychiatry requires a push toward true dual competence, as seen in the strides made by medicine and addiction (discussed in the chapter introduction) and requires all clinical staff to become skilled in the assessment and treatment of SUDs—more specifically, evidence-based treatments such as motivational enhancement therapy, relapse prevention (cognitive-behavioral therapy), and 12-step facilitation. In addition, the public-sector professional should be well-versed in integrated treatments including psychopharmacology, medical care, and empirically validated psychotherapies.[90] Miller and Brown advocate for an integration of:

> alcohol/drug problems in the core course work in psychopathology, assessment, and treatment . . . and need to be encouraged and expected from the beginning to think of substance abuse as a necessary and vital problem area to be included within their range of their professional competence, just as is the case for depression, anxiety disorders, and psychoses.[91:1275]

Integrated training programs should be the goal for medical educators. Perhaps the most crucial educational element, beyond broadening a collective treatment mindset of "whom" or "what" to treat, is to instill in students an openness, an optimism, and the desire to carry hope for patients with mental health and SUDs who are struggling to live healthier lives. It is essential, also, to focus educational efforts on developing reflective leaders within our public psychiatry settings.

SUMMARY

Public psychiatry has seen a shift in its emphasis from institution-based care to the community-as-treatment context, requiring the practitioner to take off the white coat and put on whatever hat is required. Public psychiatry calls for a compassionate human stance to the work, one in which respect and common sense prevail over traditional, rigid frames for providing care. At the same time, the field must welcome proven science into our treatment settings and actively integrate those interventions when applicable. Finally, in the authors' collective experience, leadership development of the public professional is critically essential to the health and viability of a public system poised to effectively treat mental health and SUDs.

REFERENCES

1. McGovern MP, Xie H, Segal SR. Addiction treatment services and co-occurring disorders: prevalence estimates, treatment practices, and barriers. *J Subst Abuse Treat*. 2006;31(3):267–275.
2. Substance Abuse and Mental Health Services Administration (SAMHSA). *Results from the 2009 National Survey on Drug Use and Health: Mental Health Findings*. Rockville, MD: Office of Applied Studies (OAS). http://oas.samhsa.gov/nsduh/2k9nsduh/mh/2k9mhresults.pdf. Published 2010. Accessed July 18, 2011.
3. Brunette MF, Mueser KT, Drake RE. A review of research on residential programs for people with severe mental illness and co-occurring substance use disorders. *Drug Alcohol Rev*. 2004;23(4):471–481.
4. Drake RE, et al. A review of treatments for people with severe mental illnesses and co-occurring substance use disorders. *Psychiatr Rehabil J*. 2004;27(4):360–374.
5. Mueser KT, et al. Psychosocial interventions for adults with severe mental illnesses and co-occurring substance use disorders: a review of specific interventions. *J Dual Diagn*. 2005;1(2):57–82.
6. Burnam MA, Watkins KE. Substance abuse with mental disorders: specialized public systems and integrated care. *Health Aff*. 2006;25(3):648–658.
7. Ridgely MS, Goldman HH, Willenbring M. Barriers to the care of persons with dual diagnoses: organizational and financing issues. *Schizophr Bull*. 1990;16(1):123.
8. Hoge MA, Tondora J, Marrelli AF. The fundamentals of workforce competency: Implications for behavioral health. *Adm Policy Ment Health*. 2005;32(5–6):509–531.
9. Woltmann EM, Whitley R. The role of staffing stability in the implementation of integrated dual disorders treatment: An exploratory study. *J Ment Health*. 2007;16(6):757–769.

10. White WL. Addiction medicine in America: its birth and early history (1750-1935) with a modern postscript. In Ries R, Fiellin D, Miller S, Saitz R, eds. *Principles of Addiction Medicine*. 5th ed. Baltimore, MD: Lippincott Williams & Wilkins; 2014: 327-334.
11. Huss M. *Alcoholismus Chronicus: eller Chronisk Alkoholssjukdom [Alcoholismus Chronicus: Or the Chronic Alcohol Disease]*. Stockholm, Sweden: Beckman; 1849.
12. Blumberg L. The American Association for the Study and Cure of Inebriety. *Alcoholism: Clinical and Experimental Research*. 1978;2(3):235-240.
13. Musto DF. *The American Disease: Origins of Narcotic Control*. exp ed. New York: Oxford; 1987.
14. Terry CE, Pellens M. *The Opium Problem*. Montclair, NJ: Patterson Smith; 1970 (reprint).
15. Smith B, Wilson B. *The Big Book of Alcoholics Anonymous*. Mineola, NY: Dover; 2011.
16. O'Connor PG, Nyquist JG, McLellan AT. Integrating addiction medicine into graduate medical education in primary care: the time has come. *Ann Intern Med*. 2011;154(1):56-59.
17. Hyman SE. Addiction: A disease of learning and memory. *Ann J Psych*. 2005;162(8):1414-1422.
18. Nestler EJ. Cellular basis of memory for addiction. *Dialogues Clin Neurosci*. 2013;15(4):431.
19. Robison AJ, Nestler EJ. Transcriptional and epigenetic mechanisms of addiction. *Nat Rev Neurosci*. 2011;12(11):623-637.
20. Kreek MJ, et al. Genetic influences on impulsivity, risk taking, stress responsivity and vulnerability to drug abuse and addiction. *Nat Neurosci*. 2005;8(11):1450-1457.
21. Schuckit MA. Genetics of the risk for alcoholism. *Am J Addict*. 2000;9(2):103-112.
22. National Institute of Drug Abuse. *Principles of Drug Addiction Treatment: A Research-Based Guide*. Rockville, MD: National Institute on Drug Abuse, National Institutes of Health; 2000.
23. Tetrault JM, Fiellin DA. Current and potential pharmacological treatment options for maintenance therapy in opioid-dependent individuals. *Drugs*. 2012;72(2):217-228.
24. Tetrault JM, O'Connor PG. Substance abuse and withdrawal in the critical care setting. *Crit Care Clin*. 2008;24(4):767-788.
25. Krupitsky E, et al. Injectable extended-release naltrexone for opioid dependence: a double-blind, placebo-controlled, multicentre randomised trial. *Lancet*. 2011;377(9776):1506-1513.
26. Jonas DE, et al. Pharmacotherapy for adults with alcohol use disorders in outpatient settings: a systematic review and meta-analysis. *JAMA*. 2014;311(18):1889-1900.
27. Mason BJ, et al. Gabapentin treatment for alcohol dependence: a randomized clinical trial. *JAMA Int Med*. 2014;174(1):70-77.
28. Addolorato G, et al. Ability of baclofen in reducing alcohol craving and intake: II—preliminary clinical evidence. *Alcohol Clin Exp Res*. 2000;24(1):67-71.
29. Johnson K, et al. Potential roles for new communication technologies in treatment of addiction. *Curr Psychiatry Rep*. 2011;13(5):390-397.
30. Kranzler HR, et al. Effects of ondansetron in early-versus late-onset alcoholics: a prospective, open-label study. *Alcohol Clin Exp Res*. 2003;27(7):1150-1155.
31. Cahill K, et al. Pharmacological interventions for smoking cessation: an overview and network meta-analysis. *Cochrane Libr*. 2013;31:5.
32. Center for Disease control and Prevention. Vital signs: current cigarette smoking among adults aged ≥ 18 years with mental illness-United States, 2009-2011. *MMWR*. 2013;62(5):81.
33. Fiore M, et al. Treating tobacco use and dependence: 2008 update. *Clinical Practice Guideline*. Rockville, MD: U.S. Department of Health and Human Services, Public Health Service; 2008.
34. Lawrence D, Mitrou F, Zubrick SR. Smoking and mental illness: results from population surveys in Australia and the United States. *BMC Pub Health*. 2009;9(1):285.
35. Fiore MC, Baker TB. Treating smokers in the health care setting. *N Engl J Med*. 2011;365(13):1222-1231.
36. Prochaska JJ, Delucchi K, Hall SM. A meta-analysis of smoking cessation interventions with individuals in substance abuse treatment or recovery. *J Consult Clin Psychol*. 2004;72(6):1144.
37. McCrady BS. Treating alcohol problems with couple therapy. *J Clin Psychol*. 2012;68(5):514-525.
38. McCrady BS, Epstein EE. *Overcoming Alcohol Problems: A Couples-Focused Program*. New York: Oxford University Press; 2009.
39. O'Farrell TJ, Fals-Stewart W. *Behavioral Couples Therapy for Alcoholism and Drug Abuse*. New York: Guilford; 2006.
40. Carroll KM. A cognitive-behavioral approach: treating cocaine addiction. *Therapy Manuals for Drug Addiction*. Rockville, MD: NIDA; 1998.
41. Kadden R, et al. Cognitive-behavioral Coping Skills Therapy Manual: A Clinical Research Guide for Therapists Treating Individuals with Alcohol Abuse and Dependence. *Project MATCH Monograph Series Volume 3*. Rockville, MD: NIAAA; 1992.
42. Marlatt GA, Gordon. JR. *Relapse Prevention: Maintenance Strategies in the Treatment of Addictive Behaviors*. New York: Guilford; 1985.
43. Hunt GM, Azrin NH. A community-reinforcement approach to alcoholism. *Behav Res Ther*.1973;11(1):91-104.
44. Meyers RJ, Smith JE. *Clinical Guide to Alcohol Treatment: The Community Reinforcement Approach*. New York: Guilford; 1995.
45. Meyers RJ, et al. Community reinforcement and family training (CRAFT): engaging unmotivated drug users in treatment. *J Subst Abuse*. 1998;10(3):291-308.
46. Higgins ST, Alessi SM, Dantona RL. Voucher-based incentives: A substance abuse treatment innovation. *Addict Behav*. 2002;27:887-910.
47. Petry NM. A comprehensive guide to the application of contingency management procedures in clinical settings. *Drug Alcohol Depend*. 2000;58:9-25.
48. Petry, N.M., et al., Contingency management interventions: From research to practice. *Ann J Psych*. 2001;20:33-44.
49. Stitzer, M.L., et al. Contingency management in methadone treatment: the case for positive incentives. *NIDA Res Monogr*. 1993;137:19-36.
50. Bowen S, Chawla N, Marlatt GA. *Mindfulness-Based Relapse Prevention for the Treatment of Substance Use Disorders: A Clinician's Guide*. New York: Guilford; 2010.
51. Witkiewitz K, et al. Mindfulness-based treatment to prevent addictive behavior relapse: theoretical models and hypothesized mechanisms of change. *Subst Use Misuse*. 2014;49(5):513-524.
52. Miller WR, et al. Motivational enhancement therapy manual: a clinical research guide for therapists treating individuals with alcohol abuse and dependence. *Project MATCH Monograph Series Volume 2*. Rockville, MD: NIAAA; 1992.
53. Miller WR, Rollnick S. *Motivational Interviewing: Helping People Change*. 3rd ed. New York: Guilford; 2013.
54. Nowinski J, Baker S, Carroll KM. Twelve-step facilitation therapy manual: a clinical research guide for therapists treating individuals with alcohol abuse and dependence. *Project MATCH Monograph Series Volume 1*. Rockville, MD: NIAAA; 1992.
55. Bond GR, et al. Implementing supported employment as an evidence-based practice. *Psychiatr Serv*. 2001;52(3):313-322.
56. Unger KV. Psychiatric rehabilitation through education: Rethinking the context. In: Farkas MD, Anthony WA, eds. *Psychiatric Rehabilitation Programs: Putting Theory into Practice*. Baltimore, MD: Johns Hopkins University Press; 1989:132-136, 157-161.
57. Anthony WA, Cohen MR, Farkas MD. *Psychiatric Rehabilitation*. Boston, MA: Center for Psychiatric Rehabilitation, Boston University; 1990.
58. Schottenfeld RS, Pascale R, Sokolowski S. Matching services to needs: Vocational services for substance abusers. *J Subst Abuse Treat*. 1992;9(1):3-8.

59. Azrin NH, et al. Behavior therapy for drug abuse: a controlled treatment outcome study. *Behav Res Ther*. 1994;32(8):857–866.
60. Donohue B, et al. Family behavior therapy for substance abuse and other associated problems: a review of its intervention components and applicability. *Behav Mod*. 2009;33(5):495–519.
61. Drake RE, et al. Implementing dual diagnosis services for clients with severe mental illness. *Psychiatr Serv*. 2001;52(4):469–476.
62. Najavits L. *Seeking Safety: A Treatment Manual for PTSD and Substance Abuse*. New York: Guilford; 2002.
63. Dimeff LA, Linehan MM. Dialectical Behavior Therapy for substance abusers. *Addict Sci Clin Pract*. 2008;4:39–47.
64. Project MATCH Research Group. Matching alcohol treatments to client heterogeneity: project MATCH post treatment drinking outcomes. *J Stud Alcohol*. 1997;58:7–29.
65. Project MATCH Research Group. Project MATCH secondary a priori hypotheses. *Addiction*. 1997;92:1671–1698.
66. Miller WR, Walters ST, Bennett ME. How effective is alcoholism treatment in the United States? *J Stud Alcohol*. 2001;62(2):211–220.
67. Nock MK. Conceptual and design essentials for evaluating mechanisms of change. *Alcohol Clin Exp Res*. 2007;31(10 Suppl):4s–12s.
68. Kazdin AE, Nock MK. Delineating mechanisms of change in child and adolescent therapy: Methodological issues and research recommendations. *J Child Psychol Psych*. 2003;44(8):1116–1129.
69. Kazdin AE. Evidence-based treatment research: Advances, limitations, and next steps. *Am Psychol*. 2011;66(8):685–698.
70. Morgenstern J, et al. The contributions of cognitive neuroscience and neuroimaging to understanding mechanisms of behavior change in addiction. *Psychol Addict Behav*. 2013;27(2):336–350.
71. Nutt D, Lingford-Hughes A, Nestor L. Brain imaging in addiction. In: Carter A, Hall W, Illes J, eds. *Addiction Neuroethics*. San Diego, CA: Academic Press; 2012:3–25.
72. Kiluk BD, Carroll KM. New developments in behavioral treatments for substance use disorders. *Curr Psych Rep*. 2013;15:420–429.
73. Hutchison KE. Substance use disorders: realizing the promise of pharmacogenomics and personalized medicine. *Ann Rev Clin Psychol*. 2010;6:577–589.
74. Piccart M, et al. The predictive value of HER2 in breast cancer. *Oncol*. 2001;61(Suppl 2):73–82.
75. Arranz MJ, Kapur S. Pharmacogenetics in psychiatry: are we ready for widespread clinical use? *Schizophr Bull*. 2008;34(6):1130–1144.
76. Anton RF, et al. A randomized, multicenter, double-blind, placebo-controlled study of the efficacy and safety of aripiprazole for the treatment of alcohol dependence. *J Clin Psychopharmacol*. 2008;28(1):5–12.
77. Feldstein Ewing SW, et al. Do genetic and individual risk factors moderate the efficacy of motivational enhancement therapy? Drinking outcomes with an emerging adult sample. *Addict Biol*. 2009;14(3):356–365.
78. Carroll KM, et al. Computer-assisted cognitive-behavioral therapy for addiction. A randomized clinical trial of "CBT4CBT." *Ann J Psych*. 2008;165(7):881–888.
79. Carroll KM, et al. Computer-assisted delivery of cognitive-behavioral therapy: efficacy and durability of CBT4CBT among cocaine-dependent individuals maintained on methadone. *Ann J Psych*. 2014;171:436–444.
80. Bickel WK, et al. Computerized behavior therapy for opioid-dependent outpatients: a randomized controlled trial. *Exp Clin Psychopharmacol*. 2008;16(2):132–143.
81. Hester RK, Delaney HD, Campbell W. The college drinker's check-up: outcomes of two randomized clinical trials of a computer-delivered intervention. *Psychol Addict Behav*. 2012;26(1):1–12.
82. Ondersma SJ, et al. Computer-based brief motivational intervention for perinatal drug use. *J Subst Abuse Treat*. 2005;28(4):305–312.
83. Walters ST, et al. MAPIT: Development of a web-based intervention targeting substance abuse treatment in the criminal justice system. *J Subst Abuse Treat*. 2014;46(1):60–65.
84. Dallery J, Glenn IM, Raiff BR. An Internet-based abstinence reinforcement treatment for cigarette smoking. *Drug Alcohol Depend*. 2007;86(2–3):230–238.
85. Office of Applied Studies. *National Survey of Substance Abuse Treatment Services (N-SSATS): Data on Substance Abuse Treatment Facilities*. Rockville, MD, United States Department of Health and Human Services, Substance Abuse and Mental Health Services Administration 2006.
86. Barry CL, Huskamp HA. Moving beyond parity—mental health and addiction care under the ACA. *N Engl J Med*. 2011;365(11):973–975.
87. Substance Abuse and Mental Health Services Administration. Substance abuse treatment for persons with co-occurring disorders. *A Treatment Improved Protocol Series, No.42*. Rockville, MD: US Department of Health and Human Services. Substance Abuse and Mental Health Service Administration (SAMHSA); 2005.
88. Kuehn BM. Integrated care key for patients with both addiction and mental illness. *JAMA*. 2010;303(19):1905–1907.
89. Minkoff K. An integrated treatment model for dual diagnosis of psychosis and addiction. *Psychiatr Serv*. 1989;40(10):1031–1036.
90. Ziedonis DM. Integrated treatment of co-occurring mental illness and addiction: clinical intervention, program, and system perspectives. *CNS Spectr*. 2004;9(12):892–904, 925.
91. Miller WR, Brown SA. Why psychologists should treat alcohol and drug problems. *Am Psychol*. 1997;52(12):1269.

7.

PUBLIC HEALTH CONCEPTS IN PUBLIC PSYCHIATRY

Joanne DeSanto Iennaco, Jacob Kraemer Tebes, and Selby C. Jacobs

> ### EDUCATIONAL HIGHLIGHTS
>
> Public health concepts offer a lens for public psychiatry that focuses on the importance of understanding population needs and the determinants of mental health problems and of planning for prevention, resource development, and service allocation in public psychiatry.
>
> - Attention to population-based mental health needs has resulted in the evolution of care from primarily institution-based to community-based services for those with mental illness.
>
> - Major epidemiologic studies such as the Epidemiologic Catchment Area (ECA) survey and National Comorbidity Survey (NCS) offer information about the characteristics and determinants of mental disorders. They provide a signal for problems requiring intervention and a foundation for better understanding how to promote mental health and prevent mental illness.
>
> - Understanding the risks associated with outcomes such as psychiatric morbidity, mortality, and disability allows practitioners to focus on the priority needs for service delivery.
>
> - Unique models for prevention such as the relationship between the Connecticut Mental Health Center (CMHC) and The Consultation Center (TCC) provide a model for research, service, and improvement efforts in care delivery to individuals with mental illness.

INTRODUCTION

One of the hallmarks of public psychiatry is the integration of clinical practice with epidemiologic, public health, and system perspectives. These perspectives offer a way of "seeing" clinical problems in a broader context. They enable the public psychiatry professional to understand the context of psychiatric disorders and practice, as well as set priorities for both clinical and preventive interventions and resource allocation.

Consideration of psychiatric public health is timely. Tragic events and public health problems in American society make education about public health in psychiatry of utmost importance. Public health perspectives contributed conspicuously to the community mental health movement at the dawn of the modern era of public psychiatry in 1963. Many factors contributed to the loss of that perspective over time; it is important to return to the knowledge and practice of psychiatric public health and integrate it into public-sector practice. Doing so will be critical in addressing the challenges of isolated young adults falling into psychosis and suicide and of military veterans with post-traumatic stress disorder. Public health strategies and the public system of care will help shift the focus of psychiatric practice to wellness and prevention by using population perspectives and to early intervention by bringing clinical perspectives to bear on the earliest stages of illness.

Population-focused psychiatric practice broadens the clinical lens from a focus on caring only for individuals with already present mental illness. Understanding the broader roots of illness provides a ready basis for identifying interventions that can ameliorate the effects of adversity. For example, considering activities that promote mental health or prevent mental illness includes engaging in planning, implementation, and evaluation of disaster preparedness. Such interventions may prevent the onset or lessen the severity of illness as a consequence of natural or man-made disasters. The population-focused practice frame also includes interventions for those with existing mental illness to prevent the negative consequences of chronic conditions, thus limiting disability and the effects of physical comorbidities. With a broader focus, many preventive activities impacting individuals across a continuum of health and illness are addressed. A population focus also leads to more comprehensive planning of services in public psychiatry.

This chapter includes epidemiologic and public health facts; it also illustrates how using epidemiologic data and "public health thinking" can inform public psychiatry and enhance its practice.

DEFINITIONS

WHAT IS PUBLIC HEALTH?

The American Public Health Association defines public health as "the practice of preventing disease and promoting good health within groups of people from small communities to entire countries."[1] To assess the health status of small and large populations, public health professionals use epidemiologic and other research strategies (surveillance) to understand the health concerns of specific groups. This definition defines a domain of professional practice, which involves an interdisciplinary group of professionals interested in protecting and promoting health.

WHAT IS MENTAL HEALTH?

According to the World Health Organization (WHO), mental health is "a state of well-being in which every individual realizes his or her own potential, can cope with the normal stresses of life, can work productively and fruitfully, and is able to make a contribution to his or her community."[2] Mental health, defined in relation to behavioral disorders, is an extension of the definition of public health in so far as it uses the same epidemiologic and surveillance strategies. Importantly, mental health is broader in scope, including social, behavioral, economic, and physical factors. The term "mental health" also is sometimes used as a reference to community services, and it connotes a spectrum of preventive, health-promoting, clinical, and rehabilitative services in the community. "Behavioral health" is a contemporary term used to emphasize that both mental illnesses and substance use disorders (SUDs) are within the domain of public psychiatry, which is defined in Chapter 1.

BRIEF HISTORY OF PUBLIC HEALTH IN PUBLIC PSYCHIATRY SINCE 1963

American psychiatry has a long history, starting with the mental hygiene movement in the early 20th century, of incorporating public health perspectives into psychiatric practice, or at least into the public sector of practice. In 1955, a study of treatment for individuals with mental illness was commissioned by President Dwight D. Eisenhower and led to publication of the report "Joint Commission on Mental Illness and Health: Action for Mental Health" in 1961.[3] This report ultimately ushered in a transformation of mental health care.[4] Propelled by this report, the modern era of public psychiatry opened when Congress enacted the Community Mental Health Act in 1963, which promoted construction of community-based centers for treatment and research to better understand mental illness.[5] The federally initiated community mental health movement, which spawned community psychiatry as a specialty of psychiatric practice, was predicated on public health concepts of early intervention, treatment in the community close to home, and continuity of care.[6] Based on public health concepts of primary, secondary, and tertiary prevention, the services offered by the Community Mental Health Centers Act included early identification of disease, prevention through outreach in the community to low-income and underserved populations, and action on social stresses and other environmental determinants using interdisciplinary teams to deliver care. This act spurred deinstitutionalization and initiated the delivery of public mental health care on a local level, thus improving access to care.[6] This presented unique opportunities to develop and fund community mental health centers based on interdisciplinary collaboration.

The emergence of community and social psychiatry, community psychology, public health nursing, and community-based social work, as well as growth in the field of public health to include a behavioral health focus, are examples of this influence.[7] Interdisciplinary collaboration was focal in the development of systems of care for those with mental health challenges.[8] One such community mental health center was the Connecticut Mental Health Center (CMHC) in New Haven. There, the preventive programs that originated in this period as part of general services were consolidated later into a center for prevention (The Consultation Center [TCC]), which is described later in this chapter as one example of how preventive services can be integrated into clinical practice and education.

During the 1980s, the integration of psychiatric public health into the practice of public psychiatry waned as federal and state governments focused on community-based services and rehabilitation for chronically ill people.[9] Psychiatric epidemiology and prevention pursued more independent development as investigators carried out major epidemiologic surveys such as the Epidemiological Catchment Area (ECA) study[10] and the National Comorbidity Study (NCS),[11] which provided a foundation for descriptive epidemiology. Prevention specialists continue to develop the theory and science of interventions, culminating in the Institute of Medicine (IOM) report on levels of prevention.[12]

In place of the federally driven community mental health movement, other professional, social, economic, and political forces shaped the public arena of psychiatry. Developments during these years contributed to outreach and psychosocial rehabilitation services in the community as an alternative to hospitalization, thereby reducing the disability resulting from institutionalization. Yet this determined focus was practically exclusive of anything else. Initiative for the development of community services shifted to state governments from the federal level, which continued its attenuated support through block grants. The rise of managed care and the shift to shortened hospital stays using payment based on diagnostic related groupings (DRGs) resulted in the downsizing of hospital systems and further movement of care from inpatient settings to community-based ambulatory services. Because care was constrained in hospitals and expanding rapidly in the community, it was difficult for communities with limited resources to respond to the needs of people discharged with serious and persistent mental illness.

Transinstitutionalization was a consequence; individuals with mental illness wound up in other institutions for problems associated with chronic mental illness and substance abuse problems. For example, with the development of Medicaid coverage, individuals were moved from state mental hospitals to nursing homes starting in 1965. Soon, the mentally ill represented 44% of residents, resulting in one form of transinstitutionalization.[13:10] Also, there was an increasing rate of incarceration of the mentally ill in prisons. Steadman found that patient history of incarceration for drug-related offenses increased from 12.6% in 1968 to 27.6% in 1978,[14] likely due to increased access to substances in community-based life and limited access to community-based treatment. In addition, during this same period, drug sentencing laws were tightened, thus leading to higher rates of incarceration (from 501,886 to 1,587,791 between 1980 and 1995).[15]

In the early 1990s, the balance of spending for mental health care finally tipped to greater funding for community care as opposed to state institutions.[13:1] Patients residing in state public mental institutions decreased from 559,000 to 154,000 from 1955 to 1980 and to 71,619 by 1994.[13:5] Efforts to provide care in the community were directed to both those with mental illness and those with intellectual disability. It is estimated that more than 764,000 people with SMI were living successfully in the community who would otherwise have suffered institutionalization had the changes in care never been undertaken.[15]

A public health perspective was largely lost until a Clinton White House conference in 1996 served as a prelude to a 1999 Report on Mental Health by the US Surgeon General. This public health report was the first of its kind to document the mental health of the American population and note substantial progress in establishing the efficacy of psychiatric treatments.[16] It highlighted the idea of "burden of disease," as introduced in the Global Burden of Disease study,[17] which also introduced a new metric—the Disability Adjusted Life Year (DALY) based on indirect assessments of disability combined with mortality data. Analyses of burden of disease established a high priority for mental health in mainstream public health.[17] It also underlined the need for new ways of thinking about recovery. The Surgeon General's report also advocated for better integration between mental health and general health care.[16]

Two years later, in 2001, the Surgeon General issued a call to action to reduce suicides, thereby providing the first national public health message on a major source of mortality from psychiatric disorders.[18] In another report that same year, the Surgeon General directed attention to disparities in health care outcomes for members of minority populations.[19] This report reinforced a call for culturally competent care from an earlier report to address the social factors that interfered with access to care and increased morbidity and mortality from psychiatric disorders (see Chapter 14).[16] These three reports taken together set a new course for psychiatric public health and set the stage for the New Freedom Commission (NFC) Report of 2003.[20] While defining a new public health agenda, the Surgeon General set the stage for streaming psychiatry into medicine. As the Surgeon General said in his introduction to the report, "there is no health without mental health."

In 2003, on the heels of the Surgeon General's report, the NFC noted that American society invested inadequately in programs and services at the front end of the trajectory of psychiatric illness; in contrast, enormous resources were committed to tertiary care of disabled individuals with serious mental illnesses (SMI) and addictions. The NFC report recommended more focus on the early stages of illness. As part of its call for a transformation of the American mental health system, the NFC underlined psychiatric public health as an important arena for development in public psychiatry. Specifically, the NFC report recommended in its fourth goal that mental health screening be improved to enable timely clinical assessment (early detection) and referral to continuing services if necessary to prevent chronicity. The commission intended that screening, in collaboration with primary care, become common practice. The NFC report emphasized not only early intervention but also prevention, health promotion, contingency planning for threats to the public health (such as disasters or epidemics), categorical programs for groups at high risk for burden of disease or documented as having disparate clinical outcomes, and health education. In these ways, the NFC brought modern public psychiatry full circle, back to the public health principles that guided it in its early stages of development starting in 1963.

In 2006, echoing the recommendations of the NFC, the National Institute of Mental Health (NIMH) published a report that characterized the burden of psychiatric disease on the American population as "one of the greatest public health challenges in contemporary medicine."[21,22] This article emphasized that psychiatry, in particular, faced major public health challenges, and it created a context for their solution as part of mainstream medicine. Also, 3 years later, the head of the federal Center for Mental Health Services (CMHS) highlighted the importance in the 21st century of public health in public psychiatry.[23] In her discussion, she described prevention, early intervention, attention to social variables (such as disparities in outcomes for high-risk groups), and the need to focus not only on disease but also on wellness and resilience.

We now come full circle, back to a systems-level perspective. Having furthered the science of psychiatry by identifying important brain pathways, genetic influences, and the role of personality characteristics in individuals, we can now broaden our focus to the role of these factors in the larger scope of a population-based understanding of psychiatric disorders.[24] The series of reports just described suggest areas for future research focus related to social determinants that influence health promotion, disease prevention, and intervention and that have the potential to further the evolution of public psychiatry. The policy developments in public psychiatry provide an enormous agenda for the field as it moves forward into the next decade of evolution.

PSYCHIATRIC EPIDEMIOLOGY: THE BASIC SCIENCE OF PUBLIC HEALTH.

Psychiatric epidemiology uses public health methods to provide a description of and investigate the characteristics and determinants of mental health problems and psychiatric disorders in population groups. It also evaluates the effectiveness of health services (health services research is considered in more depth in Chapter 17). Arguably, public health data serve an essential signal function in American psychiatry, monitoring progress in service development and forecasting problems needing correction. Several examples come to mind. The concept of burden of disease and data from the Global Burden of Disease study demonstrated the high burden of psychiatric disorders among all diseases and placed psychiatric disorders squarely on the agenda for state, federal, and international program initiatives.[17] The Report on Mental Health by the Surgeon General provided evidence that the mental health system was in shambles and set the stage for the NFC, which articulated a transformation agenda in mental health. Data from a report by the National Association of State Mental Health Program Directors (NASMHPD) on a shortened life expectancy of 25 years for individuals with SMI demanded a response from psychiatry and primary care.[25] Large-scale studies by services researchers exposed the misleading claims of large pharmaceutical companies that were marketing new generations of antipsychotic drugs at very high cost.[26] Finally, public health data on persistently high morbidity rates created the framework for a NIMH report calling for new directions in psychiatric research using "research domain criteria" as the dependent variable.[27]

Psychiatric epidemiology supports a population perspective on psychiatric disorders that complements a clinical focus on individuals. To grasp the mental health of the community, it is essential periodically to step back from case-by-case experience and consider the needs of and services for the whole population. A population approach considers groups of people rather than individuals. It is another way of "seeing"; for example, epidemiology tells us that the majority of people who are mentally ill do not seek or receive treatment. How do we understand that fact and incorporate the untreated person into a comprehensive picture of the disorder and need for services? And, although psychotic disorders may be the most conspicuous mental disorders in a community, they are not the most commonly occurring (incidence), nor the most disabling, given available evidence on the prevalence and burden of mental disease.

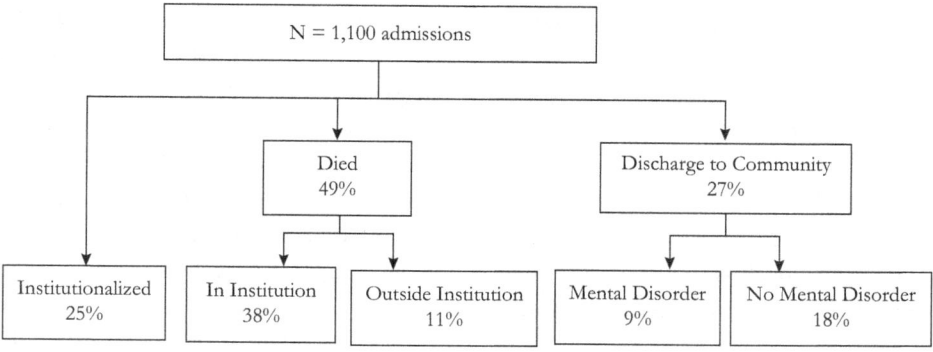

Figure 7.1 Mitchell Longitudinal Study of Institutionalized Patient Disposition (1858–70)

Epidemiologic analyses offer information about disease incidence, prevalence, and trajectory including recurrence, recovery, and comorbidity. This information is useful in a variety of ways, including in identifying risk factors important for universal prevention, in identifying high-risk groups to target with preventive interventions, and in planning for the needs of those with severe and persistent mental illness. For example, one of the earliest reports of psychiatric epidemiology that focused on psychiatric service delivery outcomes was an 1877 report of treatment at an asylum between 1858 and 1870 by Mitchell.[28] The author found that of nearly 1,100 individuals admitted over 12 years, 25% were still living in an asylum, 38% had died in the asylum, 11% had died outside the asylum, and 27% were living outside the asylum at the end of 1870 (Figure 7.1).[29] Of those living in the community, 9% continued to have a mental disorder, and 18% were identified as living "in a state of sanity."[29:26] Based on this report, attention to the causes of mortality and the need for community-based services for this cohort are highlighted.

Epidemiologic methods provide information on the effects of childhood experiences on later risk and help clinicians identify those at high risk and plan interventions to prevent future morbidity. For example, in a cohort study following children from birth to age 42 in the United Kingdom, Morgan et al. found relationships with parents in childhood predict later mental health problems: up to 24% of the studied population reported aspects of a poor relationship, resulting in a 20–80% higher risk of adult mental illness.[30:1714] These results suggest great value in wellness and health promotion strategies focused on improving parent–child relationships.

Other longitudinal studies offer psychiatry a perspective on how to intervene to prevent future morbidity. In a 24-year study, Reef et al. found specific trajectories from type of child externalizing behavior to greater risk of adult disorder as defined by the *Diagnostic and Statistical Manual of Mental Disorders* (DSM IV).[31] Children with externalizing behaviors were more likely to have substance dependence or disruptive disorders in adulthood; in addition, those with status violations (run-aways, swearing, truancy, substance abuse) were more likely to have a mood or anxiety disorder as an adult.[31:1238] Results from similar studies offer use of population-based information to inform clinical practice and planning for interventions to prevent future onset and management of psychiatric disorders.

Given the differences inherent in clinical and population perspectives on physical and mental health, there are models specific to public health that aid public psychiatry in planning for and delivery of services. These include the Levels of Prevention model, the Matrix of Intervention in Public Health model, and the Mental Health Intervention Spectrum (IOM). Each model will be briefly introduced and illustrated here.

PUBLIC HEALTH INTERVENTIONS

LEVELS OF PREVENTION

Modern public psychiatry incorporated an early framework for understanding prevention, the *levels of prevention*, which called attention to three types of prevention: primary, secondary, and tertiary.[32] These ideas still offer a useful framework for planning and implementing a range of preventive interventions. *Primary prevention* is the actual prevention of disease or disorder. Vaccinations are a good example. In the absence of known etiology, primary prevention of psychiatric disorders remains a future goal for public psychiatry. *Secondary prevention* is the reduction in morbidity from disease or disorder, usually achieved via early intervention when symptoms respond best to treatment. *Tertiary prevention* is the prevention of disability associated with disease or burden of disease. All three types of prevention are discussed here. The levels of prevention from primary to secondary to tertiary focus on the state of health or disease present, and it can be difficult to determine the point at which the disease state is present or absent. Many diseases (e.g., hypertension or depression) have a continuum of symptom severity rather than categorical thresholds that indicate a change to a disease state. Given the difficulty identifying the exact onset of mental disorders, another approach is to classify the focus of preventive intervention, which also expands the frame of targets for prevention.

MATRIX OF INTERVENTION IN PUBLIC HEALTH

This approach was first identified by Gordon[33] in regards to prevention of physical illness, and it identifies targets as universal, targeted, or selective and indicated.[12,34] The Matrix focuses on the groups of individuals involved, the costs, and the proportion of the population expected to benefit from preventive interventions.[34,35] *Universal prevention* refers to interventions provided to all individuals regardless of the presence of disorder. An example is education for all students in a school setting regarding substance abuse, mental health, or health-compromising behaviors.[36] Other examples include bullying prevention programs and social skills training in schools.[37] The intent of universal-level intervention is to either prevent problems or promote competency and impact as much as 80–90% of the population.[35:183] A smaller group, 5–15%, might benefit from *selective or targeted preventive interventions*, which are focused on those who are at risk for the onset of a disorder.[35:183] For example, children with substance-abusing parents are at higher risk for substance use and abuse and may benefit from education about this condition and supports to resist invitations for substance abuse. *Indicated preventive interventions* are for individuals with a risk factor or abnormality that constitutes an early sign of the potential for development of a disorder.[12] For example, adolescents who have experimented with substances but are not yet actively dependent may be offered a substance abuse program designed to intervene to prevent further substance use. Another example is to have a home health visitor engage new mothers to prevent postnatal depression.[38] The use of levels of prevention (primary, secondary, tertiary) helps in conceptualizing when in the course of illness an intervention might be used, whereas levels of preventive intervention from universal to indicated identify the population focus for interventions. An example of a Matrix of Intervention for Suicide Prevention is provided later in the discussion of mental health outcomes (Table 7.1).

Recent conceptual frameworks have begun to emphasize health promotion along with prevention in public psychiatry, a development that was anticipated in the landmark IOM report.[12] Reducing risks alone may be insufficient for preventing a disorder unless combined with the promotion of protective factors, such as the skills, competencies, and supports that are critical in fostering resilience to adversity.[39] Thus, both prevention and health promotion approaches function as essential tools for achieving health and well-being.[40]

Table 7.1 MATRIX OF INTERVENTIONS FOR SUICIDE PREVENTION EXAMPLES

	BIOPSYCHOSOCIAL	ENVIRONMENTAL	SOCIOCULTURAL
Universal The intervention is designed to affect everyone in a defined population.	Incorporate depression screening into all primary care practice	Promote safe storage of firearms and ammunition Package drugs in blister packs	Teach conflict resolution skills to elementary school children Provide programs that improve early parent–child relationships
Selective The intervention is designed especially for certain subgroups at particular risk for suicide.	Improve the screening and treatment of depression in the elderly in primary care practices	Reduce access to the means for self-harm in jails and prisons	Develop programs to reduce despair and provide opportunities; increase protective factors for high-risk populations, such as Native American youth
Indicated The intervention is designed for specific individuals who, on examination, have a risk factor or condition that puts them at very high risk.	Implement cognitive-behavioral therapy immediately after patients have been evaluated in an emergency department following a suicide attempt	Teach caregivers to remove firearms and old medicines from the home before hospitalized suicidal patients are discharged	Develop and promote honorable pathways for law enforcement officers to receive treatment for mental and SUDs and return to full duty without prejudice

MENTAL HEALTH INTERVENTION SPECTRUM

The IOM refers to a "mental health intervention spectrum" that ranges from prevention to treatment and maintenance for mental disorders.[12:23] *Prevention* in this spectrum refers only to preventive intervention before onset of a disorder. *Treatment* refers to both case identification (screening) and standard treatment of disorders, including interventions to reduce the risk of comorbid disorders occurring. *Maintenance* refers to interventions over time delivered to those with persistent or prolonged disorders, in whom interventions focus on relapse prevention and rehabilitation.[12:24] In the area of children's mental health, Weisz et al. identified the importance of the addition of health promotion and positive development as a population-level focus on enhancing strengths and reducing the probability of later problems.[41:632] Finally, in recent years, the SAMHSA has fully incorporated health promotion into the Mental Health Intervention Spectrum.[42]

Future approaches to prevention programs involve the use of technology in disseminating information as well as in providing screening and in understanding group-level behavior using methods such as social network analysis.[43] Dynamics of interaction, such as peer relationships and norms within a work or school group, can be better understood using methods like social network analysis to define the setting or group-level variables of importance to behavior change or disorder prevention.[43]

THREE OUTCOMES IN DESCRIPTIVE EPIDEMIOLOGY

Having provided an introduction to both epidemiology and prevention, the discussion now returns to descriptive epidemiology to review three types of outcome from mental illnesses and SUDs. These are *morbidity, mortality,* and *disability* or *burden of disease*. All of them have implications for contemporary practice in public psychiatry.

Morbidity refers to the occurrence of illness and is documented by means of descriptive, diagnostic criteria provided in criteria sets such as the DSM 5.[44] The mortality from psychiatric disorders comes from suicide and premature deaths from diabetes, hypertension, and vascular disease in people with SMI. *Burden of disease* is a term that refers to the high rate of disability associated with psychiatric disorders. The discussions presented here of each outcome offers examples of interventions that might address them.

OUTCOME 1: MORBIDITY—PREVALENCE OF PSYCHIATRIC DISORDER

Psychiatric disorders occur universally. In the past 30 years, the ECA and the NCS have described the prevalence of the major psychiatric disorders in American society.[11,45,46] The burden of disease from psychiatric disorders in American society clearly ranks among the leading causes of disability. The prevalence and disability rates are general facts that are useful background when engaging a new population or community, sizing up its special mental health needs (if any), and deciding how to allocate clinical attention.

Schizophrenia (prevalence: 1.1%), among the most conspicuous of disorders by virtue of its bizarre symptoms, although disabling, is not the most common.[45] Anxiety disorders (prevalence 18.1%) and affective disorders (prevalence 9.5%) are the most common disorders, but they tend to be less persistent and disabling.[45] SUDs (past-year prevalence of 3.8% and lifetime prevalence of 14.6%) are very common and can be acute or chronic and very disabling when addiction occurs.[45,47,48] The total prevalence of psychiatric disorders in American society is 46.4%. Comorbidity is common: 27.7% of those with a disorder have two or more disorders.[47] Only 40–60% of cases of psychiatric disorder are treated.[49] Of course, the proportion treated increases with the severity of illness (e.g., schizophrenia is more likely to require treatment vs. anxiety disorders). This chapter will not review the descriptive epidemiology of psychiatric disorders further because those data are readily accessible for clinical or evaluative purposes.

An important question that is repeatedly raised relates to the risk of aggression or violence in individuals with mental disorders (see Chapter 8). There is evidence to support the idea that individuals with mental illness are actually more likely to be victims of violence than perpetrators.[50] A recent analysis of information from the National Epidemiologic Survey on Alcohol and Related Conditions (NESARC) found that violence was associated with SMI only if substance use was involved.[51] However, this finding was called into question by Van Dorn et al. who point out that the use of lifetime diagnosis of mental illness is not focused enough to address the causal relationship of diagnosis to violent events.[52:488] In their analysis, diagnosis in the past year was used to evaluate risk of recent violence, and they found a higher risk in those with SMI (Relative Risk [RR] = 3.49); those with comorbid substance use had even higher risk (RR = 11.45), whereas those with substance use alone also had a significantly higher risk of violence (RR = 3.29).[52:490–491] Finally, those with SMI and adverse childhood events (e.g., child abuse or neglect) had more than three times the risk for violent behavior than those with SMI and no adverse childhood events.[52:492–493]

OUTCOME 2: MORTALITY

Mortality associated with psychiatric disorders manifests in two ways: suicide and premature mortality among people with SMI. The mechanisms of death for both are indirect and mediated by complex biological changes, behaviors, and social determinants. In the instance of suicide, a range of self-destructive behavior can lead to death. In the instance of premature mortality, the mechanisms are diverse, indirect, and related to the pathogenesis and course of several diseases of mid-life, but nonetheless real and devastating. The next sections consider suicide and premature mortality in that order before moving on to a discussion of disability as an outcome.

A recent analysis based on the ECA data found that of 11 disorders studied (including anxiety, depression, substance dependence, and antisocial personality disorder), only drug and alcohol dependence or abuse and antisocial personality disorder incurred significantly higher mortality risk. Five to 15 years of life were lost from these disorders.[53:1366]

Suicide

Suicide is the taking of one's own life (from the Latin, sui, of himself, caedere, to kill). Not all suicides are associated with mental disorders, but mental disorders account for the majority. It is estimated that 60–90% of suicides are associated with affective disorder. Schizophrenia, depression, and bipolar illness contribute to the number of suicides. Suicide was the tenth ranked cause of death in the United States, accounting for 38,364 deaths in 2010.[54,55] It was the seventh leading cause of death for men and the fourteenth for women. In men, suicides outnumber homicides by more than 2 to 1 and are epidemic in the sense of being common, outnumbering deaths from HIV by nearly 4 to 1.[54–56] Suicides are most common among young and middle-aged adults; however, it is important to note that rates of suicide rise sharply for men older than 70 years of age, with a rate of suicide for those aged over 75 years of 36 per 100,000.[54,57] Men have higher rates than women by a ratio of 4 to 1 and account for 79% of suicides.[56,57] The ratio increases to 6.9 to 1 in individuals older than 65, in particular Caucasian men, because men and women of color manifest lower rates of suicide in their advanced years.[57]

Suicide is the third leading cause of death among young people aged 15–24 (unintentional injuries and homicides are number 1 and 2) and second in those aged 25–34 (topping homicides).[56,57] The gender ratio for suicide is high in younger cohorts: 7.6 males to 1 female in 15-year-olds compared to 4.8 to 1 in young adults aged 20–24 years. Suicidal ideation occurs in about 16% of youth.[58] Suicide rates are much higher in the western United States (with the exception of California) and Alaska. In 2010, firearms were used in 50.5% of suicides, suffocation in 24.7%, and overdoses (poisoning) in 17.2%. Men account for 87% of firearm suicides.[56,58] Contrary to popular opinion, suicide is not more common around the winter holidays; actually, the months with the highest rates are July and August, with rates of 1.2 per 100,000 population, accounting for nearly 20% of suicides.[56:15] Attempted suicides are very unreliably reported, and it is estimated that there is one suicide death for every 25 attempted suicides.[58]

The descriptive epidemiology of suicide is the foundation for enumerating risk and protective factors. These are incorporated into the formal assessment of suicidal risk carried out in every clinical setting, most frequently emergency rooms (ERs). In the absence of a simple, single cause of suicide, an assessment of suicidal risk is predicated on a complex algebra of positive and negative factors. Factors that elevate risk are mental disorders, alcohol or substance use, pessimism, hopelessness, aggression, impulsivity, a past personal history of a suicide attempt, a family history of a suicide attempt, a past history of trauma, and the recent diagnosis of a serious medical illness.[58–62] Environmental factors increasing risk include availability of a lethal means, social isolation, recent loss, and the occurrence of "contagious" clusters. Barriers to accessing care and stigmatization also raise suicide risk.

Many protective factors are reciprocals of risk factors; these include strong family and social support, absence of a lethal means, and access to care. Other protective factors include problem-solving skills, conflict resolution skills, and religious beliefs that discourage suicide.[59,61] In addition, in every clinical assessment of suicidal risk, there is the ill-defined factor of clinical judgment, which is highly weighted. Clinical judgment incorporates the integration of risk and protective factors plus clinical experience and intuition based on a therapeutic relationship with an individual and years of practice.

Stemming from pharmaco-epidemiologic data, the use of antidepressants is a controversial factor in the risk of suicide. It is well-known clinically that a deeply depressed person who begins to feel better and more activated may act on suicidal ideation. Psychiatric clinicians are trained to monitor the early stages of antidepressant treatment for this possibility. Data from the US Food and Drug Administration (FDA) identified an elevated risk of suicide attempts in teens taking antidepressants, thus leading to a black-box warning on certain medications. In 2003, evaluation of antidepressant trial information raised concerns that antidepressants may increase the risk of suicide.[63] Other studies, mostly of an observational nature, have suggested that antidepressants actually are protective. For example, Jick et al. found that individuals on antidepressants for less than 30 days had no difference in risk of suicide than those on antidepressants for more than 30 days (Odds Ratio [OR] = 1.0, 95% Confidence Interval/CI [0.4, 2.3]).[64:217] Simon found decreasing suicide risk after antidepressant initiation in both adolescents and adults.[65] Studies suggest that with the rise in treatment of depression in youth, suicide rates declined and, with the addition of the black-box warnings about suicide, rates of suicide increased in association with declining rates of antidepressant treatment.[66] However, these were purely ecological relationships and cannot be considered causal. In the end, the use of antidepressants requires careful evaluation of risks and benefits using seasoned clinical judgment.

Prevention of Suicide

Knowledge of risk and protective factors and clinical assessments are a foundation for prevention, especially when there is an opportunity to evaluate someone with suicidal ideation. Indeed, 67% of people who commit suicide are receiving treatment at the time. The National Violent Death Reporting System (NVDRS) finds that 31% of suicides were in individuals currently receiving mental health treatment, and 44% had a currently diagnosed mental health problem.[56:18] Beyond that, a plan for prevention of suicide, given no simple cause, is a complex matrix of interventions. There is a long history of progress in trying to prevent suicide in the United States, starting with the establishment of a US Public Health Service (USPHS) Suicide Prevention Center in 1958. The culmination of developments over the years was the publication of the Surgeon General's national strategy for suicide prevention in 2001 (updated in 2012).[18,67] The 2001 plan included a matrix of activities (see Table 7.1) and called for preventing suicide over the life span, reducing the rate of suicidal behaviors, reducing the harmful after-effects of suicides, and promoting resiliency. The plan had three parts: heightening awareness of the problem, disseminating interventions, and enhancing methodologies for surveillance and studies of suicide. The Surgeon General summarized a range of interventions using the matrix of universal, selective, and indicated actions discussed earlier. The updated strategy accounts for new research results and focuses on four strategic directions: supportive environments to promote the mental health of individuals, families,

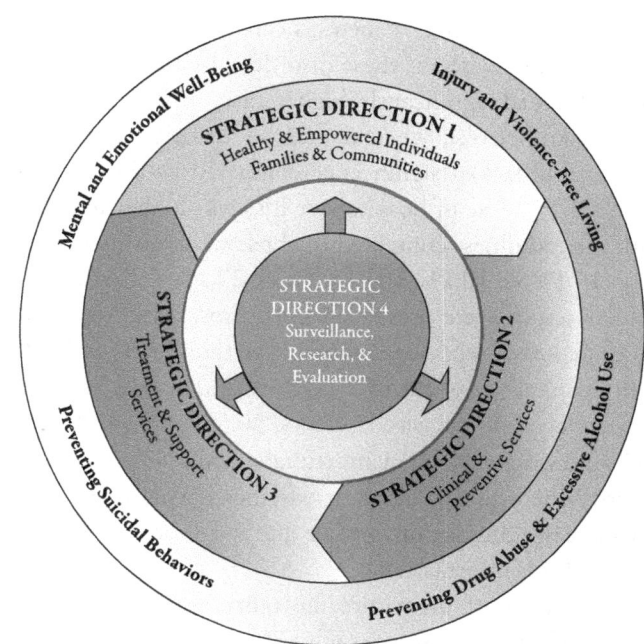

Figure 7.2 National Strategy for Suicide Prevention

and communities; enhancing preventive services; timely treatment and support; and improvement of suicide prevention surveillance, research, and evaluative activities (see Figure 7.2).

PREMATURE DEATH FROM CHRONIC DISEASES IN PEOPLE WITH SMI

The challenge of improving life expectancy among people with SMI is, perhaps, the leading public health task for psychiatry today. To achieve this objective, psychiatry must develop new ways of partnering with primary care practitioners to ensure that the comprehensive care needs of this population are met (see Chapters 5 and 10). In 2006, the NASMHPD documented a 25-year shortened life expectancy of people with SMI.[25] As a result, the National Centers for Disease Control (CDC) began to monitor mortality rates in the United States for this high-risk group.

Two major surveys provide information on the problem of comorbidity: the National Survey on Drug Use and Health (NSDUH) and the National Health Interview Survey (NHIS). The NSDUH provides information about the physical health of individuals with mental illness.[68] In addition to identifying the prevalence of mental illness, this survey also identifies comorbid conditions in those with mental illness. Nearly 20% of adults aged 18 or older had a mental illness; 6.5% had major depressive episode, and 4.6% had an SMI. Individuals with depression or any mental illness had significantly higher rates of hypertension, asthma, diabetes, heart disease, and stroke than did those without these disorders. In addition, those with SMI had significantly higher rates of hypertension, asthma, and stroke, whereas rates of diabetes and heart disease approached significance compared to those without SMI.[68:2-3] Use of hospitals or ERs was higher in those with mental illness compared to those without mental illness (15.1% vs. 10.1%; and 38.8% vs. 27.1%, respectively). Similar results were present in both those with SMI and major depressive episodes compared to those without SMI, with hospital use of 20.4% vs. 11.6% and 18.1 vs. 10.8%, respectively; ER use was 47.6% vs. 30.5% and 43.3% and 28.7%, respectively.[68:4-5] Unfortunately, this survey cannot identify the order of onset or whether having one disorder increases the risk of another due to the cross-sectional nature of this information.

The causes of premature mortality are found in the ravages of chronic diseases such as hypertension, diabetes, and vascular disease. An early harbinger of the problem is the *metabolic syndrome*, characterized by high blood pressure, high blood glucose, and high blood cholesterol. Unfortunately, the medications that have revolutionized the care and treatment of mental illness also increase the risk of metabolic syndrome, diabetes, and cardiovascular disease in those treated. Those with SMI die an average of 15–25 years earlier than the general population.[69,70] These problems are intensified by low rates of disease monitoring in those with SMI.[71] The solution to the problem requires mental health professionals and community mental health centers to address the medical care of people with SMI. The four-quadrant Behavioral Health Primary Care Integration Model is one framework that helps to distinguish ways to plan for services to provide care for both needs.[72] For example, in those with high behavioral health needs, one method is to integrate primary care into mental health services. Alternatively, within federally qualified health centers, greater integration of mental health care into primary care addresses the problem. These two major platforms of care and the issue of premature mortality are discussed in greater detail in Chapter 5.

The second source of data is the NHIS. Based on a community sample, it is a household survey of adults that provides additional information about the presence of SMI in addition to a wide range of health variables.[73] Social and economic factors contributing to the risk for chronic health problems in the seriously mentally ill include a higher frequency of living below the poverty level (35.3% SMI vs. 11.4% with no SMI, $p < 0.001$), homelessness (35.6% SMI vs. 4.8% with no SMI, $p < 0.001$), lower education (55.2% SMI vs. 44.3% with no SMI, $p < 0.001$), lower rates of working in the past year (50.2% SMI vs. 82% with no SMI, $p < 0.001$), higher rates of use of government or other assistance ($p < 0.001$), and higher frequency of having unmet care needs in the past year due to cost ($p < 0.001$).[73:1044-1045] In addition, behavior risk factors are significantly higher in those with SMI. For example, 51.4% smoke vs. 19.1% of those without SMI ($p < 0.001$); 52.1% do not exercise vs. 38.6% of those without SMI ($p < 0.001$); and 32.4% are obese vs. 26% of those without SMI ($p = 0.01$).[73:1044] Also, there were significant differences in the prevalence of heart problems (19.8% SMI vs. 11.1% with no SMI, $p < 0.001$), lung problems (24.9% SMI vs. 9.9% with no SMI, $p < 0.001$), and hypertension (31.2% SMI vs. 23.6% with no SMI, $p < 0.01$).[73:1044] Finally, there was a significant difference in the frequency of chronic conditions: 33.7% of those with SMI had one chronic condition versus 23.3% of those without SMI, and 25.7% with SMI had two or more chronic conditions versus 15.6% without SMI.[73:1044] In the past year, 47.2% had one or more ER visits, and 24.3% had one or more hospital stays versus 19.5% and 9.0% of those without SMI, respectively ($p < 0.001$ for both).[73]

Achieving the goal of reducing premature mortality will require addressing a problem identified at the dawn of modern public psychiatry as part of the community mental health movement but never successfully resolved. Although, the SAMHSA launched a "10 by 10" public awareness program (10-year improvement in shortened life expectancy by 2010), success in pursuit of this goal will take years, with not just clinical care, but also prevention and wellness programs required to make an essential contribution. Recognizing this challenge, in spring 2009, the SAMHSA issued a request for proposals for demonstration projects. The first round of these demonstration projects is completed, and a second round is well under way. (One such project is described in more detail in Chapter 5.)

OUTCOME 3: DISABILITY OR BURDEN OF DISEASE

Disability is the impact of disease on the social and occupational performance of the individual.[74] Disability is not the same as symptoms from chronic disease, although often the two are confounded. This confusion is understandable because acute psychological and behavioral symptoms can interfere with performance. This interference is temporary during the acute symptomatic phase of illness. It is well known that, given the limitations of psychiatric treatments, residual symptoms are common, thereby contributing to interference with performance and activities of daily living. Other factors, such as institutionalization or social isolation, contribute to disability as well. Psychosocial rehabilitation services are designed to target disability (see Chapter 4).

In combination, symptoms and disabilities form the broad clinical pictures encountered in public psychiatry. The distinction between symptoms and disabilities is useful not only for intellectual clarity. Understanding disability is useful for accomplishing disability assessments, which are based on assessments of capacity for self-care, social performance, and occupational behavior. Also, an understanding of disability is a foundation for planning approaches to recovery, as we now understand it in public psychiatry (see Chapter 3).

Furthermore, the concept of disability is also useful for appreciating and communicating the enormous impact of psychiatric disorders on individuals and society and comparing this with other medical, mainly physically defined diseases. The metric of the DALY placed psychiatric disorders squarely on the public health map.[17] This metric, combining years of life lost (YLL) to premature death and years of life lived with a disability (YLD) in psychiatric disorders, when compared to other medical conditions, finds that unipolar depression, self-inflicted injury, substance abuse, schizophrenia, bipolar disorder, and obsessive compulsive disorder (OCD) emerge as leading causes of disease burden. In industrialized societies, psychiatric disorders ranked in the top 10, accounting for 10.5% of the burden of disease worldwide based on findings from the Global Burden of Disease study.[17:1502]

For example, the Global Burden of Disease Study estimated that the disease burden of unipolar major depression in 1990 was fourth of 15 leading causes. It is expected that by 2020 depression will move to the second leading cause of disease burden.[75:1241] Four other mental disorders also were included in the top 10: alcohol use, bipolar disorder, schizophrenia, and OCD. In 2010, mental health and SUDs were responsible for 7.4% of all DALYs, and these disorders actually accounted for 22.9% of YLDs, the highest single proportion of all diseases.[76:1578–1579] Depression was responsible for 40.5% and anxiety disorders for 14.6% of the DALYs, followed by drug use (10.9%) and alcohol use (9.6%), whereas schizophrenia accounted for 7.4%. Of all the psychiatric disorders, SUDs resulted in 86.1% of YLLs, with alcohol use resulting in 44.4% of YLLs and drug use in 41.7% of YLLs. Globally, drug dependence is the eighth largest contributor to disability in men, with opiate dependence contributing 9.2 million DALYs or nearly half of the burden.[77:1570] This reflects a 74% increase from 1990 to 2010 for opiate dependence, with the addition of another 4 million DALYs.[77:1569] Despite the higher prevalence of SUDs in 2010 (specifically alcohol, opiates, and cocaine), mental disorders did not increase in prevalence over the same period.

Unfortunately, drug dependence takes its highest toll in the young adult years when productivity is often highest, thus further augmenting the burden of this disorder.

These epidemiologic measures are critical to justifying priorities and strategically allocating limited funds to manage public health problems. Worldwide, psychiatric disorders accounted for only 0.4% of YLLs but an enormous 26% of YLDs. In 2002, the WHO identified mental illness as the leading cause of disability in the United States and Canada.[78] This evidence is important to efforts in public psychiatry because important funding decisions often are made based on problem rank or priority.

In short, psychiatric disorders have recently emerged as major public health problems and have begun to receive the attention they deserved. Major national organizations such as the NIMH began to incorporate plans for reducing burden of disease into their strategic goals. On a service level, the recovery movement (see Chapter 3) and early intervention in psychosis (see herein and Chapter 10), two major innovations in psychiatric services, became important new directions. These programs, though not directly linked, emerged shortly after the establishment of burden of disease as a valid and essential perspective on psychiatric disorders.

One consequence of disability is unemployment, a circumstance often experienced by persons with SMI. For example, a recent analysis found that individuals had an 18% decrease in likelihood of employment for each unit increase in emotional problems causing difficulty in accomplishing goals.[79:13] The risk was greater for women (22% decrease in employment) than for men (11%). Broadhead identified that the greatest burden of all diseases on families and society are lost work days resulting from depression, with 4.78 times the risk of disability days (95% CI [1.64, 13.88]) and an average of 11 days of disability due to symptoms compared to 2 days in asymptomatic individuals.[80:2527] Individuals with major depressive disorder were more often unemployed compared to those who were asymptomatic (44.7% vs. 30.2%).[80:2526]

In this section, the discussion reviewed evidence of the importance of morbidity, mortality, and disability as essential outcomes to consider in public psychiatry. Absence of change in indicators of morbidity suggests a need for new paradigms for clinical diagnosis and research. Rates of mortality and disability of psychiatric disorders were largely ignored until 25 years ago, yet they place psychiatric disorders at the top of public health concerns in the United States and the world. Public psychiatrists need to understand these figures, not only because epidemiologic data inform practice, as in the case of suicide prediction, but also because data on these outcomes, among other indicators, reveal the "community diagnosis" of the places where they work.

EARLY INTERVENTION AND BURDEN OF DISEASE

Although early intervention is reviewed thoroughly in Chapter 10, it is mentioned here because of its role in reducing burden of disease and, conceivably, its potential for actually preventing full-blown psychotic illness. It is well known that the earlier it is possible to intervene in an incipient psychotic illness, the lower the risk of long-term disability. Strategies for the early identification of cases enable multidimensional treatment, including pharmacologic interventions, education, work-related cognitive coaching, and family psychoeducation. All of these then have a better chance of remediating the psychotic symptoms. Indeed, in some cases, the risk of a florid psychotic episode may be averted, and this may qualify as primary prevention. As we noted earlier, this type of intervention considerably rebalances the public psychiatry portfolio of services and appropriately emphasizes the prodrome of psychosis and the earliest stages of symptoms.

The concept of early intervention harkens back to central ideas of the community mental health movement, and it is intuitively convincing in a theoretical framework derived from public health. However, the efficacy of early intervention in initial episodes of psychosis is still unproved, and many studies are now under way to evaluate it (see Chapter 10). In addition, more effort is needed in the form of advocacy for health insurance benefits to cover the elements of care in an early intervention program. Success in obtaining reimbursement would provide incentive for community mental health clinics to implement the services.

PUBLIC EDUCATION

MENTAL HEALTH FIRST AID

An interesting recent initiative in public education about mental illness is Mental Health First Aid (MHFA), developed in Australia in 2001 by Anthony Jorm and Betty Kitchener.[81] It was introduced into the United States in 2008 via a national campaign that is a collaboration of the National Council for Community Behavior Healthcare (NCCBH) and the Maryland and Missouri state departments of mental health. MHFA is supported by a growing body of evidence (see website review, National Registry of Evidence Based Programs and Practices [NREPP]).[82] This program provides manualized training for people who are not mental health professionals, such as teachers or first responders. The training helps people to identify, understand, and respond to people with mental illness or addictions. MHFA is applicable to many high-risk populations such as college students, young adults, and communities suffering from traumatic occurrences. Key elements of MHFA include assisting the person facing a crisis, listening nonjudgmentally, offering support, offering information, encouraging the person to get professional help, and encouraging use of supports.[83:237] A campaign to promote MHFA nationwide is supported by a website (mentalhealthfirstaid.org). Surveys after implementation of MHFA shows improvement in beliefs about mental health professionals and treatments.[83:238]

DISASTER PREPARATION AND PREVENTION

Among the public health challenges facing public psychiatry is disaster planning in anticipation of epidemics such as influenza and natural or man-made, disasters.[84,85] Behavioral interventions are an essential part of disaster planning. These exercises are an opportunity for public psychiatry to demonstrate its role and importance in responding to the national security agenda.

Since September 11, 2001, the role of public psychiatry in preparation for response to natural and man-made disasters has been further accentuated.[84,86] Planning is usually coordinated by state government authorities in collaboration with local government and community resources. Public psychiatry, by planning and working with civil and other medical experts and resources, demonstrates its role in helping the psychiatric casualties of such events.

A common problem after disaster is the negative effects on an individual's emotional well-being, typically with psychological sequelae being greater than physical.[84,87,88] McCabe et al. identifies a need to prepare for a surge in the need for behavioral health care regardless of the kind of disaster experienced.[84] Disaster planning must address a variety of problems and groups, starting with the need of the entire population for information during events. Regular communication about the disaster event, updates about loss and resolution of services, and information about resources available in the community that support coping are essential to support healthy coping and promote health. Planning for how those with existing physical or mental health problems will receive needed services without interruption, including physical and mental health care, medications, and other resources required for normal functioning, is essential. In addition, plans must identify how psychological support and screening can be implemented in the midst of each phase of a disaster and its aftermath. Plans often include use of professionals, paraprofessionals, and lay volunteers in providing an array of needed services. Often, volunteers trained in MHFA can provide support, screening, and referral to professional services. It is well known that with disaster comes increased need for clinical services: proper planning can ensure that vital services are available when disasters strike.

One of the great challenges for US society is the prevention of future tragedies such as the Sandy Hook Elementary School shootings.[89,90] In the absence of single, high-impact solutions, some combination of public education, early intervention, improved access to clinical services, and adequate service capacity are the best, most comprehensive strategy for heading off another such incident. Health policy also plays a role in addressing risks and needs in the community, whether related to restricted access to lethal weapons as a universal precaution, the role of involuntary treatment, and the availability of professionals to provide clinical services.

SOCIAL, ENVIRONMENTAL, AND CULTURAL FACTORS AND DISPARITIES IN HEALTH CARE OUTCOMES

The future of public health in psychiatry lies in the integration of knowledge related to environmental and sociocultural factors that impact risk for mental illness. The Surgeon General's 2001 report on culture, race and ethnicity was a landmark in conceptualizing and reviewing evidence for secondary and tertiary preventive interventions to reduce burden of disease from psychiatric disorders.[19] It identified culture, race, and ethnicity as risk factors, with each defining high-risk groups for burden of disease. The documented disparities in mental health outcomes serve as a starting point. Disparities theoretically occur as a function of elevated incidence, higher risk of mortality, or chronic illness and disability—the three outcomes discussed earlier. From descriptive epidemiology, there is no evidence of differences in the incidence in psychiatric disorders among broad, national cultural groups. Rather, it is the higher risk of chronic morbidity, mortality, and burden of disease that accounts for the disparities.

Key mechanisms for the disparities are complex, operate at multiple levels, and require a transformation of the health care system.[91] For example, a recent Health and Human Services Action Plan to address racial and ethnic disparities targets systems-level factors including infrastructure and workforce development, large-scale health promotion and wellness initiatives, support for scientific innovation, and administrative accountability.[91] These systems-level efforts complement pervasive challenges of diminished access to and quality of care for racial and ethnic minorities that result in prolonged symptoms and disability.[19] Recent efforts have begun to conceptualize culture more broadly to include other social identities, such as gender, sexual orientation, social class, religion, and so on, that can result in discrimination or marginalization due to one's identity.[92,93] Adopting this broader definition of culture is likely to enhance the conceptualization of health disparities research to include the intersection of various identities (e.g., race, gender, class) to inform research and intervention.[94]

PRACTICE-BASED POPULATION HEALTH

Public health policy supports a population perspective in clinical practice in the form of practice-based population health.[95,96] Berwick's discussion of the triple aim to improve health care in the United States identifies a need for (1) a focus on high quality, (2) population-focused health care, and (3) accountability to control cost.[97] He later championed this agenda during his term as Administrator of Medicare and Medicaid Services. Promoted under the Affordable Care Act (ACA) by the Centers for Medicaid and Medicare Services (CMS) for the purpose of cost control in high-risk, high-cost patients in accountable care organizations, this model creates a new standard for clinical practice. Clinicians are responsible not only for patients who present for treatment, but also for an entire panel of potential patients, including those who do not attend the clinic.

Responsibility for the whole panel encourages service delivery systems to develop preventive and wellness interventions. This type of practice is supported by risk-based, prepaid reimbursement mechanisms in place of volume-driven, fee-for-service mechanisms. Primary care practices will have to re-engineer for this type of practice, which will be integrated through accountable care organizations (ACOs), within medical homes for people with SMI, and in community health centers and integrated care teams for patients with psychiatric illness[98] (see Chapter 5).

THE FUTURE OF PUBLIC HEALTH IN PUBLIC PSYCHIATRY

A basic premise for this chapter is that public health concepts and practices should be integrated into the clinical model of public psychiatry. A critical juncture between the two is at the forefront of the development of practice-based population health, a new service delivery model for public psychiatry and the rest of medicine (see Chapter 5).

As noted earlier, TCC is an exemplar of an academic prevention program that is part of the CMHC. We highlight it as a case example to illustrate how prevention operates and how it can support population practice.

THE CONSULTATION CENTER

In the late 1970s at the CMHC, at a time when federal, categorical community mental health funding was falling, prevention programs were consolidated into a single-unit named The Consultation Center. These programs followed a community consultation and prevention research agenda focusing on a broad range of prevention and health promotion topics. Over the years, TCC has pursued multiple grant and contract-supported projects.[7] In 2005, the National Institute on Drug Abuse (NIDA) awarded the Center and its companion research division in the Yale Department of Psychiatry (the Division of Prevention and Community Research) a training grant to support prevention research education for postdoctoral fellows. As a result of these efforts, TCC became a nationally recognized leader in prevention education that is virtually unique.

In this way, through a long fallow period for integrated public health and public psychiatry, TCC helped to maintain expertise in public health and prevention at the CMHC. This story is an example of an academic program sustaining an important stream of public psychiatry that was at risk of withering away because of funding, ideological, and service vicissitudes. When national policy discussions through the NFC report in 2003 returned to the topics of prevention and early intervention, TCC was an important building block for participation in the transformation agenda.

TCC's mission is to promote health and wellness, prevent mental health and substance abuse problems, and enhance equity and social justice (www.consultationcenter. yale.edu). This work is done in collaboration with community organizations, schools, businesses, and government agencies as well as with mental health consumers, family members, service providers, and other community stakeholders.

Center services and research target vulnerable populations, such as individuals living in poverty or those experiencing trauma or exposure to stressful family, school, or neighborhood environments. Prevention services and research include both risk reduction and health promotion strategies as appropriate, are theoretically grounded, and take into account key developmental and cultural contexts. A hallmark of the Center's research is close collaboration with key community stakeholders to effect change. Three ongoing projects are illustrative (1) the Yale-Bridgeport Gear-Up, a universal preventive intervention to reduce high school dropout and increase college entry for underrepresented minority youth[99]; (2) the Youth Development Training and Resource Center or YDTRC (http://ydtrc.org), formed more than 20 years ago as a collaboration among a network of youth-serving agencies in Greater New Haven (Connecticut) with the goal of affecting individual and systems change to promote youth development[100]; and (3) the Family Violence Program, a selected prevention intervention that provides a 9-week psychoeducational alternative to prosecution for adults arrested for domestic violence; the program, now in its twentieth year, seeks to prevent recurrence by teaching participants how to cope more effectively with anger, stress, and frustration in intimate relationships.[101] The prevention work is conceptualized less as disease prevention in individuals or as prevention of psychiatric disorders, and more broadly as community- and population-level strategies to promote behavioral health. These approaches are likely to have an impact on the socioecological conditions that cause, exacerbate, or sustain disorders and are an important focus of prevention.

Current challenges include ongoing engagement with clinical services at the CMHC to build a robust approach to practice-based population health. In contrast to the services just described, these new initiatives are disease-oriented. A range of consultations are under way, including (1) routine depression screening for the panel of patients served by the CMHC (a universal health educational and preventive intervention); (2) the indicated intervention of routine, structured screening for suicidal ideation among people with major depression during evaluation; and (3) collaborations with an early intervention program to reduce risk of metabolic syndrome (a selective prevention). Over time, the goal is to re-establish the close collaboration between prevention and clinical interventions that originally characterized the community mental health center movement and is now necessary for practice-based population health.

THE COMPLEXITY OF PREVENTION IN PUBLIC PSYCHIATRY

Psychiatry cannot be divided into "organ systems" as much of our medical system organizes care. Integrating the focus of who should be targeted for intervention with current status on a health–disease continuum offers an approach that acknowledges the complexity of the mental health–mental illness continuum. This continuum is broad enough to provide a foundation for population-based efforts at enhancing wellness; promoting health; and simultaneously preventing disease, complications, and comorbidity and limiting disability and chronicity. Although clinicians in public psychiatry may focus primarily on intervention, a scientific public health perspective can target points where prevention or intervention are most warranted. Truly methodical, comprehensive planning that weaves between levels and types of intervention is required to address the complexity inherent in mental illness. The point of public health in public psychiatry is to think broadly and in a multilevel framework and to address the structural inequalities present in our society that result in risk for mental health problems.

SUMMARY

The mental health system has changed drastically since the era of the asylum, and it currently serves individuals within their own communities. Public health approaches and tools have enhanced psychiatry's ability to identify and respond to changing needs for clinical care. The integration of clinical and public health approaches in public psychiatry provides strategies to assist in meeting future challenges in caring across the continuum of health for individuals, groups, and community populations.

A public health approach in psychiatry offers a unique lens with which to identify needs and plan to improve the health of individuals, groups, communities, and large populations. Depending on the focal length of the lens, epidemiologic methods offer ways to prioritize needs and plan, implement, and evaluate interventions. Using a broad lens, universal strategies promote mental and physical health and prevent the occurrence of physical and mental illness. With greater focus, groups at risk for mental illness are identified and strategic interventions implemented. In focusing on specific groups or individuals experiencing mental health problems, interventions home in on alleviating the symptoms and consequences of those disorders, thus preventing complications, comorbidities, and, when possible, the disability and persistence or chronicity of illness.

REFERENCES

1. American Public Health Association. 2012. *What Is Public Health?* http://www.apha.org/~/media/files/pdf/factsheets/whatisph.ashx. Accessed May 4, 2014.
2. World Health Organization. *Mental Health: A State of Well-Being.* http://www.who.int/features/factfiles/mental_health/en/. Published 2014. Retrieved May 4, 2014.
3. Ewalt JR. Goals of the Joint Commission on Mental Health and Illness. *Am J Pub Health*. 1957;47:19–24.
4. Moran M. Vision revisited: 50 years of the Community Mental Health Act. *Psychiatr News*. 2013;48(22):1. doi: 10.1176/appi.pn.2013.11b24
5. Public Law No. 88-164, 77 Stat 282.
6. Foley HH, Sharfstein SS. *Madness and Government: Who Cares for the Mentally Ill?* Washington, DC: American Psychiatric Press; 1983.
7. Tebes JK, Kaufman JS, Chinman MJ. Teaching about prevention to mental health professionals. In: Glenwick, D, Jason L, eds. *Innovative Strategies for Promoting Health and Mental Health Across the Life Span*. New York: Springer; 2002:37–60.
8. US Department of Health and Human Services. *The Road Ahead: Research Partnerships to Transform Services: A Report by the National Advisory Mental Health Council's Workgroup on Services and Clinical Epidemiology Research*. Bethesda, MD: National Institutes of Health, National Institute of Mental Health; 2006.
9. Jacobs S. *Inside Public Psychiatry*. Shelton, CT: People's Medical Publishing House; 2011.
10. Regier DA, Farmer ME, Rae DS, et al. One-month prevalence of mental disorders in the United States and sociodemographic characteristics: The Epidemiologic Catchment Area study. *Acta Psychiatr Scandinav*. 1993;88:35–47.
11. Kessler RC, Price RH. Primary prevention of secondary disorders: A proposal and agenda. *Am J Community Psychol*. 1993;21:607–634.
12. Mrazek, PJ, Haggerty RJ, eds. *Reducing Risks for Mental Disorders: Frontiers for Preventive Intervention Research*. Washington DC: National Academy Press; 1994.
13. Koyanagi C. *Learning from History: Deinstitutionalization of People with Mental Illness as Precursor to Long Term Care Reform*. Washington, DC: Kaiser Commission on Medicaid and the Uninsured; 2007.
14. Steadman HJ, Monahan J, Duffee B, et al. The impact of state mental hospital deinstitutionalization on United States prison populations, 1968–1978. *J Crim Law Criminol*. 1984;75:474–490.
15. Torrey EF. *Out of the Shadows: Confronting America's Mental Illness Crisis*. New York: Wiley; 1997. http://www.pbs.org/wgbh/pages/frontline/shows/asylums/special/excerpt.html. Accessed May 4, 2014.
16. US Department of Health and Human Services. *Mental Health: A Report of the Surgeon General*. Rockville, MD: US Department of Health and Human Services, Substance Abuse and Mental Health Services Administration, Center for Mental Health Services, National Institutes of Health, National Institute of Mental Health; 1999.

17. Murray CJL, Lopez AD. Alternative projections of mortality and disability by cause 1990-2020: the global burden of disease study. *Lancet.* 1997;349:1498–1504.
18. US Department of Health and Human Services. *National Strategy for Suicide Prevention: Goals and Objectives for Action.* Rockville, MD: US Public Health Service; 2001.
19. US Department of Health and Human Services. *Mental Health: Culture, Race, and Ethnicity—A Supplement to Mental Health: A Report of the Surgeon General.* Rockville, MD: US Department of Health and Human Services, Substance Abuse and Mental Health Services Administration, Center for Mental Health Services; 2001.
20. President's New Freedom Commission on Mental Health. *Achieving the Promise: Transforming Mental Health Care in America.* Rockville, MD: President's New Freedom Commission on Mental Health; 2003.
21. National Institute of Mental Health. *The Impact of Mental Illness on Society.* www.nimh.nih.gov/publicat/burden.cfm. Published 2006. Accessed May 4, 2014.
22. Insel TR, Fenton WS. Psychiatric epidemiology: it's not just about counting anymore. *Arch Gen Psychiatry.* 2005;62(6):590–592.
23. Power K. A public health model of mental health for the 21st century. *Psychiatr Serv.* 2009; 60(5):580–584.
24. Glass TA, McAtee MJ. Behavioral science at the crossroads in public health: extending horizons, envisioning the future. *Soc Sci Med.* 2006;62(7):1650–1671.
25. National Association of State Mental Health Program Directors. *Morbidity and Mortality in People with Serious Mental Illness.* Alexandria, VA: NASMHPD Medical Directors Council; 2006.
26. Lieberman JA. Comparative effectiveness of antipsychotic drugs. *Arch Gen Psychiatry.* 2006;63:1069–1072.
27. Insel T, Cuthbert B, Garvey M, et al. Research domain criteria (RDoC): toward a new classification framework for research on mental disorders. *Am J Psychiatry.* 2010;167(7):748–751.
28. Davey Smith G. The antecedents of epidemiological methodology in Arthur Mitchell's surveillance and care of the insane. *Int J Epidemiol.* 2010;39:25–30.
29. Mitchell A. Contribution to the statistics of insanity. *Br J Psychiatry.* 1877;22:507–515.
30. Morgan Z, Brugha T, Fryers T, Stewart-Brown S. The effects of parent-child relationships on later life mental health status in two national birth cohorts. *Soc Psychiatry Psychiatr Epidemiol.* 2012;47(11):1707–1715.
31. Reef J, Diamantopoulou S, Van Meurs I, Verhulst FC, van der Ende J. Developmental trajectories of child to adolescent externalizing behavior and adult DSM-IV disorder: results of a 24-year longitudinal study. *Soc Psychiatry Psychiatr Epidemiol.* 2011;46:1233–1241.
32. Commission on Chronic Illness. *Chronic Illness in the United States. Vol. 1.* Cambridge, MA: Harvard University Press; 1957.
33. Gordon RS. An operational classification of disease prevention. *Pub Health Rep.*1983;98(2):107–109.
34. Offord DR. Selection of levels of prevention. *Addictive Behav.* 2000;25(6):833–842.
35. Christner RW, Mennuti RB, Heim M, Gipe K, Rubenstein JS. Facilitating mental health services in schools: universal, selected, and targeted interventions. In Lionetti TM, Snyder EP, Christner RW, eds. *A Practical Guide to Building Professional Competencies in School Psychology.* New York: Springer; 2011.
36. Pettibone KG, Friend KB, Nargiso JE, Florin P. Evaluating environmental change strategies: challenges and solutions. *Am J Community Psychol.* 2013;51:217–221.
37. Durlak JA, Wells AM. Primary prevention mental health programs for children and adolescents: A meta-analytic review. *Am J Community Psychol.* 1997;25:115–152.
38. Brugha TS, Morrell CJ, Slade P, Walters SJ. Universal prevention of depression in women postnatally: cluster randomized trial evidence in primary care. *Psychol Med.* 2011;41(4):739–748.
39. Tebes JK, Kaufman JS, Adnopoz J, Racusin G. Resilience and family psychosocial processes among children of parents with serious mental disorders. *J Child Fam Stud.* 2001;10(1):115–136.
40. Miles J, Espiritu RC, Horen N, Sebian J, Waetzig E. *A Public Health Approach to Children's Mental Health: A Conceptual Framework.* Washington, DC: Georgetown University Center for Child and Human Development, National Technical Assistance Center for Children's Mental Health; 2010.
41. Weisz J, Sandler IN, Durlak JA, Anton BS. Promoting and protecting youth mental health through evidence-based prevention and treatment. *Am Psychol.* 2005;60(6):628–648.
42. Substance Abuse and Mental Health Services Administration. *Leading Change: A Plan for SAMHSA's Roles and Actions 2011–2014.* Rockville, MD: SAMHSA; 2010.
43. Gest SD, Osgood DW, Feinberg ME, Bierman KL, Moody J. Strengthening prevention program theories and evaluations: contributions from social network analysis. *Prev Sci.* 2011;12:349–360.
44. American Psychiatric Association. *Diagnostic and Statistical Manual of Mental Disorders.* 5th ed. Arlington, VA: American Psychiatric Association; 2013.
45. Kessler RC, Chiu WT, Demler O, Walters EE. Prevalence, severity, and comorbidity of twelve-month DSM-IV disorders in the National Comorbidity Survey Replication (NCS-R). *Arch Gen Psychiatry.* 2005;62(6):617–627. doi: 10.1001/archpsyc.62.6.617
46. Eaton WW, Regier DA, Locke BZ, Taube CA. The Epidemiologic Catchment Area Program of the National Institute of Mental Health. *Pub Health Rep.* 1981;96:319–325.
47. Kessler RC, Wang PS. The descriptive epidemiology of commonly occurring mental disorders in the United States. *Ann Rev Pub Health.* 2008;29:115–129.
48. National Institute of Mental Health. *The Numbers Count: Mental Disorders in America.* Bethesda, MD: National Institute of Mental Health; 2009. http://www.nimh.nih.gov/health/publications/the-numbers-count-mental-disorders-in-america/index.shtml. Accessed May 4, 2014.
49. Ormel J, Petukhova M, Chatterji S, et al. Disability and treatment of specific mental and physical disorders across the world: results from the WHO World Mental Health Surveys. *Br J Psychiatry.* 2008;192(5):368–375. doi: 10.1192/bjp.bp.107.039107.
50. Desmarais SL, Van Dorn RL, Johnson KL, Grimm KJ, Douglas KS, Swartz MS. Community violence perpetration and victimization among adults with mental illnesses [published online ahead of print February 13 2014]. *Am J Public Health.* 2014. doi: 10.2105/AJPH.2013.301680
51. Elbogen EB, Johnson SC. The intricate link between violence and mental disorder: results from the national epidemiologic survey on alcohol and related conditions. *Arch Gen Psychiatry.* 2009;66(2):152–161. doi: 10.1001/archgenpsychiatry.2008.537.
52. Van Dorn R, Volavka J, Johnson N. Mental disorder and violence: is there a relationship beyond substance use? *Soc Psychiatry Psychiatr Epidemiol.* 2012;47:487–503.
53. Eaton WW, Roth KB, Bruce M, et al. The relationship of mental and behavioral disorders to all-cause mortality in a 27-year follow-up of 4 epidemiologic catchment area samples. *Am J Epidemiology.* 2013;178(9):1366–1377.
54. Centers for Disease Control and Prevention, National Center for Injury Prevention and Control. *Web-based Injury Statistics Query and Reporting System (WISQARS).* 2010. www.cdc.gov/injury/wisqars/index.html. Accessed May 4, 2014.
55. Centers for Disease Control and Prevention. *20 Leading Causes of Death, United States 2010, All Races, Both Sexes. (WISQARS).* Atlanta, GA: Centers for Disease Control and Prevention; 2010. http://www.cdc.gov/injury/wisqars/index.html. Accessed May 4, 2014.
56. Centers for Disease Control and Prevention. Surveillance for violent deaths- National Violent Death Reporting System, 16 States, 2010. *MMWR.* 2014;63(1):15–17.

57. Centers for Disease Control and Prevention. (2012). *Death Rates for Suicide, by Sex, Race, Hispanic Origin, and Age: United States, Selected Years 1950–2010, Table 35. Health, United States, 2012.* http://www.cdc.gov/nchs/hus/contents 2012htm#35. Accessed May 4, 2014.
58. Centers for Disease Control and Prevention. *Suicide: Facts at a Glance.* Atlanta, GA: National Center for Injury Prevention and Control, Division of Violence Prevention; 2012. www.cdc.gov/violenceprevention. Accessed May 4, 2014.
59. Moscicki EK. Epidemiology of completed and attempted suicide: toward a framework for prevention. *Clin Neurosci Res.* 2001;1(5):310–323.
60. Taliaferro LA, Muehlenkamp JJ. Risk and protective factors that distinguish adolescents who attempt suicide from those who only consider suicide in the past year. *Suicide Life Threat Behav.* 2014;44(1):6–22.
61. Rodgers P, Suicide Prevention Resource Center. *Understanding Risk and Protective Factors for Suicide: A Primer for Preventing Suicide.* Newton, MA: Education Development Center; 2011.
62. Eaton D, Foti K, Brener N, Crosby A, Flores G, Kann L. Associations between risk behaviors and suicidal ideation and suicide attempts: do racial/ethnic variations in associations account for increased risk of suicidal behaviors among Hispanic/Latina 9th- to 12- grade female students? *Arch Suicide Res.* 2011;15:113–126.
63. Hammad T, Laughren T, Racoosin J. Suicidality in pediatric patients treated with antidepressant drugs. *Arch Gen Psychiatry.* 2006;63:332–339.
64. Jick SS, Dean AD, Jick H. Antidepressants and suicide. *BMJ.* 1995;310:215–218.
65. Simon G, Savarino J, Operskalski B, Wang P. Suicide risk during antidepressant treatment. *Am J Psychiatry.* 2006;163:41–47.
66. Simon G. Antidepressants and suicide. *Br Med J.* 2008;336:515–516.
67. US Department of Health and Human Services, Office of the Surgeon General and National Action Alliance for Suicide Prevention. *2012 National Strategy for Suicide Prevention: Goals and Objectives for Action.* Washington, DC: HHS; 2012.
68. Substance Abuse and Mental Health Services Administration, Center for Behavioral Health Statistics and Quality. *The NSDUH Report: Physical Health Conditions among Adults with Mental Illnesses.* Rockville, MD: Substance Abuse and Mental Health Services Administration, US Department of Health and Human Services; 2012.
69. Newcomer JW, Hennekens CH. Severe mental illness and risk of cardiovascular disease. *JAMA.* 2007;298(15):1794–1796.
70. Parks J, Svendsen D, Singer P, et al, eds. *Morbidity and Mortality in People With Serious Mental Illness.* Alexandria, VA: National Association of State Mental Health Program Directors, Medical Directors Council: 2006. http://www.nasmhpd.org/general_files/publications/med_directors_pubs/Mortality and Morbidity Final Report 8.18.08.pdf. Accessed May 4, 2014.
71. Morrato EH, Newcomer JW, Allen RR, Valuck RJ. Prevalence of baseline serum glucose and lipid testing in users of second-generation antipsychotic drugs: a retrospective, population-based study of Medicaid claims data. *J Clin Psychiatry.* 2008;69(2):316–322.
72. Mauer B. *Behavioral Health/Primary Care Integration: The Four Quadrant Model and Evidence Based Practices.* Rockville, MD: National Council for Community Behavioral Healthcare; 2006. http://www.thenationalcouncil.org/galleries/business-practice%20files/4%20Quadrant.pdf. Accessed May 4, 2014.
73. Pratt LA. Characteristics of adults with serious mental illness in the United States household population in 2007. *Psychiatr Serv.* 2012;63(10):1042–1046.
74. World Health Organization. *International Classification of Impairments, Disabilities and Handicaps.* Geneva, Switzerland: World Health Organization; 1980.
75. Lopez AD, Murray CCJL. The global burden of disease, 1990–2020. *Nature Med.* 1998;4(11):1241–1243.
76. Whiteford HA, Degenhardt L, Rehm J, et al. Global burden of disease attributable to mental and substance use disorders: findings from the Global Burden of Disease Study 2010. *Lancet.* 2013;382:1575–1586.
77. Degenhardt L, Whiteford HA, Ferrari AJ, et al. Global burden of disease attributable to illicit drug use and dependence: findings from the Global Burden of Disease Study 2010. *Lancet.* 2013;392:1564–1574.
78. World Health Organization. Annex Table 3: Burden of Disease in DALYs by Cause, Sex, and Mortality Stratum in WHO Regions, Estimates for 2002. *The World Health Report.* Geneva, Switzerland: World Health Organization; 2004. http://wwwlwho.int/whr/2004/annex/topic/en/annex_3_en.pdf. Accessed May 4, 2014.
79. Pacheco G, Webber DJ. Employment propensity: The roles of mental and physical health. *Department of Economics: Working Paper Series.* Auckland, New Zealand: Auckland University of Technology; 2011.
80. Broadhead W, Blazer D, George L, et al. Depression, disability days and days lost from work in a prospective epidemiological study. *JAMA.* 1990;264:2524–2528.
81. Kitchener BA, Jorm AF. Mental health first aid training for the public: evaluation of effects on knowledge, attitudes and helping behavior. *BMC Psychiatry.* 2002;2:10. doi: 10.1186/1471-244X-2-10.
82. Substance Abuse and Mental health Services Administration. *National Registry of Evidence Based Programs and Practices (NREPP).* Rockville, MD: Substance Abuse and Mental Health Services Administration; 2012. http://www.nrepp.samhsa.gov/ViewIntervention.aspx?id=321. Accessed May 15, 2014.
83. Jorm AF. Mental Health Literacy: Empowering the community to take action for better mental health. *Am Psychol.* 2012;67(3):231–243.
84. McCabe OL, Perry C, Azur M, et al. Guided preparedness planning with lay communities: enhancing capacity of rural emergency response through a systems-based partnership. *Prehosp Disaster Med.* 2013;28(1):8–15.
85. North CS, Pfefferbaum, B. Mental health response to community disasters: a systematic review. *JAMA.* 2013;310(5):507–518.
86. Graeff-Martins AS, Hoven CW, Wu P, Bin F, Duarte CS. Use of mental health services by children and adolescents six months after the world trade center attack. *Psychiatr Serv.* 2014;65:263–265.
87. National Institute of Mental Health. *Mental Health and Mass Violence: Evidence-Based Early Intervention for Victims/Survivors of Mass Violence. A Workshop to Reach Consensus on Best Practices.* Washington, DC: US Government Printing Office; 2002. NIH Publication No. 02-5138.
88. Norris FH, Friedman MJ, Watson PJ, Byrne CM, Diaz E, Kaniasty K. 60,000 disaster victims speak: Part I. An empirical review of the empirical literature, 1981–2001. *Psychiatry.* 2002;65(3):207–239.
89. Sedensky, SJ. *Report of the State's Attorney for the Judicial District of Danbury on the Shootings at Sandy Hook Elementary School and 36 Yogananda Street, Newtown, Connecticut on December 14, 2012.* Danbury, CT: Office of the State's Attorney Judicial District of Danbury; 2013. http://www.ct.gov/csao/lib/csao/Sandy_Hook_Final_Report.pdf. Accessed May 15, 2014.
90. Wikipedia, The Free Encyclopedia. *Sandy Hook Elementary School Shootings.* http://en.wikipedia.org/wiki/Sandy_Hook_Elementary_School_shooting. Published 2015. Accessed January 24, 2015.
91. Koh HK, Graham G, Glied SA. Reducing racial and ethnic disparities: the action plan from the department of health and human services. *Health Aff.* 2011;30(10):1822–1829.
92. Cohen AB. Many forms of culture. *Am Psychol.* 2009;64:194–204.
93. Tebes JK. Community psychology, diversity, and the many forms of culture. *Am Psychol.* 2010;65:58–59.
94. US Department of Health and Human Services, Office of Minority Health. *National Standards for Culturally and Linguistically Appropriate Services in Health and Health Care: A Blueprint for Advancing and*

Sustaining CLAS Policy and Practice. Rockville, MD: US Department of Health and Human Services; 2013. https://www.thinkculturalhealth.hhs.gov/Content/clas.asp. Accessed May 15, 2014.

95. Hodach R. *Accountable Care Organizations and Population Health Management: How Physician Practices Must Change to Effectively Manage Patient Populations*. American Medical Group Association. Phytel, Inc. 2011. http://www.amga.org/AboutAMGA/ACO/Articles/CaseStudy_final.pdf. Accessed May 15, 2014.

96. Maust DT, Oslin DW, Marcus SC. Mental health care in the accountable care organization. *Psychiatr Serv*. 2013;64(9):908–910. doi: 10.1176/appi.ps.201200330.

97. Berwick DM, Nolan TW, Whittington J. The triple aim: care, health, cost. *Health Aff*. 2008;27(3):759–769.

98. Katon W, Unutzer J. Consultation psychiatry in the medical home and accountable care organizations: achieving the triple aim. *Gen Hosp Psychiatry*. 2011;33(4):305–310.

99. Ward NL, Strambler MJ, Linke LH. Increasing educational attainment among urban minority youth: a model of university, school and community partnerships. *J Negro Ed*. 2013;82(3):312–325.

100. Tebes JK, Feinn R, Vanderploeg JJ, et al. Impact of a positive youth development program in urban after-school settings on the prevention of adolescent substance use. *J Adolesc Health*. 2007;41(3):239–247.

101. Sullivan TP. Think outside: advancing risk and protective factor research beyond the intimate-partner-violence box. *Psychol Violence*. 2013;3(2):121.

8.

THE INTERPLAY BETWEEN FORENSIC PSYCHIATRY AND PUBLIC PSYCHIATRY

Reena Kapoor, Susan Parke, Charles C. Dike, Paul Amble, Nancy Anderson, and Howard Zonana

> ### EDUCATIONAL HIGHLIGHTS
>
> - Forensic psychiatry and public psychiatry have become intertwined in the past 50 years because of important historical and legal factors, such as deinstitutionalization, mass incarceration, and changes in civil commitment criteria.
>
> - Due to the overcrowding of prisons and their inability to provide adequate psychiatric treatment, specialized mental health courts and jail diversion programs have been developed to reduce the number of persons with mental illness in correctional settings.
>
> - Community programs for forensic populations should provide individualized, recovery-oriented treatment that balances patient wishes with community safety.
>
> - Public psychiatric hospital beds are largely devoted to the management of forensic patients who often require specialized treatment and oversight by courts or quasi-judicial boards.
>
> - Because of the large proportion of forensic patients in public-sector treatment settings, all public psychiatrists should acquire some knowledge of forensic psychiatry, particularly in the areas of risk assessment and legal regulation of psychiatric practice.
>
> - Thorough risk management requires an understanding of actuarial (i.e., static) and dynamic risk factors for violence.
>
> - Forensic psychiatrists can play an important role in consulting with treatment teams about risk management. The consultation is most beneficial when teams formulate a specific question for the consultant and gather key information about the case beforehand.

INTRODUCTION

Forensic psychiatry and public-sector psychiatry were not always the intertwined specialties they are today. However, as the deinstitutionalization movement of the 1960s resulted in large-scale release of patients from state psychiatric hospitals into the community, forensic psychiatrists, with their specialized knowledge of risk assessment and legal regulation of psychiatric practice, became an essential part of public-sector mental health care. In inpatient settings, forensic psychiatrists served both as treatment providers and as risk consultants as the few remaining state psychiatric beds were largely devoted to treating forensic patients. In outpatient settings, community mental health centers were tasked with managing dangerous patients after release from long-stay forensic hospitals or prisons, and forensic expertise helped to guide treatment decisions. Furthermore, as prison populations swelled to massive proportions in the 1990s and 2000s, public sector and forensic psychiatrists joined forces with criminal justice agencies to create alternatives to incarceration for individuals with mental illness. The end result was that public psychiatry and forensic psychiatry became engaged in a long-term, multifaceted endeavor: managing persons with mental illness who exhibit dangerous behaviors or are involved with the criminal justice system.

This chapter traces the historical developments that have led to our current practice of integrating forensic and public-sector psychiatry, and it delineates the areas in which public-sector psychiatrists must acquire knowledge about forensic issues in order to practice effectively. First, we discuss the management of inpatient forensic units in state hospitals. Next, we discuss the growth of outpatient treatment programs for forensic patients, both as alternatives to incarceration and as after-care programs for individuals released from inpatient forensic units. We provide a conceptual framework for public-sector professionals interacting with the criminal justice system (court, probation, parole). Finally, we discuss violence risk assessment and management, focusing on the essential skills that public-sector psychiatrists should acquire, including when to ask for forensic and/or legal consultation.

HISTORICAL DEVELOPMENTS

In colonial times, jails, prisons, and homes were used to confine persons with mental illness. As early as 1694—long before asylums or large correctional institutions had been constructed—the Massachusetts Bay Colony passed a statute for the confinement of persons with mental illness, citing dangerousness as the major criterion for confinement.[1] A New York statute from 1790, with one section that addresses the "furiously mad," is another example of an early commitment statute[2]:

> And whereas there are sometimes persons, who by lunacy or otherwise, are furiously mad, or are so far disordered in their senses that they may be dangerous to be permitted to go abroad; Therefore, be it further enacted . . . That it shall and may be lawful for any two or more justices of the peace, where such lunatic or mad person shall be found, by warrant under their hands and seals, directed to the constables and overseers of the poor of the city or town, or some of them, to cause such person to be apprehended and kept safely locked up in some secure place within such city.

The terms "furiously mad" or "dangerous" were not defined, and justices of the peace were given broad powers to confine persons as they saw fit, including chaining them if necessary. The law also affirmed the appointment by the chancellor of guardians or family members to care for the ill person. In this era, confinement had little to do with treatment. No mention of physicians, as experts or custodians, was required. There were no explicit statutory time limits on the confinement, although some courts required judicial review after the initial confinement.[3]

The years between 1820 and 1970 saw the development of more humane prisons and mental health facilities in the United States. Psychiatric treatment centers that focused on moral treatment, such as the Friends Hospital in Philadelphia and the Hartford Retreat in Connecticut, began offering an alternative to the more austere confinement of the previous century. In 1841, Dorothea Dix began her crusade to move persons with mental illness out of jails and prisons into separate facilities where treatment could be provided. In 1881, Massachusetts gave legal recognition to the idea of voluntary admission to a mental health facility.[4] By 1924, 28 states had such laws.

Commitment laws in the first half of the 20th century were quite paternalistic, giving broad discretion to physicians. Connecticut enacted a typical law, which stated that involuntary confinement required the person to be mentally ill and a "fit subject for confinement."[5] By employing such flexible criteria, the legislature left most of the decision-making to physicians. However, by 1976, the "fit subject for confinement" criterion was replaced with a requirement to prove that the individual was either dangerous or gravely disabled. Greater procedural due process rights were also afforded to individuals facing involuntary commitment.

Stricter criteria for hospitalization, combined with President Kennedy's Community Mental Health Act of 1963, dramatically reduced the population of psychiatric hospitals. By the early 1970s, the state hospital population dropped to less than half of what it was in the 1950s. During the same time period, the prison population began to rise, leading some scholars to postulate that individuals with mental illness were being "transinstitutionalized" from mental health facilities into correctional settings.[6] This trend became clearer in the decades that followed, as prison populations continued to rise and psychiatric hospital beds fell to unprecedented levels.

Figure 8.1 depicts the phenomenon of transinstitutionalization, tracking prison and state hospital populations during the 1930s to 2000s.[7] In this study, Harcourt concluded that overall rates of institutionalization were the

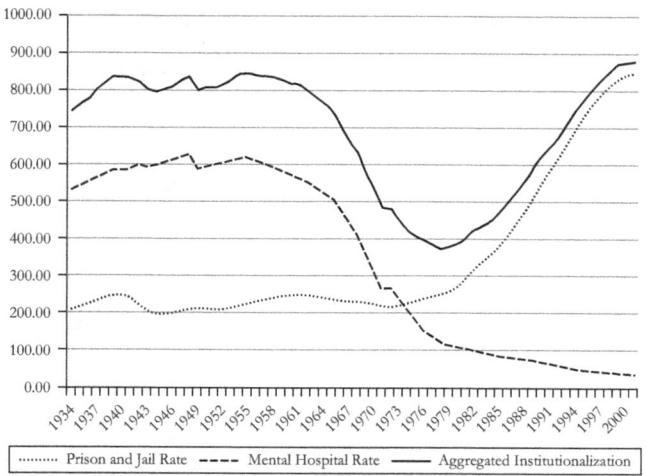

Figure 8.1 Rates of institutionalization, including jails, in the United States (per 100,000 adults), 1934-2001

same in 2001 as in the 1950s, but many more persons were in prison or jail than in hospitals.

Since 2001, the prison population has continued to grow, with the number of inmates rising from 200,000 in 1973 to more than 2 million in 2008 (approximately 1% of the US adult population). A large portion of the prison population now has symptoms of serious mental illness. Although exact numbers are difficult to calculate, in 2012, there were estimated to be more than 356,000 inmates with severe mental illness (SMI) in prisons and jails. By contrast, there were 35,000 patients with SMI in state psychiatric systems. Thus, the number of mentally ill in jails and prisons was 10 times the number remaining in state hospitals.[8]

Mass incarceration in the United States has become a hot topic of political and economic concern, in part because of the disproportionate numbers of persons with mental illness who are incarcerated. By some estimates, the Los Angeles County Jail, Rikers Island Jail in New York City, and the Cook County Jail in Chicago are now the largest mental health treatment facilities in the United States.[9] Correctional facilities are not the ideal placement for persons with mental illness. Even the US Supreme Court agreed with this position in 2011, ruling that the California prison system must reduce its population significantly in order to provide necessary mental health and medical treatment for its inmate population.[10] Many other states have also become involved in large-scale efforts to divert people out of correctional facilities and into settings more suitable for mental health treatment. These programs are discussed in the following section.

DEVELOPMENT OF ALTERNATIVES TO INCARCERATION FOR PERSONS WITH MENTAL ILLNESS

Forced to contend with a dwindling number of psychiatric inpatient beds and massive prison overcrowding, states began to look for alternative ways to manage persons with mental illness who were involved with the criminal justice system. Beginning in the 1990s, jail diversion programs gained popularity, with the goal of identifying individuals with mental illness and offering them treatment rather than punishment. Two models were initially developed: those involving specialty "mental health courts" and those in which diversion efforts occurred in "regular" criminal courts.[11] The two models used slightly different procedures to accomplish the same objective. In nonspecialty court programs, mental health clinicians were situated in the criminal courthouse and worked with patients and court personnel (prosecutors, defense attorneys, and judges) to arrange treatment programs as alternatives to incarceration. In mental health courts, a completely separate court system—one with a more therapeutic focus—was created for individuals with mental illness, in the hope of developing a system with specialized expertise.

A typical individual involved in these programs is exemplified by Mr. A:

> Mr. A had a long history of panhandling and loitering outside the local donut shop. Though he had been diagnosed with schizophrenia as a teenager, he did not believe he had a mental illness and did not take medication. He frequently used crack cocaine and drank to excess. He was homeless, alternating between local shelters and sleeping on a park bench in the town square. He was well known to law enforcement officers, who frequently responded to complaints from the donut shop owners, who reported that he harassed customers and negatively affected their business. Police offers had taken Mr. A to the emergency room for psychiatric evaluation several times, but he was released because he was not thought to be dangerous or gravely disabled. The fourth time that officers were called to the donut shop to respond to complaints about Mr. A, they arrested him and charged him with breach of peace, public intoxication, and criminal trespassing. When he arrived at the courthouse for arraignment, he was considered a candidate for jail diversion. If he agreed, he was allowed to participate in a community treatment program rather than go to jail.

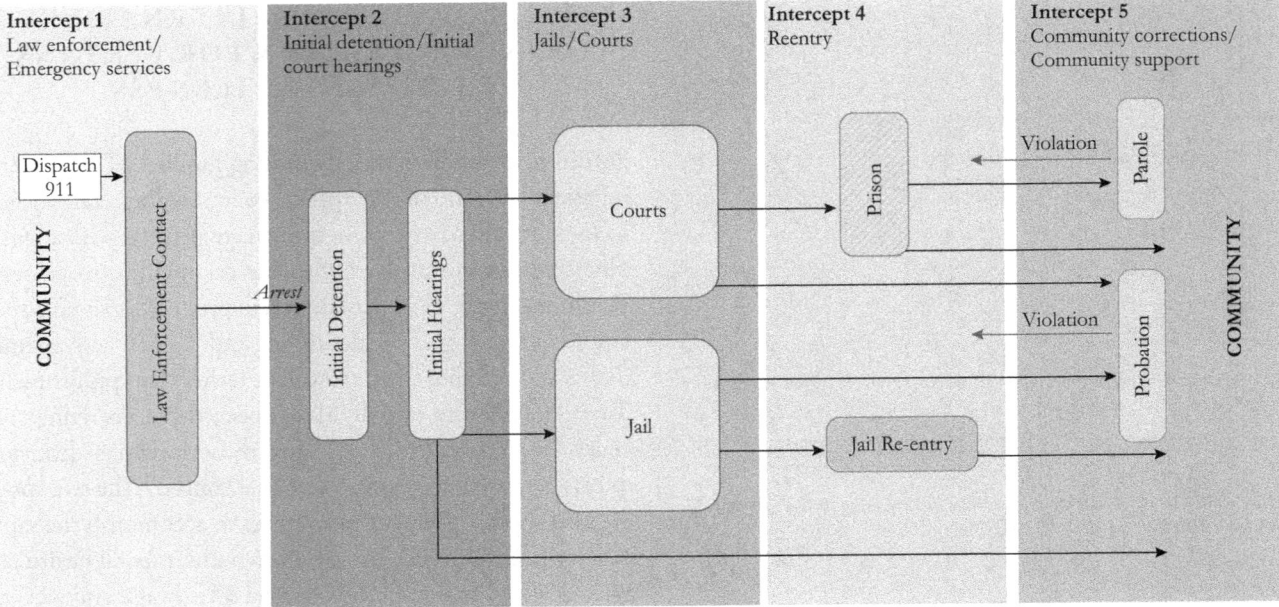

Figure 8.2 Sequential Intercept Model[16]

Early data from jail diversion programs and mental health courts were promising. Programs consistently demonstrated a reduction in jail days for persons with mental illness, and most programs showed a high retention rate in mental health treatment after 1 year. Equally compelling were the data that showed no adverse effect on public safety as a result of diversion, even for individuals with significant histories of violence.[12,13] Cost savings were also substantial. Although difficult to calculate because of the many indirect savings from jail diversion, programs were able to successfully demonstrate savings from reduced arrest/booking costs, jail days, court costs, and emergency room visits.[14] As a result, jail diversion programs and specialty courts expanded rapidly. By 2007, more than 500 jail diversion programs had been developed around the country.[11]

Efforts to divert persons with mental illness from the criminal justice system at other junctures—for example, pre-booking or post-incarceration—also flourished. Police officers received crisis intervention training to identify signs of mental illness and divert individuals to treatment instead of arresting them.[15] In addition, community reentry programs were developed for individuals with mental illness who were released after long incarcerations, with the aim of providing support and increasing their chances for successful community reintegration. Together with traditional jail diversion programs, these additional efforts make up the Sequential Intercept Model of criminal justice diversion[16] depicted in Figure 8.2.

Today, community mental health centers are common treatment settings for individuals diverted from the criminal justice system. In addition to traditional psychiatric treatment—therapy and medication—the mental health centers offer robust ancillary services, such as case management, housing, and vocational support. The nature and intensity of these services varies greatly due to patients' needs and available resources. However, most models of caring for forensic patients are based on an interdisciplinary team approach involving collaboration among physicians, other mental health clinicians, case managers, and court officers.

COMMUNITY FORENSIC TREATMENT

MODELS OF COMMUNITY FORENSIC TREATMENT

Several collaborative models of outpatient care for individuals with serious mental illness and criminal justice involvement have been developed. One of the most prevalent of these models is Forensic Assertive Community Treatment (FACT). FACT teams provide the same level of care as traditional Assertive Community Treatment (ACT) teams, but differ in a few ways. FACT programs typically have (1) enrollees with criminal justice involvement, (2) referrals primarily from a criminal justice agency, and (3) a close partnership with a criminal justice agency.[17] Although initially promising, longer-term outcomes of FACT teams have yet to be evaluated. A few studies have attempted to evaluate FACT outcomes, but methodological limitations make it difficult to draw conclusions from the data.[18] FACT programs are widely employed, but their evidence base lags far behind the pace of implementation.

Mandated outpatient treatment, sometimes referred to as "outpatient civil commitment," has also been used to manage psychiatric patients with the aim of reducing arrests, incarcerations, and psychiatric hospitalizations. As with FACT programs, data regarding outpatient commitment are mixed. The American Psychiatric Association cautiously endorsed the idea in a 1999 resource document,[19] but studies since then have indicated that the programs are not as effective in producing outpatient compliance as anticipated.[20] Some scholars now believe that the main benefit from outpatient commitment comes not from the threat of legal sanctions, but rather from the coordinated and intensive treatment efforts being provided to the committed individuals.

GOALS AND KEY FEATURES OF COMMUNITY FORENSIC TREATMENT PROGRAMS

Community treatment providers help forensic patients with serious mental illnesses and substantial violence risk to live safely in the community. The primary goal is to improve the health of the patient, but clinicians must also be mindful of additional treatment goals related to the criminal justice system:

- Reducing recidivism and rearrest
- Compliance with criminal justice mandates (i.e., probation or parole stipulations)
- Maintaining community safety

All community forensic treatment programs have several features in common. Their focus on a multidisciplinary approach involving psychotherapy, medication, case management, housing and vocational supports, and (often) legal oversight is essential for providing adequate care to this high-risk population. Many forensic programs also include:

- "In-reach" into prisons and secure hospitals, so that clinicians and patients can begin working together months (or even years) prior to community placement
- Access to varying levels of psychiatric care, from residential dual-diagnosis units to day hospitals to emergency and inpatient services
- Housing programs, because finding adequate housing can be challenging with this population, particularly for sex offenders and others with residency restrictions
- Vocational programs, because jobs are very difficult to find for those who are doubly stigmatized by a criminal record and mental illness
- Focus on risk assessment and management, with available consultation from forensic psychiatrists and/or hospital legal representatives
- Focus on staff wellness, because clinician burnout can be heightened when working with forensic patients
- Interventions to address criminogenic needs, in addition to mental health needs, because untreated mental illness is not the only cause of criminal recidivism
- Regular communication between the multiple agencies involved in different aspects of care in order to coordinate treatment efforts

When implemented correctly, community forensics programs can provide excellent, recovery-oriented mental health care to a majority of patients. However, forensic patients pose many unique clinical and administrative challenges, and the course of treatment is not always smooth.

CLINICAL CHALLENGES IN COMMUNITY TREATMENT OF FORENSIC POPULATIONS

At the outset, deciding which patients should be treated in an outpatient forensics program can be challenging because most patients in public-sector settings have at least one risk factor for violence. When screening patients for forensic diversion or re-entry programs, a diagnosis of SMI is required. However, some diagnoses—borderline personality disorder, developmental disabilities, impulse control disorders—fall into a "gray zone" of seriousness, and programs are left to make clinical judgments about whether the patient fits into the proposed treatment scheme. Depending on the availability of treatment services, the patient's level of interest, and the severity of presenting symptoms, such patients may be accepted into community forensic treatment.

Community forensic programs were originally expected to treat patients with SMI who had been arrested for relatively minor crimes. Initially, the programs did not accept patients with histories of violent crimes, sex offenses, or serious weapons charges. However, as the programs have gained experience, they have slowly expanded to serve patients with sex offenses, histories of serious assault and homicide convictions, and patients found not guilty by reason of insanity (NGRI). These patients return to the community after years of incarceration or psychiatric hospitalization, and they require a high level of monitoring and risk management, as well as additional clinical skills to provide adequate treatment.

When engaging forensic patients, risk-based and avoidance-oriented criminal justice approaches are not enough. Approaches such as the Good Lives Model (GLM) of Offender Rehabilitation,[21] a strengths-based rehabilitation model, have focused instead on building capacities and strengths in order to reduce the risk of reoffending. GLM is responsive to individuals' particular interests, abilities, and aspirations, working toward their personal goals without harming others.

Substance use is a major risk factor and treatment challenge for this population. Criminal justice agencies require abstinence to comply with legal stipulations, but many patients continue to use substances. Incarceration is usually not an option, nor does it provide the necessary treatment for substance use disorders. Forensic patients are often referred to intensive substance abuse programs for treatment, but many of them are excluded because of severe mental illness symptoms or a prolonged period of abstinence during incarceration.

Last, as community forensic programs mature, many of the patients progress in their lives and begin to take an interest in school, work, and romantic relationships. Clinicians embrace recovery-oriented care when approaching these issues, but sometimes the patient's multiple treatment goals conflict with one another. For example, a patient with a history of sexual violence involving teenagers may wish to attend high school or college classes after incarceration, and the patient's interests in getting an education must be weighed against the potential risk posed to the community. Interdisciplinary team meetings, both with and without the patient present, are often helpful in sorting through these difficult decisions.

ROLE OF PUBLIC SECTOR PSYCHIATRISTS IN COMMUNITY FORENSIC TREATMENT

Public-sector psychiatrists are involved in all aspects of recovery-oriented outpatient treatment. They join discussions about potential new referrals, reviewing prior risk assessments and consulting regarding plans for community services. When new patients are admitted, psychiatrists collaborate in comprehensive clinical assessments, interviewing patients, evaluating risk, formulating diagnostic impressions, and developing treatment plans in conjunction with patients and community providers. Psychiatrists review records of previous treatment in the community, hospitals, or correctional settings. They routinely contact providers and family members, seeking clarification of behaviors, symptoms, and efficacy of medication regimens. Forensic patients have often been treated in multiple settings in a disjointed manner, with multiple medications and diagnoses, so this type of information gathering is essential to creating a comprehensive treatment plan.

As with all complex patients, prescribing psychotropic medication for the forensic population requires close collaboration with clinicians, residential program staff, visiting nurse agencies, pharmacies, and insurance providers. Forensic patients are often mandated to comply with mental health treatment, including medication, but in most cases they cannot be forcibly medicated as outpatients. Because of this unenforceable mandate, psychiatrists must develop skills to address patients' concerns about their medications while holding a firm line about complying with recommended treatment. Discussing the consequences of medication noncompliance, including the possibility of rearrest or probation violation, is a frequent part of clinical interactions between psychiatrists and forensic patients.

Additionally, psychiatrists collaborate with medical providers to manage comorbid medical illnesses, which are frequently undiagnosed or untreated in forensic populations. An estimated 39–43% of persons returning to the community after incarceration have at least one chronic medical condition.[22] Common conditions in forensic populations include diabetes, hypertension, obesity, hepatitis, HIV, cancer, and dementia. Untreated medical illness is both a risk factor for premature death and for criminal recidivism[23] in forensic populations, so managing medical conditions is an essential part of a community treatment plan. Few patients have family or other natural supports, and they are often dependent on program staff to help them with these problems.

Psychiatrists participate in ongoing risk assessment and crisis intervention, both in the clinic and community settings. This is done in conjunction with clinicians, residential case managers, diversion program staff, and police (when indicated). Regular interagency meetings with community partners establish a collaborative working relationship and afford an opportunity to plan for crises. In addition, psychiatrists can educate and consult with the community case managers and other staff about working with high-risk individuals whose behaviors can evoke strong feelings in the staff that must be managed in order to provide adequate care.

Most importantly, community psychiatrists are clinicians, engaging and accepting people with SMIs who have committed serious crimes. They join professionals of other disciplines in treating these individuals, supporting their aspirations while helping them comply with criminal justice stipulations. Limiting the role of the psychiatrist to that of "prescriber," as has become increasingly common in outpatient clinics across the country, simply does not work when treating this high-risk, forensic population. The psychiatrist must take a more expansive role in the multidisciplinary team, including psychotherapy, risk management, and consultation and supervision of other mental health professionals.

COLLABORATING WITH COURTS, PROBATION, AND PAROLE

One of the most challenging aspects of community forensic treatment is managing the relationship between treatment providers and those involved in criminal justice oversight—police, probation, and parole officers. There are many reasons why so many individuals with mental illness find themselves on probation or parole. For some—typically those who have repeatedly committed "nuisance" crimes related to symptoms of mental illness—probation is used as a method of monitoring and encouraging compliance with mental health treatment. For others, probation and parole provide necessary oversight during the high-risk period following long incarcerations for serious violent crimes. In some states, particular crimes or legal designations, such as being a registered sex offender or a Sexually Violent Predator, are accompanied by long periods of probation and other restrictions (e.g., electronic GPS monitoring, residency and work restrictions). Thus, forensic patients are very likely to interact with probation or parole officers at some time, and community mental health clinicians must develop strategies to work collaboratively with these agencies.

A key aspect of the relationship between clinicians and probation officers is the management of patient confidentiality. Mental health treatment is typically confidential, but forensic patients are often mandated to waive the psychotherapist–patient privilege so that clinicians may communicate with the probation officer. The nature and extent of such disclosures may vary from state to state, but communicating with the patient about the limits of confidentiality is always advisable. In some states, the patient also has to waive the privilege against self-incrimination,[24] and, in those cases, it is absolutely critical for clinicians to inform patients that their statements in treatment may be disclosed to criminal justice agencies. For example, many programs for the treatment of sex offenders require that patients "take accountability" for all prior crimes. If the crimes involve prior child abuse, mandated reporting statutes may force clinicians to disclose the information to the state's child protection agency. In addition, many states also require patients to submit to polygraph tests as part of sex offender treatment programs, with the consequences of revealing information about current or past crimes governed by statute or case law. All of these exceptions to confidentiality can be confusing and frustrating to both clinicians and patients. However, in cases where mandatory disclosure statutes have been challenged as unconstitutional, courts have largely decided not to support rights to protect sex offenders' confidentiality rights because they are not viewed as a sympathetic group.[25]

In general, probation and parole officers are not considered part of the clinical treatment team, and discretion should be used in deciding how much information to disclose to them. Some probation officers are interested in bare-bones reports, requesting information only about whether the patient is in "good standing" at the treatment program. Others, however, request detailed information about medication doses, urine toxicology results, diagnoses, and treatment plans. Clinicians can weigh the risks and benefits of disclosing information on a case-by-case basis, but, given how frequently they occur, it is also prudent for mental health centers to develop institutional policies around these issues. Consultation with the Attorney General's office may be helpful for state-run institutions, and hospital attorneys can consult with private mental health centers. Forensically trained clinicians may also be helpful in developing institutional policies that aim to protect patient–clinician confidentiality as much as possible.

FORENSIC INPATIENT UNITS

Despite the large-scale movement of most persons with mental illness out of inpatient settings in the past 50 years, state psychiatric hospitals are still necessary to treat certain groups, such as insanity acquittees and those found incompetent to stand trial. Forensic hospital facilities usually comprise maximum-security units, medium- or enhanced-security units, and more secure "regular" inpatient psychiatric units. What they all have in common is an increased attention to safety and security, with the maximum-security facilities being the most restrictive and secure. In a maximum-security hospital, agency security/police officers closely monitor what patients, families, and staff bring into the facility. Security officers prohibit materials considered potentially dangerous, and they also monitor all visits—professional, social, or family.

Patients admitted into forensic psychiatric hospitals generally fall into four broad categories: those admitted for competency to stand trial-related issues (evaluation and restoration of competency), those found NGRI, transfers from the Department of Correction (DOC) for evaluation or treatment, and civil patients too dangerous to be managed in less restrictive settings. Most patients who are admitted for competency to stand trial-related issues come to the hospital for restoration to competency after the court has found them incompetent to stand trial. However, in some states, patients are also sent to forensic psychiatric hospitals for an evaluation of their competency to stand trial and restorability prior to any judicial determination. Competency restoration patients mostly come directly from correctional settings, but a small number comes from the community (those who were released on bond). Patients typically arrive at the hospital directly from court, usually after regular business hours and without any clinical information about their diagnosis or treatment in DOC. This poses a significant clinical challenge for the hospital staff because patients sometimes present with medical or psychiatric problems that require urgent attention, and the staff has insufficient information to manage the crisis.

Convicted prisoners who are transferred from DOC for evaluation or treatment of conditions that cannot be managed in the correctional setting also pose unique challenges to the hospital staff. These patients often exhibit a mixture of antisocial traits and symptoms consistent with traditional ideas of mental illness, such as psychosis or self-injury. They are at high risk of engaging in violent behavior, intimidation, and exploitation of other patients on the unit,[26] and they pose a high elopement risk. As a result, many state hospital systems are reticent to accept patient transfers from prisons into their "regular" forensic units. Some states have constructed specialized units just for prisoners because they are better able to meet these patients' needs without compromising the care of others.

A third category of forensic inpatients includes those who have been civilly committed but are too dangerous to manage in nonsecure units. Although placement of civil patients in maximum-security settings is fraught with intense scrutiny from legal and civil liberties advocates, the level of dangerousness they present sometimes makes it necessary. In such situations, strenuous effort is made to transfer patients to a less restrictive setting as soon as the level of dangerousness abates. Managing civil patients in a maximum-security forensic unit is doubly stigmatizing and makes discharge from the facility much more difficult because community providers look unfavorably upon patients with a history of maximum-security admission. Even if they present with minor symptoms in the future, they have been "marked" as too dangerous for nonforensic providers to handle.

A special group of civil patients in forensic units are DOC transfers at the end of sentence—inmates considered too ill and dangerous to be released into the community after serving a criminal sentence. In states with sexual violent predator statutes, these patients are often convicted sex offenders who have been designated Sexually Violent Predators just prior to completion of the criminal sentence. When admitted to forensic hospital units, they typically do not fit the mold of the typical psychiatric patient. For example, Sexually Violent Predator patients are more likely to be diagnosed with paraphilias and antisocial personality disorder than with psychotic or mood disorders,[27] and treatments available at the hospital may not apply to them. In addition, discharge planning is often very complicated, given the patients' serious violence histories and the reluctance of community agencies to accept them.

Forensic hospitals struggle with discharge planning for all patients, not just sex offenders. Patients can be discharged from any forensic inpatient setting, but those in maximum-security settings are usually stepped down to a less secure environment to ensure that they sustain their improvement before discharge to the community. For NGRI patients (discussed in more detail in the next section), transition back into the community is a gradual, careful, and prolonged process with incremental increases in privileges. As the patients continue to demonstrate safety and stability in the community, they have overnight leaves from the hospital, sometimes up to 7 days a week, before being conditionally released into the community.

Forensic psychiatric hospitals play a vital role in the continuum of public sector forensic services because they carry out the dual functions of treating acutely ill and often dangerous patients while also maintaining public safety. Forensic hospitals must contend with the demands of the patient, the patient's attorney, civil liberties advocates, other interested parties, and heightened public scrutiny. Navigating these dual roles (patient interest vs. public safety concerns) is a daily challenge confronting forensic mental health practitioners, and the hospitals must necessarily strike a balance between treatment and safety/security concerns.

UNIQUE OVERSIGHT OF FORENSIC PATIENTS

A large proportion of the remaining inpatient psychiatric beds in state hospitals are devoted to managing forensic populations, including individuals found NGRI of violent crimes. Pressure to discharge these patients into the community is no less than with civil patients, but this pressure must be balanced against public safety concerns. In an effort to address this tension, some states have created psychiatric security review boards (PSRBs) or similar administrative bodies to oversee the management of insanity acquittees. These boards play an integral role in all aspects of the patient's care, from initial hospital commitment to community release (typically to public-sector mental health agencies). Therefore, an understanding of their development and functioning can be helpful to psychiatrists in all public-sector settings.

The insanity defense remains an area of controversy and tension between the law and mental health. Historically, individuals involved in crimes and found NGRI were committed to institutions for the "criminally insane" with little oversight or special attention, but this began to change in the early 1970s as commitment procedures and treatment provided to acquittees came under scrutiny.[28] In 1977, the Oregon PSRB was formed. Oregon Circuit Court Judge John C. Beatty commented on the driving forces behind the board's creation[29]:

> Under the then existing law, an offender found not guilty for a crime by reason of mental disease or defect (NGI) could be committed to the Oregon State Hospital if the trial judge found him a danger to himself or others by reason of the disease or defect. At the hospital the offender was medicated until the doctors felt he was harmless and then was discharged as no longer a threat.
>
> Jurisdiction of the court terminated with the release of the offender by the hospital. Such persons, once discharged, rarely continued their medication and soon became as disturbed as they were before hospitalization. Not infrequently, they again committed serious crimes against other persons.

Following the 1982 verdict in the case of John Hinckley (who attempted the assassination of President Reagan), the American Psychiatric Association recognized PSRBs as a possible model for the management and treatment of NGRI acquittee patients.[30] Connecticut followed suit, establishing its PSRB in 1985.[31] Utah passed analogous legislation in 1989,[32] and Arizona established its PSRB in 1994.[33] These states have what has been termed "external" review boards in that they have statutory authority over NGRI acquittees with regard to their release to the community, the monitoring of conditional releases (i.e., monitored treatment in the community), and, if necessary, the revocation of releases. However, other states, such as Maryland, have established what have been referred to as "internal" review boards, with the intent to "continue judicial decision-making regarding release and revocation but seek improvement in the forensic hospital system's performance in generating recommendations to the courts."[34]

Oregon's PSRB has been written about most extensively, followed by Connecticut's PSRB, which is similarly structured. Both states' boards are made up of members appointed by their respective governors and confirmed by their legislative branches, such as an attorney, a psychiatrist, a psychologist, an individual knowledgeable about probation and parole, and lay citizens.[35,36] In addition, Connecticut's Board includes a lay citizen with victim advocacy experience.[36] Connecticut's Superior Court is responsible for committing acquittees to the Board for a specific length of time related to the sentence that might have been imposed if criminally convicted, which in turn mandates the appropriate level of supervision. The Board also recommends the treatment conditions under which an acquittee may return to the community and advises the Superior Court as to whom it deems as meeting criteria for continued commitment versus discharge from the Board.[36]

The US Supreme Court held in *Jackson v. Indiana*[37] that "due process requires that the nature and duration of commitment bear some reasonable relation to the purpose for which the individual is committed." In *Jones v. US*,[38] the US Supreme Court held that states have the right to commit a person found NGRI for an indefinite period as long as the individual remains mentally ill and dangerous. In both Oregon and Connecticut, in order for insanity acquittees to remain under the Board's jurisdiction, they must continue to be a danger to self or others because of a psychiatric disability.[39,40] In Oregon, once the maximum time that could have been served had there been a conviction is reached, the individual must either be discharged or civilly committed. However, in Connecticut, if "reasonable cause exists to believe that the acquittee remains a person with psychiatric disabilities or a person with intellectual disability to the extent that his discharge at the expiration of his maximum term of commitment would constitute a danger to himself or others, the state's attorney can petition the court for an extended commitment" under the Board.[40]

There has been some pushback and debate about how security-conscious PSRBs should be in their commitment of insanity acquittees and how much power they should possess, specifically regarding their ability to recommit end-of-term acquittees past the maximum time that could have been served had they been found guilty of the involved offense.[41] *Olmstead v. L. C. by Zimring*,[42] a US Supreme

Court case dealing with institutionalized disabled persons and the need to offer community-based treatment programs for those who qualified, has been applied to how long and where insanity acquittee patients are held and treated. It becomes a collaborative process between the hospital staff and outpatient providers to devise a treatment plan that maximizes patients' chances of remaining safe and out of the hospital, although with PSRB oversight.

Once it is recommended that NGRI patients transition back into the community, as noted earlier, the process is gradual, beginning with temporary leaves from the hospital of a few hours and progressing to include overnight leaves. During this process, acquittees begin to engage with community providers. At the point where it is determined that an acquittee patient is ready for conditional release to the community, their care is transferred to community providers who agree to follow the patient's individualized conditional release plan, which can include such provisions as continued treatment of sexual and substance abuse disorders. In addition, the provider agrees to periodically report to the PSRB regarding treatment progress and any changes in the acquittee patient's mental condition. Finding willing and qualified treatment providers can be difficult because there is often a reluctance to take these patients into treatment. Oregon provided state funding for such treatment, but Connecticut did not, forcing state facilities to provide treatment rather than the private sector. Also, in addition to providing treatment, community providers are mandated to supervise the acquittee and report any violations of release conditions. As with patients on probation, this mandate can create a difficult treatment relationship. For example, the provider maybe involved with visits to the patient's residence and be called to report violations such as finding a can of beer in the patient's refrigerator. Again, as noted earlier, the PSRB continues to closely monitor the treatment and supervision of these patients, just as it did when they were maintained in a hospital setting. At any point, the PSRB may remand the patient back to the hospital for re-evaluation if they are deemed nonadherent to the specified conditions of their conditional release plan.

Because the PSRB's prime objective is protecting the public from dangerous insanity defense acquittees, conditional release plans are often quite restrictive and conservative. In relation to the Oregon PSRB, some opined that it was risk-adverse in the management of insanity defense acquittees.[43] In response to this concern, the PSRB recently underwent a restructuring to limit its scope and power, and the insanity defense is open only to those facing felony charges or those already hospitalized insanity acquittees who have committed serious crimes.[43]

Attempting to balance the rights and treatment of individual insanity acquittee patients against the equally important task of protecting the public is difficult. Mental health professionals are mandated to maintain safety in the least restrictive treatment settings available[44] and to do so by making predictions regarding someone's future dangerousness. This task is challenging and sometimes unsuccessful,[45] but mental health professionals are currently obligated to perform it to the best of their abilities.

VIOLENCE RISK ASSESSMENT AND MANAGEMENT OF FORENSIC PATIENTS

Potentially dangerous patients are found in all public-sector treatment settings, and clinicians often struggle with how best to manage them. Forensic psychiatrists can play an important role in consulting with clinicians working with patients who are at a heightened risk for committing dangerous acts and providing education about risk management. These consultations can take many forms: regular risk management meetings, informal consultations on an as-needed basis, didactic sessions, and formal consultations with written reports. Regardless of the format, the goal is to enhance the capability of all clinicians in the mental health system to assess and manage patients at high risk for violence.

Since its inception, the field of violence risk assessment has undergone several important advancements. In *Barefoot v. Estelle*,[46] a landmark US Supreme Court case, the American Psychiatric Association wrote an amicus brief noting that psychiatrists were not particularly skilled at identifying those at risk for violence and cited that, using clinical judgment alone, psychiatrists were wrong about predictions of risk in two out of three cases. Following this decision, psychiatrists and psychologists dedicated themselves to improving the science of risk assessment. Many new tools were developed, and these are discussed herein.

ACTUARIAL TOOLS

Actuarial instruments were created to assist clinicians by identifying patients who are at high risk for committing violent acts, both physical and sexual. These instruments typically use *static factors* alone, historical information that shows little to no change over time, such as whether an adult being assessed experienced behavioral problems as an adolescent. In an attempt to find variables that both predict risk and are amenable to change through treatment, researchers have recently focused on the inclusion of *dynamic factors* into actuarial tools. Dynamic factors are those that show a greater degree of change over time, such as impulsiveness or a negative mood. To date, however, studies have not validated a dynamic variable that is correlated to a parallel change in risk with a degree of sensitivity and sensitivity that is clinically useful.[47]

Examples of static risk assessment tools are the Rapid Risk Assessment for Sex Offense Recidivism (RRASOR)[48] and Violence Risk Assessment Guide (VRAG).[49] The RRASOR asks four questions and then estimates the likelihood of a reconviction for a sexual offense over a 5- and 10-year time frame. The VRAG is a more complicated instrument that requires a detailed review of the subject's history and also incorporates scores from another actuarial instrument, the Psychopathy Checklist-Revised (PCL-R), which uses some dynamic factors and is discussed later in this section. The score from the VRAG then estimates the probability of violent recidivism at 7- and 10-year intervals.

Actuarial tools have both inherent benefits and fundamental flaws when used in clinical practice. The principal benefit is that the examiner is often required to collect detailed information on the subject's past criminal conduct and psychiatric history. This helps the examiner better understand the subject of his or her assessment, which should inevitably enhance the management of risk. These tools may also be useful for courts when considering the potential for future long-term risk to the community and in research when evaluating large populations.

However, risk predictions from actuarial tools are often not useful in clinical situations where immediate decisions are demanded. By their nature, actuarial risk assessment tools derive their data by collecting information from large groups of people. These large groups are then subdivided based on a correlation between demographic factors and criminal recidivism. For example, the VRAG has nine separate subdivisions. The evaluator who completes the tool is essentially determining into what subset the subject of his or her assessment most closely fits. By doing this, there is a potential for inaccuracy due to the study group having significant differences from the individual being assessed, such as cultural differences or the person's placement in a highly restrictive setting that lessens his likelihood of offending.

Further limitations of actuarial tools come from the nonspecific predictions of recidivism. For example, you may evaluate a patient using the VRAG and determine that the individual receives a score consistent with a probability of violent recidivism at 7 years of 44% and at 10 years of 58%. This test does not tell you whether the individual falls within the 56% of individuals who, in 7 years, will not have committed a violent crime. Furthermore, if the subject of your evaluation happens to fall in the violent 44%, this instrument will not tell you anything about who will be the subject of violence, the degree of violence, or exactly when during that 7-year time frame the violent act will be committed. Based on these limitations, there is little practical information available to psychiatrists trying to determine whether this individual should be admitted to the hospital or released into the community.

From a research perspective, there are high hurdles to overcome when developing an actuarial tool. What clinicians primarily seek from an actuarial tool is the ability to predict when a highly violent event will occur, such as a sexual assault, murder, or suicide. These are very low-frequency events, termed *low base rate* events, in the general population, and they therefore either require a very large study group for a prospective analysis or the selection of a targeted sample, such as a prison population, for a retrospective analysis. Unfortunately, retrospective analyses tend to bias findings, and the use of such information to predict future behaviors in the general population is often inaccurate.

Another hurdle in predicting behaviors that have a low base rate involves specificity and sensitivity. Finding a tool that has both a high true-positive rate (specificity) and a high true-negative rate (sensitivity) is mathematically daunting. Szmukler of King's College London[50] points out how low base rates sap the accuracy of tools to predict violent behaviors. Using a hypothetical tool that has a sensitivity and specificity of 0.7 and 0.7, which is considered high, he calculates that with a 20% base rate for the criminal conduct being predicted, the tool would be wrong 6 out of 10 times. For highly violent crimes or acts where the base rate is 1% (which is itself a high estimate), the "positive predictive value" of this same test drops to 0.03, meaning that the tool would predict wrongly 97 times out of 100.

PSYCHOPATHY

Another tool used in the consideration of risk is the PCL-R[51] developed by Robert Hare. This tool attempts to categorize elements in an individual's personality consistent with psychopathy. Although psychopathy is not a personality disorder defined in the *Diagnostic and Statistical Manual of Mental Disorders* (DSM 5), this term is often discussed in the context of risk assessments. Patrick[52] writes about the personality of an individual with psychopathy as including varying degrees of meanness, disinhibition, and boldness. Alternatively, Hare[53] describes psychopaths as "social predators who charm, manipulate, and ruthlessly plow their way through life, leaving a broad trail of broken hearts, shattered expectations, and empty wallets."

The PCL-R is a tool that looks at both static and dynamic factors in an individual and determines the relative level of psychopathy compared to control groups. The instrument has been widely studied and validated for correctional inmates, patients in forensic hospital settings, juveniles at community detention facilities, and sex offenders.[54] The PCL-R has long been considered the gold standard[55] when evaluating an individual for psychopathy. The administration of this assessment tool must be performed by a trained and qualified clinician and involves a review of an individual's past criminal conduct including police reports, an interview with a collateral source such as a family member who knows the subject well, and a semi-structured interview with the subject of evaluation.

After completing this extensive evaluation, the clinician then sums totals from 20 different factors, with responses ranging from 0 to 2. These factors assess interpersonal, affective, lifestyle, and antisocial traits possessed by the subject. If the individual scores 30 or higher, he or she is considered to meet criteria established for psychopathy. Scores on the PCL-R do not directly calculate criminal recidivism rates. The effect of this assessment is essentially to give clinicians an indication of their patient's tendency to display traits of psychopathy, which is itself a risk factor for violence. The score from the PCL-R alone is not a sufficient basis to make a determination as to whether an individual should be hospitalized or can be safely released to the community.

CORRELATION BETWEEN MENTAL ILLNESS AND VIOLENCE

Many dozens of studies have now been performed to correlate mental health and demographic factors with violence risk. Many, but not all, studies show a higher rate of violent behavior among individuals with SMI. However, when individuals with SMI are compared with others in their community, rather than with the population as a whole, the relative rates of violence show much less of a difference. Based on the current research, the following conclusions can reasonably be drawn about the correlates for violence[56]:

- Substance abuse, both alone and in combination with a mental disorder, is consistently correlated with violence.
- Sociodemographic factors (male gender, young age, low educational level, and low socioeconomic status) are strongly correlated with violence.
- Mental disorders are moderately correlated with violence but less so than either substance abuse or sociodemographic factors.
- Medication compliance in persons with SMI correlates with decreased rates of violence compared to those who are not compliant.[57]

In general, substance abuse and sociodemographic factors are more strongly predictive of violence than is mental illness. In one major study, the added risk of violence from psychosis was small; close family members and friends were the most frequent targets of violence.[57] Despite widespread media portrayals, persons with SMI are not likely to target strangers in public, and they are much more likely to be victims of violence than perpetrators.[11]

RESEARCH-INFORMED CLINICAL RISK ASSESSMENT

Clinical assessment, informed by evidence-based violence risk factors (outlined later), is the technique most utilized by psychiatrists to make decisions about dangerousness. In this approach, the clinician applies his or her knowledge of the literature and assessment skills to determine risk in a particular patient. Although this method, termed *research-informed clinical risk assessment*, does not have superior statistical accuracy to actuarial tools, the technique remains helpful to clinicians because these assessments focus directly on the patient's clinical need and treatment plan. Conclusions in these evaluations typically categorize individuals into ranges of risk, such as high, moderate, or low. Such evaluations give clinicians a reasoned basis for their clinical conclusions and justifications for interventions such as involuntary hospitalization. Several studies have shown greater-than-chance validity for clinically based risk assessments.[58] When employing this technique, it is important for clinicians to remain current in their knowledge about violence risk factors because the science is continually evolving.

In addition to identifying demographic or historical risk factors for violence, clinical assessment of violence risk should also include an assessment of *pathways to dangerousness* for a given patient. Although many individuals may have committed similar violent acts—homicide, for example—their motivations for engaging in the act are based on highly individualized factors. The judicial system has long acknowledged this individual distinction, noting that a crime requires both a guilty act (*actus reus*) and a guilty mind (*mens rea*). In managing risk and predicting dangerousness, it is important for clinicians to determine what drives violence in an individual. In the case of a person with schizophrenia who has a history of striking people when psychotic, a reasonable intervention to mitigate risk is to assure treatment compliance and perform routine mental status assessments. For an individual with schizophrenia who also has clear psychopathic traits and engages in violence to intimidate others, the intervention to reduce risk may not rest in the realm of medication compliance, and it may not be best managed in a mental health setting.

ASKING FOR A RISK MANAGEMENT CONSULTATION

Risk is a broad term that refers to the chance of an injury, damage, or loss. Although risk often refers to the danger a patient may pose to others, it may also include the danger a patient poses to himself or to property. Risk is further used in the discussion of legal liability regarding the potential fallout from a bad outcome in a challenging clinical situation. Thus, when asking for a risk assessment, it is important for the clinician to specify the type of risk being assessed and to formulate a consultation question.

Often, the clinician's question for the forensic consultant is whether or not the patient presents a risk to the community. With such a broad question, the answer often begins with, "It depends . . . ," and has little practical or clinical usefulness.

When considering a consultation question for a forensic psychiatrist, the clinician should think in terms of how the identified risk should be managed, which is why such consultations are more often referred to as a *risk management consultation* rather than a risk assessment. With this approach, the expertise of the forensic psychiatrist is directed to collaborating with the treatment team to safely manage the patient rather than simply describe the patient in terms of his or her risk of dangerousness.

Although a useful question may be "Under what community treatment would the patient pose the least risk?" an even more useful and practical consultation occurs if the provider first proposes a specific management plan for the patient and then asks for a risk management consultation based on that plan. The forensic psychiatrist can then address the details of that plan, the safety of the various elements of the plan, and what portions of the plan require revision. At that point the team is in a position to immediately offer clinical options leading directly toward a practical solution for the patient.

Psychiatrists in the public sector make risk management decisions on a daily basis. Obtaining consultation on each occasion when risk is considered is impractical and often adds limited clinical value. As risk appears to become more imminent, or the potential magnitude for dangerousness rises, the clinician should begin to consider a consultation. A first step is to consult a colleague or another member of the team. However, when the concerns for risk heighten beyond the experience or expertise of those readily available, then requesting a consultation from a forensic psychiatrist is indicated.

Circumstances warranting a risk management consultation occur in numerous clinical and medical/legal situations. Examples include:

- When the risk of harm to others is considered substantial and how to manage the case is a point of contention among the team.

- Situations when it is important to have a psychiatrist experienced with the interpretation of state or federal statutes.

- When an independent second opinion is considered necessary from a liability perspective.

- When a case involves a potentially high-profile situation.

- When testimony is required, such as for probate court, and the treating psychiatrist determines that giving testimony may negatively impact the treatment alliance.

- When the inpatient facility feels the patient is ready for discharge and the outpatient treatment team disagrees. These situations are often related to resources need to treat rather than disagreements about actual risk.

TIPS FOR BETTER RISK MANAGEMENT

Psychiatrists will enhance their ability to manage dangerous clinical situations by systematically reviewing factors contributing to risk and designing a treatment plan to address each factor. Common clinical factors that suggest a heightened risk for dangerousness are identified in Table 8.1.

When considering the potential for future dangerousness, the examining psychiatrist should carefully review each past incident of violence, including self-harm, and assess what factors contributed to that action. By doing this, the clinician can then better determine which factors are more likely to predict dangerousness in the future.

The requesting clinician is also in a position to request how the forensic consultant's findings should be reported. The requesting clinician should specify whether a verbal

Table 8.1 COMMON RISK FACTORS FOR DANGEROUSNESS

HISTORICAL FACTORS	CURRENT FACTORS
Prior violent acts	Homicidal or suicidal ideation
Suicide attempts	Delusions, especially threat/control/override themes[59,60]
Self-mutilating behaviors	Command hallucinations to act in harmful ways[61]
History of elopement	Poor coping skills
History of treatment noncompliance[62]	Recent severe disruption in the patient's life
Past substance abuse[63]	Unstable living environment[64,65]
History of fire setting	Ongoing conflicts with others
History of sexually offending behaviors	Substance abuse/intoxication

response is all that is needed or if a more formal written consultation is necessary. Typically, a written consultation is the preferred means of communication because this will provide important documentation for the provider's future treatment rationale.

An example of a typical risk management consultation:

A middle-aged man with suicidal ideation was recently psychiatrically hospitalized after an incident of domestic violence. The patient was charged with assault and released from court to the hospital without bond. His next court date is not for a month. The patient is diagnosed with major depression and an alcohol use disorder. He has no history of suicide attempts or psychiatric treatment and is no longer suicidal. The patient's spouse wants him to return home, and there is no restraining order. The treatment team is uncertain about the safety of this discharge plan.

This case represents several areas of concern: risk to self, risk to others, and the legal liability of the psychiatrist who approves the discharge plan. In addition to the ethical and moral obligations a physician holds, it is important for the psychiatrist to appreciate the elements of malpractice. These elements are that the physician has a duty to provide proper care and treatment to her patient. If there is a dereliction of that duty, damages result, and it is determined that there is a proximate cause between the dereliction of duty and the damages, liability for these damages may fall on the physician.

Based on these elements, the primary burden of the psychiatrist is to fulfill her duty to the patient. Specifically, the duty is to provide a reasonable standard of care to the patient. The duty of the psychiatrist is not to prevent all harm from occurring in the situation or to accurately predict the future, but rather to perform a proper assessment and institute treatment that represents a reasonable standard of care. In this example, if the patient is released and fatally harms his spouse, the psychiatrist may not be found liable for malpractice if a proper assessment and management plan was put into place, despite the tragic outcome.

In this example, using an actuarial tool to assess risk will have limited clinical usefulness, in part because the psychiatrist is asked to make a decision about risk in the short term. Using the clinical approach, a proper risk management assessment would be for the psychiatrist to:

1. Conduct a thorough psychiatric assessment of the patient.
2. With a valid release of information, obtain collateral records including past psychiatric treatment, substance abuse treatment, and criminal history (many states allow access to convictions on the Internet).
3. Thoroughly review with the patient his view of the violent incident and events leading up to the incident.
4. Attempt to obtain a police report for the criminal incident. The patient's lawyer may be helpful in this regard.
5. Although it may not always be appropriate to contact the victim, in this case, the victim elected to stay involved, so contacting that person to discuss the patient's history and her view of violent incident is reasonable and beneficial. A release of information from the patient is not required if information is only being obtained, but because these discussions often involve disclosures of clinical information, a valid release of information is strongly encouraged.
6. Contact the hospital attorney to determine if the court has any hold on the patient that would necessitate his return to the judicial or correctional system if discharged from the hospital.

Data collected from these sources will allow the psychiatrist to either formulate a plan for discharge that meets a reasonable standard of care or better justify the patient's need for continued inpatient treatment. The plan should address the patient's need for treatment and monitoring of compliance, support the spousal relationship in managing future conflicts, provide interventions to lessen the likelihood for future recurrences of violence (such as removal of weapons or alcohol from the home), and provide a resource for the patient and his spouse to immediately contact in the event that their relationship deteriorates.

The daily challenges confronting the public psychiatrist can be daunting, but they can be made manageable by employing techniques to identify at-risk patients and using a structured process to manage the risk. Doing so will help clinicians to provide better care to his or her patients. Although risk (and the psychiatrist's worry) can never be eliminated, it can be substantially reduced with knowledge about violence risk and appropriate consultation with forensic professionals.

SUMMARY

As a result of legal and policy changes in the latter half of the 20th century, forensic psychiatry and public-sector psychiatry have become increasingly connected. The two disciplines now collaborate in managing individuals with SMI and histories of violence because private treatment settings often lack the expertise or resources to work with these challenging patients. Forensic patients are managed in several public sector settings: secure hospitals, prisons and jails, and outpatient programs. Because of their expertise in violence assessment and risk management, forensic psychiatrists can play an integral role in all of these settings. In addition, all public-sector psychiatrists must become familiar with some aspects of forensic psychiatry, particularly the assessment and management of violence risk. With a basic understanding of actuarial and clinical risk management tools, psychiatrists can better care for these complex and challenging patients.

REFERENCES

1. Grob GN. *Mental Institutions in America*. New York: Free Press; 1973.
2. Greenleaf T. *Laws of New York (Volume II)*. New York: State of New York; 1792: 53–54.
3. *Colby v. Jackson*, 12 N.H. 526, 530–531 (1842).
4. Overholser W. The voluntary admission law: certain legal and psychiatric aspects. *Am J Psychiatry*. 1924;80(3):475–490.
5. *Mayock v. Martin*, 157 Conn. 56 (1968).
6. Lamb HR, Weinberger LE. Persons with severe mental illness in jails and prisons: a review. *Psychiatr Serv*. 1998;49(4):483–492.
7. Harcourt B. An institutionalization effect: the impact of mental hospitalization and imprisonment on homicide in the United States. *J Legal Studies*. 2011;40(1):39–83, at 56.
8. Torrey E, Zdanowicz M, Kennard A, Lamb H, Eslinger D, Biasotti M, Fuller D. *The Treatment of Persons with Mental Illness in Prisons and Jails: A State Survey*. http://tacreports.org/treatment-behind-bars. Published April 8, 2014. Accessed January 31, 2015.
9. Arceneaux M. Why are the three largest mental health providers jails? NewsOne. http://newsone.com/2744141/prisons-mental-health-providers/. Published, October, 14, 2013. Accessed January 30, 2015.
10. *Brown v. Plata*, 563 US 131 S. Ct. 1910, 2011.
11. CMHS National GAINS Center. *Practical Advice on Jail Diversion: Ten Years of Learning on Jail Diversion from the CMHS National GAINS Center*. Delmar: Author; 2007.
12. The TAPA Center for Jail Diversion. *What Can We Say About the Effectiveness of Jail Diversion Programs for Persons with Co-Occurring Disorders?* Delmar: Author; 2004.
13. Naples M, Steadman HJ. Can persons with co-occurring disorders and violent charges be successfully diverted? *Int J Forensic Mental Health*. 2005;2(2):137–143.
14. Massachusetts Department of Mental Health Forensic Services. *Pre-Arrest Law Enforcement-Based Jail Diversion Program Report July 1, 2011 to January 1, 2014*. Available at http://www.mass.gov/eohhs/docs/dmh/forensic/jail-diversion-program-2014.pdf. Accessed August 25, 2015
15. Compton MT, Bahora M, Watson AC, Oliva JR. A comprehensive review of extant research on Crisis Intervention Team (CIT) programs. *J Am Acad Psychiatry Law*. 2008;36(1):47–55.
16. Munetz MR, Griffin PA. Use of the Sequential Intercept Model as an approach to decriminalization of people with serious mental illness. *Psychiatr Serv*. 2006;57(4):544–549.
17. Lamberti SI, Weisman R, Faden DI. Forensic assertive community treatment: Preventing incarceration of adults with serious mental illness. *Psychiatr Serv*. 2004;55(11):1285–1293.
18. Morrissey JP. *Forensic Assertive Community Treatment: Updating the Evidence*. SAMHSA GAINS Center. http://gainscenter.samhsa.gov/cms-assets/documents/141801-618932.fact-fact-sheet---joe-morrissey.pdf. Published January 21, 2014. Accessed January 31, 2015.
19. American Psychiatric Association. *Mandatory Outpatient Treatment Resource Document*. http://www.psychiatry.org/learn/library-archives/resource-documents. Published December 1999. Accessed January 31, 2015.
20. Kisely SR, Campbell LA. Compulsory community and involuntary outpatient treatment for people with severe mental disorders. *Cochrane Database Syst Rev*. 2014;12:CD004408. doi: 10.1002/14651858.CD004408.pub4. Epub December 4, 2014.
21. Siegert RJ, Ward T, Levack WM, McPherson KM. A Good Lives Model of clinical and community rehabilitation. *Disabil Rehabil*. 2007;29(20–21):1604–1615.
22. Binswanger IA, Krueger PM, Steiner JF. Prevalence of chronic medical conditions among jail and prison inmates in the USA compared with the general population. *J Epidemiol Community Health*. 2009;63(11):912–919.
23. Kinner SA, Wang EA. The case for improving the health of ex-prisoners. *Am J Public Health*. 2014;104(8):1352–1355.
24. *People v. Friday*, 225 Cal. App. 4th 8 (2014).
25. *McKune v. Lile*, 122 S. Ct. 2017 (2001).
26. Coid J, Ullrich S. Prisoners with psychosis in England and Wales: diversion to psychiatric inpatient services? *Int J Law Psychiatry*. 2011;34(2):99–108.
27. Smith JT, Baranoski MV, Kapoor R. *After Commitment of Sexual Predators: A Survey of States*. Presented at: the 41st Annual Meeting of the American Academy of Psychiatry and the Law. Tucson, AZ, October 23, 2010.
28. Bonnie RJ, Coughlin AM, Jeffries JC, Low PW. *Criminal Law: Cases and Materials*. 3rd ed. New York: Foundation Press; 2010.
29. Beatty JC. *The Politics of Public Ventures: An Oregon Memoir*. Bloomington, IN: Xlibris (self-published); 2010:341.
30. Appelbaum PS. *Almost a Revolution: Mental Health Law and the Limits of Change*. New York: Oxford University Press; 1994.
31. Scott DC, Zonana HV, Getz MA. Monitoring insanity acquittees: Connecticut's psychiatric security review board. *Hosp Community Psychiatry*. 1990;41(9):980–984.

32. Bloom JD, Williams MH, Bigelow DA. Monitored conditional release of persons found not guilty by reason of insanity. *Am J Psychiatry*. 1991;148(4):444–448.
33. Arizona Department of Health Services. *About Us*. http://www.azdhs.gov/azsh/psychiatric-security-review-board/index.php?pg=about-us. Last updated August 18, 2015.
34. Patterson RF, Wise BF. The development of internal forensic review boards in the management of hospitalized insanity acquittees. *J Am Acad Psychiatry Law*. 1998;269(4):661–664.
35. Bloom JD, Buckley MC. The Oregon Psychiatric Security Review Board: 1978–2012. *J Am Acad Psychiatry Law*. 2013;41:560–567.
36. Connecticut's Psychiatric Security Review Board. *Our Mission*. http://www.ct.gov/psrb/cwp/view.asp?a=2502&q=312772. Last updated on April 29, 2015.
37. *Jackson v. Indiana*, 406 US 715, 738 (1972).
38. *Jones v. United States*, 463 US 354 (1983).
39. ORS § 161.351: http://www.oregonlaws.org/ors/161.351. Accessed May 18, 2014.
40. CGS § 17a-593c: http://www.cga.ct.gov/current/pub/chap_319i.htm#sec_17a-593. Accessed May 17, 2014.
41. Resnick PJ. Continued civil commitment of insanity acquittees. *J Am Acad Psychiatry Law*. 2013;41(4):578–581.
42. *Olmstead v. L. C. by Zimring*, 527 US 581 (1999).
43. Bloom JD. CRIPA, Olmstead, and the transformation of the Oregon Psychiatric Security Review Board. *J Am Acad Psychiatry Law*. 2012;40:383–389.
44. European Committee for the Prevention of Torture and Inhuman or Degrading Treatment or Punishment (CPT). The CPT standards. In: Davoren M, Abidin Z, Naughton L, et al., eds. *Prospective Study of Factors Influencing Conditional Discharge From a Forensic Hospital: The DUNDRUM-3 Programme Completion and DUNDRUM-4 Recovery Structured Professional Judgement Instruments and Risk. BMC Psychiatry*. 2013;13:185.
45. Bloom JD, Williams MH, Bigelow DA. Monitored conditional release of persons found not guilty by reason of insanity. *Am J Psychiatry*. 1991;148(4):444–448.
46. *Barefoot v. Estelle*, 463 US 880 (1983).
47. Kraemer HC, Kazdin AE, Offard DR., et al. Coming to terms with the terms of risk. *Arch Gen Psychiatry*. 1997;54:337–343.
48. Hanson RK. *The Development of a Brief Actuarial Scale for Sexual Offense Recidivism*. (User Report No. 1997-04.) Ottawa: Solicitor General of Canada; 2007.
49. Quinsey VL, Grant TH, Rice ME, Cormier CA. *Violent Offenders: Appraising and Managing Risk*. Washington DC: American Psychological Association; 1998.
50. Szmukler G. Violence risk prediction in practice. *Br J Psychiatry*. 2001;178:84–85.
51. Hare RD. *The Psychopathy Checklist—Revised*. North Tonawanda, NY: Multi-Health Systems; 1991.
52. Patrick C. *Handbook of Psychopathy*. New York: Guilford; 2005.
53. Hare RD. (1993). *Without Conscience: The Disturbing World of the Psychopaths Among Us*. New York: Pocket Books.
54. Hare RD. *PCL-R, Technical Manual*. 2nd ed. North Tonawanda, NY: Multi-Health Systems; 2003.
55. Acheson SK. Review of the Hare Psychopathy Checklist-revised. 2nd ed. In: Spies RA, Plake BS, eds. *The Sixteenth Mental Measurements Yearbook*. Lincoln: University of Nebraska; 2005:429–431.
56. Norko MA, Baranoski MV. The prediction of violence: detection of dangerousness. *Brief Treatment and Crisis Intervention*. 2007;8(1):73–91.
57. Steadman HJ, Mulvey EP, Monahan J, et al. Violence by people discharged from acute psychiatric inpatient facilities and by others in the same neighborhoods. *Arch Gen Psychiatry*. 1998;55:393–401.
58. Mulvey EP, Lidz CW. Clinical prediction of violence as a conditional judgement. *Soc Psychiatry Psychiatr Epidemiol*. 1998;33:S107–S113.
59. Link BG, Stueve A, Phenal J. Psychotic symptoms and violent behaviors: probing the components of "threat/control override" symptoms. *Soc Psychiatry Psychiatr Epidemiol*. 1998;33:S55–S60.
60. Teasdale, B, Silver, E, Monahan, J. Gender, threat/control-override delusions and violence. *Law Hum Behav*. 2006;30:649–658.
61. McNeil DE, Eisner JP, Binder RL. The relationship between command hallucinations and violence. *Psychiatr Serv*. 2000;51:1288–1292.
62. Swartz MS, Swanson JW, Hiday VA, Borum R, Wagner R, Burns BJ. Taking the wrong drugs: the role of substance abuse and medication non-compliance in violence among severely mentally ill individuals. *Soc Psychiatry Psychiatr Epidemiol*. 1998;33: S75–S80.
63. Swanson JW, Holzer CE, Ganju VK, Jono RT. Violence and psychiatric disorder in the community: evidence from the epidemiologic catchment area surveys. *Hosp Community Psychiatry*. 1990;41:761–770.
64. Mulvey EP, Lidz CW. Clinical considerations in the prediction of dangerousness in mental patients. *Clin Psychol Rev*. 1984;4:379–401.
65. Swanson JW, Swartz MS, Meador KG. The social-environmental context of violent behavior in persons treated for severe mental illness. *Am J Pub Health*. 2002;92:1523–1531.

PART III

SERVICES AND CLINICAL COMPETENCIES OF PUBLIC PSYCHIATRY

9.

CHILDREN, ADOLESCENTS, AND YOUNG ADULTS IN THE PUBLICLY FUNDED SYSTEM OF CARE

Thomas J. McMahon, Nakia M. Hamlett, Christy L. Olezeski, Timothy C. Van Deusen, Natasha Harris, and Doreen J. Flanigan

INTRODUCTION

Amid calls for a comprehensive, continuous, coordinated, compassionate, and culturally competent system of health care that is developmentally informed and technically sophisticated,[1] children and adolescents usually receive health care services from professionals in a pediatric system located in one setting, and adults usually receive health care services from professionals in an adult system located in another setting. In public psychiatry, the system of care for children and adolescents exists relatively independent of the system of care for adults in ways that mirror differences present throughout the health care system. Children and adolescents with serious emotional-behavioral difficulty are typically treated in one system by professionals working from one perspective, whereas adults with serious psychiatric difficulty are typically treated in another system by professionals working from a somewhat different perspective. Although there are similarities across the two systems, there are important differences that should be outlined in any textbook for behavioral health professionals interested in public psychiatry. Consequently, this chapter provides an overview of the publicly funded system of care for children and adolescents experiencing serious emotional-behavioral difficulty. Although professionals entering the system of care for children and adolescents may find this summary helpful, the discussion focuses most clearly on the needs of professionals entering the system of care for adults. Educational highlights of this chapter and definitions of key terms are outlined in Box 9.1.

When considered from an educational perspective, there are a number of reasons that adult clinicians should have a basic understanding of developmental psychopathology and the publicly funded system of care for children and adolescents. First, epidemiologic research indicates that adult psychopathology tends to be characterized by developmental precursors that first become evident during childhood or adolescence.[2] Understanding adult clients from a developmental perspective can inform their assessment and treatment. Second, research on the nature of child and adolescent psychopathology often informs understanding of adult psychopathology.[2] Again, current understanding of developmental trajectories associated with specific adult presentations can inform the differential diagnosis of clients who appear similar when examined from a symptomatic perspective but may differ in important ways when examined from a developmental perspective.

Moreover, many clients in the publicly funded system of care for adults have also been clients in the publicly funded system of care for children and adolescents. Understanding the pediatric system may help clinicians understand the pathway their clients took to their current position in the service delivery system. Next, adult clinicians may have to assist with the transition of adolescents from the pediatric to the adult system. Understanding the publicly funded system of care for children and adolescents will facilitate movement of clients into the publicly funded system of care for adults. Finally, many clients in the adult system are parents with children at risk for psychiatric difficulty. Understanding the publicly funded system of care for children and adolescents will help clinicians support parents who have to seek services for their children and then work with other providers to coordinate services being provided to the family across the two systems.

Box 9.1

Educational Highlights

- Clinicians working in the publicly funded system of care for adults need to have a basic understanding of child and adolescent psychopathology and the publicly funded system of care for children and adolescents.
- Although the child study and child guidance movements served as the foundation of the publicly funded system of psychiatric treatment for children and adolescents, the concept of a system of care formally introduced in 1986 has influenced the development of the publicly funded system of psychiatric treatment for children and adolescents for more than 25 years.
- The guiding principles supporting the development of the publicly funded system of care for children and adolescents dictate that psychiatric services and supports be (1) population-based, (2) developmentally oriented, (3) child-centered, (4) family-driven, (5) strength-based, (6) community-based, and (7) culturally sensitive. Within the publicly funded system of care, there is also an emphasis on (1) empirically based practice, (2) interdisciplinary treatment, and (3) interagency collaboration.
- The publicly funded system of care needs to consider ways to offer developmentally informed approaches to engagement and intervention designed to better support adolescents with serious psychiatric difficulty as they make the transition from the pediatric to the adult system of care.
- The four traditional behavioral health disciplines of psychiatry, clinical psychology, nursing, and social work need to consider ways to recruit and train the next generation of professionals to further develop the publicly funded system of care for children, adolescents, and young adults.

Key Terms

Throughout this chapter, the terms *child, adolescent*, and *young adult* are used to refer to an individual from birth to 11 years old, 12 to 17 years old, and 18 to approximately 25 years old. The term *transitioning youth* is used to refer to an individual 16 to approximately 25 years of age leaving the mental health, child welfare, juvenile justice, special education, or other system of care as eligibility for services expires.

A BRIEF HISTORY OF THE PUBLICLY FUNDED SYSTEM OF CARE FOR CHILDREN AND ADOLESCENTS

Many historians believe that the origins of contemporary child psychiatry can be traced back to the child study and child guidance movements that began as the 1800s came to a close. Although remnants of both movements can be found in the publicly funded system of care for children and adolescents, the system has, over more than 100 years, been redefined and reorganized by a number of other influences. Other important influences include (1) worldwide expansion of child psychoanalysis, (2) the introduction and expansion of Medicaid, (3) the community mental health movement, and (4) ideas about a system of care. The concept of a system of care for children and adolescents with serious emotional-behavioral difficulty has, more than anything else, shaped the development of the publicly funded system of care. It is important to note, however, that some policy analysts[3] have argued that the development of a comprehensive system of appropriate, accessible psychiatric services for children and adolescents has been slowed by the absence of a national policy on child mental health. These critics complain that, rather than being directed by a coherent, consistent national policy, the development of psychiatric services for children and adolescents has been driven by policy and program developments in the areas of social welfare, child welfare, special education, juvenile justice, and adult mental health.

CHILD STUDY MOVEMENT

G. Stanley Hall, the first president of Clark University and the first president of the American Psychological Association, is frequently credited with starting the child study movement, which contributed to the evolution of developmental psychology, educational psychology, and child psychiatry.[4] Directly influenced by Hall, several pediatricians established child study centers throughout the country to study normative child development.[5] Arnold Gesell, for example, established the Clinic of Child Development within the Yale University School of Medicine in 1911, before completing his medical degree. Subsequently, financial support from the Laura Spelman Rockefeller Memorial helped to establish a national network of child study centers. The Iowa Child Welfare Research Station; the Institute of Child Welfare at the University of California, Berkeley; the Saint George School for Child Study at the University of Toronto; the Institute for Child Development at the University of Minnesota; and the Child Welfare Institute at Teachers College, Columbia University were some other early child study centers.[5] Although originally developed to promote the study of normative child development with the intent to generate empirical knowledge for use in the education of parents, teachers, and pediatricians, some of the early child study centers moved toward the study of aberrant development. As the focus of the research being done in child study centers linked with academic institutions shifted over time, they gradually became important components of an early publicly funded system of care for children and adolescents.

CHILD GUIDANCE MOVEMENT

Without dismissing the influence of the child study movement, the publicly funded system of care for child and adolescents can also clearly be linked with the child guidance movement. Conceptually, the child study versus child guidance movements represented an early distinction between the medical tradition of studying normative and aberrant child development in an academic setting and the social work tradition of providing services to socially and economically disenfranchised individuals in a community setting. Many historians[6] believe that the child guidance movement was grounded in the work of William Healy, who founded the Juvenile Psychopathic Institute in 1909. Concerned about juvenile delinquency in Chicago, a group of philanthropists opened what many people believe to be the first child guidance clinic with a conceptual model of service delivery clearly grounded in a commitment to interdisciplinary collaboration. In 1922, the Commonwealth Fund began its Program for the Prevention of Juvenile Delinquency that supported the development of child guidance clinics designed to provide preventive services to school-aged children of normal intelligence exhibiting behavioral difficulty.[6]

From the beginning, the child guidance movement drew on the values of social work and clinical psychology, and the medical control of the child guidance clinics was actively resisted.[6] Over years, the original goal of preventing juvenile delinquency waned, and child guidance clinics became outpatient treatment programs for children and adolescents experiencing psychiatric difficulty.[6] Although the early child guidance clinics provided services to low-income families on a sliding-fee basis, there was no clear mechanism to ensure that child guidance services were widely available and easily affordable. With public support, the extensive network of child guidance clinics established before 1960 did, however, eventually become a cornerstone of the publicly funded system of care for children and adolescents.[6] Although a sensitive issue with historical evidence of battles over professional turf,[7] the child guidance movement, more than anything else, advanced the idea of an interdisciplinary approach to the assessment and treatment of children and adolescents experiencing serious emotional-behavioral difficulty.

CHILD PSYCHOANALYSIS

Both the child study and child guidance movements of the early 1900s were also influenced by the introduction of child psychoanalysis. Psychoanalytic work with children began in 1909, when Sigmund Freud summarized his consultation with the father of a little boy suffering with an irrational fear of horses that Freud interpreted using his theory of the Oedipus complex.[8,9] Child psychoanalysis then emerged as an extension of adult psychoanalysis advanced by Anna Freud, Melanie Klein, Margaret Mahler, Edith Jacobson, Erik Erikson, and Donald Winnicott.[8,9] Anna Freud and Melanie Klein developed the two most prominent schools of thought on child psychoanalysis and engaged in rigorous debate about the specifics of their approaches during a series of meetings sponsored by the British Psychoanalytical Society between October 1942 and February 1944.[8] Anna Freud also helped to open the Hampstead War Nursery in London and then the Hampstead Child Therapy Course and Clinic following the end of World War II. Historians[10,11] often identify the Hampstead Child Therapy Course and Clinic as the first psychoanalytic institute devoted exclusively to research, training, and treatment being pursued with children. Much of the work done in the nursery and the clinic focused on the needs of children affected by World War II.[10,11] After her death, the Hampstead Child Therapy Course and Clinic was renamed the Anna Freud Centre, and the center continues to serve low-income children and adolescents with links to the publicly funded system of care in the United Kingdom.[11]

As the child psychoanalytic movement expanded, service delivery within child guidance clinics in North America and Europe began to integrate ideas outlined in the psychoanalytic literature on children and adolescents.[12] Building on the early work of Anna Freud, child guidance clinics became more enthusiastic about understanding psychopathology as deviance from normative development, and the concept of a developmental diagnosis became popular.[9] Likewise, the concepts of a holding environment, a transitional object, and good-enough mothering outlined by Donald Winnicott; the concept of separation-individuation presented by Margaret Mahler; and ideas about attachment advanced by John Bowlby became influential.[9] Consistent with child psychoanalysis, child guidance clinics also began to emphasize the use of close observation in the clinical assessment and the use of play in treatment.[9] The emphasis on the developmental sequelae of early psychological trauma, the emphasis on early intervention with infants and preschool children, and the concept of collateral intervention with parents were also integrated into the evolving publicly funded system of care.[9]

COMMUNITY MENTAL HEALTH MOVEMENT

Although the final report called for the continued development of psychiatric clinics for children and adolescents, the first major public policy initiative outlined by the Joint Commission on Mental Health and Illness,[13] in 1961, focused largely on the needs of adults, and there was early debate about whether child guidance services should be located within a community mental health center.[14] Consequently, the subsequent funding of community mental health centers did not have a dramatic impact on the publicly funded system of care for children and adolescents.[3] Part F of the Mental Retardation Facilities and Community Mental Health Center Construction Act did, however, include funding for special projects designed to better meet the needs of children and adolescents.[3,15] With the success of these demonstration projects, the government required that community mental health centers offer services to children and adolescents on a limited basis.[15] Despite these early efforts, a general lack of attention to the needs of children and adolescents during the early community mental health movement led to a report by the Joint Commission on the Mental Health of Children titled, *Crisis in Child Mental Health*.[16] The final report of the commission did not result in a national policy or program, but it did articulate the principles of child advocacy that became the basis for the articulation of the concept of a system of care.

Some 10 years later, the Mental Health Systems Act of 1981 that was passed during the Carter Administration with intent to continue financing of community mental health centers listed children and adolescents with serious emotional-behavioral difficulty as an underserved population deserving special attention, but the act was repealed by the Reagan Administration before it was implemented.[3] Block grant funding of psychiatric and substance abuse services during the Reagan Administration reduced funding to the states, but the process eventually required that the states set aside a certain percentage of block grant funding for psychiatric services designed to better meet the needs of children and adolescents.[3] As federal financing for community mental health declined, the states did not provide community mental health centers with the funding necessary to support special programming, and services for children and adolescents disappeared from many community mental health centers.

MEDICAID

Although the community mental health movement did not have a dramatic impact on the publicly funded system of care for children and adolescents, simultaneous passage of the Social Security Amendments of 1965 did have a dramatic impact by creating Medicaid.[17] By matching state funding for health care with federal funds, Medicaid dramatically expanded access to health care for children living in low-income families. It also included a formal mandate that the states offer psychiatric services, including psychiatric services for children and adolescents. After Medicaid was operated on a fee-for-service basis for several decades, active management of Medicaid benefits during the 1990s dramatically reduced utilization of inpatient resources and dramatically increased the development and utilization of intensive outpatient programs and other alternatives to inpatient hospitalization.[18] Its impact on the utilization of outpatient services was equivocal.

The State Children's Health Improvement Plan that was introduced in 1997 increased access to health care for children living in low-income families by expanding eligibility for Medicaid and retaining an expectation that, with qualification, benefit plans include provisions for psychiatric services.[18] Historically, approximately 33% of Medicaid recipients who receive psychiatric services are children and adolescents.[19] Children in foster care and children with serious developmental difficulty account for a disproportionate percent of Medicaid spending on psychiatric services, and the largest portion of Medicaid funds spent on psychiatric services supports outpatient treatment.[20] Although Medicaid may have dramatically increased access to services for children and adolescents experiencing serious emotional-behavior difficulty, low rates of Medicaid reimbursement for psychiatric services probably contributed, over time, to the separation of the public and private systems of care.

CONCEPT OF A SYSTEM OF CARE

In 1982, Jane Knitzer[21] highlighted the need for a national system of psychiatric services for children and adolescents in a report commissioned by the Children's Defense Fund. Following publication of her report, the National Institute of Mental Health initiated the Child and Adolescent Service System Program that provided financial and technical assistance for the development of systems of care for children and adolescents with psychiatric difficulty.[3] From the beginning, the initiative recognized that children and adolescents with serious emotional-behavioral difficulty are often involved with several service delivery systems such that planning for effective intervention requires interagency collaboration. In 1986, Beth Stroul and Robert Friedman[22] formally and broadly defined a system of care as a comprehensive continuum of services and supports organized into a coordinated network to meet the complex needs of children and adolescents with psychiatric difficulty, and they began to outline a set of principles to guide the development of local systems of care for children and adolescents experiencing serious emotional-behavioral difficulty.

In 1992, Congress passed legislation creating the Comprehensive Community Mental Health Services for Children and Their Families Program to provide funding to build systems of care. Today, the program continues to be an important source of federal funding to support the development of a comprehensive array of community-based services grounded in the concept of a system of care.[23] Over more than 25 years, the concept of a system of care for children and adolescents has evolved,[24-28] and it served as the basis for many of the recommendations made by the Subcommittee on Children and Families for the New Freedom Commission on Mental Health.[29] Although debate about the most appropriate definition of the concept continues,[30] Stroul, Blau, and Friedman[31] last updated it by defining a system of care as a broad array of community-based services and supports organized into a coordinated network to help children and adolescents with serious emotional-behavioral difficulty function better at home, in school, and in the community. As implementation of the Patient Protection and Affordable Care Act and the Health Care and Education Reconciliation Act of 2010 (ACA) continues, policy analysts[32] have begun to explore ways that health care reform may influence further development of the concept of a system of care for children and adolescents with psychiatric difficulty.

CHARACTERISTICS OF THE PUBLICLY FUNDED SYSTEM OF CARE FOR CHILDREN AND ADOLESCENTS

As noted earlier, the concept of a system of care first outlined by Stroul and Friedman[22] continues, more than anything else, to influence the development of the publicly funded system of care for children and adolescents. Within the federal government, the Child, Adolescent, and Family Branch of the Center for Mental Health Services within the Substance Abuse and Mental Health Services Administration (SAMHSA) supports ongoing development of the publicly funded system. However, many policy analysts and child advocates[33-35] believe that the development of effective systems of care occurs largely at the state, county, tribal, and local level. Consequently, the Center for Mental Health Services sponsors a National Technical Assistance Center for Children's Mental Health[36] that strives to sustain, expand, and improve local systems of care for children and adolescents experiencing serious emotional-behavioral difficulty. The guiding principles that have directed development of the publicly funded system of care over more than 25 years are outlined in Table 9.1. As noted, these guiding principles dictate that psychiatric services and supports be (1) population-based, (2) child-centered, (3) developmentally oriented, (4) family-driven, (5) strength-based, (6) community-based, (7) minimally restrictive, and (8) culturally sensitive. Within the publicly funded system of care, there is also an emphasis placed on (1) empirically based practice, (2) interdisciplinary collaboration, (3) interagency collaboration, and (4) accountability.

CHARACTERISTICS OF CHILDREN AND ADOLESCENTS IN THE PUBLICLY FUNDED SYSTEM OF CARE

Epidemiological data suggest that, across technologically oriented cultures, 10–15% of children meet diagnostic criteria for a lifetime episode of psychiatric difficulty, with evidence that there is a degree of specificity and consistency in the presence of specific signs and symptoms over time, particularly for girls.[37-39] By adolescence, 20–25% of teens meet diagnostic criteria for a lifetime episode of psychiatric difficulty.[40] Much of this psychopathology represents developmental precursors of serious and persistent psychiatric difficulty as an adult,[2] and policy analysts[41] argue that psychiatric disorders are among the most frequently occurring and most costly of pediatric health problems. Consistent with this, the National Research Council and Institute of Medicine[42] estimate that psychiatric difficulty in children and adolescents costs more than $250 billion annually. This estimate is, however, complicated by the fact that, despite national attention to the publicly funded system of care for children and adolescents, most children with serious

Table 9.1 GUIDING PRINCIPLES FOR THE DEVELOPMENT OF THE PUBLICLY FUNDED SYSTEM OF CARE FOR CHILDREN AND ADOLESCENTS

CHARACTERISTIC	COMMENT
Population-based	Services and supports for children and adolescents with serious emotional-behavioral difficulty should be grounded in a thorough understanding of the target population.
Child-centered	Services and supports for children and adolescents with serious emotional-behavioral difficulty should be configured and delivered to meet the unique needs of each child or adolescent.
Developmentally oriented	Services and supports for children and adolescents with serious emotional-behavioral difficulty should be designed, developed, and delivered with intent to promote normative child development.
Family-oriented	Services and supports for children and adolescents with serious emotional-behavioral difficulty should allow for active participation of family in all aspects of service delivery.
Strength-based	Services and supports for children and adolescents with serious emotional-behavioral difficulty should be designed, developed, and delivered to draw upon strengths present in the child, family, and community.
Community-based	Services and supports for children and adolescents with serious emotional-behavioral difficulty should be designed, developed, and delivered in a community setting.
Minimally restrictive	Services and supports for children and adolescents with serious emotional-behavioral difficulty should be offered in the least restrictive setting possible.
Empirically based	The design, development, and delivery of services and supports for children and adolescents with serious emotional-behavioral difficulty should be grounded in the best available empirical evidence.
Culturally sensitive	Services and supports for children and adolescents with serious emotional-behavioral difficulty should be designed, developed, and delivered in ways that promote sensitivity to the needs of all segments of the target population and minimize risk for discrimination against any segment of that population.
Interdisciplinary collaboration	The administration and delivery of services and supports for children and adolescents with serious emotional-behavioral difficulty should promote interdisciplinary collaboration with professionals with different expertise working cooperatively with one another to better meet the needs of children and adolescents.
Interagency collaboration	Services and supports for children and adolescents with serious emotional-behavioral difficulty should be designed, developed, and delivered in ways that promote coordination and collaboration across organizations serving the diverse needs of children and adolescents.
Accountability	The performance of systems, organizations, and clinicians providing services and supports to children and adolescents with serious emotional-behavioral difficulty should be evaluated to provide data that inform a process of continuous quality improvement.

Note. This list of guiding principles was extracted from the evolving literature on the concept of a system of care for children and adolescents with serious emotional-behavioral difficulty.[22–31]

emotional-behavioral difficulty do not receive adequate services.[43,44]

Data from the Comprehensive Community Mental Health Services for Children and Their Families Program[23] and similar federal initiatives characterize, better than most sources of information, the children and adolescents being served in the publicly funded system of care. These data suggest that almost all children and adolescents receiving services in the publicly funded system of care are living in low-income settings. Approximately 60% of the children and adolescents receiving services are living in urban or rural poverty. Almost all the children and adolescents entering the publicly funded system of care are in the custody of a biological parent or other biological relative, but, relative to the general population, children and adolescents in the legal custody of both biological parents are dramatically underrepresented. Approximately 50% of the children and adolescents are in the custody of their biological mother. Up to 85% of the children and adolescents begin services with a family history of psychiatric and substance use problems. A family history of depression or substance abuse is very common. Unemployment among their parents is also relatively common.

Data collected from this federally funded system-of-care initiative[23] suggest that, relative to their distribution in the general population, boys tend to be overrepresented throughout the publicly funded system of care. Likewise, children of African American, Hispanic, and Native

American heritage are usually also overrepresented, but they are still underserved. Children of European and Asian heritage are usually underrepresented. Undoubtedly a consequence of the criteria for admission, children aged 6–15 years tend to be overrepresented in the publicly funded system of care, whereas infants and preschool children, along with transitioning youth, tend to be underrepresented.

Data collected from this federal initiative[23] also indicate that children and adolescents entering the publicly funded system of care present with significant exposure to psychological trauma and family adversity. They average four to seven traumatic life events. Emotional, physical, and sexual abuse is common. Exposure to physical, emotional, educational, and medical neglect tends to be even more common. Diagnostically, they present with varying patterns of both internalizing and externalizing difficulty. Internalizing difficulty in the form of anxiety, depression, and somatization is common. Externalizing difficulty in the form of angry affect, oppositional-defiant behavior, hyperactivity, aggressive behavior, and conduct problems is equally common. Some data suggest externalizing difficulty may be more common, but there does not appear to be consensus about the predominance of externalizing over internalizing difficulty. Children and adolescents presenting with a mix of internalizing and externalizing difficulty may actually be most common. Although not represented in the most recent version of the *Diagnostic and Statistical Manual of Mental Disorders*,[45] some scholars[46] argue that the mix of internalizing and externalizing difficulty common among children and adolescents entering the publicly funded system of care can be best understood as the consequence of repeated exposure to interpersonal trauma.

Looking beyond internalizing versus externalizing pathology, federal data[28] also suggest that a history of suicidal thoughts, deliberate self-harm, and suicidal behavior is common among children and adolescents entering the publicly funded system of care. Problems with school attendance, academic performance, and classroom behavior are also common. Although most typically present with low average to average intelligence, children and adolescents with attentional problems, specific learning problems, intellectual disability, and autism spectrum disorders are disproportionately represented in the publicly funded system of care. Running away, substance use, and early sexual activity are not unusual among the adolescents. Children and adolescents entering this system also present with disproportionately higher rates of asthma, allergy, and obesity. A minority present with other serious medical problems.

Finally, children and adolescents entering the publicly funded system of care are usually involved with other publicly funded systems of care. For example, up to 40% of the children and adolescents may be involved with the child welfare system, up to 35% may be involved with the special education system, and up to 30% may be involved with the juvenile justice system.[47,48] Although children and adolescents entering this system are frequently involved with other service delivery systems, policy analysts[47,48] argue that rates of engagement in psychiatric services are actually still lower than the documented need among children and adolescents engaged with the child welfare, juvenile justice, and special education systems. That is, although children and adolescents seeking psychiatric services are frequently involved with these other service delivery systems, a substantial segment of children and adolescents involved with those systems have a need for psychiatric services that is not being met. The clinical vignettes presented in Box 9.2 illustrate ficitionalized presentations of children and adolescents entering the publicly funded system of care.

Box 9.2

A Family Entering the Publicly Funded System of Care

Jennifer and Robert (Bobbie) were a pair of siblings born to the same mother but different fathers. They were referred to the child and adolescent service at a small community mental health clinic by their protective services worker shortly after they were removed from the care of their biological mother because of concern about persistent physical, educational, and medical neglect.

Jennifer was an 8-year-old, Caucasian girl of Italian heritage. At the time of her admission, she was living in North Somewhere, Connecticut, with her therapeutic foster parents. Prior to this therapeutic foster placement, she had two brief, unsuccessful foster placements with extended family. She was attending Main Street Elementary School as a third-grade student assigned to a mainstream classroom with social work support. Presenting problems included depressed mood, anxiety about separation from her mother and older brother, preoccupation with her return home, suicidal threats, and aggressive outbursts at home and in school. After having attended school sporadically for several years, she was socially isolated, and she was struggling academically. Although visiting with her mother regularly, Jennifer had been refusing to visit with her biological father who had recently been located by her protective services worker.

Robert (Bobbie) was a 13-year-old, Caucasian boy of Italian and Hispanic heritage. At the time of his admission, Bobbie was living in East Somewhere, Connecticut, with his foster mother and an 11-year-old foster sister, and he was doing very well academically and socially as an eighth-grade student assigned to a mainstream classroom at Main Street Middle School. In addition to the substantiated accusations of serious neglect, there were questions about whether Bobbie had also been physically abused by a man who briefly lived with his mother. Because of his age, Bobbie also had a juvenile court case pending for failure to attend school regularly. Presenting problems included anxiety about separation from his mother and younger sister, guilt about his failure to attend school regularly, and difficulty sleeping. Although visiting with his mother regularly, he was upset with his mother because she could not tell him who his biological father was.

Their mother, Donna, was a 31-year-old, single Caucasian woman of Italian heritage who has a high school diploma but no significant work history. Shortly before her children were admitted to the clinic, she had referred herself to the adult service at the same community mental health clinic. Upon admission, she was homeless and living in West Somewhere, Connecticut, with extended family. Her psychosocial history was notable for a history of childhood trauma, residential placement as an adolescent, early pregnancy in the context of an unstable romantic relationship, failure to adequately support herself financially, and difficulty maintaining stable housing for her family. In the context of the child welfare proceedings, she presented with depressive symptoms and signs of serious personality disturbance characterized by avoidant, dependent, and compulsive traits. Although there were initially questions about limited intelligence, she demonstrated low average to average cognitive ability on standardized assessments.

A Preschool Child Entering the Publicly Funded System of Care

Gabriel was a 4-year-old boy of Hispanic heritage who was referred to the child and adolescent service at a small community mental health clinic by the preschool special education team within the Safe Haven Public School System. The referral represented the second effort school staff had made to help his father secure a comprehensive psychiatric evaluation. At the time of his referral, Gabriel was living with his biological father and 2-year-old biological sister whose cognitive, emotional, and social development appeared to be appropriate for a child her age. He was enrolled in an inclusion program for preschool children with special needs. His father was a 24-year-old Hispanic man of Puerto Rican heritage whose primary language is Spanish. He was unemployed and stressed by the demands of caring for two children with limited vocational skills and minimal social support. Gabriel's mother was a 23-year-old woman of Colombian heritage whose primary language was also Spanish. She reportedly left the family to return to Colombia to resume a romantic relationship with a man she knew as a child. During an initial meeting, Gabriel's father complained about being very depressed and anxious because the family faced eviction from their apartment for failure to pay rent.

When seen for an initial assessment, Gabriel presented with signs of intellectual disability, hyperactivity, limited attentional capacity, poor impulse control, and pica. School staff were concerned that, when not closely supervised, Gabriel was eating inedible objects in ways that were jeopardizing his health. They were also concerned about what appeared to be reactive aggression directed at peers in school that left them at risk for serious injury. He also presented with signs of attachment difficulty characterized by indiscriminate pursuit of caregiving from strange adults. His pediatric records documented a history of lead poisoning, inadequate well-child care, and an absence of repeated screening for lead poisoning in the context of his pica. There was also a note that Gabriel had been referred for a pediatric neurological consultation, but the family had not kept two appointments arranged by his pediatrician. His school records documented excessive absenteeism during his first 2 years of school that the educators thought had compromised his capacity to benefit from his program of special education. As the treatment team completed his admission evaluation, there was agreement that the clinic had an obligation to make a mandated report to child protective services because of concern about educational and medical neglect.

A School-Age Child Entering the Publicly Funded System of Care

Melanie was a 9-year-old biracial girl of European and African American heritage whose mother referred her to the child and adolescent service at a small community mental health clinic. She had been encouraged to do so by school staff and her protective services worker. At the time of her referral, Melanie was living in West Somewhere, Connecticut, with her biological mother, maternal grandmother, and an older sister. She was registered as a second-grade student at Main Street Elementary School, but she was not attending school regularly. Child protective services was involved with the family because, during kindergarten and first grade, Melanie had missed more than 50% of the school year. Because there was no evidence that Melanie had any medical problem that would warrant her missing so much school, the school social worker had made a mandated report of educational neglect to child protective services during the previous school year.

Upon admission, school staff reported that her mother frequently kept Melanie home from school, reporting she was sick. When she did not attend, her mother would consistently call the school nurse to report that Melanie was ill with some minor illness or injury. Occasionally, she would also provide a note indicating that Melanie had been seen by her pediatrician, but the notes never documented any clear signs of illness at the time of the visit. Because she had missed so much school, Melanie had been retained twice and was two grades behind her age cohort. A special education evaluation completed by school staff failed to document any emotional or learning problems. When in school, Melanie was described as a pleasant, cooperative child who was doing her school work as best she could and getting along well with her teacher and her peers.

When first seen at the clinic, Melanie was still not attending school regularly, she was at risk to be retained again, and there was a pending legal petition to remove her from her mother's care. Melanie presented as a quiet, compliant child who did not demonstrate any signs or symptoms of serious emotional-behavioral difficulty. She indicated that she enjoyed being in school and did not identify any problems at school. She also reported that she sometimes did not feel sick when her mother kept her home from school, but she also indicated that she knew she had to do what her mother told her to do. Her mother presented as a very anxious, cooperative woman who reported she was supporting her family with disability benefits and financial assistance from her mother. She confirmed a long list of medical problems, acknowledged a serious sexual assault as an adolescent, and reported that her father had died unexpectedly approximately 5 years ago. She seemed to be hypervigilant about Melanie's health and offered a long list of childhood illnesses and injuries that she believed warranted keeping Melanie out of school. Although she faced losing custody of Melanie in several months, she insisted that the judge would understand her need to keep her child home from school when she was sick.

An Adolescent Entering the Publicly Funded System of Care

Khalid was a 15-year-old boy from Morocco who was referred to the child and adolescent service of a small community mental health clinic by his older brother who was also his legal guardian. His was of Muslim faith, and Arabic was his first language. Upon referral, he was living with his 28-year-old brother in an apartment in West Somewhere, Connecticut, where he attended Safe Haven High School as a tenth-grade student. He was enrolled in mainstream classes with English as a Second Language (ESL) supports. Approximately 1 year prior to his admission, Khalid, who was the youngest of six children, had immigrated precipitously to the United States to live with his oldest brother after he had witnessed the death of his parents in a motor vehicle accident. His brother's work visa allowed them to live in the country legally, but Khalid was not eligible for Medicaid benefits, and his family could not afford to pay for private insurance.

Presenting problems included complaints of sadness, difficulty sleeping, and myriad somatic complaints involving headaches, dizziness, joint pain, pressure in his chest, and double vision. For more than a year, Khalid had attempted to cope with his somatic complaints by praying, but when that did not prove helpful, he asked that his brother bring him to a doctor for a medical evaluation. Because he had no medical insurance, Khalid did not have a primary care physician and eventually went to the local emergency room for a physical examination and laboratory studies during an episode of dizziness. When his medical evaluation proved negative, the physician in the emergency room suggested that his complaints were psychosomatic in nature and referred him to the clinic for a psychiatric evaluation.

Although Khalid and his brother reported that psychiatric treatment is frowned upon in their culture, they agreed to seek services because Khalid was so distressed. His psychosocial history suggested that the sudden death of his parents had triggered a cascade of other interpersonal losses for Khalid as he left his home in Morocco with a simultaneous increase in psychosocial stress associated with his need to live with his brother, attend school, and make new friends in a country where he did not know the culture or the language. Anti-Arab sentiment within his new high school and his need to immediately learn English added to the stress. His family history was positive for difficulty with anxiety and depression in several first-degree relatives, and a standardized trauma screen suggested that he was experiencing symptoms of traumatic grief related to the unexpected death of his parents.

CHALLENGES IN THE PUBLICLY FUNDED SYSTEM OF CARE FOR CHILDREN AND ADOLESCENTS

Despite more than 100 years of ongoing development, the publicly funded system of care for children and adolescents has always been confronted with a number of challenges. Some of these challenges, like access to services and engagement in treatment, have been long-standing and the subject of empirical investigation. Others, like concern about the use of psychiatric medication, are relatively new and shaped by independent review of the system. Still others, like the validity of psychiatric diagnoses, concern about the empirical basis for practice, and the need for empirically validated treatments, are relatively new and shaped by concerns evolving from within the behavioral health professions. To illustrate some of these challenges, seven issues currently facing the system are briefly described here.

ACCESS

Despite the prevalence of developmental psychopathology, most minors with a documented need for psychiatric treatment do not, as noted earlier, receive treatment.[37,44] Although overrepresented in the publicly funded system of care, children and adolescents from low-income families have disproportionately higher rates of unmet need.[47,48] Likewise, African American, Hispanic, and Native American children and adolescents living in poverty have even higher rates of unmet need.[47,48] Demographic groupings of children and adolescents with specific patterns of emotional-behavioral difficulty also tend to have more unmet need. For example, girls with externalizing difficulty and boys with internalizing difficulty are less likely to receive psychiatric services.[49]

Kimberly Hoagwood and her colleagues[50] have defined three clusters of potential influences that may limit access to services: (1) structural characteristics of the system of care, (2) perception of the psychiatric difficulty, and (3) perception of the services. Research indicates that influences easily sorted to each cluster do, in fact, influence access to behavioral health services. Structural characteristics of the service delivery system known to influence access include a lack of providers, wait-lists, lack of insurance, inadequate insurance, transportation problems, inconvenient location, inconvenient hours, and lack of culturally and linguistically competent clinicians. Perceptions of the psychiatric difficulty known to influence access include failure to identify serious emotional-behavioral difficulty, denial of problem severity, denial of the need for professional services, and belief that the problem will resolve without treatment. Perceptions of services known to influence access include lack of trust in behavioral health professionals, negative experiences with behavioral health professionals, child or adolescent reluctance to seek services, social stigma, and parental concern about mandated reporting of potential child abuse and neglect. Limited research done with this conceptual model suggests that, despite a historical focus on structural characteristics of the service delivery system, access to services will only improve with concurrent attention to perceptions of the psychiatric difficulty and perceptions of psychiatric services.[50]

ENGAGEMENT

Although problems with access to services persist for children and adolescents, engagement in treatment is a persistent problem when caregivers do seek services. Consequently, there are high rates of failure to keep an initial appointment, failure to attend treatment sessions, early withdrawal from treatment, and administrative discharge for failure to attend regularly. Although there has been extensive discussion about the potential reasons for poor attendance in the face of high need and limited access, systematic review of the literature[51] suggests that locating help elsewhere, competing demands at the time of the scheduled appointment, length of wait time for the appointment, dissatisfaction with the initial contact, improvement in the presenting problem, and child or adolescent refusal may contribute to failure to keep an initial appointment. Unfortunately, the results of research are not consistent, and no single influence emerges as particularly robust across investigations.[51]

Similarly, Alan Kazdin and his colleagues[52] argued that no single characteristic or condition appears to sufficiently explain failure to attend treatment once enrolled. Research on early withdrawal suggests that family crisis, conflict with a significant other about treatment, problems with other children, conflict with other appointments, situational stressors associated with poverty, quality of the relationship with the clinician, perceived relevance of the treatment, and rate of clinical improvement may be some of the contributing factors.[52] More recently, Bruce Chorpita[53,54] has argued that conceptual models of engagement need to involve more than just documentation of simple attendance, and Chorpita and his colleagues[53,54] have begun to more clearly document how different approaches to engagement affect three dimensions of engagement: (1) attendance at treatment, (2) readiness for treatment, and (3) adherence to treatment.

PSYCHIATRIC DIAGNOSIS

Comprehensive psychiatric evaluation poses many conceptual and practical challenges for behavioral health clinicians working with children and adolescents. Conceptually, for many years, there has been tension between advocates of a categorical medical diagnosis grounded in the *Diagnostic and Statistical Manual of Mental Disorders* (DSM)[45] or International Classification of Diseases (ICD)[55] and advocates of a developmental diagnosis grounded in the principles of developmental psychopathology.[56] Within the psychiatric community, there has also been controversy about the reliability and validity of psychiatric diagnoses used with children and adolescents. More recently, there has, for example, been controversy about the incorrect, inconsistent, and excessive use of diagnoses like attention deficit hyperactivity disorder, bipolar mood disorder, and posttraumatic stress disorder in children and adolescents.[57-59] With the introduction of the latest revision (DSM 5)[45] in 2013, there has been concern about (1) the reliability of specific child and adolescent diagnoses,[60] (2) the reorganization of autistic spectrum diagnoses,[61] (3) the inclusion of disruptive mood regulation disorder,[62] and (4) the exclusion of developmental trauma disorder.[46]

PSYCHOPHARMACOLOGY

Medication can be effective in the treatment of psychiatric disorders of childhood and adolescence. However, there is consensus that treatment with psychiatric medication should only be initiated after a comprehensive psychiatric evaluation and as one component of a comprehensive treatment plan.[63] Over the past 10 years, there has been concern about the recent and very dramatic increase in the number of children and adolescents receiving specific classes of psychiatric medications.[64-66] Concern about the use of psychiatric medications with children and adolescents has been complicated by the fact that only a few large clinical trials document the safety and efficacy of psychiatric medications when used in the treatment of children or adolescents. Moreover, most psychiatric medications approved by the US Food and Drug Administration (FDA) for use with children and adolescents have been approved following safety and efficacy testing done over relatively brief periods of time with relatively small samples. Unfortunately, relatively little is presently known about the long-term use of these medications with children and adolescents.

Although the Pediatric Research Equity Act (PREA) and the Best Pharmaceuticals for Children Act (BPCA) have promoted safety and efficacy research on drugs when used with children and adolescents,[67] pediatric drug trials involving psychiatric conditions have been limited,[68] and much of the psychiatric medication prescribed to children and adolescents, particularly second-generation antipsychotic medication, is being prescribed for the treatment of pediatric conditions without approval of the FDA.[65,66,69] Moreover, it is important to note that independent reviews of the existing research suggest that the evidence supporting federal approval of specific drugs for use in the treatment of specific conditions can vary significantly.[70] Consequently, the American Academy of Child and Adolescent Psychiatry has urged prescribers to consider the quality of the safety and efficacy data along with the status of federal approval when choosing psychiatric medications for children and adolescents. Examples of psychiatric medications with demonstrated efficacy and federal approval for use in the treatment of children and adolescents with specific conditions are listed in Table 9.2.

For reasons that are not clear, children and adolescents with Medicaid receiving psychiatric services in the public sector are more likely to receive psychiatric medication than are children and adolescents with commercial insurance receiving services in the private sector.[71] For children and adolescents in the publicly funded system of care, there has also been concern about (1) the use of psychiatric medications at an increasingly early age,[72] (2) use of more than one psychiatric medication simultaneously,[73] and (3) use of psychiatric medications without psychosocial intervention.[74] Similarly, there has been concern about children and adolescents involved with the child welfare system being more likely to receive psychiatric medication[75,76] and relatively consistent ethnic differences in the likelihood that children and adolescents will receive psychiatric medication.[69,72,77,78] For reasons not entirely clear, children and adolescents of African American and Hispanic heritage are less likely than children of European heritage to receive psychiatric medication in the publicly funded system of care.[69,72,77,78]

EMPIRICALLY BASED PRACTICE

Building on concepts concerning the empirical basis for pharmacologic intervention, there is ongoing interest in other dimensions of evidence-based practice within the publicly funded system of care for children and adolescents.[79,80] Throughout the health care system, evidence-based practice is defined as the integration of the best available research with clinical expertise after consideration of the characteristics of the client, cultural factors, and client preference.[81] The goals associated with implementation of evidence-based practice include improving accountability, quality of care, and cost-effectiveness by enhancing clinical assessment, case formulation, the

Table 9.2 EXAMPLES OF PSYCHIATRIC MEDICATIONS WITH FEDERAL APPROVAL FOR USE WITH CHILDREN AND ADOLESCENTS

DISORDER	MEDICATION	TRADE NAME	MINIMUM AGE
Attention deficit hyperactivity disorder	Methylphenidate	Ritalin®	6 years
		Concerta®	6 years
		Daytrana®	6 years
	Dexmethylphenidate	Focalin®	6 years
	Lisdexamfetamine	Vyvanse®	6 years
	Amphetamine	Adderall®	3 years
	Atomoxetine	Strattera®	6 years
	Guanfacine	Intuniv™	6 years
Depressive disorders	Fluoxetine	Prozac®	8 years
	Escitalopram	Lexapro®	12 years
	Amitriptyline	Elavil®	12 years
Obsessive-compulsive disorder	Sertraline	Zoloft®	6 years
	Fluvoxamine	Luvox®	8 years
	Clomipramine	Anafranil®	10 years
Bipolar disorder	Aripiprazole	Abilify®	10 years
	Quetiapine	Seroquel®	10 years
	Lithium	Eskalith®	12 years
Schizophrenia	Risperidone	Risperdal®	13 years
	Paliperidone	Invega®	12 years
	Chlorpromazine	Thorazine®	6 months
Tourette's disorder	Haloperidol	Haldol®	3 years
	Aripiprazole	Abilify®	10 years
Enuresis	Imipramine	Tofranil®	6 years

therapeutic relationship, and clinical intervention.[82] The main elements of evidence-based practice involve (1) the use of evidence-based approaches to engagement, (2) the selection of clinical interventions that have empirical support for use with the target population, (3) formal assessment of targeted outcomes, and (4) ongoing monitoring of response to treatment with sensitivity to the developmental status of the client, cultural beliefs of the family, and treatment preferences of the family.[82]

It is important to note that evidence-based practice is a widely encompassing concept. Narrower concepts involving empirically validated approaches to assessment and treatment are also emphasized within the publicly funded system of care for children and adolescents. Empirically validated assessments and treatments are evaluative and treatment procedures that have undergone standardization, empirical testing, and rigorous review to document their validity when used with a particular population presenting with a particular problem.[83] The two dimensions on which assessments are judged are reliability and validity. Three dimensions on which clinical interventions are judged are (1) clinical utility or the extent to which the treatment is applicable, feasible, and useful; (2) clinical efficacy or the extent to which the treatment works in a research setting; and (3) clinical effectiveness or the extent to which the treatment works when delivered by clinicians in a system of care. The Society for Clinical Child and Adolescent Psychology[84] and SAMHSA[85] maintain resource lists of empirically validated psychosocial treatments for use with children and adolescents experiencing specific forms of emotional-behavioral difficulty. Examples of empirically validated psychosocial treatments for use in the treatment of specific conditions common among children and adolescents are listed in Table 9.3. Although principles of evidence-based practice are more widely accepted, there is ongoing controversy about how to best integrate empirically validated assessments and treatments into the publicly funded system of care for children and adolescents.[86]

SYSTEMIC INTEGRATION

As noted earlier, children and adolescents entering the publicly funded system of care typically present with involvement in other publicly funded service delivery systems. Moreover, the concept of a system of care also values interagency collaboration in the assessment and treatment of serious emotional-behavioral difficulty and seeks ways to actively promote collaboration across service delivery systems.[22,24] Consequently, behavioral health professionals working in the publicly funded system of care for children and adolescents must communicate and collaborate with professionals working in school readiness programs, pediatric clinics, educational settings, juvenile justice programs, child welfare systems, and other community-based programs. When parents also need behavioral health services, there must also be communication and collaboration across the pediatric and adult systems of care. Despite the long-standing emphasis on interagency collaboration,[22,24] repeated calls have been made for better collaboration across service delivery systems that intersect to serve children and adolescents with serious emotional-behavioral difficulty.[30,31] Although policy initiatives, pilot projects, and systemic reforms have been pursued, communication, collaboration, and integration across service delivery systems remain some of

Table 9.3 EXAMPLES OF EMPIRICALLY VALIDATED PSYCHOSOCIAL INTERVENTIONS FOR CHILDREN AND ADOLESCENTS

MODALITY	INDICATION	EXAMPLE
Individual psychotherapy	Traumatic stress	Trauma-Focused Cognitive Behavioral Therapy
	Depression	Interpersonal Psychotherapy for Depressed Adolescents
		TADS Cognitive-Behavioral Therapy
	Social phobia	Coping Cat
Parent intervention	Externalizing difficulty	Parent Management Training
		Parent-Child Interactional Therapy
		Triple P Positive Parenting Program
Family therapy	Externalizing difficulty	Brief Strategic Family Therapy
	Substance abuse	Functional Family Therapy
	Mood disorders	Multi-Family Psychoeducational Psychotherapy
Home-based intervention	Early autism	Lovaas Approach to Applied Behavior Analysis
	Externalizing difficulty	Multidimensional Treatment Foster Care
Multisystemic intervention	Externalizing difficulty	Incredible Years
	Conduct problems	Multisystemic Therapy
	Substance abuse	Multidimensional Family Therapy

Note. This list of examples was extracted from databases maintained by the Society for Clinical Child and Adolescent Psychology[84] and the Substance Abuse and Mental Health Services Administration.[85]

the more daunting challenges facing the publicly funded system of care for children and adolescents.

CAUGHT BETWEEN TWO WORLDS: THE SPECIAL CHALLENGE OF TRANSITIONING YOUTH

As the health care system has become increasingly specialized, gaps between pediatric and adult systems have grown to the extent that Healthy People 2020[87] includes a national goal that calls for adolescents with chronic conditions to receive the services they need to make a successful transition from the pediatric to the adult system of care. For adolescents with serious emotional-behavioral difficulty, this transition from the pediatric to the adult system of care is as complicated as it is for adolescents with other chronic, recurring health problems. As the concept of a system of care has evolved, the sensitive transition of adolescents with serious psychiatric difficulty from the pediatric to the adult system of care has become one of the important principles of effective service delivery.[88]

Given the focus of this textbook, it is important to highlight four trends that have converged in the public sector to make young adults with psychiatric difficulty a special population within the publicly funded systems of care. First, social and economic influences have changed the transition from adolescence to early adulthood. Second, epidemiologic research has more clearly documented the risk for psychiatric difficulty during this transition from adolescence to early adulthood. Third, developmental research has better documented patterns of continuity and discontinuity in psychopathology that begins during childhood, frequently escalates during adolescence, and then continues into early adulthood. Fourth, service delivery systems have, as noted, become more sensitive to the needs of transitioning youth.

CONCEPT OF EMERGING ADULTHOOD

Noting that social, economic, and technological changes have redefined the transition from adolescence to early adulthood, Jeffrey Arnett[89] has argued for the conceptualization of a new period of biopsychosocial development that occurs between 18 and 25–30 years of age when, despite being granted legal status as an adult, young people do not think of themselves as either adolescents or adults. Over approximately 40 years, widespread availability of effective contraception, changing values about premarital sexual relations, demands for postsecondary education, broad acceptance of cohabitation, the high cost of living, and other social forces have contributed to a dramatic delay in the age at which young people meet the traditional developmental milestones of early adulthood,[90,91] thus creating a period during which young people report feeling as if—despite having reached the age of majority—they are still preparing for adulthood.[89] Given these changes, Arnett has argued that this time is substantial enough and distinct enough to now be considered a specific stage of development in technologically advanced cultures. Rejecting other labels in favor of a new description of a new phenomenon, Arnett[89] began calling this phase of life *emerging adulthood* to capture the idea that young people use this time to develop the social and psychological resources they need to successfully negotiate the demands of adulthood in an increasingly complex, technologically oriented culture. Although there has been debate about elements of his position,[92–94] Arnett,[89,95,96] more than anyone else, has focused the attention of developmental researchers on this phase of life, and they are identifying important markers of biopsychosocial development in the areas of neurological development, affective regulation, cognitive capacity, identity development, psychosexual development, vocational-educational planning, and family functioning.[97–101]

CLINICAL EPIDEMIOLOGY

Across the life span, epidemiologic research clearly indicates that risk for the onset of chronic recurring anxiety, mood, and psychotic disorders peaks during emerging adulthood.[102] When substance use disorders are included, the highest rate of behavioral health disorders occurs among young adults aged 18–25 years.[103] Much of the risk within this age group is accounted for by much higher rates of substance use disorders and higher rates of concurrent substance use and psychiatric disorders. Risk for major depression and suicidal ideation are most clearly highest during this developmental period. Epidemiologic data also suggest that substance use, high-risk sexual behavior, sexually transmitted infections, unplanned pregnancy, unemployment, homelessness, and death due to accident, homicide, and suicide rise, peak, and then begin to decline during this developmental period.[104] Within this age group, rates of behavioral health disorders appear to be highest among young people of Native American heritage followed by young people of European, African American, Hispanic, and Asian heritage. Within this age group, approximately 4% of the general population has a serious psychiatric disorder, and serious psychiatric disorders are more common among young women than young men. Consistent with other age groups, substance use disorders are more common among young men. Despite the higher prevalence of behavioral health problems during this phase of life, young adults are less likely than other adults to seek treatment.

DEVELOPMENTAL PERSPECTIVES ON PSYCHOPATHOLOGY

Developmental perspectives on psychopathology have provided a more comprehensive understanding of psychiatric difficulty during emerging adulthood. Longitudinal research done with large samples of children followed through childhood and adolescence into early adulthood suggests that, although serious emotional-behavioral difficulty evident during childhood and adolescence attenuates for many young adults, there can also be a consolidation of psychiatric difficulty, personality disturbance, and social problems during this phase of life that represents risk for persistent difficulty as an adult.[102] As noted earlier, risk for the onset of chronic recurring anxiety, mood, and psychotic disorders peaks during this time of life. Regardless of the course of the psychopathology, developmental research suggests that young adults with a history of psychiatric difficulty are more likely to experience difficulty negotiating developmental challenges associated with the transition to adulthood.[105] They are, for example, less likely to complete high school, less likely to successfully pursue postsecondary education, and less likely to secure stable employment. They are also more likely to be estranged from an unstable, conflictual family of origin without access to the emotional, instrumental, and financial support from family that continues to be important during the transition to adulthood.[106] Relative to their peers, young adults with psychiatric difficulty are also more likely to experience difficulty in sexual partnerships, more likely to marry early, and more likely to become parents early without the social and economic resources necessary to adequately support children. Box 9.3 contains a fictional clinical vignette illustrating the typical presentation of a young adult making the transition from the pediatric to the adult system of care.

GAPS IN SERVICE DELIVERY SYSTEMS

In 2005, the MacArthur Foundation Research Network on Transitions summarized its findings on transitions from child and adolescent to adult systems of care in a book aptly titled, *On Your Own Without a Net*. In that document, D. Wayne Osgood and his colleagues[105] identified seven overlapping groups of transitioning youth at risk to fall through gaps in the human service system during the transition to adulthood: (1) youth involved with the child mental health system, (2) youth in foster care, (3) youth receiving special education services, (4) homeless youth, (5) youth with special medical needs, and (6) youth involved with the juvenile justice system. During this transition to adulthood, vulnerable youth with complex service needs are likely to find that services they need are no longer available, services they need are less available, eligibility for services is defined differently, and the scope of services is dramatically different.[105]

Because young adults leaving the publicly funded system of care for children and adolescents are more likely to have been receiving services in several service delivery systems, disruptions in social support during this transition to early adulthood are likely to have a significant impact on the stability of their social situation. As noted by Osgood and his associates,[105] difficulty managing systemic transitions often increases the risk for educational failure, unemployment, early parenthood, homelessness, criminal activity, victimization, and poverty. Difficulty negotiating systemic issues may also contribute to an escalation of psychiatric difficulty. Moreover, even when young adults make the systemic connections they need, they often find themselves in systems of care oriented to the needs of middle-aged adults working with clinical staff who, because of shortcomings in patterns of professional training, do not fully understand their development as a young adult.[105]

Despite growing interest in the needs of transitioning youth, there are few conceptual models of service delivery for young adults experiencing serious psychiatric difficulty. Policy-makers, researchers, and clinicians have, however, begun efforts to better address gaps in the publicly funded system of care to better address the special needs of transitioning youth with psychiatric difficulty. For example, the US Government Accountability Office[107] undertook a study of transitioning youth with psychiatric difficulty in 2008. A year later, SAMHSA funded the Emerging Adults Initiative,[108,109] which provided funding for seven states to create developmentally informed systems of care designed to better address the needs of transitioning youth. As the first round of grants came to an end, SAMHSA issued another call for proposals to continue the program as part of the *Now Is the Time Plan*[110] to reduce gun violence. As they begin to evolve, the primary goal of specialized services for transitioning youth is to stabilize them, as much as possible, in a community-based system of care for adults in an effort to reduce the personal and social costs of the psychiatric difficulty by promoting developmental

Box 9.3

A Young Adult Entering the Publicly Funded System of Care

Shamika was an 18-year-old, single African American woman who was referred for admission to a special young adult program at a large, urban community mental health center. At the time of her referral, she was living in a group home for teenage girls in the custody of child protective services, and she had just completed her high school education in a special education program for students with serious emotional disturbance.

Shamika had an extensive history of emotional-behavioral difficulty associated with a long history of childhood trauma. Her mother was reportedly a loving parent with a history of recurrent major depressive episodes that frequently required she be hospitalized for psychiatric treatment. Her father was reportedly an angry, alcoholic man who provided financial support for the family through his job as a long-haul truck driver. He was reported to be emotionally and physically abusive with his wife. When 11 years old, Shamika had been removed from the care of both her biological parents after her older sister reported that she, Shamika, and a younger sister were being physically and sexually abused by their father. Although there were early signs of psychosexual difficulty, Shamika had always insisted that, although she knew her father was mistreating her older sister, he had never mistreated her. After removal from her parents' care, Shamika had been placed with a friend of her mother, several other foster placements, and a residential school. As she moved through this series of placements, she acknowledged that she had been sexually abused by a foster mother's boyfriend and a residential counselor.

Presenting problems at the time of her admission to the young adult service included hypervigilance, referential thinking, emotional lability, verbally and physically aggressive behavior with peers, and sexually provocative behavior with male peers and older men. Throughout her medical records, there was documentation that Shamika also suffered from dissociative episodes during which she would behave in sexually provocative ways with limited memory of what had happened. During some of these episodes, she would engage in high-risk sexual behavior with men she did not know. Although interested in monogamous romantic relationships with young men, these encounters had been marked by reciprocal verbal, physical, and sexual aggression. Her relationships with young women were, by her report, generally poor. Upon admission, Shamika was referred for residential placement in a transitional living program, individual psychotherapy, vocational-educational services, occupational therapy, social and recreational activity, and psychiatric consultation. By her report, she was motivated to be responsible for her behavior as an adult, be more independent, leave the child welfare system, have a better relationship with her boyfriend, get a job, attend community college, see her mother more often, and move into her own apartment.

competence. Given current understanding of the target population, evolving programs for transitioning youth need to also develop clear mechanisms to reduce risk for substance abuse, high-risk sexual behavior, vocational-educational failure, homelessness, and premature death by an accident, suicide, or homicide.

With acknowledgment of the early efforts, it is important to note that there are relatively few specialized programs for transitioning youth that have been proved clinically and cost-effective. Although the literature on clinical and systemic outcomes is limited, findings from several federal initiatives suggest that transitioning youth enrolled in specialized programs can make substantial gains.[108,109] Specifically, the SAMHSA reported that 28% of transitioning youth in a special program confirmed significant improvement in emotional-behavioral difficulty during the first 6 months of enrollment, and 38% reported significant improvement in emotional-behavioral difficulty within the first 12 months of enrollment. Rates of homelessness also dropped by 36% over the first 6 months of enrollment for those participants older than 18 years of age, and participants of all ages reported having more confidence in their ability to independently perform important life tasks. Although there is obviously a great deal of conceptual and empirical work to be done as the development of comprehensive programs designed to reduce the psychiatric difficulty and promote normative development during this transition to early adulthood continues, policy-makers, administrators, and clinicians on both sides of the pediatric-to-adult transition in the publicly funded system of care need to consider how to better address the developmental needs of young adults with psychiatric difficulty.

PROFESSIONAL TRAINING: THE SPECIAL CHALLENGE OF WORKFORCE DEVELOPMENT

As policy-makers pay close attention to the education, credentialing, and orientation of the next generation of behavioral health clinicians to work in public psychiatry, there have been consistent calls for more professionals and paraprofessionals competent to work with children, adolescents, and young adults in the publicly funded system of care.[111] Nationally, there are particular needs for child and adolescent psychiatrists and substance abuse counselors prepared to work with adolescents and young adults.[112,113] Although there are clear mechanisms for professional training in clinical work with children and adolescents, there are relatively few structured opportunities for graduate or postgraduate training in clinical work with transitioning youth. Following the general structure of public psychiatry, professional training programs typically identify themselves as focusing on the mental health needs of either children and adolescents or adults. With increased attention to the needs of transitioning youth with serious psychiatric difficulty, there are, however, new programs designed to introduce clinicians to clinical work with transitioning youth entering the publicly funded system of care for adults. The rest of this section focuses on professional preparation in the traditional behavioral health disciplines of psychiatry, psychology, nursing, and social work. It is, however, important to note that marriage and family counselors, licensed professional counselors, occupational therapists, other credentialed professionals, and an array of paraprofessionals also work within the publicly funded system of care for children, adolescents, and young adults.

CHILD AND ADOLESCENT PSYCHIATRY

Career paths to child and adolescent psychiatry typically involve completion of medical school, a general psychiatry residency, a child and adolescent psychiatry fellowship, a license to practice medicine, and board certification in child and adolescent psychiatry. The American Council on Graduate Medical Education accredits general psychiatry residency programs and child and adolescent psychiatry fellowships. At this time, there are approximately 130 accredited child and adolescent psychiatry fellowships.[114] Traditionally, this involves 2 years of specialty training after 3 or 4 years of a general psychiatry residency. Some programs also offer an integrated program in which both adult and child and adolescent training are completed in 5 years, and there are combined programs in pediatrics and child and adolescent psychiatry. Psychiatric residency training programs are, however, most frequently based on traditional ideas about psychosocial development that hold that adolescence ends and adulthood begins at 18 years of age. Consequently, neither adult nor child and adolescent programs typically include focused training in the delivery of developmentally informed services to young adults. With the ongoing development of clinical programming to better meet the needs of transitioning youth with serious psychiatric difficulty, special rotations on young adult services are beginning to be offered on a limited basis to child and adolescent and adult psychiatry residents. Following completion of residency, the American Board of Psychiatry and Neurology offers specialty certification in child and adolescent psychiatry,[115] and the American Academy of Child and Adolescent Psychiatry has a program to recognize distinguished fellows for their contribution to the specialty.[116]

CLINICAL CHILD AND ADOLESCENT PSYCHOLOGY

Career paths to clinical child and adolescent psychology typically involve a doctoral degree in professional psychology, a doctoral internship and postdoctoral fellowship in clinical child and adolescent psychology, and licensure as a professional psychologist. Most often, students earn a doctoral degree in clinical psychology in a program that allows for a focus on clinical child and adolescent psychology. There are also some combined programs in clinical and school psychology or clinical and developmental psychology. Students usually earn either a doctor of philosophy or doctor of psychology degree. The American Psychological Association (APA) accredits both doctoral training programs and doctoral internships.[117,118] The Society for Clinical Child and Adolescent Psychology maintains a list of APA-accredited doctoral internships and postdoctoral fellowships in clinical child and adolescent psychology,[119] and the American Board of Clinical Child and Adolescent Psychology offers board certification for advanced practice with children and adolescents.[120] Although not systematically addressed in doctoral training programs in clinical psychology, doctoral internships and postdoctoral fellowships focusing on clinical work with young adults have begun to emerge,[121] and the Society for Clinical Child and Adolescent Psychology recently began a special interest group for clinicians, researchers, and educators interested in clinical work with young adults.[122]

ADVANCED PRACTICE NURSING

Career paths to psychiatric nursing typically involve a bachelor of science degree in nursing, a master of science or doctorate of nursing practice degree in psychiatric-mental health nursing, national certification, and licensure as an advance practice registered nurse or nurse practitioner.[123] Requirements for licensure vary from state to state. Although the American Association of Colleges of Nursing recommends the entry-level credential for advanced practice nursing be the doctorate of nursing practice degree by 2015,[124] most states have not changed the minimum requirements for licensure. The Commission on Collegiate Nursing Education accredits graduate training programs,[125] and the American Nurses Association provides board certification for psychiatric-mental health nurse practitioners with a life span focus and child and adolescent psychiatric-mental health clinical nurse specialists through the American Nurses Credentialing Center.[126] Although board certification as a psychiatric-mental health nurse practitioner allows for practice across the life span, psychiatric nursing does not yet have any professional initiatives devoted specifically to meeting the needs of young adults.

PSYCHIATRIC SOCIAL WORK

Career paths to psychiatric social work with children and adolescents typically involve a master of social work degree involving 2 years of graduate study with field placements in a system of care. Under some circumstances, a bachelor and master of social work degree can be completed in 5 years. Programs of study are accredited by the Council on Social Work Education,[127] and some programs offer a specialty track or specialty concentration for students interested in working with children, adolescents, and their families in a variety of settings. Students interested in clinical work with children and adolescents can also usually choose field placements in settings that offer psychiatric services to children and adolescents. Following graduation, most states require a period of supervised practice before licensure. Again, professionals interested in establishing credentials as a child and adolescent clinician can complete that period of supervised practice in a setting that offers psychiatric services to children and adolescents. Some clinical settings offer a postgraduate fellowship in psychiatric social work with children and adolescents. The National Association of Social Workers has a specialty section on practice with children, adolescents, and young adults,[128] and the organization offers an advanced certification in practice with children and adolescents.[129]

SUMMARY

Over more than 100 years, the publicly funded system of care for children and adolescents with serious emotional-behavioral difficulty has evolved from historical roots that differ rather dramatically from those of the publicly funded system of care for adults. Despite the historical differences, the publicly funded systems of care for children, adolescents, and adults share some guiding principles. Within the publicly funded system of care for children and adolescents, the concept of a system of care has, more than anything else, influenced the development of the service delivery system. Despite efforts to develop a coordinated system of care for children and adolescents, problems with access and engagement continue, and most children and adolescents experiencing psychiatric difficulty do not receive appropriate services.

When caregivers do seek services, children and adolescents entering the publicly funded system of care typically present with both acute and chronic difficulty characterized by internalizing pathology, externalizing pathology, and substance abuse. Psychopathology is typically complicated by social problems associated with poverty, and concurrent involvement with other service delivery systems is common. Although the system of care for children and adolescents faces a number of challenges emanating from within and outside the system, there are special challenges associated with workforce development and the need to better bridge systems of care for adolescents whose psychiatric difficulty persists during the transition to early adulthood. To better serve adults seeking assistance within the publicly funded system of care, behavioral health professionals need to have a good basic understanding of developmental perspectives on psychopathology and the publicly funded system of care for children, adolescents, and young adults so that they are in a better position to provide empirically based assessment and intervention in a complex health care system that typically separates the care of children and adolescents from the care of adults.

REFERENCES

1. American Academy of Pediatrics, American Academy of Family Physicians, American College of Physicians: American Society of Internal Medicine. A consensus statement on health care transitions for young adults with special health care needs. *Pediatrics*. 2002;110(6 pt 2):1304–1306.
2. Rutter M, Kim-Cohen J, Maughan B. Continuities and discontinuities in psychopathology between childhood and adult life. *J Child Psychol Psychiatry*. 2006;47(3–4):276–295.
3. Lourie IS, Hernandez, M. A historical perspective on national child mental health policy. *J Emot Behav Disord*. 2003;11(1):5–9.
4. White SH. G. Stanley Hall: From philosophy to developmental psychology. *Dev Psychol*. 1992;28(1):25–34.
5. Smuts AB. *Science in the Service of Children, 1893–1935*. New Haven, CT: Yale University Press; 2006.
6. Horn M. *Before It's Too Late: The Child Guidance Movement in the United States, 1922–1945*. Philadelphia: Temple University Press; 1989.

7. Levy DM. Critical evaluation of the present state of child psychiatry. *Arch Gen Psychiatry.* 1952;108(7):481-494.
8. Geissman C, Geissmann P. *A History of Child Psychoanalysis.* New York: Psychology Press; 1998.
9. Reubins BM. *Pioneers of Child Psychoanalysis: Influential Theories and Practices in Healthy Child Development.* London: Karnac; 2014.
10. Ludwig-Körner C. Anna Freud and her collaborators in the early post-war period. In: Malberg NT, Raphael-Leff J, eds. *The Anna Freud Tradition: Lines of Development. Evolution of Theory and Practice over the Decades.* London: Karnac; 2012:17-29.
11. Pretorius IM. From the Hampstead War Nurseries to the Anna Freud Centre. In: Malberg NT, Raphael-Leff J, eds. *The Anna Freud Tradition: Lines of Development. Evolution of Theory and Practice over the Decades.* London: Karnac; 2012:30-37.
12. Friedlander K. Psychoanalytic orientation in child guidance work in Great Britain. *Psychoanal Study Child.* 1945;2:343-357.
13. Joint Commission on Mental Health and Illness. *Action for Mental Health.* New York: Basic Books; 1961.
14. Rosenblum G. Can children's services flourish in a comprehensive community mental health center program? *J Am Acad Child Adolesc Psychiatry.* 1969;8(3):485-492.
15. Lourie IS, Katz-Levy J, DeCarolis G, Quinlan W. The role of the federal government. In: Stroul BA, ed. *Children's Mental Health: Creating Systems of Care in a Changing Society.* Baltimore, MD: Paul H. Brooks; 1996:99-114.
16. Joint Commission on the Mental Health of Children. *Crisis in Child Mental Health.* New York: Harper and Row; 1969.
17. Howell EM. *Access to Children's Mental Health Services under Medicaid and SCHIP.* Washington, DC: Urban Institute; 2004. http://www.urban.org/uploadedpdf/311053_b-60.pdf. Accessed January 24, 2015.
18. Hutchinson AB, Foster EM. The effect of Medicaid managed care on mental health care for children: a review of the literature. *Ment Health Serv Res.* 2003;5(1):39-54.
19. Rowland D, Garfield R, Elias R. Accomplishments and challenges in Medicaid mental health. *Health Aff.* 2003;22(5):73-83.
20. Pires SA, Grimes K, Gilmer T, Allen K, Mahadevan R, Hendricks T. *Identifying Opportunities To Improve Children's Behavioral Health Care: An Analysis of Medicaid Utilization and Expenditures.* Hamilton, NJ: Center for Health Care Strategies; 2013. http://www.chcs.org/media/identifying-opportunities-to-improve-childrens-behavioral-health-care2.pdf. Accessed January 24, 2015.
21. Knitzer J. *Unclaimed Children: The Failure of Public Responsibility to Children and Adolescents in Need of Mental Health Services.* Washington, DC: Children's Defense Fund; 1982.
22. Stroul BA, Friedman R. *A System of Care for Children and Youth with Severe Emotional Disturbances.* Washington, DC: National Technical Assistance Center for Children's Mental Health, Georgetown University Child Development Center; 1986.
23. Center for Mental Health Services, Substance Abuse and Mental Health Services Administration Center for Mental Health Services, US Department of Health and Human Services. *The Comprehensive Community Mental Health Services for Children and Their Families Program: Evaluation Findings (Report to Congress 2011).* Rockville, MD: Center for Mental Health Services; November 2013. PEP13-CMHI2011. https://store.samhsa.gov/shin/content/pep13-cmhi2011/pep13-cmhi2011.pdf. Accessed January 20, 2015.
24. Stroul BA, Friedman RM. The system of care concept and philosophy. In: Stroul BA, ed. *Children's Mental Health: Creating Systems of Care in a Changing Society.* Baltimore, MD: Paul H. Brookes; 1996:3-21.
25. Stroul BA. *System of Care: A Framework for System Reform in Children's Mental Health.* Washington, DC: National Technical Assistance Center for Children's Mental Health, Georgetown University Child Development Center; 2002. http://gucchd.georgetown.edu/products/socissuebrief.pdf. Accessed January 20, 2015.
26. Stroul BA, Blau G, Sondheimer D. Systems of care: A strategy to transform children's mental health care. In: Stroul BA, Blau G, eds. *The System of Care Handbook: Transforming Mental Health Services for Children, Youth, and Families.* Baltimore, MD: Paul H. Brookes; 2008:3-24.
27. Pires SA. *Building Systems of Care: A Primer.* 2nd ed. Washington, DC: National Technical Assistance Center for Children's Mental Health, Georgetown University Child Development Center; 2010.
28. Center for Mental Health Services, Substance Abuse and Mental Health Services Administration, US Department of Health and Human Services. *Helping Children and Youth with Serious Mental Health Needs: Systems of Care.* Rockville, MD: Center for Mental Health Services; January 2006. SMA06-4125.
29. Huang L, Stroul BA, Friedman R, et al. Transforming mental health care for children and their families. *Am Psychol.* 2005;60(6):615-627.
30. Hodges S, Ferreira K, Israel N, Mazza J. Systems of care, featherless bipeds, and the measure of all things. *Eval Program Plann.* 2010;33(1):4-10.
31. Stroul BA, Blau G, Friedman R. *Updating the System of Care Concept and Philosophy.* Washington, DC: National Technical Assistance Center for Children's Mental Health, Georgetown University Center for Child and Human Development; 2010.
32. Pires SA. *Customizing Health Homes for Children with Serious Behavioral Health Challenges.* Rockville, MD: Substance Abuse and Mental Health Services Administration; March 2013. http://gucchdgeorgetown.net/data/issues/2013/0413_article.html. Accessed January 20, 2015.
33. Pires SA, Ignelzi, S. The role of the state in system development. In: Stroul BA, ed. *Children's Mental Health: Creating Systems of Care in a Changing Society.* Baltimore, MD: Paul H. Brooks; 1996:115-130.
34. Stroul BA. Profiles of local systems of care. In: Stroul BA, ed. *Children's Mental Health: Creating Systems of Care in a Changing Society.* Baltimore, MD: Paul H. Brooks; 1996:149-176.
35. Hoagwood KE, Olin SS, Horwitz S, et al. Scaling up evidence-based practices for children and families in New York State: toward evidence-based policies on implementation for state mental health systems. *J Clin Child Psychol.* 2014;43(2):145-157.
36. Georgetown University Center for Child and Human Development. *National Technical Assistance Center for Children's Mental Health.* http://gucchd.georgetown.edu/67211.html. Published September 8, 2009. Updated July 22, 2014. Accessed January 20, 2015.
37. Merikangas KR, He JP, Brody D, Fisher PW, Bourdon K, Koretz DS. Prevalence and treatment of mental disorders among US children in the 2001-2004 NHANES. *Pediatrics.* 2010;125(1):75-81.
38. Centers for Disease Control and Prevention, US Department of Health and Human Services. Mental health surveillance among children: United States, 2005-2011. *Morb Mortal Wkly Rep Surveill Summ.* 2013, May 17;62(Suppl 2):1-35.
39. Costello EJ, Mustillo S, Erkanli A, Keeler G, Angold A. Prevalence and development of psychiatric disorders in childhood and adolescence. *Arch Gen Psychiatry.* 2003;60(8):837-844.
40. Merikangas KR, He JP, Burstein M, et al. Lifetime prevalence of mental disorders in US adolescents: results from the National Comorbidity Survey Replication-Adolescent Supplement (NCS-A). *J Am Acad Child Adolesc Psychiatry.* 2010;49(10):980-989.
41. Roemer M. *Health Care Expenditures for the Five Most Common Children's Conditions, 2008: Estimates for US Civilian Noninstitutionalized Children, Ages 0-17.* Rockville, MD: Agency for Healthcare Research and Quality; December 2011. http://www.meps.ahrq.gov/mepsweb/data_files/publications/st349/stat349.pdf. Accessed January 20, 2015.
42. National Research Council, Institute of Medicine. *Preventing Mental, Emotional, and Behavioral Disorders among Young People: Progress and Possibilities.* Washington, DC: National Academies Press; 2009.
43. Kataoka SH, Zhang L, Wells KB. Unmet need for mental health care among US children: variation by ethnicity and insurance status. *Am J Psychiatry.* 2002;159(9):1548-1555.

44. Costello EJ, He JP, Sampson NA, Kessler RC, Merikangas KR. Services for adolescents with psychiatric disorders: 12-month data from the National Comorbidity Survey-Adolescent. *Psychiatr Serv.* 2014;65(3):359–366.
45. American Psychiatric Association. *Diagnostic and Statistical Manual of Mental Disorders.* 5th ed. Arlington, VA: American Psychiatric Association; 2013.
46. D'Andrea W, Ford J, Stolbach B, Spinazzola J, van der Kolk BA. Understanding interpersonal trauma in children: why we need a developmentally appropriate trauma diagnosis. *Am J Orthopsychiatry.* 2012;82(2):187–200.
47. Masi R, Cooper J. *Children's Mental Health: Facts for Policymakers.* New York: National Center for Children in Poverty, Mailman School of Public Health, Columbia University; 2006.
48. Stagman SM, Cooper JL. *Children's Mental Health: What Every Policymaker Should Know.* New York: National Center for Children in Poverty, Mailman School of Public Health, Columbia University; 2010.
49. Zimmerman FJ. Social and economic determinants of disparities in professional help-seeking for child mental health problems: evidence from a national sample. *Health Serv Res.* 2005;40(5):1514–1533.
50. Owens PL, Hoagwood K, Horwitz SM, et al. Barriers to children's mental health services. *J Am Acad Child Adolesc Psychiatry.* 2002;41(6):731–738.
51. Benway CB, Hamrin V, McMahon TJ. Initial appointment nonattendance in child and family mental health clinics. *Am J Orthopsychiatry.* 2003;73(4); 419–428.
52. Kazdin A, Holland L, Crowley M, Breton S. Barriers to treatment participation scale: evaluation and validation in the context of child outpatient treatment. *J Child Psychol Psychiatry.* 1997;38(8):1051–1062.
53. Lindsey MA, Brandt NE, Becker KD, et al. Identifying the common elements of treatment engagement interventions in children's mental health services. *Clin Child Fam Psychol Rev.* 2014;17(3):283–298.
54. Becker KD, Lee BR, Daleiden EL, Lindsey M, Brandt NE, Chorpita BF. The common elements of engagement in children's mental health services: which elements for which outcomes? *J Clin Child Psychol.* 2015;44(1):30–43.
55. World Health Organization. *International Classification of Diseases.* http://apps.who.int/classifications/icd10/browse/2015/en. Published November 4, 2014. Updated August 11, 2015. Accessed September 6, 2015.
56. Sameroff AJ. Developmental systems and psychopathology. *Dev Psychopathol.* 2000;12(3):297–312.
57. Carlson GA, Klein DN. How to understand divergent views on bipolar disorder in youth. *Annu Rev Clin Psychol.* 2014;10:529–551.
58. James A, Hoang U, Seagroatt V, Clacey J, Goldacre M, Leibenluft E. A comparison of American and English hospital discharge rates for pediatric bipolar disorder, 2000 to 2010. *J Am Acad Child Adolesc Psychiatry.* 2014;53(6):614–624.
59. Moreno C, Laje G, Blanco C, Jiang H, Schmidt AB, Olfson M: National trends in the outpatient diagnosis and treatment of bipolar disorder in youth. *Arch Gen Psychiatry.* 2007;64(9):1032–1039.
60. Narrow WE, Clarke DE, Kuramoto SJ, et al. DSM-5 field trials in the United States and Canada: development and reliability testing of a cross-cutting symptom assessment for DSM-5. *Am J Psychiatry.* 2013;170(1):71–82.
61. Ghaziuddin M. (2010). Brief report: should the DSM V drop Asperger syndrome? *J Autism Dev Disord.* 2010;40(9): 1146–1148.
62. Axelson DA, Birmaher B, Findling RL, et al. Concerns regarding the inclusion of temper dysregulation disorder with dysphoria in the Diagnostic and Statistical Manual of Mental Disorders. *J Clin Psychiatry.* 2011;72(9):1257–1262.
63. American Academy of Child and Adolescent Psychiatry. *Guide for Community Child Serving Agencies on Psychotropic Medications for Children and Adolescents.* Washington, DC: American Academy of Child and Adolescent Psychiatry; February 2012. http://www.aacap.org/app_themes/aacap/docs/press/guide_for_community_child_serving_agencies_on_psychotropic_medications_for_children_and_adolescents_2012.pdf. Accessed January 20, 2015.
64. Zuvekas SH, Vitiello B. Stimulant medication use in children: a 12-year perspective. *Am J Psychiatry.* 2012;169(2):160–166.
65. Olfson M, Blanco C, Liu SM, Wang S, Correll CU. National trends in the office-based treatment of children, adolescents, and adults with antipsychotics. *Arch Gen Psychiatry.* 2012;69(12):1247–1256.
66. Matone M, Localio R, Huang YS, dosReis S, Feudtner C, Rubin D. The relationship between mental health diagnosis and treatment with second-generation antipsychotics over time: a national study of US Medicaid-enrolled children. *Health Serv Res.* 2012;47(5):1836–1860.
67. Institute of Medicine. *Safe and Effective Medicines for Children: Pediatric Studies Conducted Under the Best Pharmaceuticals for Children Act and the Pediatric Research Equity Act.* Washington, DC: National Academies Press; 2012.
68. Murthy S, Mandl KD, Bourgeois F. Analysis of pediatric clinical drug trials for neuropsychiatric conditions. *Pediatrics.* 2013;131(6):1125–1131.
69. Zito JM, Burcu M, Ibe A, Safer DJ, Magder LS. Antipsychotic use by Medicaid-insured youths: impact of eligibility and psychiatric diagnosis across a decade. *Psychiatr Serv.* 2013;64(3):223–229.
70. Lorberg B, Robb A, Pavuluri M, Chen DTW, Wilens T. Pediatric psychopharmacology: Food and Drug Administration approval through the evidence lens. *J Am Acad Child Adolesc Psychiatry.* 2014;53(7):716–718.
71. US Government Accounting Office. *Children's Mental Health: Concerns Remain about Appropriate Services for Children in Medicaid and Foster Care.* Washington, DC: US Government Accounting Office; December 2012. GAO-13-15. http://www.gao.gov/assets/660/650716.pdf. Accessed January 20, 2015.
72. Chirdkiatgumchai V, Xiao H, Fredstrom BK, et al. National trends in psychotropic medication use in young children: 1994–2009. *Pediatrics.* 2013;132(4):615–623.
73. Comer JS, Olfson M, Mojtabai R. National trends in child and adolescent psychotropic polypharmacy in office-based practice, 1996–2007. *J Am Acad Child Adolesc Psychiatry.* 2010;49(10):1001–1010.
74. Harris E, Sorbero M, Kogan JN, Schuster J, Stein BD. Concurrent mental health therapy among Medicaid-enrolled youths starting antipsychotic medications. *Psychiatr Serv.* 2012;63(4):351–356.
75. Burcu M, Zito JM, Ibe A, Safer DJ. Atypical antipsychotic use among Medicaid-insured children and adolescents: duration, safety, and monitoring implications. *J Child Adolesc Psychopharmacol.* 2014;24(3):112–119.
76. US Government Accounting Office. *Foster Children: HHS Guidance Could Help States Improve Oversight of Psychotropic Prescriptions.* Washington, DC: US Government Accounting Office; December 2011. GAO-12-270T. http://www.gao.gov/products/gao-12-270t. Accessed January 20, 2015.
77. Zito J, Safer DJ, dosReis, S, Riddle MA. Racial disparity in psychotropic medications prescribed for youths with Medicaid insurance in Maryland. *J Am Acad Child Adolesc Psychiatry.* 1998;37(2):179–184.
78. Raghavan R, Brown DS, Allaire BT, Garfield LD, Ross RE, Snowden LR. Racial/ethnic differences in Medicaid expenditures on psychotropic medications among maltreated children. *Child Abuse Negl.* 2014;38(6); 1002–1010.
79. Hoagwood K, Burns BJ, Kiser L, Ringeisen H, Schoenwald SK. Evidence-based practice in child and adolescent mental health services. *Psychiatr Serv.* 2001;52(9):1179–1189.
80. Kazak AE, Hoagwood K, Weisz JR, et al. A meta-systems approach to evidence-based practice for children and adolescents. *Am Psychol.* 2010;65(2):85–97.

81. Evidence-Based Medicine Working Group. Evidence-based medicine: a new approach to teaching the practice of medicine. *JAMA*. November 1992;268(17):2420–2425.
82. American Psychological Association Presidential Task Force on Evidence-Based Practice. Evidence-based practice in psychology. *Am Psychol*. 2006;61(4):271–285.
83. Chorpita BF, Daleiden EL, Ebesutani C, et al. Evidence-based treatments for children and adolescents: an updated review of indicators of efficacy and effectiveness. *Clin Psychol*. 2011;18(2):154–172.
84. Society for Clinical Child and Adolescent Psychology. *Effective Child Therapy: Evidence-Based Mental Health Treatment for Children and Adolescents*. http://effectivechildtherapy.com. Published January 4, 2003. Updated December 20, 2014. Accessed January 20, 2015.
85. Substance Abuse and Mental Health Services Administration, US Department of Health and Human Services. *National Registry of Evidence-Based Programs and Practices*. http://www.nrepp.samhsa.gov/Index.aspx. Published September 22, 2006. Updated December 24, 2014. Accessed January 20, 2015.
86. American Psychological Association Task Force on Evidence-Based Practice for Children and Adolescents. *Disseminating Evidence-Based Practice for Children and Adolescents: A Systems Approach to Enhancing Care*. Washington, DC: American Psychological Association; 2008. http://www.apa.org/practice/resources/evidence/children-report.pdf. Accessed January 20, 2015.
87. US Public Health Service, US Department of Health and Human Services. *Healthy People 2020*. https://www.healthypeople.gov. Published October 3, 2000. Updated January 4, 2015. Accessed January 20, 2015.
88. Cooper JL, Aratani Y, Knitzer J, et al. *Unclaimed children revisited: The status of children's mental health policy in the United States*. New York: National Center for Children in Poverty, Mailman School of Public Health, Columbia University; November 2008. http://www.nccp.org/publications/pdf/text_853.pdf. Accessed January 20, 2015.
89. Arnett JJ. Emerging adulthood: a theory of development from the late teens through the twenties. *Am Psychol*. 2000;55(5):469–480.
90. Furstenberg FF. On a new schedule: transitions to adulthood and family change. *Future Child*. 2010;20(1):67–87.
91. Settersten RA, Ray B. What's going on with young people today? The long and twisting path to adulthood. *Future Child*. 2010;20(1):19–41.
92. Hendry LB, Kloep M. Examining emerging adulthood: investigating the emperor's new clothes? *Child Dev Perspect*. 2007;1(2):74–79.
93. Kloep M, Hendry LB. A systemic approach to the transitions to adulthood. In: Arnett JJ, Kloep M, Hendry LB, Tanner JL, eds. *Debating Emerging Adulthood: Stage or Process?* Oxford: Oxford University Press; 2011:53–76.
94. Kloep M, Hendry LB. Rejoinder to chapters 2 and 3: critical comments on Arnett's and Tanner's approach. In: Arnett JJ, Kloep M, Hendry LB, Tanner JL, eds. *Debating Emerging Adulthood: Stage or Process?* Oxford: Oxford University Press; 2011:107–120.
95. Arnett JJ. Emerging adulthood: what is it, and what is it good for? *Child Dev Perspect*. 2007;1(2):68–73.
96. Tanner JL, Arnett JJ. Presenting "emerging adulthood:" what makes it developmentally distinctive? In: Arnett JJ, Kloep M, Hendry LB, Tanner JL, eds. *Debating Emerging Adulthood: Stage or Process?* Oxford: Oxford University Press; 2011:13–30.
97. Halpern-Meekin S, Manning WD, Giordano PC, Longmore MA. Relationship churning, physical violence, and verbal abuse in young adult relationships. *J Marriage Fam*. 2013;75(1):2–12.
98. Masten AS, Desjardins CD, McCormick CM, Kuo SI, Long JD. The significance of childhood competence and problems for adult success in work: a developmental cascade analysis. *Dev Psychopathol*. 2010;22(3):679–694.
99. Schulenberg JE, Bryant AL, O'Malley PM. (2004). Taking hold of some kind of life: how developmental tasks relate to trajectories of well-being during the transition to adulthood. *Dev Psychopathol*. 2004;16(4):1119–1140.
100. Tanner JL. Recentering during emerging adulthood: a critical turning point in life span human development. In: Arnett JJ, Tanner JL, eds. *Emerging Adults in America: Coming of Age in the 21st Century*. Washington, DC: American Psychological Association; 2006:21–55.
101. Tsai, KM, Telzer, EH, Fuligni AJ. Continuity and discontinuity in perceptions of family relationships from adolescence to young adulthood. *Child Dev*. 2013;84(2):471–484.
102. Schulenberg JE, Zarrett NR. Mental health during emerging adulthood: continuity and discontinuity in courses, causes, and functions. In: Arnett JJ, Tanner JL, eds. *Emerging Adults in America: Coming of Age in the 21st Century*. Washington, DC: American Psychological Association; 2006:135–172.
103. Substance Abuse and Mental Health Services Administration, US Department of Health and Human Services. *Results from the 2013 National Survey on Drug Use and Health: Mental Health Findings*. Rockville, MD: Substance Abuse and Mental Health Services Administration; 2014. SMA 14-4887. http://www.samhsa.gov/data/sites/default/files/nsduhmhfr2013/nsduhmhfr2013.pdf. Accessed January 26, 2015.
104. National Research Council, Institute of Medicine. *Improving the Health, Safety, and Well-Being of Young Adults: Workshop Summary*. Washington, DC: National Academies Press; 2013.
105. Osgood DW, Foster EM, Flanagan C, Ruth GR, eds. *On Your Own without a Net: The Transition to Adulthood for Vulnerable Populations*. Chicago: University of Chicago Press; 2005.
106. Schoeni RF, Ross KE. *Material Assistance from Families During the Transition to Adulthood*. Chicago: University of Chicago Press; 2005.
107. US Government Accountability Office. *Young Adults with Serious Mental Illness: Some States and Federal Agencies Are Taking Steps to Address Their Transition Challenges*. Washington, DC: US Government Accountability Office; June 2008. GAO-08-678. http://www.gao.gov/assets/280/277167.pdf. Accessed January 20, 2015.
108. Substance Abuse and Mental Health Services Administration, US Department of Health and Human Services. *Promoting Recovery and Independence for Older Adolescents and Young Adults Who Experience Serious Mental Health Challenges*. Rockville, MD: Substance Abuse and Mental Health Services Administration; May 2013. SMA-13-4756. http://www.samhsa.gov/sites/default/files/samhsa_short_report_2013.pdf. Accessed January 20, 2015.
109. Substance Abuse and Mental Health Services Administration, US Department of Health and Human Services. From youth to adulthood: offering help. *SAMHSA News*. Summer 2014;22(3). http://www.samhsa.gov/samhsanewsletter/volume_22_number_3/successful_transition. Accessed January 20, 2015.
110. Substance Abuse and Mental Health Services Administration, US Department of Health and Human Services. *"Now is the Time" Healthy Transitions: Improving Life Trajectories for Youth and Young Adults with, or at Risk for, Serious Mental Health Conditions*. SM-14-017. http://www.samhsa.gov/grants/grant-announcements/sm-14-017. Published April 11, 2014. Accessed January 20, 2015.
111. Huang L, Macbeth G, Dodge J, Jacobstein D. Transforming the workforce in children's mental health. *Adm Policy Ment Health*. 2004;32(2):167–187.
112. Kim WJ. Child and adolescent psychiatry workforce: a critical shortage and national challenge. *Acad Psychiatry*. 2003;27(4):277–282.
113. Thomas CR, Holzer CE. The continuing shortage of child and adolescent psychiatrists. *J Am Acad Child Adolesc Psychiatry*. 2006;45(9):1023–1031.
114. Accreditation Council for Graduate Medical Education. *ACGME Graduate Medical Education Data Resource Book: Academic Year 2013–2014*. Chicago: Accreditation Council for Graduate Medical Education; September 2014. http://acgme.org/acgmeweb/

tabid/259/graduatemedicaleducation/graduatemedicaleducationdataresourcebook.aspx. Accessed January 20, 2015.
115. American Board of Psychiatry and Neurology. *Child and Adolescent Psychiatry.* http://www.abpn.com/sub_cap.html. Published October 5, 2011. Updated August 21, 2014. Accessed January 20, 2015.
116. American Academy of Child and Adolescent Psychiatry. *How to Become an AACAP Distinguished Fellow.* http://www.aacap.org/aacap/member_resources/fellowship/how.aspx. Accessed January 20, 2015.
117. American Psychological Association. Accredited doctoral programs in professional psychology: 2014. *Am Psychol.* 2014;69(9):911–926.
118. American Psychological Association. Accredited internship and postdoctoral programs for training in psychology: 2014. *Am Psychol.* 2014; 69(9):881–910.
119. Society of Clinical Child and Adolescent Psychology. *Internship and Postdoctoral Positions.* https://www.clinicalchildpsychology.org/internships_postdocs. Published April 27, 2015. Accessed September 6, 2015.
120. American Board of Clinical Child and Adolescent Psychology. *American Board of Clinical Child and Adolescent Psychology: A Member of the American Board of Professional Psychology.* http://www.clinicalchildpsychology.com. Published June 28, 2002. Updated December 19, 2014. Accessed January 20, 2015.
121. Psychology Section, Department of Psychiatry, Yale University School of Medicine. *Young Adult Services.* http://medicine.yale.edu/psychiatry/psychology/predoc/sites/cmhc/youngadult.aspx. Published June 30, 2014. Updated September 3, 2014. Accessed January 20, 2015.
122. Society of Clinical Child and Adolescent Psychology. *Emerging Adulthood Special Interest Group.* https://www.clinicalchildpsychology.org/emerging-adulthood-special-interest-group. Accessed January 20, 2015.
123. American Psychiatric Nurses Association, International Society of Psychiatric-Mental Health Nurses. *Psychiatric-Mental Health Nursing: Scope and Standards of Practice, 2014 Edition.* Falls Church, VA: Author; 2014.
124. Auerbach DI, Martsolf G, Pearson ML, et al. *The DNP by 2015: A Study of the Institutional, Political, and Professional Issues that Facilitate or Impede Establishing a Post-Baccalaureate Doctor of Nursing Practice Program.* Santa Monica, CA: Rand Corporation; 2014. http://www.aacn.nche.edu/dnp/dnp-study.pdf. Accessed January 20, 2015.
125. American Association of Colleges of Nursing. *Find Accredited Programs.* http://www.aacn.nche.edu/ccne-accreditation/accredited-programs. Published October 15, 2011. Updated January 16, 2015. Accessed January 20, 2015.
126. American Nurses Credentialing Center. *Psychiatric-Mental Health Nurse Practitioner (Across the Lifespan).* http://www.nursecredentialing.org/familypsychmentalhealthnp. Published June 8, 2013. Updated July 11, 2014. Accessed January 20, 2015.
127. Council on Social Work Education. *Directory of Accredited Programs.* http://www.cswe.org/17491.aspx. Published July 18, 2013. Updated June 28, 2014. Accessed January 20, 2015.
128. National Association of Social Workers. *Specialty Practice Sections.* http://www.naswdc.org/sections. Published February 24, 2003. Updated July 16, 2014. Accessed January 20, 2015.
129. National Association of Social Workers. *The Certified Advanced Children, Youth, and Family Social Worker (C-ACYFSW).* http://www.naswdc.org/credentials/specialty/C-ACYFSW.asp. Published December 21, 2003. Updated October 3, 2013. Accessed January 20, 2015.

10.

EARLY INTERVENTION AND PREVENTION FOR PSYCHOTIC DISORDERS

Jessica M. Pollard, Cenk Tek, Scott W. Woods, Thomas H. McGlashan, and Vinod H. Srihari

EDUCATIONAL HIGHLIGHTS

- Psychotic disorders like schizophrenia are costly and, historically, have typically been disabling.
- Treatments earlier in the course of psychotic disorders have a greater impact on illness trajectory and long-term functioning.
- Duration of untreated psychosis (DUP) is the length of time between onset of active psychotic symptoms and connection to appropriate psychiatric care.
- Long DUP is associated with negative outcomes, including suicide, poor functioning, diminished response to antipsychotic medication, and reduced quality of life.
- Early detection (ED) aims to shorten DUP and includes outreach and education campaigns that can reduce harmful delays in accessing care after psychosis onset.
- Early intervention (EI) includes both ED and programs that attempt to systematically deliver empirically based treatments to those presenting with a first episode of psychosis.
- Predicting who is at ultra-high risk of developing psychotic disorders and preventing or delaying their onset has been demonstrated. Accuracy is improving with the accumulation of large datasets and biological measures.

INTRODUCTION

Psychotic disorders are a source of significant distress, disability, and cost under usual systems of care. Each year in the United States, approximately 100,000 young persons will experience the onset of a chronic psychotic disorder.[1] Schizophrenia spectrum disorders rank among the top 20 sources of Years Lived with Disability (YLD) worldwide and constitute the single largest driver of health care costs among serious mental illnesses in the United States.[2] Despite advances in treatment, the majority of patients with schizophrenia endure partial remission of positive symptoms with enduring negative symptoms and cognitive dysfunction. In usual systems of care, this can translate to limited functional recovery. Persons with chronic schizophrenia are more likely to be single, unemployed, without health insurance, and homeless. In addition, individuals with chronic psychotic disorders die on average 20 years before their peers, with much (>80%) of this excess mortality attributable to cardiovascular disease.[3-5] The common lack of insight into psychotic symptoms by persons with these illnesses can threaten engagement with and adherence to treatment and challenge the establishment of collaborative therapeutic relationships. For every person affected by psychotic illness, there are many more around them—friends, family, and other supports—who are also impacted, and perceived caregiver burden is high among those who have a relative with schizophrenia.[6]

Psychotic disorders typically emerge during an already vulnerable period of life. With a peak onset between the ages of 15 to 25, psychosis can disrupt developmentally important transitions from adolescence to adulthood and derail evolving instrumental capacities. Furthermore, many potentially modifiable prognostic factors emerge soon after psychosis onset including suicidality, symptomatic relapses and rehospitalization, violence, substance misuse, social isolation, negative symptoms, and cognitive dysfunction.[7]

Despite the complicated challenge of effectively treating psychotic disorders, there are strong grounds for optimism. Over the past two decades, innovative efforts by research groups around the world have yielded a wealth of information relevant to the prediction, prevention, and early treatment of psychotic illnesses. This chapter provides an overview of these efforts to empower the recent entrant to public psychiatry to participate in this exciting area of research, education, clinical care, and health care policy.

BRIEF HISTORY

A diagnosis of schizophrenia can generate undue pessimism. Poor outcome became part of the diagnostic description in *Diagnostic and Statistical Manual of Mental Disorders* (DSM III), although this was supported by circular reasoning (i.e., if people diagnosed with schizophrenia recovered functioning, they must not have had the illness). However, early intervention (EI) research and other improvements in the treatment of psychosis have challenged that outlook.

In 1992, researchers and clinicians in Melbourne, Australia, established the Early Psychosis Prevention and Intervention Centre (EPPIC). Long-term outcomes for EPPIC were better than for individuals with chronic schizophrenia, including higher rates of employment, symptomatic remission, and lower suicide rates.[8] Researchers at EPPIC then began systematically assessing and following young people presenting with low-grade or subthreshold psychotic symptoms who were believed to be at risk for psychosis. They developed an assessment tool, the Comprehensive Assessment of At Risk Mental States (CAARMS)[9] and opened the Personal Assessment and Crisis Evaluation (PACE) clinic in 1995 to serve and study this population.

In Norway, in 1997, the Treatment and Intervention in Psychosis early detection (ED) study (TIPS) began testing a duration of untreated psychosis (DUP) reduction strategy that coupled rapid response teams with massive information campaigns to educate health care providers and the general public about the warning signs of psychosis and the importance of early treatment. The resulting ED was associated with significant advantages in cognitive, negative, and depressive symptoms compared to usual detection over 5 years[10] and superior functioning over 10 years.[11] Concurrently, McGlashan and colleagues at Yale developed the Scale of Prodromal Symptoms (SOPS) and an accompanying semi-structured interview to elicit and rate prepsychotic phenomenology, the Structured Interview for Prodromal Syndromes (SIPS).[12] An International Early Psychosis Association (IEPA) was formed, and numerous prediction, prevention, and first-episode treatment and research programs began to appear around the world.

The Connecticut Mental Health Center (CMHC) has played an important role in the development of EI and prevention in psychotic disorders. The Yale programs of Psychosis Risk Identification, Management, and Education (PRIME) and Specialized Treatment Early in Psychosis (STEP) have a history of developing cutting-edge assessment and treatment strategies for emerging psychotic disorders. PRIME was founded in 1996 and consists of an interdisciplinary team proficient in both clinical practices and research methodology. Representing the "patchwork" funding still largely necessary in the United States for development of EI services, the work of the clinic is supported largely by research grants, mostly from the National Institute of Mental Health (NIMH), but also from the pharmaceutical industry (for clinical trials of medication treatment) and from private donors (e.g., the Staglin Music Festival). In addition to conducting research, the tasks of the clinic include educating the potential referring community about the signs and symptoms of psychosis risk and developing a network of clinicians and educators who refer potential at-risk candidates for evaluation at the clinic.

PRIME is dedicated to the diagnosis, study, and treatment of patients who meet psychosis risk criteria (see Table 10.1). Clientele includes the patients, their families, and members of the referring network and can also include key people from the patient's educational system. Each of the numbers comprising our published group statistics represent an individual struggling with the immense daily task of growing up, of negotiating the last major phase of neurological development. Our patients illustrate, often painfully, that this developmental trajectory can suddenly and sometimes without warning swerve sideways from its expected path. Sometimes this liability toward slippage is foreshadowed by prior expressions of vulnerability, such as early childhood deficits in social or cognitive capacity or psychotic-like perceptual experiences. However, the neurodevelopmental processes that appear to lead to the majority

Table 10.1 PSYCHOSIS RISK SYNDROME CRITERIA

Attenuated Positive Symptoms Syndrome (APS):
1. Abnormal unusual thought content, suspiciousness, and/or organization of communication that is below the threshold of frank psychosis, AND
2. These symptoms have begun or worsened in the past year, AND
3. These symptoms occur at least once per week for the last month on average, AND
4. Psychosis can be ruled out.

Brief Intermittent Psychotic Symptoms Syndrome:
1. Frankly psychotic unusual thought content, suspiciousness, grandiosity, perceptual abnormalities, and/or organization of communication, AND
2. These symptoms have begun in the past 3 months, AND
3. The symptoms occur currently at least several minutes per day at least once per month, AND
4. Psychosis can be ruled out.

Genetic Risk and Functional Deterioration Risk Syndrome:
1. First-degree relative with history of any psychotic disorder OR
2. Schizotypal personality disorder in the patient, AND
3. Substantial functional decline in the past year as measured by GAF, AND
4. Psychosis can be ruled out.

Psychosis:
1. Frankly psychotic unusual thought content, suspiciousness, grandiosity, perceptual abnormalities, and/or organization of communication, AND
2. Symptoms are disorganizing or dangerous, OR
3. Symptoms occur more than 1 hour per day more than four times per week in the past month.

of cases of psychotic disorder (e.g., aberrations in the management of synaptic pruning) do not become biologically online and active until adolescence.

To address the concern of previous psychosis risk studies being underpowered, PRIME, along with similar clinics in the United States and Canada, formed a research consortium, the North American Prodrome Longitudinal Study (NAPLS). In its first iteration, NAPLS produced the largest sample of longitudinally followed psychosis risk subjects ($N = 291$) worldwide and a large dataset, producing an algorithm with high positive predictive power for conversion to psychosis (~80%), albeit modest sensitivity (~40%).[13,14] These efforts led to a second NIMH-funded iteration with the original eight sites, known as NAPLS 2, which is anticipated to recruit a large enough sample of subjects to address fundamental questions regarding neurobiological correlates in the development of psychosis.[15]

When conversion to full-blown psychosis occurred, the PRIME staff experienced considerable difficulty finding providers to care for these patients, especially when family income or insurance status made them ineligible for public-sector care. The notion of creating a clinic for first-episode psychosis patients was raised. We expected that many individuals experiencing an initial psychotic episode would require lower intensity, longer term treatment that could accommodate active work or school schedules. Several other arrangements had been previously attempted locally but failed because of the mismatch between ideal clinical care and available reimbursement structures. We concluded that financial incentives within the local private sector were not favorable and thus focused on public-sector options. As part of this planning process, the workgroup identified three relevant barriers to constructing an optimal EI service in the Connecticut public sector. First, our state mental health centers are under no obligation to accept privately insured patients. Our clinical experience indicated that such individuals often lost employment-based coverage after a psychotic break or aged out of parental coverage and thus represented an important target group for any EI program. Many of these patients were eventually treated in the state mental health system but often after a long period of poor access to treatment and after too much time had elapsed for EI to be clinically meaningful. Any EI service that excluded these patients would thus miss an important opportunity for indicated prevention. Second, Connecticut cares for adolescents and young adults via separate agencies, thereby fragmenting potential interventions aimed at the peak ages of onset of psychotic illnesses. Third, the division of public mental health care services by geographic catchment areas would limit the collection of a critical mass of early-psychosis patients around which to organize care.

The CMHC presented an excellent location to pilot an EI service. The center has a long history of supporting clinical research programs, including PRIME. Given our interest in developing a nationally relevant model of care, we saw that CMHC offered three distinct advantages. First, it is owned by the Connecticut Department of Mental Health and Addiction Services (DMHAS), which is one of 50 nationwide single state agencies (SSAs) for mental health that together constitute a de facto national mental health system. Although the degree of state funding and the role of the SSAs in mental health care vary across states, these agencies provide a link to administrative structures and personnel who are experienced in treating serious mental illnesses. These resources could serve as a platform for national implementation of early intervention. Second, the SSAs bear the brunt of the financial burden and thus have the greatest incentive to reduce disability from psychotic illnesses. Third, through Medicaid, each of the SSAs already participates in cost-sharing arrangements with the federal government that could be adapted to an EI initiative.

In 2006, the CMHC and the DMHAS agreed to support a pilot project by accepting a limited number of patients who were early in their illness course and for whom the center had no statutory obligation to provide care (i.e., individuals who were privately insured or living outside the catchment area or under age 18). This decision removed the three barriers identified by the workgroup, and the STEP clinic was established. Over the years, STEP has been staffed by many talented clinical providers: academic psychiatrists, psychologists, and trainees from Yale's Department of Psychiatry and DMHAS-employed social workers, nurses, and mental health workers. All clinical personnel were drawn from the existing chronic psychosis ambulatory team at CMHC. With funding from the NIMH and a private foundation (Donaghue Foundation), STEP conducted the first US randomized controlled trial (2007–13) to test the effectiveness of this first-episode service. The results demonstrated that EI and well-organized care is cost-effective and can have significant benefits for individuals experiencing early psychosis (study details are presented later in this chapter). Despite very limited recruitment efforts, the STEP clinic received referrals at the rate of about two per week within the first few months, with many more inquiries by phone and e-mail from area clinicians, families, and patients. Given evidence of high clinical need and the effectiveness of the service, the leadership of DMHAS committed funding to convert STEP from a research pilot program into a regular clinical service at CMHC in 2013. This allowed for the recruitment of full-time staff for the service, including a clinical director. Additional funding from the Substance Abuse and Mental Health Services Administration (SAMHSA) allowed further expansion of vocational services. In 2014, STEP began a new National Institutes of Health (NIH)-funded initiative to test a campaign to reduce the duration of untreated psychosis in eight surrounding towns and modeled on the TIPS project described earlier. This campaign will use a variety of mass and social media outlets combined with professional outreach to hasten access to care and enable STEP to model a population-based approach to improving outcomes for psychotic disorders.[16]

Public–academic collaboration has been pivotal for the development of PRIME and STEP. Specifically, state DMHAS support enabled initial resourcing of clinical services to allow outcomes assessments and subsequent grant-funded projects. Such data will contribute to an evaluation of the cost-effectiveness of early intervention in a "real-world" US setting. The final outcomes, as well as the implementation experience from demonstrations such as these, can provide a reasoned basis from which the various payers in our health care system can determine the allocation of scarce health care dollars.

The work described here has contributed to a growing consensus toward implementing EI in the United States. This represents a growing alignment of psychiatry with mainstream health care, in which practical strategies to prevent morbidity have greater acceptance. Widespread adoption of EI has not been achieved, however, and much work remains to reduce stigma and pessimism regarding the outcomes of psychotic disorders in both public perception and within psychiatry. Some countries, such as the United Kingdom, now have nationwide ED and treatment programs; others have little or none. In the United States, EI has typically been in the form of research programs at academic centers. However, in 2009, the NIMH announced funding for a large-scale study of first-episode services (FES)—Recovery After an Initial Schizophrenia Episode (RAISE)—to determine the efficacy of a package of interventions designed to be readily adoptable in "real-world settings." The NIMH has advocated that the question is "not *whether* early intervention works for FEP, but *how* specialty care programs can be implemented in community settings throughout the United States" (emphasis added).[17] In January 2014, President Obama signed into law the Consolidated Appropriations Act, which acknowledges that most persons with serious mental illnesses experience symptoms in adolescence and young adulthood, that there are long delays in accessing evidence-based care, and that other countries have viable EI models for reducing symptoms, illness relapse, and deteriorations in functioning. This legislation was accompanied by an approximately $25 million set-aside in the SAMHSA block grant funding program to support the development of evidence-based EI programming across the United States.

REVIEW OF TOPICS

WHAT DO THE TERMS "EARLY INTERVENTION" AND "PREVENTION" MEAN IN PSYCHOSIS?

EI for psychotic illnesses can be conceptualized as including one or more of two interlocking elements. First are ED efforts that seek to minimize delay in initiating treatment of manifest illness. This delay has been operationalized internationally in various measures of the DUP. The second element is the provision of "phase-specific" interventions that are adapted to younger patients and their families who are confronting the recent onset of a psychotic illness. Although several trials of individual pharmacologic and psychological treatments—often adapted from studies of chronic patient samples—have been mounted, the myriad needs of patients and their caregivers necessitate services that deliver packages of such empirically supported treatments. Such comprehensive FES typically provide care for the first 2–5 years after onset of a diagnosable psychotic disorder. The work of the STEP program is best understood as serving these related aims, first in testing a model of FES and, more recently, in launching an ED initiative.[16]

In chronic illnesses, "prevention" refers to interventions for persons who are not currently affected by a disease, and these interventions are intended to decrease future manifestation of the disease. This conception of prevention demands that cost-benefit analyses inform the application of interventions to appropriate populations so as to reduce overall morbidity and/or mortality. Thus, *universal* prevention (e.g., wearing of seat belts) is recommended for all, whereas *selective* prevention (e.g., influenza vaccination for high-risk groups such as elderly adults) can only be justified for subpopulations. Finally, *indicated* preventions (e.g., medications for control of high blood pressure) often involve professional expertise and entail more risk but can be justified based on their ability to prevent the onset or significantly ameliorate the course of subsequent disease (in this case, stroke or myocardial infarction). In this view, interventions for adolescents and young adults who are discovered to be at significantly increased risk for a psychotic disorder might be seen as closely following upon indicated prevention. The help-seeking samples currently presenting to prodromal clinics are typically already suffering the effects of mental disorder and have a variety of poor psychosocial outcomes even when they do not convert to psychosis.[18,19] Although no effective preventive approaches have yet been substantiated for psychotic illnesses, there is a strong argument for proactive efforts to offer low-risk psychosocial interventions for these high-risk patients and their families and to continue to test a variety of interventions that might survive a cost-benefit analysis to prevent morbidity. Such efforts, led by clinics such as PRIME, would optimally be seamlessly connected to early detection and treatment for manifest psychotic illness (see Box 10.1).

WHEN TO INTERVENE

Typically, a pre-illness period of 1–5 years exists when symptoms begin to emerge but are not yet diagnosable. This is known as the *prodromal phase*. Already present during this phase are functional decline, gray matter volume loss, distressing subthreshold psychotic symptoms, neuropsychological impairment, and often comorbid mood, anxiety, and substance use disorders. Insight and willingness to engage in treatment, however, typically remain intact and provide a window of opportunity for engagement into treatment. Among patients with an established diagnosis of schizophrenia, the majority retrospectively identify a prodrome. Prospective identification is a greater challenge. However, assessment tools have been developed to predict who may be at "ultra-high risk" or "clinical high risk" for developing a psychotic disorder, now known as *psychosis risk syndrome*. The psychosis risk syndrome is most commonly characterized by subthreshold positive symptoms with at least partially intact insight or reality testing, the symptoms have not reached a disorganizing or dangerous level, and the frequency of symptoms is less than in frank psychosis (several minutes per day at least once a month).[12] Instruments such as the Structured Interview for Psychosis Risk Syndrome (SIPS) developed by Woods, McGlashan, and colleagues in PRIME[12] or the CAARMS[9] are used to assess level of risk for schizophrenia. Three types of psychosis risk syndromes have been defined: *attenuated positive symptoms syndrome* (APS), *brief intermittent psychotic syndrome* (BIPS), and *genetic risk and functional deterioration psychosis risk syndrome* (GRD) (see Box 10.4 for diagnostic criteria[12] and Figure 10.1).

The prodrome ends with the onset of frank psychotic symptoms, typically referred to as the first episode of psychosis or "first break." This transition is often characterized by a loss of reality testing and insight along with some combination of severe disorganization, hallucinations, or delusions. Entry to care at this stage can occur in the context of a behavioral crisis involving emergency services or law enforcement, and it frequently results in a forced (involuntary) psychiatric hospitalization that is often traumatic for patients and their families.

Although investigators have variably operationalized "first-episode" or "early psychosis," the first 5 years are typically considered to be a critical period or "window of opportunity" for EI. Without timely connection to care, this period is characterized by repeated psychotic episodes; cognitive impairment; multiple hospitalizations; severe functional decline, often accompanied by comorbid substance use, mood, and anxiety disorders; and substantial stress on the family and social networks. The odds for developing a severely symptomatic and functionally compromised state are substantially elevated.

Box 10.1

Early Intervention for Psychosis

Tony is a 19-year-old African American male who presented to a FES in an urban community mental health center at the urging of his parents, who had become increasingly alarmed at his unusual behavior. He had a history of good academic and social function, earning above average grades, participating in sports, and spending time with friends in music-related activities. However, during his senior year of high school, his parents and friends noticed that he had become somewhat quiet, spending more time in his room alone than with others; his grades began to slip; and he did not sign up for spring baseball—a first for him—despite his team's likelihood of a championship year. Tony's parents chalked this up to typical adolescent moodiness and perhaps anxiety about transitioning to college in the fall, although they also wondered if he had started abusing substances. When his friends tried to talk to Tony about what was wrong, he became uncharacteristically suspicious of their motives and accused them of collecting information for a secret website about him. He graduated high school and began attending a local university. A few weeks into the semester, Tony stopped going to class, his hygiene became noticeably poor, and he got into a verbal altercation with a professor. When his parents asked him about being home rather than at class, he became agitated, and, in the ensuing argument, his speech was difficult to follow: he made statements about being constantly monitored by video cameras, a conspiracy involving everyone he knew, and that he could hear them talking about him over radio waves. Unable to calm their son, Tony's parents called an ambulance, and he was taken to a local emergency department for psychiatric evaluation. Because he was not an imminent danger to self or others and not grossly disorganized, Tony was not admitted for inpatient treatment. The psychiatric resident in the emergency department referred Tony to a local FES.

The FES contacted Tony and got permission to meet with him and his parents at their home after Tony expressed reluctance to come in to the mental health center. A thorough assessment was completed by the team's psychologist who determined that Tony had been suffering from auditory hallucinations of multiple voices commenting on his behavior, ideas of reference, paranoia, and disorganization at a psychotic level for 2 months with a prior prodromal period of 1 year. A diagnosis of Psychotic Disorder, Not Otherwise Specified was made until the psychiatrist worked in collaboration with Tony's primary care physician (PCP) to consider secondary etiologies. Tony was also experiencing negative symptoms in the form of social withdrawal, decreased energy, and avolition and cognitive symptoms of decreased executive functioning. Tony's key clinician, a social worker, took care to engage with him around his interests in sports and music, balancing clinical material with conversations about leisure activity and social and occupational goals in their meetings. Tony identified that he would like most to go back to school, go back to spending time with friends, and get a girlfriend. His key clinician used cognitive behavioral therapy to address his delusional ideation and teach coping mechanisms to reduce secondary anxiety. The resulting improvement in rapport allowed her to connect him with the psychiatrist and supported education specialist. He was also encouraged to join a Social Cognition and Interaction Training (SCIT) group, and he began meeting the family clinician with his parents. A second-generation antipsychotic was started at a low dose, which Tony responded to and tolerated well. His psychiatrist and nurse carefully monitored his weight and other cardiac risk factors in collaboration with his PCP. Tony and his parents participated in Family Focused Treatment, their communication and problem-solving skills improved, and they began to better understand Tony's illness and the diathesis-stress model. He began to feel more competent in social situations and gradually resumed going out with his friends. Tony got a part-time job and returned to school the following semester. He continued with the FES for 2 years, and, as his symptoms and functioning improved, his visits were reduced in frequency. He was subsequently transitioned to the care of a psychiatrist and therapist in his town, at which point Tony and his family felt well-educated in how to monitor for early signs of relapse and comfortable with their new caregivers.

HOW TO INTERVENE?

Care for the Psychosis Risk Syndrome

In this phase of engagement, when the presence of an illness is not established, a staging approach is favored. Progressively more intensive interventions with a higher risk of potential adverse effects are introduced as functional impairment and severity increase. Programs can tailor treatments to subthreshold symptoms and behavioral deficits and aim to delay or prevent the onset of a first episode of active psychosis. For example, mild symptoms may be treated with case management while moderate symptoms are treated with cognitive behavioral therapy (CBT). Treatment typically involves monitoring families and providing education about psychosis risk and symptoms, the diathesis stress model, and sometimes expressed emotion. Comorbid depression and/or anxiety may be treated pharmacologically and/or with evidence-based psychotherapies (see Table 10.2).

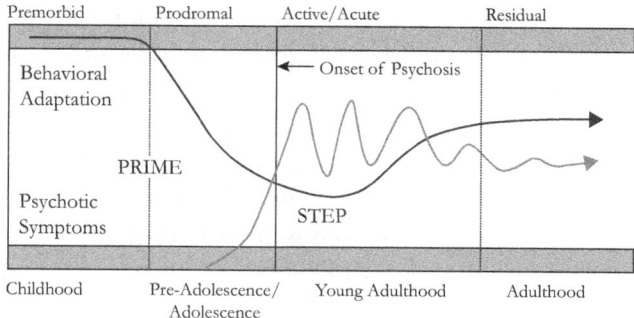

Figure 10.1 Typical course of psychotic illness and targets for early intervention

Only a handful of randomized controlled trials (RCTs) have been published that focus on the psychosis risk syndrome population, although there are numerous naturalistic and open label studies. The RCTs have been of antipsychotic medications, CBT, and omega-3 fatty acids. First, in 2002, McGorry and colleagues in Melbourne compared 6 months of active treatment (risperidone 1–3 mg/d plus modified CBT) to needs-based intervention and found that significantly fewer individuals in active treatment progressed to a first episode of psychosis after 6 months; however, the difference was no longer significant after 1 year.[20] McGlashan and Woods led the first double-blind, randomized, placebo-controlled trial of an antipsychotic medication (olanzapine) to prevent or delay the onset of psychosis.[21] In this North American trial, help-seeking patients who met criteria for clinical high risk of psychosis were randomized to medication or placebo for 1 year, followed by no medications for the second year. After 1 year, more than twice as many placebo-treated participants than olanzapine-treated subjects had converted to psychosis, although this difference was not statistically significant; after 2 years, the rate of psychosis onset did not differ significantly between the groups. Olanzapine was associated with significantly reduced psychosis risk symptoms compared to placebo; however, weight gain was also substantially higher, leading the authors to conclude that the benefits did not outweigh the risks. Multiple RCTs have compared time-limited CBT to an alternative nonpharmacologic intervention (e.g., supportive therapy, befriending) with variable findings regarding the superiority of CBT.[22] In these studies, CBT followed an empirically validated cognitive model of psychosis, was problem-oriented, collaborative, and included use of homework tasks and guided discovery. In one single, blind, controlled trial, CBT significantly reduced the likelihood of progression to psychosis and antipsychotic prescription over 1 year.[23] Whereas one trial comparing CBT to supportive therapy found no difference between treatment groups at 18 months[24] (both treatments were effective in reducing attenuated positive symptoms, anxiety, and depression, thus suggesting the clinical relationship as the potentially key variable), a Dutch study comparing routine care to routine care with add-on CBT found CBT to be superior for reducing conversion to psychosis and for cost saving.[25] CBT interventions have several advantages: they are acceptable to psychosis risk patients, make sense within a stress-vulnerability model of psychosis development, offer coping strategies that buffer against environmental stressors that are likely to precipitate conversion to psychosis, have shown efficacy for associated comorbidities (mood, anxiety, substance use), and target metacognition and self-schemas that are impaired in the prodrome. A RCT by Amminger compared 12 weeks of omega-3 fatty acid supplementation with placebo.[26] After 1 year, significantly few subjects in the omega-3 group developed psychosis, and there were significant improvements in positive and negative symptoms in favor of the treatment group. Although these results are encouraging, overall, trials thus far for preventative interventions have tended to be underpowered.

The large sample sizes of NAPLS, and its second iteration NAPLS 2, address questions of power by combining data across multiple sites. A recent meta-analysis including 1,112 subjects from 10 trials with at least 1-year follow-up concluded that preventative interventions are effective at reducing conversion rates to active psychosis among those considered to be at high risk and that this effect diminishes but does not disappear over time.[22] Of note, subjects who do not transition to psychosis are help-seeking individuals suffering from a range of mental and social role functioning problems and cannot simply be considered healthy false positives.[19]

Table 10.2 EVIDENCE-BASED AND PROMISING INTERVENTIONS

Psychosis Risk Syndrome:
- Cognitive behavioral therapy (CBT)
- Antidepressant medications as indicated
- Family education and support
- Family-Focused Therapy (FFT)
- Family-Assisted Assertive Community Treatment (FACT)
- Supported Employment/Individual Placement and Support
- Omega-3 fatty acids

First-Episode Psychosis:
- Cognitive behavioral therapy (CBT)
- Low-dose antipsychotic medications
- Family education and support
- Assertive Community Treatment (ACT)
- Vocational/Educational Rehabilitation
- Cognitive Remediation

Early Detection

Two systematic reviews reported a consistent association across countries between DUP and clinical outcomes.[27,28] There has thus been much interest in finding ways to decrease the time between onset of psychotic symptoms and entry into appropriate psychiatric care. The most successful initiative to date has been the Norwegian TIPS study. A potentially key element of the TIPS campaign to reduce DUP was its multifaceted approach. While other studies tested single outreach interventions (e.g., educating general practitioners/primary care providers), TIPS targeted both professionals who come in contact with young people as well as the general public with messages regarding how to recognize signs of psychosis, the importance and effectiveness of early treatment, and a simple referral number, and it debunked myths regarding psychosis and treatment. The campaign utilized a variety of media and other methods, such as mailings to every household in their geographic area and mailing items with TIPS branding to general practitioners. ED teams based in emergency departments rapidly responded to referrals and also assessed patients in their preferred community settings. The TIPS campaign shortened DUP and improved long-term functioning. When the campaign was discontinued, DUP began to rise again, further supporting the conclusion that the outreach and education campaign was essential for reducing and maintaining shortened DUP.

The authors of this chapter are currently undertaking a replication of TIPS in the United States. We are interested in whether ED using similar methods, with an updated media component, can succeed in the more fragmented US health care system, with its long and complicated pathways to care. The STEP Early Detection (STEP-ED) study[16] will employ a social-ecological model of pathways to care that envisions multiple sources of DUP including individual, interpersonal, institutional/organizational, community, and social structures, policies, and systems. A key component is the use of social marketing tools to facilitate help-seeking behavior by patients and families and prompt referral by professionals. A branding approach was used to generate a name and logo for the campaign—MindMap: A Clear Path to Mental Health (for sample materials, see www.mindmapct.org). Aside from the use of mass and social media, the campaign will include intensive professional outreach to various stakeholders including educational, health care, judicial, social welfare, and religious organizations. Additionally, a rapid access approach at STEP will screen and initiate engagement within a few days of referral and offer meetings at the point of referral, including community settings (e.g., in primary care or school counseling centers). STEP-ED will compare a baseline year of usual detection to a 3-year campaign and a control site, a demographically and clinically similar FES in Boston affiliated with Harvard (also an academic–public partnership), on our main outcome of DUP, as well as functional and clinical outcomes. We seek to reduce DUP through ED, gain a better understanding of pathways to care for psychosis in the United States, and determine whether or not ED improves outcomes beyond those already achieved by our FESs.

Professionals within the public sector can play a key role in outreaching and providing education to other professionals who come into contact with young people, as well as participate in the development of media campaigns. ED work presents unique opportunities for psychiatrists outside of traditional clinical, academic, and research roles and represents a clear intersection between psychiatry and public health.

FES

Four RCTs have demonstrated the efficacy of FES in the United Kingdom, Denmark, Norway, and the United States. In the United Kingdom, the Lambeth Early Onset (LEO)[29] study randomized individuals with early psychosis to a package of interventions including CBT, family counseling, vocational services, and low-dose antipsychotic medication all provided within community-based teams. Those receiving these more intensive services had improved social and vocational functioning, satisfaction, quality of life and medication adherence, and lower rates of relapse and dropout at 18-month follow-up. The Danish OPUS[30] study offered home-based assertive case management integrated with pharmacotherapy that favored lower dose antipsychotics and included family and individual psychoeducation with social skills training and vocational assistance as needed compared to involvement with a standard community mental health team. OPUS demonstrated benefits in positive and negative symptom control, secondary substance abuse, treatment adherence, and higher satisfaction with care in the EI condition. A Norwegian study of a similar home-based integrated approach compared to standard office-based care reported 2-year improvements in the number and duration of hospitalizations, symptom relapse, and treatment adherence in enriched care group.[31,32]

The US study compared an office-based integrated service package (STEP) that included structured family psychoeducation, cognitive behavioral individual and group therapy, antipsychotic medications, and vocational and educational supports compared to treatment as usual (TAU) in the community.[33] Patients early in the course of a psychotic illness were randomized to STEP care or TAU. STEP patients had significantly fewer hospitalizations and hospital days and greater vocational engagement. This study demonstrated the feasibility and effectiveness of a public-sector model of FES. The STEP FES was significantly less resource-intensive than those used in the OPUS and Lambeth studies and was still able to engender significant benefits for individuals and their families.

The FES in the OPUS and LEO trials were offered for 2 years. Their positive impact on a variety of outcomes was not detectable 3 years after specialized care was discontinued. This has focused attention on an important question: how long should specialized care be offered? STEP has implemented a less resource-intensive approach that can be sustained longer than Assertive Community Treatment (ACT) levels of care, but has also had to transfer patients after establishing long-standing therapeutic alliances. A Canadian public-sector program successfully extended the effects of EI by using stepped reductions in intensity to prolong care through 5 years after entry. This is an area ripe for innovation and further study.

HOW ARE FES DELIVERED?

Just as important as *what* interventions are offered is *how* services are offered. The culture and values of EI teams are essential. It is important to maintain optimism and focus on recovery toward personal goals and a collaborative therapeutic alliance. Often, patients presenting for FES may not believe that they are in need of mental health treatment, thus making engagement one of the most critical elements of care. Avoiding power struggles, connecting with patients around their interests, discussing their understanding of their experiences or illness, emphasizing patients' goals for treatment and their definition of recovery, flexibility, and patience are some of the essential ingredients to engagement. The initial assessment can facilitate engagement by expanding the discussion beyond symptoms to include patient-centered metrics of quality of life, including social and vocational goals, and communicating (verbally and nonverbally) comfort with discussing unusual or bizarre material. Patients may present with disorganization or agitation that clinicians would do well to respond to with patience and validation of what that experience is like for the patient rather than immediately debating the content or explanation of those experiences. Despite initial resistance and limited or absent insight, many patients respond well if they are given an opportunity to feel heard and if the clinician's perspective is only offered after careful assessment and, preferably, with the patient's permission. Clinicians should emphasize what the program or clinic can offer to match the patients' priorities and be prepared to address confusion, stigma, or pessimism about the causes or treatment of mental illness.

Inclusion of family members and other naturalistic supports is an essential component of FES. Families will often be able to provide invaluable historical information during the assessment process, collaborate in monitoring the patient between clinic visits, and notice early warning signs of psychotic relapse. The emotional environment they provide the patient is one of the strongest predictors of psychiatric relapse and hospitalization. Reducing high levels of "expressed emotion"—criticism, lack of warmth, hostility, and emotional overinvolvement—is likely to have tremendous benefit. Families should be treated as allies and members of the treatment team. They may present with incorrect attributions regarding illness, be frightened, grieving the loss of a relative's health, or agitated toward staff or the patient. It is important to keep in mind that initial meetings with families may come at what is the worst time for them. Many may have recently had a frustrating experience seeking help for their ill relative, and empathic and patient responses to their initial requests can go a long way. Reassurance, education, and communication of optimism from the clinician are useful and appropriate.

Following implementation of the RAISE Project, the NIMH issued a white paper providing guidelines for FES, "Coordinated Specialty Care." Several treatment manuals have recently been published or are forthcoming. Consistent across most FES is the use of interdisciplinary teams to provide an array of services. Various disciplines bring diverse perspectives to understanding and treating patients in a collaborative manner. Psychiatry, psychology, social work, nursing, occupational therapy, and persons with lived experience with psychosis (peers) are some of the relevant actors in the interdisciplinary team. Weekly interdisciplinary team meetings and frequent communication ensure fidelity to treatment principles, facilitate morale, and encourage high-quality service delivery. Roles are clarified rather than rigidly assigned along disciplinary lines. For example, depending on their strengths, interests, and training, any of the disciplines can serve in the primary clinician role and assist patients in navigating the care pathway. Alternative or additional roles for the same clinician can include education and support of the family or therapy for patients in an individual or a group modality. However, the supported employment and education role requires specialized skills and significant time in the community to develop and to assist clients in seeking work. This role is thus less likely to be interchangeable among the clinicians. Psychiatrists or advanced practice nurses typically provide medication management, coordinate with primary care, and play a pivotal role in health and wellness monitoring and intervention. The team leader role serves to coordinate clinic activities, lead team meetings, provide supervision, fulfill administrative functions, oversee development and implementation of services, ensure adherence to treatment philosophies, and, sometimes, carry a caseload as primary clinician.

Many FES provide treatment in the community, similar to or following an ACT model of care. Patients are treated primarily in settings outside the clinician's office, treatment teams are interdisciplinary, the staff-to-patient ratio is low, and a menu of interventions aimed at maximizing functioning is offered. However, unlike ACT, treatment is typically time limited (of 2–3 years duration in most programs), with step-down to less specialized services at that time. Ongoing supervision and continuing education are also important components to ensuring continued focus on FES principles and specialization.

EVIDENCE-BASED PRACTICES

Many treatments have demonstrated efficacy; these include CBT and low-dose atypical antipsychotic medications, and inclusion of supported employment/education and family education and involvement in a FES. Multifamily Group Psychoeducation and Support (MFG), Family Assisted Assertive Community Treatment (FACT), and Family-Focused Therapy (FFT) are models for family intervention. Social Cognition and Interaction Training (SCIT), developed and tested in chronic schizophrenia, is a promising approach for improving social functioning in early psychosis. Cognitive remediation studies have shown improved memory, social functioning, and self-esteem among first-episode samples. Providers of FES should consider making available a menu of interventions that can be matched to patient priorities. Participation rates in group-based interventions in early-psychosis samples tend to be low, and, ideally, patients will be returning to work or school and social involvement so that enrollment in all interventions offered within a FES may not be realistic or desirable (Table 10.3).

CHALLENGES AND CLINICAL CONSIDERATIONS IN EI

EI services are designed to assertively engage and treat primary psychotic disorders. Although recognizable by their characteristic symptoms and natural history, these are diagnoses of exclusion. A multitude of medical conditions and drug-induced states can present with psychotic symptoms.

Table 10.3 PSYCHOSIS RISK TREATMENT GUIDELINES

- It is essential to have a specialized assessment carried out to determine whether the person actually meets criteria for the ultra-high-risk phase or psychosis risk syndrome.
- Monitor closely for progression to full psychosis (monthly assessments).
- Treat co-existing conditions (e.g., anxiety, depression) as appropriate.
- Provide psychosocial support, including the family.
- Recognize that youth meeting psychosis risk criteria are help-seeking and in need of care whether or not they develop a full psychotic disorder.

In these cases, psychosis is "secondary" to an identifiable cause that often requires distinct treatment and sometimes referral away from an FES. Professionals working in an FES may be the first to conduct a diagnostic assessment for a first episode of psychosis and should remain vigilant for these secondary causes. A comprehensive medical history and examination, targeted follow-up for unusual presentations or treatment resistance, and, perhaps most important, continued vigilance for the emergence of signs or symptoms suggestive of neurologic or other medical illnesses can reduce the risk of misdiagnosis. After careful exclusion of secondary causes, considerable ambiguity is to be expected in classifying early-course primary psychosis. The variability in expression of symptoms and lack of an extended or reliable longitudinal history in young patients can make it difficult to distinguish between depressive or bipolar disorder with psychotic features and schizophrenia spectrum disorders. It is helpful not to wed oneself to a diagnosis with too much certainty and to encourage patients and their families to exercise the same caution while focusing on symptom control, rehabilitation of functional disabilities, and continued longitudinal diagnostic clarification (see Table 10.4 for early warning signs of psychosis).

Working effectively within EI requires specialized knowledge of common problems encountered in early-course psychotic disorders but also a more general understanding of the developmental psychology of adolescence and young adulthood. Samples of FEP have disproportionately high percentages of immigrants, trauma, substance use, suicidality, anxiety, and, particularly, obsessive compulsive disorder (OCD). For example, roughly 10% of the TIPS sample had comorbid OCD, which was associated with higher rates of suicide plans or attempts compared to FEP without OCD.[34] Patients and their families will likely have questions regarding substance use and its relationship to psychosis risk; providers would do well to become familiar with the literature on cannabis use in particular. Substance

Table 10.4 EARLY WARNING SIGNS OF PSYCHOSIS

Increased difficulty at school or work
Withdrawal from friends or family
Difficulty concentrating or thinking clearly
Suspiciousness or mistrust of others
Changes in the way things look or sound
Odd thinking or behavior
Emotional outbursts or lack of emotion
Poor personal hygiene

use in FEP is associated with higher rates of hospitalization and more severe psychopathology.

As with any aspect of public psychiatry, cultural context must be considered when evaluating and treating persons in the early stages of psychosis (see Chapter 14 for a review of cultural competence). Understanding how treatment options fit within the patient's beliefs, values, attributions, and interpretation of symptoms is an important component of culturally competent EI.

In addition to elevated rates of trauma and stressful life events among FEP populations, the experience of becoming psychotic is often frightening and potentially traumatizing in itself. Entry into treatment can involve aversive experiences including interactions with police, physical restraint, and involuntary hospitalizations. Assessing for and attempting to alleviate fears about treatment through reassurance, education, and a patient, therapeutic stance is essential. For example, a patient may be reluctant to engage and particularly guarded due to anxiety regarding involuntary hospitalization, but may be forthcoming if the criteria for emergency commitment are provided along with reassurance from the professional that this is a last resort. As always, careful consideration must be given when considering involuntary commitment. Although safety is the top priority, the risk of disengagement from outpatient treatment following inpatient discharge and the threat to the therapeutic alliance must also be considered. If hospitalization is necessary, clinicians can mitigate damage by exercising principles of procedural justice (e.g., being treated fairly and respectfully, feeling heard, getting a chance to tell one's side of the story, being included in the decision process) and, if possible, working with the inpatient treatment team and the patient on the unit. As described earlier, engagement is a significant challenge in treating FEP, and addressing treatment-related fears in the context of establishing a trusting therapeutic relationship is an important task.

After connection with FES, the overall prevalence of violence among FEP gradually drops to rates close to those of the general population except for patients with persistent comorbid substance use.[35] Paranoia and persecutory delusions may also increase risk for aggressive behavior because patients may believe they are acting in self-defense. Although the majority of those in the early stages of psychosis will not be violent, they may still come into contact with the criminal justice system for behaviors related to symptoms, such as trespassing or disorderly conduct, and professionals working within public psychiatry will likely find themselves interacting with the legal system regarding their patients. Understanding the local criminal justice system, as well as the ethical considerations of working with patients with legal charges or court-mandated treatment, will prove useful (see Chapter 8 for a review).

Although positive symptoms often respond adequately to antipsychotic medication, the symptoms that can have the greatest impact on functional recovery—negative and cognitive symptoms—typically do not. Few interventions have shown efficacy in alleviating negative symptoms. Cognitive remediation programs have shown promise in reducing the intellectual deficits that typically develop in schizophrenia and, in combination with other approaches, like supported employment, might have particular promise in improving functional outcomes.[36] Professionals working within EI should familiarize themselves with the common cognitive symptoms associated with psychosis, such as executive functioning deficits, and consider referral for neuropsychological assessment. Such an assessment can both evaluate the extent of dysfunction compared to population norms, monitor for changes over time, and suggest strategies to reduce their impact on school and work function.

SALIENCE OF EI AND PREVENTION FOR PUBLIC PSYCHIATRY

The work described in the preceding sections is better seen not as a specific set of interventions but rather as a paradigm of approaching a set of diseases that, like many other serious mental illnesses, have their onset in late adolescence and early adulthood. Although the primary psychotic disorders are believed to be heterogeneous in etiology and pathophysiology, the organizing exemplar of schizophrenia provides a rational focus for this paradigm. Specifically, efforts to investigate and care are guided by the knowledge of these as neurodevelopmental illnesses with possible in utero causal factors, identifiable but imprecise markers in childhood, and reliable recognition in full-blown psychosis during early adulthood. Although the needs of patients and families can now be anticipated and outcomes demonstrably improved after the FEP, much work needs to be done to better predict and prevent the onset of psychosis in those at risk. Furthermore, the identification of biomarkers that predict illness onset could provide opportunities for selective and even universal prevention. These aspirational goals illustrate the goals of this paradigm, one that brings psychiatry into the mainstream of public health and medical practice.

This paradigm requires close relationships between the activities of research and clinical care. Both PRIME and STEP have enabled the recruitment of patients and families into a variety of investigations across the translational continuum—from genetics to policy—while also allowing patients access to cutting-edge interventions and knowledge. This platform for innovative research and care has also been an attractive training site for social work, psychology, anthropology, and psychiatry trainees. While possible in other settings, the public–academic collaboration at the core of this work has been pivotal in allowing innovative models of care and research to be supported in ways that are not yet possible in fee-for-service environments.

EI clinics also provide the opportunity to prevent comorbidities associated with shortened life span in chronic schizophrenia. Relative to their peers without serious mental illness, patients with schizophrenia experience a threefold increase in cardiovascular mortality between the ages of 18 and 49 and an almost twofold increase in mortality between the ages of 50 and 75 years. Although this increased disease burden is likely multifactorial, persons with schizophrenia have a higher prevalence of several modifiable risk factors for cardiovascular disease including smoking, obesity, diabetes, dyslipidemia, and hypertension. Long-term use of antipsychotic medications may play an important role in the increased risk for cardiovascular diseases because antipsychotic medication use is associated with significant weight gain, dyslipidemia, and insulin resistance. In contrast to the consistently poor cardiovascular risk in chronic schizophrenia, studies of first-episode psychosis samples have been inconsistent. Given discrepancies in the reported prevalence of cardiovascular risk factors in early-psychosis samples, STEP compared FEP patients with minimal prior antipsychotic exposure with age-, gender-, and race-matched peers drawn from the National Health and Nutrition Survey on 10-year cardiac risk. Although indistinguishable from peers at entry, patients suffered pervasive adverse trajectories of cardiovascular risk factors over the subsequent year due to higher rates of nicotine dependence and obesity. Similar adverse trends in blood pressure, lipids, and fasting glucose led to an increase in prevalence of the metabolic syndrome.[37] These findings provide a rational focus for prevention of premature cardiovascular mortality. The first year of treatment constitutes the beginning of a critical period for such preventive efforts. Public psychiatrists have the opportunity to intervene early with young patients on health and wellness behaviors before harmful habits set in, collaborate with primary care to assure that their patients do not follow the typical pattern of disengagement, and play a role in reducing premature cardiovascular mortality (see Chapter 5 for a review of health promotion strategies).

FUTURE CHALLENGES

Much progress has been made over the past quarter century in understanding how to implement the two major domains of EI in psychosis: the early detection and effective care of young patients and their families. The goals of prevention have so far been limited to exploration of possible indicated prevention in selected high-risk samples, and the state of the art might better be conceptualized as early treatment for those who are seeking help for significant psychological distress or social dysfunction that only in some cases will result in the diagnosis of a psychotic disorder but in most cases merits clinical attention.

Outcomes for psychosis are indeed better when interventions are delivered early or when they are delivered by a specialized team, but this is not usually the case on transfer to regular care systems. Also, EI is not widely available in the United States. In other words, there is still a long way to go for the goals of EI to be realized. What tasks and questions remain for future public psychiatry professionals?

We will answer this question by addressing two other broad questions that we hope will engage the novice entrant to public psychiatry. First, how can we continue to increase our understanding of how to prevent and, when this is not possible, rapidly intervene to meaningfully improve outcomes for patients with psychotic disorders? Second, how can we engage with stakeholders outside the health care community to extend the reach and impact of empirically validated service models on public health?

The NIH focus on mechanisms and circuits that are agnostic to current phenomenology-based classification (e.g., DSM 5) might deliver new insights on common vulnerabilities (e.g., working memory deficits, social cognition impairments) and mechanisms of disease progression. This could lead to better causal discrimination of various psychotic illnesses and provide rational targets for preventive approaches and more targeted pharmacologic and psychosocial treatments. The psychosis risk syndrome was not included in the DSM 5 as a diagnostic category due to controversy surrounding false positives and concerns that assigning this diagnosis would be both stigmatizing and lead to even greater inappropriate prescribing of antipsychotic medication. The countervailing argument is that prodromal psychosis may currently be misdiagnosed as depression or attention deficit disorder, and inappropriate treatments might be worsening clinical outcomes. The question of how best to categorize developing and heterotypic adolescent psychopathology is thus ripe for empirical investigation. The large sample sizes in the NAPLS studies continue to contribute to this debate and have already facilitated improved models of prediction.[13] Improving our ability to predict the onset of psychosis will allow us opportunities to reach back earlier in the trajectory of disease progression and test approaches to indicated and, theoretically, perhaps even to selective or universal prevention.

In the domain of treatment of manifest illness, even the most effective EI services cannot succeed unless youth in early stages of psychosis are reached and engaged. In Australia and the United Kingdom, EI research programs have advocated for and are seeking to embed themselves within broader youth mental health service models (e.g., Headspace, Youthspace). The United States also may need to consider this approach. In keeping with the reality that most serious mental illnesses are chronic diseases of the young,[38] this model could lift all boats by providing a less stigmatizing entry point into care not just for schizophrenia spectrum disorders, but also for bipolar disorder, substance use disorders, and depression. At the federal level, the SAMHSA has recently shown an interest in such an approach with its Healthy Transitions initiative in support of the President's "Now Is the Time Plan." Healthy Transitions places emphasis on engagement and aims to improve access to treatment and support services for youth at risk for serious mental illness.

Another unresolved issue is how long FES services should be continued or how their benefits can be sustained on transition to less intensive models of care. Given that these disorders, like most chronic illnesses, are not cured by current treatments, it should not be a surprise that some effects are not durable after 2–3 years of specialized care, and different health care systems will have to test models that allow more tailored and economically sustainable transitions into less intensive services that can maintain and even advance the positive trajectories delivered by EI services.

Although there is much to learn about disease mechanisms, best clinical practices, and models of service delivery to improve our success at prevention and EI, there is already much in the "toolbox" that clinicians and administrators can draw upon to improve population outcomes today. Described by some commentators as the challenge of knowledge translation,[39] this involves work further "up" a translational continuum that begins at the genetic level and ends in public policy. The developing professional in public mental health would do well to be at least conversant with the multiple languages spoken at the different levels of analyses. Of particular relevance to public psychiatry is the ability to communicate the public health benefits of treatments or service delivery models to a wide variety of stakeholders with distinct and valuable perspectives and roles in human well-being. The novice in this heterogeneous arena should guard against two common seductions that can oversimplify into ideology what is better accomplished by negotiated and empirically driven change. On the one hand, the logic of bureaucracy might weigh in the direction of stasis and resist disinvestment and reallocations of resources from legacy services to make way for newer approaches. On the other hand, the logic of the marketplace can confuse an overly narrow emphasis on financial cost to one stakeholder (e.g., hospital bed days) with true health economic merit, which requires a broad societal perspective (loss to the labor market, judicial costs, entitlement costs). Although health care "cost" has rightfully become an important focus in US health care policy, the mental health professional would do well to familiarize him- or herself with the broad societal perspective of health economics.[40] Between these two extreme positions, novel programs might be asked to answer to a higher standard of evidence than legacy practices or present a cost-saving solution to one agency while ignoring wider economic benefits. To be an informed advocate, the young professional can draw on her clinical skills in building rapport and listening to diverse points of view to engage and educate herself about how to interact within complex organizations.[41] She might also educate herself on current concepts of value in health care that seek to orient resource allocation decisions toward those services that maximize "health outcomes achieved per dollar spent"[42] and extend the focus beyond existing patients to population health,[43] which is in keeping with the ethos of public psychiatry. In the United States, where the presence of multiple payers creates incentives for the cost-shifting of non-reimbursable but high-value activities, creative financial mechanisms will be necessary to realize health care value. A recent proposal for funding EI in the United States is illustrative of how these challenges might be addressed.[43]

Although the funding mechanisms for EI are clearly in their infancy in the United States, there are grounds for

Table 10.5 ESSENTIAL QUALITY METRICS—BENCHMARKS

DOMAIN	MEASURE	STANDARD
A. Access		
A.1 Rapidity	DUP 1 <3 months	Achievable (30%); Aspirational (75%)
	DUP 2 <12 months	Achievable (50%); Aspirational (75%)
A.2 Equity	Proportion of females, ethnic groups, town of residence, age	Demographics will match 2010 Census for local region served
A.3 Coverage	Number annually offered STEP/Expected annual incidence	Achievable (15%); Aspirational (80%)
A.4 Pathway to care	Proportion admitted after hospital admission	Achievable (60%), Aspirational (30%)
B. Engagement		
B.1 Overall	In contact with STEP at 1 year	Achievable (70%); Aspirational (90%)
B.2 Quality	Service Engagement Scale	Assess along 4 domains and across A.2 groupings for disparities
B.3 Exposure to family education	Exposure to FFT	Achievable 75%; Aspirational 90% of patients will have had at least one caregiver attend at least one meeting
B.4 Exposure to peer/social skills	Exposure to SCIT	Achievable 75%; Aspirational 90% of patients will attend at least one meeting
C. Outcomes		
C.1 Hospitalization	Admission to Psych unit in 1st year	Achievable (<25%); Aspirational (<10%)
C.2 Remission	Positive psychotic symptoms	PANSS 8-item score <3 at 6 months: Achievable (50%–70%); Aspirational (85%)
		PANSS 8-item score <3 at 1 year: Achievable (80%); Aspirational (90%)
C.3 Recovery	Global Functioning-Role & Social scale	75% are at level 8 or better on both
C.2 Vocational Engagement	In at least part-time school or work or actively looking for vocational opportunities (e.g., engaged in supported employment)	Achievable (85%); Aspirational (90%)
C.3 CV Risk		
(a) Smoking	New smokers at 1 year	Achievable (20%); Aspirational (10%)
	Smoking rate at 1 year	Achievable (60%); Aspirational (30%)
(b) Overweight or obesity	BMI < 25 at 1 year	Achievable (30%); Aspirational (75%)
	Retain BMI WNL at 1 year	Achievable (60%); Aspirational (75%)

optimism. The UK National Health Service, which has pioneered the use of cost-utility analyses to inform investment in health care interventions, has already made a significant commitment to FES and adds credibility to the economic rationale for EI. Also, in the United States, the SAMHSA, for the first time in 2014, required 5% of its mental health block grants to be allocated to FEP in all states, thus signaling a small but significant indication that such services may become part of the landscape of usual care in this country.

ESSENTIAL QUALITY METRICS

As EI services mature, so should the standards for measuring success. Clinical trials provide opportunities to examine in great detail areas of symptom severity, social and occupational functioning, duration of untreated psychosis, quality of life, physical health, adverse effects, treatment engagement, and so on. However, routine clinical practice should also examine effectiveness in an ongoing manner to allow for course corrections and examination of potential shortcomings in treatment delivery. A benchmark model whereby FES would regularly audit and compare itself to international standards is advocated by the authors of this chapter. Although traditional assessments of fidelity to a particular model of care can be useful for the purposes of training in technical interventions and disseminating appropriate cultures of practice, these process-oriented approaches do not directly address value; that is, the degree to which population outcomes are improved for a specific investment in resources. In STEP, we favor ongoing examination of benchmarks as a way of alerting us that changes to our service delivery or interventions may be necessary. See Table 10.5 for a putative sample of benchmarks based on STEP's past outcomes and a review of the international outcomes literature. These are not meant to be comprehensive or even prescriptive, but to illustrate what a standard of care might mean for an EI service and allow transparent communication to patients and families: for example, "If you come to our service you can expect a higher than 85% chance that you will be vocationally engaged in 1 year."

SUMMARY

It is an exciting time to be entering the field of public psychiatry. The promise of early intervention in schizophrenia is being realized, yet much work remains in order to fully achieve prevention of illness and its harmful effects. Public psychiatry plays an important role in EI, where much of the services are likely to take place, and in addressing a tremendous public health and human burden. Professionals who decide to specialize in EI will be rewarded with participating in their patients' recovery to more satisfying lives than previously thought possible, and they will assist in the development of cutting-edge treatments and their implementation.

Although the evidence base for EI is compelling, more work is needed to refine and extend the impact of EI models. This includes studying and adding refinements to existing FES that are informed by a better understanding of disease pathophysiology but also improving the rate at which empirically supported models are implemented to reduce morbidity and mortality. The varieties of professions within public psychiatry, including social work, nursing, psychology, and psychiatry, can play an important role in advocating for the delivery of existing best practices to this vulnerable population. Optimism is warranted, given growing success by many developed economies in realizing the promise of EI and the more recent focus by the NIH and SAMHSA in disseminating FES across the United States. The building of robust systems of care for early psychosis will reduce suffering now, but can also provide a valuable platform from which to study and develop improved approaches to treatment and even prevention. For the trainee in public psychiatry, this is an excellent time to enter an area that offers opportunities for meaningful engagement in clinical work, research, policy, and workforce education.

REFERENCES

1. McGrath J, Saha S, Chant D, et al. Schizophrenia: a concise overview of incidence, prevalence, and mortality. *Epidemiol Rev.* 2008;30:67–76.
2. Murray CJL, Lopez AD. Alternative projections of mortality and disability by cause 1990–2020: Global Burden of Disease Study. *Lancet.* 1997;349(9064):1498–1504.
3. Rossler W, Salize HJ, van Os J, et al. Size of burden of schizophrenia and psychotic disorders. *Eur Neuropsychopharmacol.* 2005;15(4):399–409.
4. Juckel G. [Psychiatric disorders and their effects on mortality and morbidity]. *Versicherungsmedizin/herausgegeben von Verband der Lebensversicherungs-Unternehmen eV und Verband der Privaten Krankenversicherung eV.* 2014;66(4):184–187.
5. Laursen TM, Munk-Olsen T, Vestergaard M. Life expectancy and cardiovascular mortality in persons with schizophrenia. *Curr Opin Psychiatry.* 2012;25(2):83–88.
6. Caqueo-Urizar A, Miranda-Castillo C, Lemos Giraldez S, et al. An updated review on burden on caregivers of schizophrenia patients. *Psicothema.* 2014;26(2):235–243.
7. Srihari VH, Shah J, Keshavan MS. Is early intervention for psychosis feasible and effective? *Psychiatric Clin N Am.* 2012;35(3):613–631.
8. Henry LP, Harris MG, Amminger GP, et al. Early Psychosis Prevention and Intervention Centre long-term follow-up study of first-episode psychosis: methodology and baseline characteristics. *Early Interv Psychiatry.* 2007;1(1):49–60.
9. Yung AR, Yuen HP, McGorry PD, et al. Mapping the onset of psychosis: the Comprehensive Assessment of At-Risk Mental States. *Austral New Zeal J Psychiatry.* 2005;39(11–12):964–971.
10. Larsen TK, Melle I, Auestad B, et al. Early detection of psychosis: positive effects on 5-year outcome. *Psychol Med.* 2011;41(7):1461–1469.
11. Hegelstad WT, Larsen TK, Auestad B, et al. Long-term follow-up of the TIPS early detection in psychosis study: effects on 10-year outcome. *Am J Psychiatry.* 2012;169(4):374–380.
12. McGlashan TH, Walsh, BC, Woods, SW. *The Psychosis-Risk Syndrome: Handbook for Diagnosis and Follow-Up.* New York: Oxford University Press; 2010.
13. Cannon TD, Cadenhead K, Cornblatt B, et al. Prediction of psychosis in youth at high clinical risk: a multisite longitudinal study in North America. *Arch Gen Psychiatry.* 2008;65(1):28–37.
14. Addington J, Cadenhead KS, Cannon TD, et al. North American Prodrome Longitudinal Study: a collaborative multisite approach to prodromal schizophrenia research. *Schizophr Bull.* 2007;33(3):665–672.
15. Addington J, Cadenhead KS, Cornblatt BA, et al. North American Prodrome Longitudinal Study (NAPLS 2): overview and recruitment. *Schizophr Res.* 2012;142(1–3):77–82.
16. Srihari VH, Tek C, Pollard J, et al. Reducing the duration of untreated psychosis and its impact in the US: the STEP-ED study. *BMC Psychiatry.* 2014;14(1):335.
17. National Institutes of Medicine. *Evidence-Based Treatments for First Episode Psychosis: Components of Coordinated Specialty Care.* Bethesda, MD; 2014.

18. Tarbox SI, Addington J, Cadenhead KS, et al. Functional development in clinical high risk youth: prediction of schizophrenia versus other psychotic disorders. *Psychiatry Res.* 2014;215(1):52–60.
19. Addington J, Heinssen R. Prediction and prevention of psychosis in youth at clinical high risk. *Ann Rev Clin Psychol.* 2012;8:269–289.
20. McGorry PD, Yung AR, Phillips LJ, et al. Randomized controlled trial of interventions designed to reduce the risk of progression to first-episode psychosis in a clinical sample with subthreshold symptoms. *Arch Gen Psychiatry.* 2002;59(10):921–928.
21. McGlashan TH, Zipursky RB, Perkins D, et al. Randomized, double-blind trial of olanzapine versus placebo in patients prodromally symptomatic for psychosis. *Am J Psychiatry.* 2006;163(5):790–799.
22. van der Gaag M, Smit F, Bechdolf A, et al. Preventing a first episode of psychosis: meta-analysis of randomized controlled prevention trials of 12 month and longer-term follow-ups. *Schizophr Res* 2013;149(1–3):56–62.
23. Morrison AP, French P, Walford L, et al. Cognitive therapy for the prevention of psychosis in people at ultra-high risk: randomised controlled trial. *Br J Psychiatry.* 2004;185:291–297.
24. Addington J, Epstein I, Liu L, et al. A randomized controlled trial of cognitive behavioral therapy for individuals at clinical high risk of psychosis. *Schizophr Res.* 2011;125(1):54–61.
25. van der Gaag M, Nieman DH, Rietdijk J, et al. Cognitive behavioral therapy for subjects at ultrahigh risk for developing psychosis: a randomized controlled clinical trial. *Schizophr Bull.* 2012;38(6):1180–1188.
26. Amminger GP, Schafer MR, Papageorgiou K, et al. Long-chain omega-3 fatty acids for indicated prevention of psychotic disorders: a randomized, placebo-controlled trial. *Arch Gen Psychiatry.* 2010;67(2):146–154.
27. Perkins DO. Review: longer duration of untreated psychosis is associated with worse outcome in people with first episode psychosis. *Evidence-Based Mental Health.* 2006;9(2):36.
28. Marshall M, Lewis S, Lockwood A, et al. Association between duration of untreated psychosis and outcome in cohorts of first-episode patients: a systematic review. *Arch Gen Psychiatry.* 2005;62(9):975–983.
29. Tempier R, Balbuena L, Garety P, et al. Does assertive community outreach improve social support? Results from the Lambeth Study of early-episode psychosis. *Psychiatr Serv.* 2012;63(3):216–222.
30. Secher RG, Hjorthoj CR, Austin SF, et al. Ten-year follow-up of the OPUS specialized early intervention trial for patients with a first episode of psychosis. *Schizophr Bull.* 2014;41(3):617–626.
31. Malla A, Norman R, Schmitz N, et al. Predictors of rate and time to remission in first-episode psychosis: a two-year outcome study. *Psychol Med.* 2006;36(05):649–658.
32. Malla A, Norman R, Bechard-Evans L, et al. Factors influencing relapse during a 2-year follow-up of first-episode psychosis in a specialized early intervention service. *Psychol Med.* 2008;38(11):1585–1593.
33. Srihari VH TC, Kucukgoncu S, et al. First-episode service for psychotic disorders in the US public sector: a pragmatic randomized controlled trial [published online January 15, 2015]. *Psychiatr Serv.* 2015;66(7):705–712.
34. Hagen K HB, Joa I, Larsen TK. Prevalence and clinical characteristics of patients with obsessive-compulsive disorder in first-episode psychosis. *BMC Psychiatry.* 2013;13:156–162.
35. Langeveld J, Bjorkly S, Auestad B, et al. Treatment and violent behavior in persons with first episode psychosis during a 10-year prospective follow-up study. *Schizophr Res.* 2014;156(2–3):272–276.
36. Allott KA, Cotton SM, Chinnery GL, et al. The relative contribution of neurocognition and social cognition to 6-month vocational outcomes following individual placement and support in first-episode psychosis. *Schizophr Res.* 2013;150(1):136–143.
37. Srihari VH, Phutane VH, Ozkan B, et al. Cardiovascular mortality in schizophrenia: defining a critical period for prevention. *Schizophr Res.* 2013;146(1–3):64–68.
38. Insel TR, Fenton WS. Psychiatric epidemiology: it's not just about counting anymore. *Arch Gen Psychiatry.* 2005;62(6):590–592.
39. Straus SE, Tetroe J, Graham I. Defining knowledge translation. *CMAJ: Can Med Assoc J.* 2009;181(3–4):165–168.
40. Meltzer D. Perspective and the measurement of costs and benefits for cost-effectiveness analysis in schizophrenia. *J Clin Psychiatry.* 1999;60(Suppl. 3):32–35; discussion 36–37.
41. Perrow C. *Complex Organizations: A Critical Essay. Echo Point Books & Media*; Second Edition. Glencoe, IL; Sott, Foresman. USA. 2014.
42. Porter ME. What is value in health care? *N Engl J Med.* 2010;363(26):2477–2481.
43. Gray JA. Better value healthcare—the 21st century agenda. *Zeitschrift fur arztliche Fortbildung und Qualitatssicherung.* 2007;101(5):344–346.

11.

HOSPITAL SERVICES

*Charles C. Dike, Marc Hillbrand, Richard Ownbey, Daniel Papapietro,
John L. Young, Srinivas Muvvala, and Selby C. Jacobs*

EDUCATIONAL HIGHLIGHTS

- From the late 19th century to the mid-20th century, state hospitals, most with thousands of residents, provided accommodation and treatment for all hospitalized individuals with mental illness.

- A combination of political and legal mandates, in addition to the discovery of chlorpromazine, led to deinstitutionalization of state hospitals, with a corresponding precipitous decline in both the number and population of state hospitals.

- State hospitals now serve as the receptacle for the most challenging patients from community mental health agencies and general and tertiary hospitals.

- State hospitals house the most severely ill patients who present a high risk of danger to others or themselves, are gravely disabled by their illness, or are under legal commitment or hold to the hospital.

- Treatment planning is by a multidisciplinary team of professionals with the patient and his or her advocates or family members at the center of decision-making regarding the patient's treatment.

- Individualized, recovery-oriented, patient-centered treatment driven by legal and patient advocates has limitations for a select group of patients.

- Agencies such as the Joint Commission, the Center for Medicare and Medicaid Services, the Department of Public Health, and the US Department of Justice monitor and regulate treatment practices in state hospitals.

- State hospitals should develop metrics for evaluating and monitoring the quality of care provided.

BRIEF HISTORY

In the 1840s, human rights activist Dorothea Dix proposed that the mentally ill should be treated in a more therapeutic and humane manner than was the current practice, which was primarily custodial. Her influence was considerable. By the beginning of the 20th century, dozens of state psychiatric hospitals had been built in the United States, some populated by thousands of persons with severe psychiatric disabilities. In the United States and much of the Western world, these men and women were from then on treated according to an institutional model of often life-long inpatient care. The legal foundation for these commitments, most of them involuntary, was often questionable.

State psychiatric hospitals were self-sufficient communities where land was farmed by staff and residents and where cattle were raised. Most staff resided in hospital housing. Many hospitals were built at some distance from existing towns. An important function of this arrangement was ridding the community of its most unruly citizen, a function not unlike that served by jails and prisons.[1,2] For instance, at Connecticut Valley Hospital in Middletown, Connecticut,

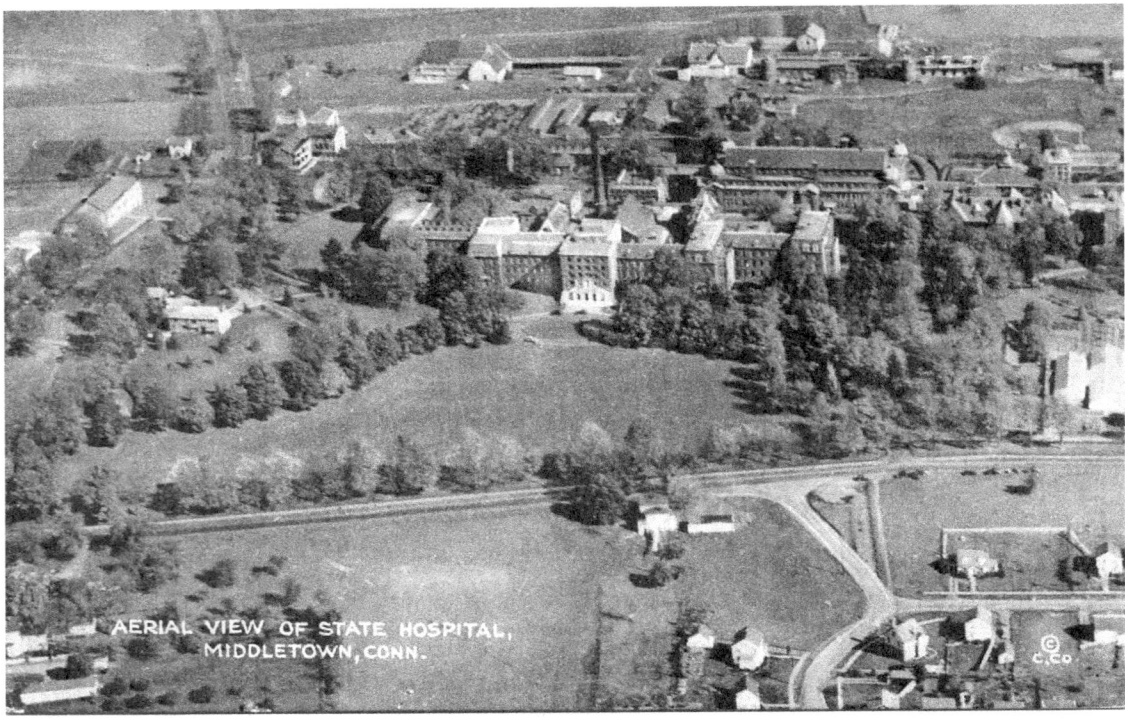

Figure 11.1 Connecticut Valley Hospital, in Middletown Connecticut: Aerial View of the Campus

built in the 1870s, the 5,000-plus residents and staff were early "locavores." Each ward and each department received fresh, warm (unpasteurized) cow's milk daily, delivered by residents who had a job on the hospital farm. The same was true of fresh bread, baked daily in the hospital's oversized kitchens. This practice did not end until the late 1950s, when the ethics and legality of employing hospital residents without adequate compensation came into question (Figures 11.1 and 11.2).

In spite of some strengths, such as the focus on rehabilitation through work, this system of institutionalization suffered from uneven care, inadequate staffing, and often poor living conditions.[3] Deinstitutionalization emerged as an outgrowth of the National Mental Health Act of 1946.[4] The efforts to humanize the care of the severely mentally ill were made possible by the discovery of the antipsychotic benefits of chlorpromazine and other drugs. The National Mental Health Act funded the newly created National Institute of

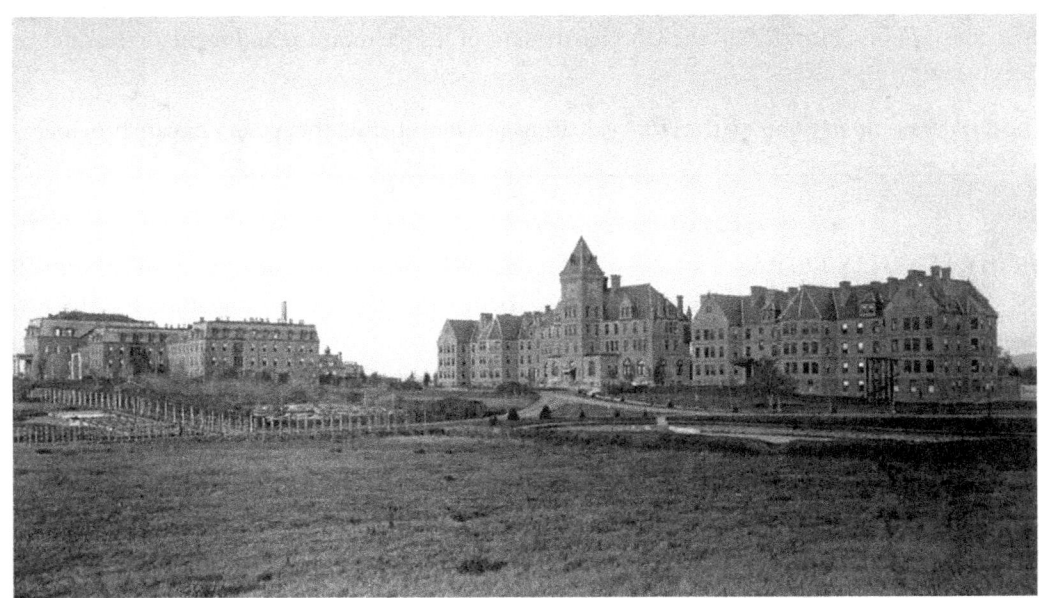

Figure 11.2 Architectural Designs of State Hospital Buildings

Mental Health and set the research agenda of uncovering the causes of mental illness and developing treatments for it. The Mental Health Study Act of 1955[5] then led to the establishment of the Joint Commission on Mental Illness and Mental Health. The Commission's 1961 report listed concerns about civil rights violations and poor living conditions in state hospitals and became the basis of the Mental Retardation Facilities and Community Health Centers Construction Act of 1963,[6] also referred to as the Community Mental Health Act. The Act is the foundation of the community mental health model of care, one of President Kennedy's New Frontiers. Prior to the era of community psychiatry, which began in 1963, state psychiatric hospitals provided virtually all hospital-based care, both acute and long-term. In the past 60 years, as a result of deinstitutionalization, bed capacity in state hospitals has declined precipitously as states redirected their resources to community-based care.[7] Consequently, state hospitals currently devote few if any of the currently available beds to acute care. Coincident with this decline in acute state hospital beds, the enactment of Medicare[8] and Medicaid in 1965[9] financed an enormous expansion of acute care psychiatric beds in general and community hospitals (Medicare and Medicaid Title XVIII, and Title XIX of the Social Security Act). In 2008, Congress also enacted parity of insurance coverage for mental disorders through Medicare and private commercial insurance, thus reinforcing this development (Mental Health Parity and Addiction Equity Acts of 2008).[10]

On the other hand, managed care, utilization review, and fiscal problems in hospitals over the past 20 years have considerably eroded the number of acute beds in general hospitals (see Chapter 2; AHA reports 2007[11], 2012[12]). Furthermore, managed care, sometimes in violation of the federal law parity provisions, reduced the length of stay in acute beds to an average of 7.2 days by 2010, according to the national hospital discharge survey conducted by the National Center for Health Statistics.[13] In response to these fiscal and management pressures, as well as a function of "services research" testing their efficacy, alternatives to hospitalization have emerged such as partial hospital units, intensive outpatient programs, and crisis-respite programs. All these are frequently paired with residential services (see Chapter 4 on Housing). In short, the net result, first noted in an appendix of the New Freedom Commission Report in 2003[14] and heralded in American Hospital Association publications since 2007, is that there is now a shortage of acute psychiatric beds across the United States, and this presents a crisis for general hospital emergency departments (EDs) that struggle to find suitable therapeutic settings to admit acutely ill psychiatric patients.

The Affordable Care Act of 2010[15] reinforces many of the trends discussed briefly so far. Health services research must be directed toward globally assessing both inpatient and outpatient mental health capacitates, developing clinical standards and protocols for each level of service and reducing gaps within the system of care, and improving development of effective interventions to prevent and manage behavioral crises in the community, such as investing in expansion of urgent care and crisis intervention programs.[16] A reason to be hopeful about general hospitals' future investment in psychiatric care is the recent change in attitude within hospitals, aptly captured by the dictum of the Surgeon General of the United States: "there is no health without mental health."[17]

ACUTE HOSPITAL SERVICES

As a result of the developments just reviewed, over the past two decades, acute hospital care essentially has become intensive care. It focuses on rapid evaluation, prompt institution of treatment, management of risk, and concomitant discharge planning to transition patients to step-down care as soon as possible.

The clinical competencies required to work on acute care units are core clinical skills learned in basic professional training. These are refined to address the needs of people with serious mental illnesses and addictions at the height of symptomatic severity. Given the nature of admissions to acute care units, risk assessment is essential (see Chapter 8). In order to step-down care, clinicians must exercise professional judgment to assure that the risk of danger to oneself or others is manageable. Also, given the number of involuntary admissions, issues of informed consent about treatment are common, and efforts to establish cooperative, voluntary, clinical relationships are essential. In addition, on specialized units such as those treating children and young adults or individuals with eating disorders or traumatic brain injury (TBI), expertise in those diagnostic categories or age groups is vital.

Professional staffing of acute care hospital units includes physicians, psychologists, nurses, social workers, counselors, and other support staff who work as members of an interdisciplinary team (IDT). Medical staff guidelines for the hospital, including policies of hospital nursing and social work departments, define the roles of behavioral professionals. These roles include traditional hospital functions such as special diagnostic services, prescribing treatments, 24-hour nursing care, and discharge planning. Given the time pressures created by short lengths of stay, the IDT must function efficiently, usually with a division of labor and often under the eye of a hospital administrator monitoring its productivity and quality. Despite these constraints, skilled, acute-care professionals strive to develop person-centered plans of care that take into account the wishes of people with serious mental illnesses and addictions and set the direction for continuing ambulatory care (see Chapter 3). Consistent with person-centered care, acute-care professionals in hospitals are incorporating the recovery model and patient- and family-centered care (PFCC) approaches into the planning and delivery of mental health care (see Chapter 3 on Recovery model).[18,19] PFCC improves the experience of care and outcomes by ensuring that this care revolves around the needs and wishes of patients and their families. This is achieved by actively involving patients and their families both in clinical care planning and in policy and program development within the organization.

For acute hospital units to operate effectively and maintain safe, therapeutic, and efficient flow of referrals and discharges, they must establish collaborative interfaces with a variety of clinical programs both within the general hospital and in the public arena of community services. Regarding admission, the acute care hospital must be responsive to its own ED, which is often working over census, with high demand and slow transfers into the hospital. Some EDs are equipped with observation beds/units that serve as an intermediate placement while awaiting disposition. Although urgent care services (also known as *crisis intervention units*) are a frequent source of referrals into the hospital, they also help to avoid hospitalizations through the provision of effective, early interventions and placement into respite and residential care. Sometimes this diversion is critical in managing periods of heavy demand, and it is always useful in considering less costly yet safe, effective plans of care.

During hospitalization, the psychiatric consultation service, backed up by the acute inpatient service, responds to other hospital medical units on which acute psychiatric problems arise, sometimes transferring patients to the psychiatric unit when a behavioral problem cannot be managed in a scatter bed. Reciprocally, when a psychiatric admission develops an acute medical crisis, transfer to a medical unit for treatment may occur. The possible synergy between medical care and behavioral health care rarely leads to mutually supportive programs in recognizing and effectively treating the co-occurring conditions on both sides of the health divide. Going forward, the increasing co-occurrence of medical illnesses among psychiatric patients and behavioral health problems among medical patients demands creative approaches to the co-management of these conditions.[20]

At the end of a hospitalization, it is essential for the acute care unit to have well-developed links to the systems of ambulatory and community-based care.[21] Often, acute care units step-down to partial hospital or intensive outpatient programs. Discharge into ambulatory care typically occurs to a community behavioral health center or community health center (federally qualified health center). In each of these cases, the person being transferred enters a difficult transitional period that must be managed as well as possible by both sides of the continuum of care.

Sometimes, in cases with unremitting acute symptoms or an unabating risk of danger to self or others, it is impossible to step-down care. In these cases, the acute care unit must maintain a boundary with long-term care beds, typically in public hospitals or in specialized units for forensic problems, substance abuse rehabilitation, or residential programs for youth.

ACUTE HOSPITAL EMERGENCY SERVICES

Emergency services provide care for those in extreme states of distress or emergent changes in mental status. They congregate a variety of essential capacities that make them unique entities in general hospital function. They are one of the few places where the full range of the technical and personnel resources of the institution can be focused quickly and efficiently on the needs of patients and where decisions about flow and destination can be made. Not only do the ED and colocated behavioral health emergent services have the personnel to address major and urgent physical needs, they also have the mental health resources to handle the evaluation, brief treatment, and dispositional needs of a variety of mental health and substance abusing patients. The ED functions as the valve regulating flow to scarce resources, holding patients who require admission until a bed comes free, diverting patients to appropriate community and institutional outpatient services, and coordinating care by helping patients make the connection to the next best level of care for their needs.

As such, with a diversity of tasks, the ED must have a diversity of personnel with the expertise to carry out those tasks required. Physicians need to be present or quickly available, and advance practice nurses and physician assistants must also handle evaluations and therapeutic needs. It is essential to have specialized psychiatric nursing staff with psychiatric back-up skilled in handling behavioral emergencies. Social workers help manage the collateral contact and the dispositional resources for community-based referrals. Other ancillary staff and protective services also help keep the milieu safe and therapeutic despite the acuity of the presentations to the ED. These behavioral health professionals, drawing in part on psychiatric consultation skills, work in close collaboration with medical colleagues in the ED to ensure that the patient's essential medical needs are taken care off along with his or her mental health needs.

LONG-TERM HOSPITAL SERVICES

People with serious mental illnesses and addictions tend not to respond rapidly to acute interventions. Those who do not respond to acute hospitalization, who cannot be referred into community care, and who require longer term care are referred to the state hospital. The majority of people are admitted under emergency physician orders or probate commitment, for substance abuse-related issues, or for identified forensic issues such as restoration to competency, not guilty by reason of insanity (NGRI), or other court-mandated issues. Although attempts are made to address these patients' needs on an outpatient basis, the population in need of inpatient care presents increasingly with multiple and significant challenges in multiple domains. As with the general population, they are aging and have more medical comorbidities. Many suffer from comorbid substance abuse, personality disorders, and medical illnesses such as obesity or renal, hepatic, cardiac, and pulmonary disorders. Many are treatment nonadherent or frankly treatment-resistant. They are challenged with a lack of resources, cognitive impairments (either as a result of their illness or secondary to medication side effects), social and familial estrangement, housing and employment deficits, and negative symptoms of chronic psychosis that make cooperative access to care challenging.

The patients in state hospitals usually enter because of imminent risk of danger toward self or others or because of grave disability leading to an inability to care for themselves. Even with patients who are not in imminent danger of acting aggressively, frequently, the significance of their aggression history creates challenges for discharge from the hospital. Problematic clinical presentations include repetitive self-injurious acts or suicide attempts; a past history of having acted on dangerous command hallucinations, especially if the psychotic disorder is treatment refractory; a sex-offending history with ongoing sexual urges that are ego-syntonic in a patient without treatable psychotic or mood disorder; and dangerous and severe personality disorders.

TREATMENT PROGRAMS IN LONG-TERM HOSPITALS

By virtue of state hospitals being the repository of refractory mental illnesses of all kinds, subspecialty areas have developed. These include dual-diagnosis units for substance abuse and mental illness, geriatrics, child and adolescent, and forensic subspecialties. In addition, some hospitals have traumatic or acquired brain injury treatment units, and sexual offenders' treatment units. Although not a predictable cohort, there are the inevitable admissions of people who do not fit in other systems. This group is almost always very violent, cognitively challenged, and poorly responsive to psychopharmacologic or psychotherapeutic interventions. Some do not present with diagnosable major mental illness but instead are impaired by severe character pathology that makes them violent and unmanageable in settings other than prison; intermittent short-lived symptoms of psychosis or mood disorder that accompany their character pathology leads to their incarceration in state hospitals rather than prison.

The common characteristic of the special population of patients needing hospitalization in the state hospitals is the long period of time needed to manage their symptoms sufficiently enough to ameliorate the risks of danger that they pose to others in the community (as well as risks of danger to themselves). With the exception of those patients admitted for competency restoration who must be returned to court as soon as they regain competency, state psychiatric inpatients often require specialized and prolonged treatment interventions and, even then, show only incremental improvement of symptoms at a slow pace. Some may never recover enough to be considered safe in the community, whereas some others, such as sex offenders, evoke such negative response from the community that discharge to the community becomes a nearly impossible task. As a result, the length of stay in state hospitals varies widely from several months to decades. Although most of the longest stay patients are those under some form of legal mandates to be hospitalized (e.g., NGRI), some civil patients remain so difficult to manage in any other setting that they require inpatient treatment for many years.

ANCILLARY SERVICES

Given the long duration of stay in state hospitals, ancillary services such as internal medicine, dentistry, neurology, gynecology, optometry, and podiatry play an important role. Ideally, the services are provided on-site, given the patient population's resistance to or refusal of care and the risk of transporting them to medical centers or local hospitals. Additionally, the specter of patients arriving or sitting in waiting rooms of medical centers or acute care general hospitals in restraints and with security staff in close attendance due to their risk of danger to others or of elopement further tarnishes the image of psychiatric patients and decreases the willingness of outside medical staff to treat them. It would, therefore, be prudent for state hospitals to contract with specialty medical services to provide care for these patients on the grounds of the state hospital where they can be safely managed. In that vein, some state psychiatric hospitals have dialysis and nephrology services available on site. Furthermore, a psychiatric hospital will inevitably have emergency situations that necessitate access to a general hospital ED for assessment and treatment. In such situations, the presence of a general hospital nearby is invaluable because transporting the patients long distances could pose additional safety as well as medical risks (Figure 11.3).

THE IDT

PSYCHIATRISTS

As a general rule, the attending psychiatrist is the clinical leader of the treatment team[22] in the state hospital. The psychiatrist's role is to coordinate the care of the patients by integrating the assessments of the various disciplines into generating a differential diagnosis and a coherent plan of care that incorporates the findings of other members of the team. During the treatment planning meeting, the psychiatrist assumes primary responsibility for the individual's treatment; requires that the treatment team function in an interdisciplinary fashion; ensures that the patient's advocates, other clinical staff, and outside agencies (as necessary) have been invited to participate; and ensures that the individual patient is treated with dignity and respect. The psychiatrist ensures that the patient has a substantial and identifiable input into the treatment plans, is informed about the purposes and side effects of prescribed medication, is informed of pertinent results of investigations and consults ordered, and is an active participant in the discharge planning process.

The psychiatrist ensures that all team members participate in the development, monitoring, and, as necessary, revision of treatments. In addition to the patient, any family members present or other advocates are encouraged to participate in the discussion of treatments, and all discharge-related objectives are reviewed and required changes to interventions are considered. In addition, factors that might affect treatment outcomes, including age, gender, culture, and treatment adherence, should be discussed as relevant in the plan of care.

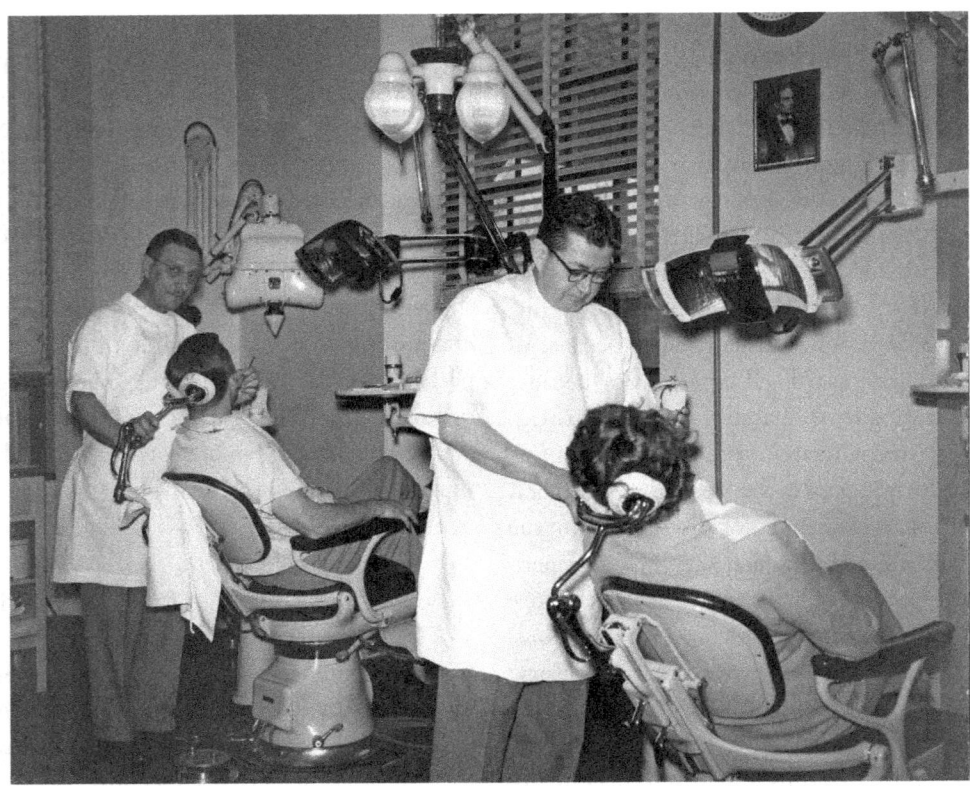

Figure 11.3 Dental Department within the Grounds of a State Psychiatric Hospital

The psychiatrist works collaboratively with a general medicine practitioner (including family practitioners, advanced practice psychiatric nurses [APRNs], etc.) for the treatment and monitoring of medical issues, including side effects of psychotropic medications. It is important to note that the psychiatrist is the physician of record in charge of patients under his or her care, and the role of the general medicine practitioner is consultative. The psychiatrist must be alert to consult the services of the general medicine practitioner as needed and ensure that recommendations are promptly carried out. If the psychiatrist is not satisfied with the recommendation of the general medicine practitioner, the psychiatrist is obliged to seek additional consultation from other providers and communicate with them as necessary in order to address a patient's physical health needs. There should be no confusion as to who bears the ultimate responsibility for the care of the patients: the attending psychiatrist. Of course, the general medical practitioner also bears some responsibility if a negative outcome related to physical health issues occurs.

With regard to risks, the psychiatrist has statutory responsibility and liability risks for judgments about suicide and risk of danger to others. Sometimes, other professionals with a license to practice, such as nurses and social workers, may share in the risk of liability depending on the specifics of the case. Risk assessment is a critical function of the attending psychiatrist (in conjunction with other members of the treatment team), the results of which determine a patient's access to privileges and movement within and outside the hospital. Some state hospitals employ the services of consulting forensic psychiatrists experienced in risk assessment to assist the attending psychiatrist in decisions regarding the movement of dangerous and often legally involved patients into the community or to community placements.

NURSES

Nursing as a discipline coordinates all aspects of the patient's care, reviews issues that arise in the milieu, actively engages with the individual in providing treatment interventions as outlined in the patient's plan of care, and provides support and empathic listening. These interventions further assist in the development of a therapeutic relationship. The nurse continues to assess the individual's response to actual and potential health concerns and provides evaluative data derived from the nursing process prior to the development of the treatment/recovery plan.

Essential nursing interventions include counseling, including crisis intervention; management of the therapeutic environment; assisting with self-care activities; administering and monitoring psychobiological treatments; health teaching, including psychoeducation; providing culturally relevant health promotion, maintenance, and disease prevention strategies; case coordination; and assisting with skill acquisition.

The nurse documents nursing interventions planned to facilitate goals and objectives. The interventions take into consideration the individual's likes, dislikes, and personal preferences. The interventions are specific enough to provide concrete directions for the patient's nursing care providers.

THE APRN

The APRN functions in an increasingly important role on the inpatient unit. The APRN can function as a colleague to the psychiatrist in prescriptive treatment as well as psychotherapeutic (group or individual) interventions. As clinical nurse specialists, advanced practice nurses may also serve as a resource for the clinical education and supervision of the nursing staff, even as they serve an important bridging function between the nursing staff and other members of the team.

REHABILITATION THERAPISTS

The rehabilitation therapist assigned to the treatment team is responsible for presenting the information derived from the rehabilitation assessment, including the patient's education level; employment status; cognitive skills; social, recreational, and leisure activities; life skills; interpersonal and communication skills; coping skills (problem-solving, stress management, and anger/impulse control); substance abuse; and support systems. The rehabilitation therapist is also responsible for providing treatment updates with regard to the patient's progress toward his treatment goals in his assigned individual/group sessions. They ensure that psychosocial rehabilitation services are provided as prescribed in each individual's treatment plan. Rehabilitation therapists include art therapists, recreation therapists, music therapists, and pet therapists.

CLINICAL SOCIAL WORKERS

The role of the clinical social worker is to involve the patient, his or her family and significant others, and the relevant community agencies in both the assessment process and throughout treatment. The clinical social worker conducts a thorough analysis of the person's past life experiences prior to hospitalization (including historical information and past community experience), analyzes the material found, and develops a plan for discharge that includes making specific recommendations to the treatment team regarding relevant discharge-specific interventions based on level of care required in the community or the next level of care. The clinical social worker brings to the team a distillation of specific factors that contributed to the person's hospitalization including history, past successes and failures, community contacts, strengths, supports, and goals that will lead to a formulation of discharge requirements that will increase the likelihood of the person's successful return to the community.

The clinical social worker, in conjunction with the psychiatrist, will address those factors that will likely foster successful discharge, including the individual's strengths, preferences, and personal life goals, as well as the individual's level of psychosocial functioning and failures at lower levels of care. The clinical social worker will identify the skills and supports necessary for the individual to live in the setting into which the individual may be placed, will note progress being made toward discharge and the aftercare plan, and will assess the individual's needs during transitioning to the next level of care.

PSYCHOLOGISTS

The psychologist plays a role in treatment planning and shares an important part of clinical leadership with the attending psychiatrist. General clinical psychologists and other psychologists with specific subspecialty training or certification, such as cognitive and behavioral psychology, neuropsychology, psychoanalytic/psychodynamic psychology, and geriatric psychology (which is comprised of cross-training in geriatrics, organic/neurological disorders, and cognitive-behavioral psychology), make up the psychology staff of a state hospital. Although the ideal is for each unit to have an assigned psychologist, resource constraints often make this difficult to achieve. In most instances, the psychologist and psychiatrist "split" responsibilities between treatment modalities, such as individual and group psychotherapy and pharmacological treatment or physical health work-ups. The psychologist takes responsibility for evaluation and provision of required psychotherapeutic interventions, while the psychiatrist focuses on medication management and, in collaboration with a general medicine practitioner, physical health interventions. In situations where there is no psychologist assigned to a unit, the attending psychiatrist should have a low threshold for seeking the input of a psychologist to manage the challenging patients who form the bulk of individuals admitted to state hospitals today.

All newly admitted patients should undergo an initial psychological assessment, which is an evaluation leading to a basic psychological profile of adaptive, intellectual, or personality functioning and characteristics. The primary responsibility of the psychologist then is to identify individuals whose complex or difficult presentation warrants specialized testing (psychological or neuropsychological) to better ensure the most comprehensive approach to engaging them in treatment. These tests also assist in providing treatment in the format that specifically suits the individual's particular need or impairment.

A psychological evaluation involves the assessment of those various phenomenological, behavioral, and/or cognitive components that underlie one's emotional states and personality. A neuropsychological evaluation, on the other hand, involves the assessment of a variety of cognitive and behavioral functions, such as intelligence, attention and concentration, problem-solving, reasoning, conceptualization, planning and organization, mental speed and flexibility, verbal skills, language, academic skills, perceptual and visuo-spatial skills, new learning and memory, and/or motor skills. Neuropsychological evaluation is indicated whenever brain-based impairments and/or deficits in any of the listed functions are suspected. Psychological testing may be utilized alone or in combination with neuropsychological testing in order to better understand how affective and personality variables may influence one's cognitive skills and functions. Both psychological and neuropsychological evaluations are consultative/assessment procedures. By virtue of the chronicity or intractability and the overall difficult nature of the illness presentation of most patients in state hospitals, it is prudent to conduct psychological or neuropsychological testing on all challenging patients, especially if one has not been done in more than 2 years. The results serve as a useful adjunct in formulating the care of these patients.

Psychologists also conduct specialized assessments and treatment such as positive behavioral support plans (PBSP) or problem sexual behavior evaluation and treatment. The criteria for PBSP include that (1) there is no diagnostic clarity even following psychological and/or neuropsychological evaluations, (2) there is lack of clarity regarding the specific function of a behavior of concern, (3) there is failure to respond to medication trials, or (4) there is a high intensity and high frequency of severe maladaptive behavior such as aggression and self-harm. These assessments are indicated to provide comprehensive functional analyses of the behavior of concern.

In the absence of a behavioral psychologist on a unit, some hospitals establish a mobile behavioral intervention team (BIT) that can be deployed to requesting units to assist in developing behavioral plans as needed and to train staff in their implementation. The behavioral plans range from basic behavioral management techniques or guidelines to more comprehensive (and sometimes complex) positive behavior support plans. The BIT then monitors the implementation and effectiveness of the behavioral plan and makes adjustments as necessary.

The most challenging issue with behavioral plans in state hospitals is the consistent application of the plan by the front-line staff members charged with implementing them. With chronic staff shortages common in state hospitals, staff members untrained in applying specific behavioral plans are often "floated" or reassigned from other units to provide coverage. Even when there is no "float" staff on the unit, the application of the plans often varies across the three shifts. Usually, the unit staff on first shift, by virtue of being in direct contact with the professional, clinical staff, will more likely be better at implementing the behavioral plan than will staff on the other two shifts. One way to overcome this problem is to designate several units as specialty behavioral units, such as a social learning program unit or a unit for other forms of behavioral intervention, in which a token economy system and other behavior re-enforcements techniques and shaping groups are at the core of unit's functioning. Staff will ultimately become steeped in the behavioral techniques by immersion and will be, therefore, more likely to consistently apply the interventions. This is useful for a select group of patients identified as needing behavior modification to manage their aggressive behavior or to improve their social functioning in the community.

Psychologists also take responsibility for psychotherapy programs in state hospitals. It is not infrequent that patients are moved from one unit to another, sometimes several times while in the hospital, but retain the same psychotherapist. Some state hospitals have developed a mobile psychotherapy service (or person) to provide psychotherapy across all units of the hospital. In this situation, all referrals for psychotherapy are assigned (to interns or other trainees and to regular staff) by the psychotherapy service. The psychologist in turn supervises the interns and other trainees.

Psychoanalytic, psychodynamic, and personality theory can be useful in the state hospital to understand and manage individual psychopathology and the milieu. Although all professional staff may draw on this knowledge, often the psychologist is best prepared to use these approaches. In any event, all professional staff must attend to the problems posed by having severely ill people living together for prolonged periods of time in closed environments.

MENTAL HEALTH ASSISTANT (MHA)

The MHAs (frequently called *psychiatric technicians*) play an important role in care and treatment planning. Because the MHA spends as much, if not more time with the patient than most other members of the treatment team and has the opportunity to observe the patient across the three shifts and in different treatment and leisure settings, the MHA presents to the team a more complete description of the patient's behavior and response to treatment interventions. Information garnered through regular (weekly) formal meetings between MHAs and patients often informs treatment, too. The skills of individual MHAs can be harnessed to engage patients in activities during off-shifts, weekends, and holidays; keeping patients busy decreases opportunities for mischief and aggressive behaviors. For example, sports-loving MHAs can be encouraged to run sports groups, watch various sports with patients, and engage them in discussions about them. Other group activities include games group, cooking group, news group, women's and men's grooming group, and so on. Some hospitals train MHAs to use simple manuals developed to teach basic social skills to the most regressed patients in small groups. Although these are not psychoeducational groups, they do teach appropriate social skills and nonviolent interactions, and they complement the more structured groups run by psychologists, rehabilitation therapists, and, sometimes, social workers. Most importantly, they improve communication and positive interaction between patients and MHAs, foster mutual respect, and ultimately decrease opportunities for aggressive behavior by patients.

THE PATIENT

Although the patient is not a formal member of the treatment team, he or she is not a passive recipient of treatment decisions made by the IDT; in fact, the patient is the most important member of the "treatment team." Patient advocacy groups increasingly assert that treatment decisions be driven by the patient, with professional advice only from clinicians; hence, programs and interventions to encourage patient empowerment are on the rise. Most state hospitals have patient advocates on staff, and some have additional legal advocates, often imposed on the hospital through legal mandates or consent decrees, whose role is to protect the civil rights of hospitalized patients. Patients have free and easy access to these advocates and are encouraged to present their grievances to them if they are unable to resolve them with their treatment team. To further foster a collaborative relationship between patients and the state hospital, some hospitals have established patient–staff steering committees with representatives from patients across the hospital, front-line staff members, and some members of the hospital administrative leadership, such as the program manager and the medical director. Patients on the steering committee run the meeting with the support of staff. Because patients are housed in the hospital for months and even decades, the hospital becomes their home by default. Patients are therefore encouraged to present issues that would improve their comfort in the hospital, including environmental issues (e.g., more water fountains, chairs, dustbins in the courtyard, more lighting and heat, etc.) and household issues such as type of toiletries, clothing, laundry times, frequency of showers, and so on. The steering committee also requests and plans activities for special holidays and events (e.g., July 4th, Christmas, and the Super Bowl). In turn, patients are informed of new interventions and proposed changes in the hospital early enough to allow for their input before the changes or interventions are introduced. In most hospitals, a patient representative is included in the planning of such proposed changes and interventions.

State hospitals also empower patients through their involvement in publishing a newsletter on a regular basis, developing and participating in a patient–staff-run radio station, and including patients in the training of new staff.

Before the advent of the recovery movement, the idea of chronically ill and disabled psychiatric patients being active participants in decision-making regarding their well-being and self-maintenance was not always seen as possible or necessary. Now, however, patients are empowered to view themselves as able and capable of managing various aspects of their lives, and they are encouraged to not be afraid to pursue their desires and goals. To that effect, the treatment/recovery planning process is increasingly focused on creating opportunities for patients to manage their lives and on developing resources to enable them to do so. As such, patient-centered care in a state psychiatric hospital must necessarily integrate both treatment and rehabilitation.

MULTIDISCIPLINARY TREATMENT/RECOVERY PLANS

The treatment plan is essentially a written contract between a person and his treatment team that maps out the supports and interventions that the patient will receive to resolve his reasons for admission so that he can be discharged as quickly as possible to a less restrictive setting in the community.[22] The treatment plan describes a complex set of clinical interventions designed to address an array of biological, psychological, and social challenges, as well as to provide a conceptual framework for coordinating services.

One of the most salient influences of the recovery movement (see Chapter 3) in inpatient care lies in its influence on the process of treatment planning. Recovery-oriented treatment planning is a collaborative process, directed by patients (consumers) and produced in partnership with care providers and natural supporters with the goal of encouraging consumer preferences. It aims to identify the specific steps a person can take, within a specific time frame, along with the interventions that can be provided to enable and support those steps, for the purpose of improving his or her life and moving it toward the individual's long-term aspirations.

Recovery-oriented care focuses on goals that are quite different from traditional treatment goals. Rather than focusing only on reducing symptom severity, increasing insight, and strengthening adherence, all of which remain important, recovery-oriented care values goals such as managing one's own life, promoting satisfying relationships and spiritual fulfillment, facilitating access to educational and occupational outlets, assisting in access to permanent housing, and contributing to other quality-of-life indices that emphasize community integration. As such, treatment interventions including social skills training, money management, navigating the challenges of transportation, conflict resolution, vocational skills, and leisure skills that would enhance the chances of success in the community are emphasized in individual and group therapy sessions, irrespective of impairments imposed by the patient's symptoms. These "core groups" are graded so that patients progress from the basic level to a more sophisticated level as they improve.

Personal strengths play a prominent role in recovery-oriented care. They are deliberately incorporated in the treatment plan. In traditional care, they are acknowledged rather than actively used. In recovery-oriented care, strengths and assets are leveraged toward achievement of the individual's stated goal. Treatment should be tailored to the patients' strengths and assets to improve the chances of success.

In a traditional, medical model treatment plan, patients' presenting symptoms are identified as problems; a problem list is subsequently generated, and these form the foundation of the treatment plan. In contrast, recovery-oriented care focuses on the patients' hopes and aspirations and on the barriers (not problems) preventing them from achieving their goals. Hence, the recovery-oriented care is person-centered; it requires that, to the extent possible, the person in treatment identify life goals that set the treatment plan into motion. The focus of treatment planning in this model is not the eradication of problems or symptoms, but rather the mitigation of the barriers that interfere with a person's quality of life. Therefore, unlike in the traditional treatment model, patients with identical diagnoses are likely to have distinctly different treatment plans.

Distinguishing barriers from problems has the benefit of acknowledging that symptom elimination is not always possible—and indeed is often elusive in individuals who are long-term residents of public mental health hospitals. This reconceptualization of problems makes it possible to focus treatment on a wider range of factors that interfere with reaching life goals. Examples of such factors include both deficits, such as limited skills in a given life domain (e.g., social, self-care, safety), paucity of social supports, or hopelessness/helplessness, or excesses, such as interpersonal violence, self-injury, or institutional dependence. From this perspective, treatment aims at ensuring that barriers to life goals are effectively overcome so that the individual can transition to a less restrictive level of care. The patient's input must be adequately represented in the treatment plan, and it must be written in language easily understood by the patient and his or her natural support.

The treatment/recovery plan is based on a foundation of partnership, in which there is mutual respect between the patient and the caregiver. The model recognizes that the person seeking care is an autonomous individual who deserves respect and that the ultimate decision-making rests with the autonomous individual. However, the expertise of the caregiver is also recognized, and high regard is given to his or her professional opinion.

It must be acknowledged, however, that for a subset of patients, especially those mandated by the legal system into the hospital, the concept of autonomy as described here may be circumscribed by external factors. These include individuals involuntarily admitted to the hospital due to risk of danger to self or others, those legally deemed to not have the capacity to give informed consent to treatment, those admitted for restoration to competency, patients found NGRI and whose subsequent treatment and movement are determined by a body or system outside of themselves or their advocates, and those transferred from the Department of Correction (DOC) for psychiatric stabilization after which they will be returned to DOC custody. For these special classes of patients, recovery-oriented, patient-centered care should be pursued with caution. As noted in Chapter 3, a patient-centered plan should allow for uncertainty, setbacks, and disagreements because these are inevitable steps on the path to greater self-determination. Additionally, in their path to recovery, a patient's "dignity of risks" and "right to fail" should be recognized. Understandably, the autonomy of a patient who, in response to untreated paranoid psychosis, killed another person, would be restricted. Any setback or uncertainty regarding her recovery would attract much concern, thereby further limiting her autonomy; she would be seen as having lost her "right to fail" because any failure could lead to unacceptable consequences. However, regardless of legal status, all patients should be encouraged to actively participate in the treatment planning process and exercise choices that will impact their treatment and life, even if such choices are from a restricted range of options.

PARTIAL HOSPITALIZATION

Partial hospitalization is a treatment program for individuals who do not require psychiatric inpatient hospitalization but who need an extended period of observation and treatment during the day. If provided in a timely manner, it can avert inpatient hospitalization. Partial hospitalization also can be used to transition inpatients into the community while still receiving intensive treatment and monitoring.

The first psychiatric day hospital opened in Moscow, during the 1930s, to be followed a decade later in Montreal and London.[23,24] The British Mental Health Act of 1959 encouraged the spread of the modality in England and similarly, in the United States, the 1963 Mental Health Centers Act mandated this form of service.[25] Two years later, the American Association for Partial Hospitalization became established, forming chapters in most states. Annual meetings (with well-prepared proceedings) began in 1976, and 1983 saw the inauguration of the quarterly *International Journal of Partial Hospitalization*.

Although the use of day hospitals may appear to be waning in state hospitals in the United States,[26] a recent report from Scotland has demonstrated their effectiveness for returning forensic patients from the forensic hospital to the community.[27]

It remains to be seen whether this trend is affected by the implementation of the Affordable Healthcare Act of 2010. Although not many mental health professionals have experience with this treatment modality, it has worked well for such challenging groups as individuals with substance use disorders and those living with borderline personality problems. It is especially relevant as a means of safely reducing length of stay for inpatients.

The use of partial hospitalization for the restoration of competency to stand trial has not been systematically demonstrated in the literature so far. It may be of some ethical concern that inpatient hospitalizations for competency restoration increased by 20% between 1968 and 1978, a decade that saw a 20% decrease in admissions overall. The implication is that, as hospitalization becomes less available, more patients are being treated in departments of correction, more by default than by design, and more for nonwhites than for whites.[28] These numbers at least suggest that little or no use of day hospitals is being made for the treatment of patients found incompetent to stand trial and, moreover, that correcting this anomaly may be an effective way to decrease the tendency to criminalize the mentally impaired.

Partial hospitalization has played some role in the evaluation and treatment of insanity acquittees. This application has taken place in Oregon, which for many years has entrusted its insanity acquittees to the jurisdiction of its Psychiatric Security Review Board. An early report pointed to the importance of community programs for successful rehabilitation based on legal, clinical, and financial results.[29] One of the program's major elements was a large day treatment center in a major urban setting, described in a later report.[30] The program provides individualized treatment for its long-term mentally ill clients including suitably qualified insanity acquittees. Between 1980 and 1983, it accepted 110 referrals; most of the rejections were due to the patients' perceived inadequate interest or motivation. Once having entered treatment, after an average of 9 months, half of the patients were returned to the state mental hospital unit for more intensive inpatient treatment. The authors noted difficulty in achieving a transition to independent living among the unsuccessful patients. Among the successful individuals, any new offenses were few and less serious than their original charges.

Other case study or small series reports include the application of partial hospitalization for adolescents in a rural setting,[31] mentally disturbed adolescent offenders from the Court Referred Project in Brooklyn,[32] and aggressive adult psychiatric patients in a rural setting.[33]

SYSTEMIC CHALLENGES IN HOSPITAL PSYCHIATRIC CARE

Conflicts among the various parts of the complex public system sometimes play out in the clinical care of a patient in the hospital. A range of organizations that include community agencies that provide outpatient care (be they public, private, or publicly supported), patients rights organizations, state bureaucracies such as the departments that oversee adult and child public mental health services, public mental health services for individuals with developmental disorders, regional and federal regulatory agencies (such as the Joint Commission, the Department of Public Health, the Centers for Medicare and Medicaid Services [CMS], and US Department of Justice), professional organizations (such as the American Psychiatric Association and the American Psychological Association), and hospital employee unions, are parts of the system that can influence care. The state hospital is only one part of a large and complex system. It is useful to think of each of these agencies as constituencies that have "needs" that must be taken into account as treatment in the microcosm of the hospital is being planned for an individual. A few examples follow.

COMMUNITY MENTAL HEALTH AGENCIES

Many state mental health departments have only one or two inpatient facilities. Community agencies serving individuals with severe psychiatric disabilities are, by contrast, numerous. Some are freestanding and for-profit; others are state-supported through various funding mechanisms such as grants. Each has a unique culture, a unique way of doing business, and a unique history. For example, a community agency may have experienced the loss of a patient to suicide soon after discharge from the hospital. The recollection of this traumatic outcome flavors not only the clinical decisions made at that agency (e.g., greater focus on suicide risk management) but also the anxieties of agency clinicians about accepting patients recently discharged from the hospital.

To ensure continuity of care between the inpatient and outpatient settings, it is necessary for inpatient clinicians to be familiar with the culture of the various community agencies to which they discharge their patients. Without such knowledge, mismatches occur. This task of matching the individual with the appropriate community agency has become so complex that it has largely become a full-time job, one often assigned to a psychiatric social worker on the IDT.

HOSPITAL EMPLOYEE UNIONS

Public psychiatric hospitals are similar to other organizations with respect to their relationship with unions. Sometimes, the missions of the two clash. The basic mission of a union is the protection of its members, both with respect to their safety and their rights. The basic mission of a psychiatric hospital is ensuring the proper care and safety of its patients. At times, good patient care entails placing an employee at some risk for the benefit of a patient. For example, a psychiatric technician may be asked by a supervisor to accompany a patient to a therapeutic activity off the ward, even though the patient recently had an episode of behavioral dyscontrol and therefore poses some risk of harm to that employee. A tension thus exists between ensuring the employee's safety and ensuring optimal care. In the example just mentioned, the technician may refuse to do so, sensing that his union would support him.

In our experience, negotiating dilemmas of this sort is best addressed in the context of a history of labor–management collaboration. This collaboration is best fostered through regular (perhaps monthly) meetings between the hospital administration staff and the leadership of the union to discuss issues with a view of resolving them expeditiously. If the union leadership and its members are convinced that the hospital leadership and the professional staff truly care about the union members and their safety and well-being, then it is possible that the patient will be accompanied to the gym, even though he fairly recently threw a chair against the wall, acknowledging that this intervention poses a risk to the accompanying staff.

REGULATORY AGENCIES

Public mental health facilities frequently receive visits by unexpected site visitors from the Joint Commission, the state department of public health, the CMS, and the US Department of Justice, among others. These agencies often visit in response to a complaint by a patient, a friend or family member of a patient, or a disgruntled employee.

With the exception of the Joint Commission, interactions with regulatory agencies are often adversarial in nature because their involvement can result in litigation or other untoward consequences, including loss of funding for the state hospital. If litigation ensues, all parties lose.

Again, in our experience, with rare exceptions, conflicts between regulatory bodies and hospitals usually are resolved and often with benefit for hospital services. The hospital may have to do some things differently (e.g., use physical restraints less frequently), secure more resources (e.g., hire more nurses), improve the physical plant (e.g., renovate aged wards), or discontinue a practice (e.g., no more two-point ambulatory restraints), among others. In the end, a solution exists that allows both parties to accomplish their mission; namely, for regulatory agencies, to regulate, and, for hospitals, to deliver high-quality patient care. It is worth noting that the oversight provided by these regulatory agencies ultimately leads to improvement and more humane care for patients that otherwise would be lacking.

In conclusion, the following principles emerge from this brief overview of the systemic challenges in state psychiatric hospitals:

1. The task of the public mental health professional is the competent and compassionate delivery of treatments that are evidence-based, in a manner that acknowledges the complex nexus of systemic forces that exert either a facilitating or a complicating influence on patient care.
2. Synergies exist in these systemic conflicts that can be used in a beneficial or harmful way. For example, a regulatory agency review that points out a shortage of nurses empowers hospital leadership to secure funding to hire more nurses.
3. Good outcomes are more likely with an approach that is sensitive to all the complexities of the clinical environment. When bad outcomes occur, it would be comforting to know that the hospital acted professionally and took all the steps necessary to avoid them by incorporating the principles described throughout this chapter.
4. Finally, it comes down to relationships among all the players within and outside the institution. A professional attitude, respect, sensitivity, humility, validation, positivity, and collaboration are all essential ingredients to navigate successfully the seas of inpatient care.

QUALITY METRICS FOR HOSPITALS

Hospitals carefully monitor the quality of care via several mechanisms and metrics. Hospitals must comply with the Joint Commission requirements in order to maintain certification. The Joint Commission has developed a set of core performance measures for Hospital-Based Inpatient Psychiatric Services (HBIPS), which went into effect in 2008. In 2012, the CMS later adopted these measures into its Inpatient Psychiatric Facilities Prospective Payment System (IPF PPS). Also, given recent attention paid to iatrogenic errors, hospitals monitor major treatment events and outcomes. A basic concern in acute care, perhaps more than in any other part of practice in public psychiatry, is the use of restraints and seclusion. Quality assurance teams review restraint and seclusion episodes and pursue treatment strategies that minimize their use. Furthermore, morbidity and mortality conferences review all fatal or other high-risk outcomes, which fortunately are rare. Standard metrics (such as readmissions within 30 days of discharge) are a measure of the success of the hospital service. Another largely independent dimension of outcome is patient satisfaction, as measured in routine surveys. A variety of process measures related to person-centered care also contribute to the overall picture of quality. Other important metrics include the use and justification of polypharmacy, adequate management of side effects of psychotropic medications (e.g., metabolic syndrome and neuromuscular abnormalities), and identification and tracking of individuals deemed by the treatment team to be discharge-ready but for whom there are no appropriate placements in the community.

SUMMARY

This chapter has reviewed hospital services as a major domain of clinical practice in public psychiatry. A sea change has occurred in the past 50 years as the public system swung from almost exclusive hospital care to community care as the basic premise, backed up by specialized, acute, and chronic hospital services. In the hospital setting, a recovery model and practice in IDTs are consistent with other parts of the public system. Excellent communication with all parts of the system enhances hospital care.

REFERENCES

1. Foucault M. *Madness and Civilization: A History of Insanity in the Age of Reason*. London: Tavistock; 1963.
2. Lamb HRL, Weinberger LE. The shift of psychiatric inpatient care from hospitals to jails and prisons. *J Am Acad Psychiatry Law*. 2005;33:529–534.
3. Novella EJ. Mental health care and the politics of inclusion: a social systems account of psychiatric deinstitutionalization. *Theor Med Bioeth*. 2010;31:411–427.
4. National Mental Health Act of 1946, HR 4512, 79th Cong, 2nd Sess (1946).
5. Mental Health Study Act, HR 3458, 84th Cong, 1st Sess (1955).
6. Mental Retardation Facilities and Community Health Centers Construction Act, 88–164, 77 Stat 282 (1963).
7. Glover RW, Miller JE, Sadowski SR. *Proceedings on the State Budget Crisis and the Behavioral Health Treatment Gap*. Washington, DC: National Association of State Mental Health Program Directors; 2014.
8. Medicare and Medicaid: Keeping us healthy for 50 years. Available at http://www.medicare.gov/. Accessed on September, 14, 2015.
9. Medicare and Medicaid: Keeping us healthy for 50 years. Available at http://www.medicare.gov/. Accessed on September, 14, 2015.
10. Mental Health Parity and Addiction Equity Act, 2008. Available at dol.gov/ebsa/newsroom/fsmhpaea.html. Accessed on September 14, 2015.
11. Community Hospitals: Addressing Behavioral Health Care Needs. Available at http://www.aha.org/research/reports/tw/twfeb2007behavhealth.pdf. Accessed on September 14, 2015.
12. Bringing behavioral health into the care continuum: opportunities to improve quality, costs, and outcomes. Available at http://www.aha.org/research/reports/tw/12jan-tw-behavhealth.pdf. Accessed on September 14, 2015.
13. Hospital Utilization (in non-Federal short-stay beds). Available at www.cdc.gov/ncha/fastats/hospital.htm. Accessed on September 14, 2015.
14. President's New Freedom Commission Report. *Achieving the Promise: Transforming Mental Health Care in America*. Rockville, MD: President's New Freedom Commission on Mental Health; 2003.
15. Affordable Care Act, HR 3590, 111th Congress, 2nd Sess (2010).
16. Salinsky E, Loftis C. Shrinking inpatient psychiatric capacity: cause for celebration or concern? *Issue Brief Natl Health Policy Forum*. 2007;(823):1–21.
17. US Department of Health and Human Services, US Public Health Service. *Mental Health: A Report of the Surgeon General*. Rockville, MD; USDHHS, SAMHSA, CMS, NIH, NIMH; 1999.
18. Patient and Family Centered Care Innovation Center. www.pfcc.org. Accessed on September 14, 2015.
19. Institute for Patient and Family-centered Care. www.ipfcc.org. Accessed on September 14, 2015.
20. Bronheim HE, Fulop G, Kunkel EJ, et al. The Academy of Psychosomatic Medicine practice guidelines for psychiatric consultation in the general medical setting. *Psychosomatics*. 1998;39(4):S8–S30.
21. Vigod SN, Kurdyak PA, Dennis CL, et al. Transitional interventions to reduce early psychiatric readmissions in adults: systematic review. *Br J Psychiatry*. 2013;202(3):187–194. doi:10.1192/bjp.bp.112.115030.
22. Connecticut Valley Hospital. *Treatment Planning Manual*. Middletown, CT: Author; 2012.
23. Goldman DL, Arvanitakis K. Ewen Cameron's day hospital and the day hospital movement. *Can J Psychiatry*. 1981;26:365–368.
24. Editorial. Day hospitals for psychiatric care. *Lancet*. 1985;2:1106–1107.
25. DiBella GAW, Weitz GW, Poyntner-Berg D, Yurmkark JL. *Handbook of Partial Hospitalization*. New York: Brunner/Mazel; 1982.
26. Hoge MA, Davidson L, Hill L, Turner VE, Ameli R. The promise of partial hospitalization: a reassessment. *Hosp Community Psychiatry*. 1992;43:345–354.
27. Alcock D, White T. Study of the clinical and forensic outcome of admission to a forensic psychiatry day hospital at one, two, and three years. *J Forensic Psychiatry Psychology*. 2009;20:107–129.
28. Arvanites TM. The differential impact of deinstitutionalization on white and nonwhite defendants found incompetent to stand trial. *Bull Am Acad Psychiatry Law*. 1989;17:311–320.
29. Rogers JL, Bloom J, Manson SM. Oregon's new insanity defense system: a review of the first five years, 1978–1982. *Bull Am Acad Psychiatry Law*. 1984;12(4):383–403.
30. Bloom JD, Williams MH, Rogers JL, Barbur P. Evaluation and treatment of insanity acquittees in the community. *Bull Am Acad Psychiatry Law*. 1986;14:231–244.
31. Gaylor ML. Treating the adolescent offender in a rural partial hospitalization program. In: *Proceedings of the Annual Conference on Partial Hospitalization*. 1978;3:107–116.
32. Jacobs BJ, Schweitzer R. Conceptualizing structure in a day treatment program for delinquent adolescents. *Am J Orthopsychiatry*. 1979;49:246–251.
33. Straussman J. The aggressive client in day treatment—mad and bad. *Proceedings of the Annual Conference on Partial Hospitalization*. 1980;5:107–116.

12.

OUTPATIENT BEHAVIORAL CARE SERVICES

Deborah Fisk, Joanne DeSanto Iennaco, Donna LaPaglia, and Aniyizhai Annamalai

---

EDUCATIONAL HIGHLIGHTS

- Clinical care of persons with serious mental illnesses (SMIs) has shifted from state-funded inpatient psychiatric hospitals to community mental health centers.

- Community mental health centers provide a broad range of clinical and rehabilitative services of varying intensity to people who have SMI and co-occurring disorders.

- The 2010 Affordable Care Act improves the delivery of mental health and substance abuse services, including integrating primary, acute, and behavioral services and creating patient-centered medical homes for people who have chronic diseases.

- Outpatient services in community mental health centers include walk-in services, continuing care treatment, hospital liaison, and specialty teams.

- Effective delivery of outpatient mental health care requires the development of essential core competencies.

- Outpatient mental health treatment services in community mental health centers are delivered by interdisciplinary staff groups, which include psychiatrists, social workers, psychologists, social and vocational rehabilitation workers, peer workers, and case managers.

DEFINITION AND PURPOSE OF AMBULATORY CARE

Ambulatory behavioral health services are mental health and substance use treatment services that are provided for people outside of institutional settings who have disorders that range from mild to severe, including those who have comorbid mental health and substance use disorders (SUDs). In a given year, approximately 26% of Americans who are over the age of 18 suffer from a diagnosable behavioral health disorder. Of these individuals, an estimated 6% have disorders classified as severe, which denote substantial disability and include schizophrenia, bipolar disorder, and severe depression.[1]

When compared to the general population, people who have a psychiatric disorder have higher rates of a co-existing SUD.[2] Studies have found lifetime prevalence rates for SUDs among people with schizophrenia or bipolar disorder of about 50%.[3-5] Integrated care—the treatment of the psychiatric disorder in tandem with the SUD—is increasingly recognized as being the most effective treatment option for these individuals.[6]

Behavioral health services are provided in a wide variety of primary care and specialty care settings and by a range of different providers. Individuals who have mild and moderate disorders receive mental health care from primary care practitioners and community health clinics. Individuals who have serious mental illnesses (SMI) and co-occurring SUDs largely receive mental health and case management services from public-sector community mental health centers. These publicly funded mental health agencies are uniquely staffed and designed to provide a wide range of intensive clinical and rehabilitative services to people who have SMIs and co-occurring SUDs.

HISTORY

Before the passage of the Community Mental Health Centers Act of 1963, ambulatory mental health care for people with SMIs and co-occurring SUDs was provided in private practice offices, very small outpatient clinics, and state hospitals. The Community Mental Health Center Act provided $150 million in federal funds to build new community mental health centers. The primary goal of this expansion was to facilitate the transition of people with SMIs and co-occurring SUDs out of state-funded institutions and back into the community where they would receive their mental health care. Advances in Medicare and Medicaid provided federal government financing for outpatient mental health care, inpatient psychiatric services at general hospitals, and nursing homes. Rather than focusing their attention on treating people with SMIs and co-occurring SUDs in hospital settings, state mental health authorities began to design and deliver a range of clinical and rehabilitative services in outpatient settings.

In 1980, President Jimmy Carter established the Mental Health Systems Act, which was designed to increase and strengthen links between local, state, and federal governments to support and develop community mental health services. This pivotal legislation reoriented ambulatory care to include community mental health, case management, and Assertive Community Treatment (ACT) services. One year later, President Ronald Reagan passed the Omnibus Budget Reconciliation Act (OBRA), which rescinded or redesigned all the items passed in the Mental Health Systems Act. By this time, however, many innovative and intensive community-based mental health care programs were already established as an intrinsic part of the range of services offered by these community mental health agencies.

Mental health outpatient care delivered by federally qualified health care centers (FQHC) was also expanded under the OBRAs of 1989 and 1990. This legislation provided enhanced Medicare and Medicaid payments to health centers via cost-based reimbursement for services. Although FQHCs receive funds from other sources, federal entitlements provide a solid base of health and mental health funding for these organizations.

The 2010 Affordable Care Act (ACA) expands and improves the quality of outpatient mental health services for the uninsured. First, this landmark health care law requires that all individual market and group plans provide coverage for mental health and substance abuse services. Second, the coverage that these insurers provide for mental health and substance abuse care must achieve parity with covered services for medical or surgical care. Third, insurance coverage for behavioral health care is extended to a large group of Americans who are uninsured. Fourth, new funding will support the construction and expansion of services at community health centers, allowing these centers to serve more individuals, offer expanded hours, and hire additional staff. Finally, additional funding is offered to states that strategically integrate primary, acute, and behavioral services, thus creating patient-centered medical homes for people who have chronic diseases.

Despite the passage and implementation of federal mental health parity legislation in 2008 and the provisions for behavioral health in the ACA, challenges remain in developing services that are responsive to the comprehensive needs of people with serious mental health difficulties and co-occurring SUDs. These challenges include timely access to services and referrals, appropriate organization and coordination of services, and a commitment to provide high-quality evidence-based treatment.

COMMUNITY MENTAL HEALTH CENTERS

Originally funded in 1963, community mental health centers were designed to account for a changing locus of care in mental health services. Advances in psychopharmacology enabled many people with psychiatric disorders to live self-sufficiently outside of institutions and in community settings. As these individuals were moved out of institutional settings, their psychiatric care was shifted to these newly constructed community mental health centers. Strategically located in high-poverty areas, community mental health centers provided a range of outpatient, partial hospital, and emergency services to residents of defined geographical areas, known as *catchment areas*. The legislation also defined a role for state mental health authorities in planning and coordinating mental health funding and developing and implementing a wide range of housing, social, and vocational support services for those with SMIs and co-occurring SUDs.

As these agencies grew in size and complexity around the mid-1980s, they faced challenges in engaging, retaining, and effectively serving people with SMIs and co-occurring SUDs. First, many people who needed psychiatric treatment services had trouble navigating large bureaucratic agencies and did not always follow traditional treatment recommendations. Second, many people with SMIs and co-occurring

SUDs have impairments across multiple domains and, as such, need intensive assistance (information, transportation, and brokering) to obtain the community services they require (entitlements, housing, and medical care). Third, the agencies that offered necessary services were often themselves too complex to navigate effectively. This led to a need for case managers to help people with SMIs and co-occurring SUDs obtain the full range of services they needed and support their engagement in ongoing mental health care.

The broad and complex needs of persons with mental illness require that community-based mental health agencies develop collaborative relationships across multiple service sectors, including both within and outside the health care system (income supports, education, employment, housing, police departments, probation and parole offices, correctional system, primary care centers, and general hospitals). Managing a serious illness in which people have myriad social, housing, and vocational impairments requires case management services that are individualized and flexibly deployed.

The specialized outpatient and case management services that are provided to people with people with SMIs and co-occurring SUDs are broader in scope than the care provided through other mental health agencies. Given this, the population of individuals served by community mental health centers is relatively small and the services reflect the type of intensive care required by those individuals.

FEDERALLY QUALIFIED HEALTH CARE CENTERS

Compared to community mental health centers, FQHC serve a larger group of persons with SMIs and co-occurring SUDs; however, the focus of care is routine and preventative. The majority of people with mild or moderate psychiatric conditions such as mood and anxiety disorders and SUDs receive their outpatient mental health care in private doctor's offices or FQHCs.[7]

FQHCs are community-based public and private nonprofit health care organizations that provide a range of primary and preventative care, including health and behavioral health care services. Care is provided regardless of age or income. These agencies must meet certain criteria under the Medicare and Medicaid programs and receive funds for certain health care initiatives under the Public Health Service Act. These initiatives include:

- Community Health Centers, serving federally defined underserved populations.

- Migrant Health Centers, providing preventative medical services to migrant and seasonal workers.

- Health Care for the Homeless Programs, offering outreach, medical, and substance abuse treatment to homeless individuals and families.

- Public Housing Primary Care Programs providing services to residents of public housing buildings in or near their communities.

Primary care providers in FQHCs receive consultation from behavioral health providers related to the mental health needs of individuals presenting for care and offer assistance with assessment and screening, psychopharmacologic management, and, when needed, referral to behavioral health services providers in the community.

Some FQHCs offer full-service mental health clinics. These clinics can accept internal referrals from the primary care providers of people with comorbid psychiatric needs who require more complex management than the primary care setting is able to manage. For example, common referrals might include individuals who do not improve after psychopharmacologic treatment is initiated or who had unexpected responses to treatment. Additionally, behavioral health clinicians in FQHCs offer substance abuse screening and treatment, as well as individual, group, and family psychotherapy.

There are benefits to providing both primary care and behavioral health services in one FQHC setting. First, the medical and psychiatric providers are able to more freely exchange information about persons with SMIs and co-occurring SUDs. Second, consultation may be initiated by the psychiatric provider for medical staff to address chronic health conditions, lab work, and other procedures. These advantages are most evident in serving particular subgroups such as individuals being treated for chronic pain and those who have multiple medical problems as well as comorbid psychiatric symptoms (which may include anxiety and depression). The ability to freely communicate and coordinate care between medical and psychiatric providers enhances the quality of both services.

Depending on the size of the mental health unit of the FQHC, services available can be similar to those offered in community mental health clinics. Smaller FQHCs may be limited in the scope of after-hour psychiatric care. These behavioral health programs may have after-hour coverage, but it is often limited to medical care. This limits the kind of psychiatric emergency support that is available to persons with SMIs and co-occurring SUDs. In turn, FQHCs may not be able to accept and/or treat individuals who are unable to consistently attend clinic appointments and who have complex comorbidities. These individuals would be referred for more comprehensive and intensive services at local community-based mental health agencies.

INTEGRATION OF MENTAL HEALTH AND MEDICAL CARE

People who have serious behavioral health and substance use disorders often have co-existing chronic medical conditions that lead to increased mortality when compared to the general population.[8] These comorbid medical problems are often due to side effects of psychiatric medications, inadequate diet, a sedentary lifestyle, or some combination of these. These individuals often do not receive the medical services they need in a timely manner. They either do not seek preventative medical care or have challenges navigating the complex medical care service system. Additionally, there is a lack of bridged care across the behavioral health and health care sectors. Recognition of this fact has led to a shift toward integrating primary care services into the mental health sector. As a result, multiple integrated care models are being developed. (Refer to Chapter 5 for more information on these models, such as on-site health care and illness prevention services.)

CLINICAL SERVICES

WALK-IN SERVICES

An integral part of any continuum of mental health care is the provision of walk-in services. This is when behavioral health staff members assess and develop service plans for individuals who are referred or present to the agency. These encounters are either crisis-oriented or routine. Crisis services are designed to help individuals manage acute symptoms of emotional distress. This care is designed for those having difficulty coping with a current life event or stressor. People are more amenable to support and intervention during times of crisis, thus making it crucial that crisis intervention services are easily accessible.

When individuals present in a crisis situation, the clinician should focus on understanding the current presenting problem rather than on obtaining a comprehensive and detailed life history. Clinical sessions are focused on helping persons with SMIs and co-occurring SUDs understand the current stressor that prompted them to seek support. Crisis services are brief and problem-focused. If the individual presents with symptoms and is unable to clearly define a problem, the clinician can explore his or her current life circumstances (personal, family, work, and social) to help the individual identify the key issue(s). Crisis intervention is a critical service that demands a high level of clinical skill. In order to fully understand an acute situation, the worker needs to access the person's present behavior and social stressors, but also understand how the person functions when he or she is not in crisis.

Walk-in services also accommodate individuals who are either referred to or present to the agency for routine mental health treatment. These cases involve an intake and assessment in which comprehensive information about the person is collected and evaluated including:

- Demographic data, which includes age, sex, marital status, veteran status, education, and occupation
- Chief complaint, often in the person's own words
- Present episode of illness, including current stressors
- Psychiatric history
- Past and current substance use
- Current medical history
- Personal and social history
- Family history
- Thoughts about suicide, including details about past attempts
- Aggressive thoughts, including details about past incidents
- Present and past legal involvement
- Trauma history
- Adequacy of environmental resources (finances, food, clothing, and shelter)
- Protective factors, including personal coping strategies

Table 12.1 COMPETENCIES FOR WALK-IN SERVICE CLINICIANS

- Conduct a complete evaluation including a mental status examination.
- Develop a clinical formulation.
- Develop an initial treatment plan.
- Assess for capacity for self-harm.

Throughout the initial interview, the clinician is conducting a mental status examination and observing the following:

- Appearance, behavior, and speech
- Consciousness
- Psychomotor functions
- Affect and mood
- Thought content
- Cognitive functions (orientation, memory, intelligence, and executive functions)
- Insight and judgment

The clinician prepares a written case formulation, which is a summary of key psychological, social, and medical factors and their contribution to the person's current psychiatric presentation. The case formulation often includes differential diagnoses. Of critical importance is the development of an initial treatment plan, which includes the length of recommended treatment, frequency of visits, and the provider.

Walk-in units serve as an access point to continuing mental health care both at the agency and in the catchment area. A comprehensive and efficient evaluation may be needed before individuals can be referred to agencies in the community for their ongoing mental health care. While serving as a gateway to continuing treatment within its own walls, the public mental health center also serves as a clearinghouse for information about community agencies that provide continuing mental health treatment services and how to access them.

Many walk-in services also operate mobile crisis teams, telephone crisis services, and actively liaison with local police departments. Mobile crisis teams provide community-based assessments of individuals who are experiencing acute symptoms of mental illness or emotional distress who are unwilling or unable to come to the agency for an evaluation. Mobile crisis staff members also provide immediate response to situations in the community in which there is the potential for self-harm or aggressive behavior directed at others. Mobile crisis services are provided to individuals who are not engaged in ongoing mental health care with the agency, as well to those enrolled persons with SMIs and co-occurring SUDs. Generally, mobile crisis units work in collaboration with officers from the local police department.

Critical competencies for walk-in clinicians include the ability to engage and develop rapport, to convey a nonjudgmental attitude, to listen, to convey genuine empathy, and the ability to build an alliance and form a trusting relationship. Other important competencies include the ability to conduct a mental status examination, develop a clinical formulation, and form an initial diagnostic impression.

CONTINUING CARE TREATMENT SERVICES

In community mental health centers, continuing care treatment teams deliver ongoing mental health and case management services to people with SMIs and co-occurring SUDs. It is essential that these services are evidence-based, person-centered, and recovery-oriented.

In its 2001 report, *Crossing the Quality Chasm*, the Institute of Medicine (IOM) defined evidence-based practice as the integration of the best clinical research, patient values, and clinical expertise. The *best clinical research* is determined by systematic reviews that synthesize the results of multiple studies or individualized controlled trials. *Patient values* refer to the individualized concerns, preferences, and expectations that individuals have for their treatment. These values are essential in guiding all clinical decisions.[9] *Clinical expertise* refers to the proficiency and judgment that comes from clinical experience and clinical practice (Table 12.2).

In continuing care treatment teams, the primary interventions include medication management and psychosocial treatments. Medication management is an important component of care for those who have serious and persistent psychiatric and substance use disorders. Many psychiatric disorders necessitate the use of medications for acute symptom control, stabilization, and relapse prevention. Thus persons with SMIs and co-occurring SUDs often require psychotropic medications for extended periods of time. Additionally, there are subgroups of persons with SMIs and co-occurring SUDs for whom medications are not effective in reducing or stabilizing psychiatric symptoms. For example, it is estimated that 25–50% of people who

Table 12.2 COMPETENCIES FOR CONTINUING TREATMENT CLINICIANS

- Ability to work as a member of a multidisciplinary team
- Knowledge of evidence-based treatment models
- Ability to provide individualized, person-centered, and recovery-oriented care

have schizophrenia have persistent residual symptoms,[10-12] even when they do adhere to a prescribed medication regimen. Clozapine, an antipsychotic medication with superior efficacy in treating refractory symptoms of schizophrenia, is limited in that only 30% of persons with SMIs and co-occurring SUDs show an adequate response to the medication.[13,14]

Many other biologic treatments, some of which are still under development, are also used with treatment-refractory persons with SMIs and co-occurring SUDs, especially those with mood disorders. Electroconvulsive therapy, one of the oldest somatic treatments, can be effective for the aforementioned individuals who have major depressive disorders or for acute symptom control in many psychiatric conditions.[15] Examples of other somatic treatments include vagal nerve stimulation and transcranial magnetic stimulation for refractory depression and other mood disorders.[16] However, symptom reduction with medications or other biologic treatments is only part of the overall self-management plan. A collaborative discussion of the person's goals, treatment targets, and barriers to self-management is necessary for effective care. Pharmacologic treatment, in particular, should always be within a person-centered context. Shared decision-making about use of psychiatric medications—*patient-centered medicine*—is being advocated as an ethical imperative[17] that also has been shown to increase medication adherence and improve outcomes.[18]

An important aspect of patient- or person-centered medicine is an understanding of the risks and benefits associated with the use of medications. It is important that persons with SMIs and co-occurring SUDs understand the risks and benefits associated with prescribed medications so that they can make an informed choice about whether or not to take these medications, as well as to participate in effective monitoring to minimize side effects and thereby improve long-term outcomes. Many second-generation antipsychotics are associated with weight gain and metabolic disturbances and require persons with SMIs and co-occurring SUDs to appropriately manage these conditions with the support of outpatient behavioral health clinicians. Also, adherence to treatment is improved if specific treatment targets are identified by individuals rather than predetermined by clinicians. Also, somatic-based treatments are more likely to be effective if based within a person-centered, recovery-oriented model of care.

Shared decision-making can be difficult to implement in circumstances in which the individual's judgment is impaired due to symptoms of mental illness. Also, stigma surrounding mental illness is an important reason why people are resistant to acknowledging and accepting treatment. There are also situations in which treatment is involuntary, such as when a physician commits someone to a hospital. In these circumstances, it is still possible to find commonly agreed upon goals between the provider and the patient. In cases where coercion is required, such as in forensic and acute care settings, these coercive measures should be undertaken in ways that the person's remaining degree of autonomy is maintained. The ultimate goal is always recovery and self-management. The following principles are helpful in attaining goals of self-management:

- Elicit the person and family's perspectives on the issues that brought the person to care.

- Assess the person and family's perceived needs and priorities, including cultural preferences (e.g., ethnic, sexual, spiritual).

- Identify the person's short- and long-term goals.

- Identify medication targets that indicate that people are overcoming barriers to life goals or increasing their quality of life (over and above symptom reduction).

- Prescribe medication as one component of an overall self-management plan that builds on the person's and his or her family's strengths.

- Identify and address barriers to self-management, including the need for additional supports (e.g., transportation, child care, reminders, environmental modifications).[19]

Empirical evidence exists for the use of several psychosocial treatment interventions for people who have schizophrenia. These include intensive case management, assertive community treatment, family psychoeducation, and supported employment services. These psychosocial interventions, evaluated in randomized clinical trials, have been found to be effective in various ways for those with schizophrenia:

- Intensive case management is associated with reduced use of psychiatric hospital services, higher rates of employment, lower rates of homelessness, and overall improvements in general functioning.[20]

- Assertive community treatment is associated with reduced use of psychiatric hospital services and higher rates of maintaining involvement with outpatient mental health care.[21]

- Family interventions, including those that educate families about schizophrenia, and provide family support, offer families training in effective problem-solving and communication and are associated with fewer rates of relapse.[22]

- Supported employment services are associated with improved vocational outcomes.[23,24]

Empirical evidence has also found that cognitive behavior therapy is an effective treatment for people who have anxiety disorders[25] and for those who are severely depressed, provided that it is conducted by well-trained therapists.[26] Additionally, there is empirical evidence that dialectical behavior therapy is an effective treatment for people with borderline personality disorder,[27] and motivational interviewing is an effective treatment for people who have alcohol or drug use disorders.[28]

Many states, including Connecticut, have implemented the evidence-based practice of integrated dual disorders treatment (IDDT). This allows for the provision of treatment for both illnesses within one program conducted by a multidisciplinary team. Integrated treatments, in addition to ensuring that both mental health and substance abuse issues are addressed in one setting, also allow for comprehensive person-centered recovery planning. This is optimal because it avoids placing the burden on persons with SMIs and co-occurring SUDs who formerly had to seek services from two separate systems of care (the public mental health system and the specialty substance abuse treatment system). Drake and colleagues have found that the three most effective psychosocial interventions for improving substance use outcomes in integrated service systems are group counseling, contingency management, and longer term residential services.[29]

It is important that clinicians receive education and training in psychosocial treatment approaches that meet best practice standards, including the therapeutic techniques used in these approaches. Clinical supervision from more experienced staff members is also an essential tool in supporting and monitoring clinicians as they implement these techniques in practice.

To complement the range of evidence-based psychosocial treatments, supportive individual counseling, medication management, group treatment, resocialization groups, and other specialized groups (clozapine, relapse prevention, trauma groups) can be offered. Since serious psychiatric disorders can have a substantial impact on activities of daily living, case management, social rehabilitation, and vocational rehabilitation services are important additional components to outpatient behavioral health treatment for many individuals. These support services are designed to assist people with serious behavioral health disorders develop basic skills in various activities of daily living. Some of these skill areas are in money and medication management, as well as in health and wellness, social and interpersonal skills, vocational assistance, and entitlement and housing supports.

The care of many persons with SMIs and co-occurring SUDs by behavioral health treatment teams requires contact with a range of agencies and providers outside of the mental health service system. This includes a range of housing supports including local housing authorities, board-and-care facilities, homeless shelters, and local landlords. Additionally, entitlement workers, probation and parole workers, visiting nurses, social and vocational workers, and health care personnel are also involved in the care of people who have SMIs and co-occurring SUDs (see Box 12.1).

Continuing mental health treatment teams in community mental health centers are often interdisciplinary and include psychiatrists, social workers, psychologists, social and vocational rehabilitation workers, peer workers, and case managers. These teams are responsible for providing a broad range of treatment services including pharmacotherapy, individual, group and family psychotherapy, brief treatment, crisis management, case management, social and vocational rehabilitative services, housing supports, and psychoeducation. Guided by recovery-oriented principles, individual and group treatments are person-centered. They are designed for persons with SMIs and co-occurring SUDs based on their clinical and current psychosocial situations as well as their individual preferences.

Box 12.1 COMMUNITY MANAGEMENT OF A MAN WITH MULTIPLE NEEDS

Mr. W. is a 48-year-old man who has a long history of schizophrenia. He has resided in mental health-supported housing for two decades. Despite taking psychiatric medication, he continues to have paranoid delusions. After a bout of enuresis, he allowed the case management staff of the housing program to take him to a medical doctor where he was found to have a small mass on one of his kidneys. He refused to consider the doctor's recommendation to have it removed because he believed that his internal organs were not his and that God told him that he did not need surgery. An additional case manager was assigned to coordinate care with all involved providers. His clinician worked with the psychiatrist to apply for conservatorship, which was awarded to the person's sister. After having been estranged from the family for some time, his sister worked with the providers and convinced Mr. W to have what was a successful surgical procedure.

Essential competencies for continuing treatment team clinicians include the ability to work as a member of an interdisciplinary team, knowledge of evidence-based treatment models, the ability to flexibly provide case management services or collaborate with case managers, and the ability to provide individualized, person-centered, and recovery-oriented care.

INPATIENT HOSPITAL ADMISSIONS AND DISCHARGES

Deinstitutionalization refers to an international reorientation in the provision of treatment for peoples with SMIs and co-occurring SUDs in which the psychiatric treatment provided to these individuals was shifted from state hospitals to community settings. This involved three interrelated and evolving forces. The first is the release of long-term hospitalized persons with SMIs and co-occurring SUDs from institutions into the community. The second is the diversion of new hospital admissions and readmissions, and the third is the development of a wide array of community mental health treatment and residential care services.

Prior to the mid-1950s, people with SMIs and co-occurring SUDs were predominately treated in public mental hospitals. In 1955, the number of individuals in these hospitals peaked with a total of 558,922 people in state facilities. Between 1955 and 1965, there was a 15% reduction in these hospitals, and, after the passage of Medicare in 1965, these rates dropped a dramatic 65%. By 1980, the total number of public state hospital residents declined to 137,810.

This historical shift in care is the result of a complex set of interrelated factors, was led by the introduction of Medicaid, which paid for nursing home care for people with SMI. As a result, many individuals were directly transferred from state hospitals to nursing homes, and, through screening processes, many more prospective state hospital residents with SMIs and co-occurring SUDs were diverted to nursing care facilities, thus shifting the cost of psychiatric care for these individuals from the states to the federal government.[30]

Deinstitutionalization was further fueled by the discovery of antipsychotic medications, lobbying by families and human rights groups, the expansion of federal disability income, and federal reimbursement for inpatient psychiatric services at general and private hospitals.

The implication of deinstitutionalization for psychiatry is that access to psychiatric inpatient beds is more restricted, hospital admissions are of a relatively short duration, and inpatient hospital psychiatric beds are located across different agencies (i.e., general hospitals, private psychiatric hospitals, and state hospitals). Despite the restricted access to acute psychiatric beds, inpatient psychiatric care remains an essential and important component of the mental health service system. Inpatient psychiatric treatment is used for acute stabilization of psychiatric symptoms. Examples of people who are admitted to inpatient psychiatric beds include individuals who are experiencing severe psychiatric symptoms and have difficulties with behavioral control, are at serious risk for self-harm, pose serious physical risk to others, or have complex comorbid medical and psychiatric problems or neuropsychiatric impairment.

Local emergency rooms serve as the main portal of entry to inpatient psychiatric beds in specified geographic areas. This makes it important that community mental health agencies develop and maintain a close working alliance with their local emergency departments, thus affording efficient sharing of the clinical information necessary for a thorough evaluation of persons with SMIs and co-occurring SUDs. This is particularly important for making the important decision as to whether or not to hospitalize a particular individual. This cross-agency collaboration helps optimize the use of available psychiatric inpatient beds, the majority of which are now located in local general hospitals (see Box 12.2).

An important strategy for monitoring and supporting peoples who are transitioning out of hospitals to outpatient behavioral health care involves establishing a liaison role. A liaison can provide an important bridge for people to

---

Box 12.2 **A TRANSITION ACROSS LEVELS OF CARE**

Mr. L. is a 39-year-old man who has a long history of schizophrenia and persistent delusions that he has had children with several women who have kidnaped them. He insisted that a woman who worked at a local public elementary school was the woman who kidnapped one of his daughters. He started stalking her, calling the school and telling them to fire her because she was a danger to children, and visiting the school playground during school hours looking at the children and hoping to find his daughter. He was involuntarily hospitalized on the psychiatric unit of the local general hospital. Three days later, one of the covering social workers called the agency's hospital liaison to say that they planned to discharge the patient because he had baseline psychotic symptoms. The liaison reminded the staff of the circumstances that preceded the admission. The social worker conveyed this information to the hospital treatment team who decided to hold the patient for a longer admission and invited the outpatient clinician to the hospital to assess the patient further

Table 12.3 COMPETENCIES FOR HOSPITAL LIAISON STAFF

- Facilitation and collaboration skills
- Willingness to participate in shared planning and decision-making
- Demonstration of mutual respect and conflict resolution skills
- Knowledge of both private and public psychiatric systems, including emergency rooms and inpatient units

Table 12.4 COMPETENCIES FOR STAFF WHO WORK ON SPECIALIZED TEAMS

- Flexibility
- Persistence
- Ability to work on interagency and interdisciplinary teams

the community, whether they are leaving general hospital psychiatric units after short-term admissions or state hospitals after longer term admissions. The liaison can establish a relationship with the individual's treatment team, thus facilitating communication between the inpatient and outpatient teams. Additionally, the liaison can visit the person in the hospital, help create an individualized transition plan, link these individuals to community services, and schedule after-care appointments for mental health care prior to their discharge from the hospital. A successful transition from inpatient to outpatient treatment may involve reinstatement of entitlements, securing housing, a referral to social rehabilitation services, and helping to ensure family support.

The liaison can arrange for newly assigned outpatient clinicians to meet individuals before they leave the hospital. Rates of follow-up after discharge have been enhanced by direct communication between individuals and newly assigned clinicians.[31,32]

Essential competencies for liaison staff include knowledge of both private and public psychiatric systems including emergency rooms and inpatient units and facilities, facilitation and collaboration skills, willingness to participate in shared planning and decision-making, the ability to cooperate and work together, demonstration of mutual respect, and conflict resolution skills.

SPECIALTY TEAMS

Several intensive and innovative programs exist in the mental health sector including ACT teams, jail diversion programs, crisis intervention teams (CITs), and homeless outreach teams, among others. Each of these programs or teams provides specific services to a particular subgroup of people with SMIs and co-occurring SUDs. These programs are offered as part of a continuum of care, with people flexibly moving between outpatient behavioral health services and specialized care teams.

ACT is an evidence-based treatment model that provides assertive and community-based clinical and case management services to individuals who have serious behavioral health disorders and co-occurring SUDs who have not otherwise engaged in outpatient treatment. Interdisciplinary teams provide psychiatric care and case management services to these individuals in community settings, including their own living environments. ACT teams maintain a low client-to-staff ratio and provide services beyond the typical workday. These services are reserved for people who are severely ill and who use intensive services such as inpatient and emergency psychiatric care.[33] Given the volume of the services provided by ACT teams, there are often waitlists for this effective service, and, in some agencies, the service is not available. In these circumstances, severely ill individuals receive outpatient treatment services (see Chapter 13 for a more detailed summary of the ACT team model).

In many community mental health clinics, forensic services have been designed in response to concern about the high prevalence of people with mental illness in criminal justice and correctional settings. It is estimated that people with SMI comprise between 6% and 18% of the inmates in jails and prisons across the United States, a rate that is two to five times higher than that of the general population.[34] Rates of arrest among people with SMI are also high: between 28% and 52% of persons with SMI in the United States have been arrested at least once.[35–37]

Jail diversion programs target people with SMIs and co-occurring SUDs who have committed nonviolent crimes or probation offenses. This is beneficial in diverting such individuals from jail to community mental health programs. These programs screen individuals for the presence of a mental illness and evaluate them or collaborate with mental health professionals who conduct these evaluations. Furthermore, diversion programs seek to negotiate with attorneys and the courts for a disposition that links these individuals with psychiatric and substance abuse treatment rather than continued confinement, an important component of follow-up procedures. There is recent evidence that jail diversion programs lead to reduced days spent in jail and increased connections to community-based services for those who have SMIs and co-occurring SUDs.[38]

Pinals (2014) suggests that expanding community-based psychiatric and case management services for people with SMIs and co-occurring SUDs in all phases of criminal justice involvement is important in helping these individuals remain connected with psychiatric care and providing assistance in securing tangible supports, including entitlement and housing services[39] (See Chapter 8 for a more detailed discussion of forensic services for people with SMIs and co-occurring SUDs.)

A CIT is a collaborative model between mental health staff and local police. A CIT is designed to enhance the ability of police officers to respond to situations in the community that involve people with SMIs and co-occurring SUDs. Although the goals of these programs vary from one site to the next, overarching goals include providing improved safety for officers and the disordered individual, linking individuals to psychiatric services, and diverting those with SMIs and co-occurring SUDs to hospital settings rather than jails. Research on CIT has found that it improves officers' confidence in interacting with citizens with mental illness,[40–42] enhances their knowledge about mental illness,[41,42] improves the ability to divert those with SMIs and co-occurring SUDs from arrests, and improves rates of referrals to psychiatric clinics for follow-up services.[43]

Homeless outreach teams (refer to Chapter 13 for more detail on this model) are designed to locate people with mental illnesses or co-occurring disorders who are not receiving behavioral or medical health care and provide intensive case management to link them with mental health resources, substance abuse treatment, medical services, and housing. Developing collaborative relationships with a continuum of community providers, particularly public housing agencies designed to extend subsidized housing services for people with serious behavioral health disorders, is particularly important in the effective delivery of homeless services (refer to Chapter 13 for more detail on homeless outreach team models).

Competencies that are essential for staff members who work in these specialty teams will vary based on the specific team, but often include persistence, the ability to broker services between agencies or service systems, and the ability to work on interagency and interdisciplinary teams.

BEHAVIORAL HEALTH CARE COMPETENCIES

The outpatient behavioral health workforce is large and interdisciplinary. The adoption of core competencies necessary for outpatient staff supporting patients with psychiatric disorders is complex, dynamic, and ongoing. Competence in outpatient behavioral health care has been defined as "attitudes, values, knowledge, and skills needed to deliver quality services to people with SMI".[44] A competency is a measurable human capability required for effective delivery of evidence-based and recovery-oriented outpatient care in public-sector psychiatry.

In 1998, the Substance Abuse and Mental Health Services Administration (SAMHSA) commissioned a consensus group that articulated 12 general core competencies for providing outpatient services to adults with behavioral health disorders. These include the knowledge and skills necessary to (1) develop a person-oriented service delivery system; (2) engage and provide relevant services to those close to the patient (i.e., family and friends); (3) develop psychosocial knowledge about SMI; (4) develop basic biological and pharmacological knowledge about mental illness and psychiatric medications; (5) develop and implement a range of effective psychosocial interventions; (6) provide individualized treatment approaches, including the ability to design, deliver, and document their interventions; (7) maintain a thorough understanding of community resources, entitlements, and benefit programs in order to assist persons with SMIs and co-occurring SUDs in obtaining them; (8) understand relevant laws and legal issues; (9) demonstrate the ability to collaborate within and across multiple funding, governing, and service agencies; (10) ensure that agency providers adhere to professional and ethical standards and pursue professional development; (11) understand the elements of culturally competent mental health treatment; and (12) be aware of the importance of research and other types of feedback to improve personal and agency outcomes.[44]

In 1999, the Surgeon General's Report on Mental Health first introduced the concept of *recovery*. The SAMHSA's working definition of recovery is a process of change through which individuals improve their health and wellness, live self-directed lives, and strive to reach their full potential.[45] Some key components of recovery include involvement in fulfilling activities and having a sense of purpose in one's life, as well as hope, dignity, respect, choice, and social support. Recovery-oriented care is a collaborative model that identifies and incorporates a person's goals, interests, and strengths in order to support him or her in living a full and meaningful life in the community. Additionally, it promotes person-centered care or shared decision-making in which the provider includes the person in any and all aspects of his or her treatment.

All aspects of clinical outpatient services, including medication management, psychosocial interventions, walk-in and crisis services, liaison to inpatient hospital units, and specialty services, require competencies that are evidence-based and recovery-oriented. Ongoing training and supervision are essential tools for sustaining these essential competencies.

SUMMARY

Community mental health centers provide person-centered and recovery-oriented clinical and rehabilitative services to persons with SMIs and co-occurring SUDs. These specialty care services are provided to a relatively small group of eligible individuals who have a range of needs, at times intensive in nature. Interdisciplinary teams provide outpatient behavioral health care services that include walk-in and crisis services, continuing care treatment, hospital liaison services, and specialty teams. Evidence-based medication management and psychosocial treatments are offered in tandem with case management and rehabilitative services. Designed to provide a range of supports, these services help individuals to lead independent and full lives in the community. Particular emphasis is placed on the staff member's ability to see the person beyond his or her illness and believe in his or her potential for recovery.

REFERENCES

1. Kessler RC, Berglund P, Demler O, Jin R, Walters EE. Lifetime prevalence and age-of-onset distributions of DSM-IV disorders in the National Comorbidity Survey Replication. *Arch Gen Psychiatry.* 2005;62(6):593–602.
2. Kessler RC, Crum RM, Warner LA, Nelson CB, Schulenberg J, Anthony JC. Lifetime co-occurrence of DSM-III-R alcohol abuse and dependence with other psychiatric disorders in the national comorbidity survey. *Arch Gen Psychiatry.* 1997;54(4):313–321.
3. Mueser KT, Yarnold PR, Rosenberg SD, Swett C Jr, Miles KM, Hill D. Substance use disorder in hospitalized severely mentally ill psychiatric patients: Prevalence, correlates, and subgroups. *Schizophr Bull.* 2000;26(1):179–192.
4. Kavanagh DJ, Waghorn G, Jenner L, et al. Demographic and clinical correlates of comorbid substance use disorders in psychosis: Multivariate analyses from an epidemiological sample. *Schizophr Res.* 2004;66(2–3):115–124.
5. Regier DA, Farmer ME, Rae DS, et al. Comorbidity of mental disorders with alcohol and other drug abuse. Results from the epidemiologic catchment area (ECA) study. *JAMA.* 1990;264(19):2511–2518.
6. Drake RE, Mueser KT, Brunette MF. Management of persons with co-occurring severe mental illness and substance use disorder: program implications. *World Psychiatry.* 2007;6(3):131–136.
7. Kessler RC, Wang PS. The descriptive epidemiology of commonly occurring mental disorders in the United States. *Ann Rev Pub Health.* 2008;29:115–129.
8. Colton C, Manderscheid R. Congruencies in increased mortality rates, years of potential life lost, and causes of death among public mental health clients in eight states. *Prevent Chronic Dis.* 2006;3(2):1–14. http://www.cdc.gov/pcd/issues/2006/apr/05_0180.htm. January 4, 2015.
9. Institute of Medicine. *Crossing the quality chasm: A new health system for the 21st century.* Washington, DC: National Academy Press; 2001.
10. Kane JM, Marder SR. Psychopharmacologic treatment of schizophrenia. *Schizophr Bull.* 1993;19(2):287–302.
11. Pantelis C, Barnes TRE. Drug strategies and treatment-resistant schizophrenia. *Austral New Zeal J Psychiatry.* 1996;30(1):20–37.
12. Wiersma D, Nienhuis FJ, Slooff CJ, Giel R, Davies TW. 15 Years of follow-up of nonaffective functional psychotic disorders showed a high risk for relapse, suicide, and chronicity. *Evidence-Based Medicine.* 1998;3(5):159.
13. Kane JM, Honigfeld G, Singer J, Meltzer H. Clozapine for the treatment-resistant schizophrenic: results of a US multicenter trial. *Psychopharmacology.* 1989;99(1 Suppl.):S60–S63.
14. Essali A, Al-Haj Haasan N, Li C, Rathbone J. Clozapine versus typical neuroleptic medication for schizophrenia. *Cochrane Database Syst Rev.* 2009;21(1): CD000059.
15. Geddes J, Carney S, Cowen P, et al. Efficacy and safety of electroconvulsive therapy in depressive disorders: a systematic review and meta-analysis. *Lancet.* 2003;361(9360):799–808.
16. Rosa MA, Lisanby SH. Somatic treatments for mood disorders. *Neuropsychopharmacology.* 2012;37(1):102–116.
17. Drake RE, Deegan PE. Shared decision making is an ethical imperative. *Psychiatr Serv.* 2009;60(8):1007.
18. Davidson L, Roe D, Andres-Hyman R, Ridgway P. Applying stages of change models to recovery from serious mental illness: contributions and limitations. *Isr J Psychiatry Rel Sci.* 2010;47(3):213–221.
19. SAMHSA. *Guiding Principles for Person-Centered Psychopharmacology and the Promotion of Patient Self-Management.* Rockville, MD: Substance Abuse and Mental Health Services Administration; 2013.
20. Dieterich M. Intensive case management for severe mental illness. *Cochrane Database Syst Rev.* 2010; (10): CD007906
21. Scott JE, Dixon LB. Assertive community treatment and case management for schizophrenia. *Schizophr Bull.* 1995;21(4):657–668.
22. Dixon LB, Lehman AF. Family interventions for schizophrenia. *Schizophr Bull.* 1995;21(4):631–643.
23. Drake RE, McHugo GJ, Bebout RR, et al. A randomized clinical trial of supported employment for inner-city patients with severe mental disorders. *Arch Gen Psychiatry.* 1999;56(7):627–633.
24. Lehman AF, Goldberg R, Dixon LB, et al. Improving employment outcomes for persons with severe mental illnesses. *Arch Gen Psychiatry.* 2002;59(2):165–172.
25. Gelernter CS, Uhde TW, Cimbolic P, et al. Cognitive-behavioral and pharmacological treatments of social phobia. A controlled study. *Arch Gen Psychiatry.* 1991;48(10):938–945.
26. DeRubeis RJ, Hollon SD, Amsterdam JD, et al. Cognitive therapy vs medications in the treatment of moderate to severe depression. *Arch Gen Psychiatry.* 2005;62(4):409–416.
27. Linehan MM, Comtois KA, Murray AM, et al. Two-year randomized controlled trial and follow-up of dialectical behavior therapy vs therapy by experts for suicidal behaviors and borderline personality disorder. *Arch Gen Psychiatry.* 2006;63(7):757–766.
28. Burke BL, Arkowitz H, Menchola M. The efficacy of motivational interviewing: A meta-analysis of controlled clinical trials. *J Consult Clin Psychol.* 2003;71(5):843–861.
29. Drake RE, O'Neal EL, Wallach MA. A systematic review of psychosocial research on psychosocial interventions for people with co-occurring severe mental and substance use disorders. *Journal of Substance Abuse Treatment.* 2008;34(1):123–138.
30. Mechanic D. The challenge of chronic mental illness: A retrospective and prospective view. *Hosp Community Psychiatry.* 1986;37(9):891–896.
31. Olfson M, Mechanic D, Boyer CA, Hansell S. Linking inpatients with schizophrenia to outpatient care. *Psychiatr Serv.* 1998;49(7):911–917.
32. Boyer CA, McAlpine DD, Pottick KJ, Olfson M. Identifying risk factors and key strategies in linkage to outpatient psychiatric care. *Am J Psychiatry.* 2000;157(10):1592–1598.

33. Lehman AF, Dixon LB, Kernan E, DeForge BR, Postrado LT. A randomized trial of assertive community treatment for homeless persons with severe mental illness. *Arch Gen Psychiatry.* 1997;54(11):1038–1043.
34. Ditton PM. Mental health and treatment of inmates and probationers. *US Department of Justice, Bureau of Justice Statistics Special Report.* 1999:1–14. http://www.ojp.usdoj.gov/bjs/pub/pdf/mhtip.pdf. December 12, 2014.
35. Fisher WH, Roy-Bujnowski KM, Grudzinskas AJ Jr, Clayfield JC, Banks SM, Wolff N. Patterns and prevalence of arrest in a statewide cohort of mental health care consumers. *Psychiatr Serv.* 2006;57(11):1623–1628.
36. Holcomb WR, Ahr PR. Arrest rates among young adult psychiatric patients treated in inpatient and outpatient settings. *Hosp Community Psychiatry.* 1988;39(1):52–57.
37. McFarland BH, Faulkner LR, Bloom JD, Hallaux R, Bray JD. Chronic mental illness and the criminal justice system. *Hosp Community Psychiatry.* 1989;40(7):718–723.
38. Steadman HJ, Naples M. Assessing the effectiveness of jail diversion programs for persons with serious mental illness and co-occurring substance use disorders. *Behav Sci Law.* 2005;23(2):163–170.
39. Pinals DA. Forensic services, public mental health policy, and financing: Charting the course ahead. *Journal of the American Academy of Psychiatry and the Law.* 2014;42(1):7–19.
40. Borum R, Deane MW, Steadman HJ, Morrissey J. Police perspectives on responding to mentally ill people in crisis: perceptions of program effectiveness. *Behav Sci Law.* 1998;16(4):393–405.
41. Compton MT, Esterberg ML, McGee R, Kotwicki RJ, Oliva JR. Crisis intervention team training: changes in knowledge, attitudes, and stigma related to schizophrenia. *Psychiatr Serv.* 2006;57(8):1199–1202.
42. Compton MT, Bakeman R, Broussard B, et al. The police-based Crisis Intervention Team (CIT) model: I. effects on officers' knowledge, attitudes, and skills. *Psychiatr Serv.* 2014;65(4):517–522.
43. Compton MT, Bakeman R, Broussard B, et al. The police-based Crisis Intervention Team (CIT) model: II. effects on level of force and resolution, referral and arrest. *Psychiatr Serv.* 2014;65(4):523–529.
44. Coursey RD, Curtis L, Marsh DT, Campbell J, Harding C. Competencies for direct service staff members who work with adults with severe mental illnesses in outpatient public mental health/managed care systems. *Psychiatr Rehabil J.* 2000;23(4):370–377.
45. SAMHSA. Recovery and recovery support. *Substance Abuse and Mental Health Administration.* http://www.samhsa.gov/recovery. Published 2014. January 6, 2015.

13.

CLINICAL COMPETENCE IN OUTREACH AND FOR SPECIAL POPULATIONS

Anne Klee, Lynette Adams, Neil Beesley, Deborah Fisk, Marcia G. Hunt, Monica Kalacznik, Howard Steinberg, and Laurie Harkness

> ### EDUCATIONAL HIGHLIGHTS
>
> When working with special populations, practitioners must:
>
> - Understand the culture and specific needs of each special population.
>
> - Identify and understand the barriers to care that the population may experience.
>
> - Be aware of one's own biases and develop one's multicultural competence through continuing education, consultation, and personal reflection.
>
> - Work within interdisciplinary care teams to engage these individuals in welcoming and recovery-oriented care.

Hospitals and clinics provide acute and traditional outpatient treatment, but many special populations require enhanced services in the home, on the streets, or in other settings like transitional living facilities. Providing community-based mental health, psychotherapy, case management, and psychosocial rehabilitation services requires a unique set of skills. When working with special populations in the community, it takes a seasoned practitioner with sophisticated clinical knowledge and skills to apply his or her expertise and provide comprehensive quality mental health care. When a practitioner goes into the community, boundaries and the locus of control change, and often the predictability of how the encounter will unfold varies. The practitioner must attend to environmental and behavioral cues and then creatively, comfortably, and seamlessly provide quality care. The ability to readily assess physical safety by examining the environment is paramount to the success of a community-based intervention for both the client and the practitioner. Utilizing an interdisciplinary team (IDT) approach is critical to this work. Each discipline brings its unique training and education, but also a different set of skills, treatment interventions, and perspectives. In a non-structured setting, successful community-based practitioners possess solid clinical skills, self awareness, the ability to utilize a team approach, and know when to call for support or even the police or emergency services. In this chapter, we review the important clinical skills and technical knowledge that a practitioner must possess to be effective in working with special populations and in community settings. These special populations include people with serious mental illness (SMI), homelessness, and traumatic brain injuries (TBI) who often require residential and/or community wrap-around services to live outside of a hospital setting. This chapter also focuses on the impact that culture and life experiences have on mental health, with a specific focus on special populations such as veterans, older adults, and lesbian, gay, bisexual, and transgender (LGBT) individuals. Understanding the diverse experiences and person-centered needs of these populations is critical in providing effective quality care.

WORKING WITH INDIVIDUALS EXPERIENCING HOMELESSNESS

Homelessness is a persistent economic and social problem in the United States, although accurate estimates of the population are difficult to produce. Every 2 years on a single night in January, the Department of Housing and Urban Development (HUD) collects point-in-time (PIT) counts of homeless people in communities in every state; participation in the PIT count is a requisite for qualifying for federal homeless assistance dollars (see Box 13.1). The January 2013 PIT count determined that 610,042 people were experiencing homelessness in the United States. On that night, 394,698 (65%) were staying in emergency shelters or transitional housing programs, and 215,344 (35%) were in unsheltered locations (e.g., vehicles, the street, parks, sidewalks, bus stops or stations, abandoned buildings, and tents). Approximately, 36% (222,197) were people in families, and 387,845 (64%) were individuals.[1] One-night and one-week surveys miss individuals who are intermittently homeless or those who are homeless for short periods of time. They also do not count individuals or families living in motels or those doubled up with family or friends. Homeless individuals who are not living in shelters or transitional housing programs are often difficult to find and, even when located, may refuse to disclose that they are homeless.

Whereas veterans comprise approximately 9.5% of the US population over the age of 18,[1,2] in January 2013 about 12% of homeless adults were veterans, a percentage that has declined by 24% since 2009.[3] In 2014, there was a further drop in the number of homeless veterans in the United States by 33% since 2010. Most homeless veterans are 55 years or older, but a growing proportion are younger service members who served in Iraq and Afghanistan, including women and families. Although homeless veterans are more likely to be older than the general homeless population, in both the general and veteran homeless populations, black race significantly predicts homelessness.[4] Although any one individual's descent into homelessness is multidetermined, many suffer from mental illness, substance abuse, and unemployment and/or underemployment; some of these conditions may be military service-related.

The problem of contemporary homelessness captured federal attention in the 1980s; homeless people became visible beyond skid row, and a large number of homeless people had behavioral health disorders. In 1987, Congress passed the Stewart B. McKinney Homeless Assistance Act, which provided funding for a range of services to homeless adults, including emergency shelter, transitional housing, job training, primary health care, and some permanent housing.

These programs emphasized the importance of assertive outreach in nontraditional settings (on the streets, in shelters, and in soup kitchens), the process of engagement, intensive and long-term case management (including smaller caseloads and community-based care), mental health and substance abuse treatment, and rehabilitative services.[6]

Over the past three decades, there has been substantial progress in developing evidence-based practices for serving homeless people with behavioral health disorders. Permanent supported housing (permanent housing with mental health and wrap-around case management services) has emerged as a central strategy for improving housing outcomes for persons who have been chronically homeless, most often with behavioral health disorders. Two evidence-based practices that are effective in treating homeless people with behavioral health disorders are (1) the Assertive Community Treatment (ACT) model, a team-based model of care that involves providing services to people in community settings; and (2) Critical Time Intervention, a time-limited and intensive case management program designed to assist people through transitions from homelessness to housing.

According to the Substance Abuse and Mental Health Services Administration (SAMHSA), approximately 30% of individuals who are chronically homeless have a serious psychiatric disorder, and about 50% have a co-occurring substance abuse problem.[7] Although studies on the prevalence of comorbid psychiatric and substance use disorders (SUDs) among homeless adults are limited due to small sample sizes and limited geographical areas, there is evidence of a high rate of comorbid psychiatric and SUDs among homeless persons. Sullivan and colleagues[8] examined data on a course-of-homelessness study of 520 homeless persons in Los Angeles over a 15-month follow-up period and found that people with psychiatric disorders, compared to those without psychiatric disorders, were more likely to

---

Box 13.1 **HUD'S DEFINITION OF CHRONIC HOMELESSNESS**

"Either (1) an unaccompanied homeless individual with a disabling condition who has been continuously homeless for a year or more, OR (2) an unaccompanied individual with a disabling condition who has had at least four episodes of homelessness in the past three years."[5]

have a comorbid SUD. Furthermore, approximately half of homeless veterans have SMI,[3] and both general and veteran population studies demonstrate that SUDs are among the strongest predictors of homelessness.[9,10] With high rates of post-traumatic stress disorder (PTSD), TBI, and sexual trauma among veterans, all three are risk factors for homelessness.[3]

Community mental health agencies must provide a range of treatment, housing, and rehabilitative services that integrate medical, mental health, and social services. Since public-sector agencies are often overburdened with individuals already receiving services, it is often a challenge to prioritize services to homeless people who are not seeking treatment, particularly when they only want community resources (see Chapter 6 on Community Supports and Inclusion).

COMPETENCIES FOR STAFF WORKING WITH PERSONS EXPERIENCING HOMELESSNESS

During an initial assessment of a person experiencing homelessness, the goal is to triage for safety and then connect the person with the most appropriate community resources and services. Assessments will differ based on where the person experiencing homelessness is encountered. When assessing a homeless person in the community, it is important to pay attention to the physical safety of his or her living conditions (e.g., in condemned buildings), exposure to extreme temperatures, and interpersonal violence risks such as being victimized or preyed upon by others (e.g., domestic violence, gang violence, decreased cognitive abilities, living in a dangerous neighborhood). In these situations, there also may be a limited window of time in which the person will feel comfortable speaking with a practitioner. When assessing a homeless individual, there is also less need to conduct an intensive diagnostic assessment. It may take several visits to collect detailed clinical information and engage the person in services. The practitioner may determine that the individual is in need of behavioral health treatment, but he or she may not want any services at the time. Meeting the person "where they are at" is essential in the engagement process. Building trust and rapport are often the critical first steps, helping the person access safe and affordable housing will often be the next steps, and engaging the person in treatment may be a longer term process. Although there may be some discernible patterns among homeless individuals, there is also significant heterogeneity among this population;

each person requires a care plan to meet his or her individual needs and preferences. Comprehensive services are needed that address (1) health care, (2) mental health services, (3) housing assistance, (4) life skills training, and (5) employment training.

When engaging a person experiencing homelessness, it is important to determine if the person is a veteran. For eligible veterans, rapid referral to the local US Department of Veterans Affairs Veterans Health Administration (VA) medical center will facilitate engagement in medical, mental health, substance abuse, housing, and other social services. (The US Department of Veterans Affairs is a federally sponsored public system of care for military veterans. It has three main subdivisions known as Administrations. They include the Veterans Health Administration, Veterans Benefits Administration, and the National Cemetery Administration. In this chapter, we use the acronym VA to refer to services provided by the Department of Veterans Affairs.) In November 2009, the VA launched a campaign to end homelessness among veterans by investing significant resources in outreach and engagement, transitional and permanent housing, homeless primary care services, specialized programs for veterans involved with the criminal justice system, and vocational services for chronically homeless veterans and their families. The VA also funded support services to assist with rental assistance, benefits, and other basic social service needs to prevent homelessness and facilitate rapid rehousing.[11] As part of this campaign, all VA medical centers are mandated to track veterans experiencing homelessness to ensure they are offered an array of resources and programs and housed as quickly as possible. Although this effort has greatly reduced homelessness among veterans, unemployment and underemployment continue to be major obstacles that place many veterans at risk for homelessness. Many veterans distrust the VA and other federal government agencies and choose to receive their medical and mental health services through the state system of care, such as at a local clinic or community mental health center. It is important to be mindful of these issues when engaging homeless veterans in needed services.

ASSERTIVE COMMUNITY TREATMENT

ACT is a widely accepted method of delivering intensive services in the community to people with serious psychiatric illness who have not responded well to treatment in traditional outpatient clinics. In this section, we outline the history of ACT, describe some of its crucial elements, discuss some of the important competencies required of staff in the program, and highlight current issues and possible future directions of ACT programs.

The movement to deinstitutionalize hospitalized psychiatric patients that began in the 1950s was discussed in Chapter 2 of this book. In the 1970s, in Madison, Wisconsin, when large numbers of patients from Mendota Mental Health Institute were discharged to the community, a group from the hospital, spearheaded by Drs. Stein and Test, listened carefully to front-line staff who thought they had found a way to engage and transition patients with long hospital stays to the community.[12] From their efforts, ACT was born and has grown to be a widely accepted evidenced-based treatment for people with serious psychiatric illness.[13] The premise of this program, radical for the time, was that comprehensive clinical, rehabilitative, and case management services should be delivered to people where they lived, in their own communities (see Table 13.1).

ACT programs have been disseminated widely, both nationally and internationally, and there have been many studies of the efficacy of ACT programs.[15-17] Studies demonstrate that ACT is an effective model in engaging people with SMI who are often resistant to coming in for traditional outpatient services and/or have long inpatient hospital stays.[17] In a review article by Bond et al.,[15] the authors conclude "that ACT substantially reduces psychiatric hospital use, increases housing stability and moderately improves symptoms and subjective quality of life, but has little effect on social functioning."

Standards for the operation of ACT programs define admission criteria, staffing requirements, the nature of the services delivered, and program organization.[18] Scales for the measurement of fidelity to those standards are used both for programmatic reviews and for research.[19] The Dartmouth ACT (DACT) scale has been used as the metric in many of these studies.[20] Multiple studies show that programs with higher fidelity have better outcomes.[21]

COMPETENCIES FOR ACT STAFF

Specific competencies are required for the staff of ACT programs. The work is, by its nature, team-oriented. Although traditional outpatient mental health teams meet weekly and typically discuss a portion of their clients, interdisciplinary ACT teams meet daily and discuss each of the clients in the program. IDT members on ACT teams work closely together to address the diverse needs and preferences of the clients. The team carries lower caseloads than traditional outpatient teams in order to provide more intensive services. The teams are also truly multidisciplinary, with psychiatrists, nurses, social workers, psychologists, mental health workers, substance abuse specialists, employment specialists, and peer workers all working in concert. Each staff member is first a generalist, involved in treatment planning, crisis intervention, and case management; this includes helping with transportation, housing and benefits applications, and daily living errands like shopping and banking. And yet each is also a specialist. Nurses educate about medication issues. Peer specialists provide role models and practical advice. Psychiatrists manage psychopharmacologic treatment. Social workers and psychologists provide housing resources and offer counseling and evidence-based psychotherapies. A psychologist on the team can also provide psychological testing and program evaluation. The staff on an ACT team need to be skilled in working in an interdisciplinary model. Structures such as daily rounds facilitate the different disciplines in working together.

Clients on ACT teams are people who have serious psychiatric illness, often with comorbid substance abuse and medical issues. Many have not found mental health treatment helpful, and they have little insight into the need for treatment. An important staff competency is the ability to engage "reluctant" clients into treatment.[22] Engagement techniques include the ability to work collaboratively with clients by addressing practical needs first, working flexibly, and offering optimism and hope in difficult situations. For staff prescribing medication on an ACT team, it can be challenging when people with severe psychiatric illnesses choose not to take medication or to take doses that would be considered subtherapeutic. Here, too, skills in collaborative, patient-centered approaches are important.

It is also important for staff to be "trauma-informed." Many of these clients have past experiences of trauma and abuse.[23] To some, the mental health treatment system has

Table 13.1 ELEMENTS OF ASSERTIVE COMMUNITY TREATMENT[14]

- A team approach using a multidisciplinary staff with shared responsibility for clients and shared governance of the team
- Integrated services, in which the team is the provider of clinical and rehabilitative services
- An assertive, individualized approach to treatment, with many services provided "in vivo," whether during home visits or in various community locations
- Low patient-to-staff ratios (12:1)
- Rapid access to services and crisis services that are available 24 hours a day
- A commitment to providing services as long as the client needs them

been experienced as traumatizing. Many have been hospitalized against their will, have had difficult experiences on psychiatric inpatient units, or have experienced coercive measures to ensure adherence to outpatient treatment. It is important for staff to be sensitive to hearing the trauma histories of clients and to be aware of the potential for retraumatization.[24]

Another critical competency is the ability to provide clinical and rehabilitative services to clients in community settings. Seeing a person outside of the office, in his or her home, or in a public place in the community such as a coffee shop presents particular challenges. Staff always need to be cognizant of issues of privacy and confidentiality. Whether it is to take a table in the back of a restaurant, to check with the person if he or she would like the staff member to ask family members to move to another room during a home visit, or to defer a particular conversation to another time, the staff member needs to be adept at preserving confidentiality. Boundary issues are also more challenging in settings outside of the office.[25] The informality of a coffee shop may certainly help with engagement, but maintaining professional boundaries cannot be compromised. Supervision and team discussions are critical to address issues of confidentiality and boundaries. For example, many community-based programs have hired peer specialists who are living examples that recovery is possible. Peer specialists are encouraged to discuss their recovery journeys, but, in the context of helping the client and like other staff, they must learn to ask themselves how their personal information will help or hurt the client. Peer specialists often encounter clients in community meetings such as Alcoholics Anonymous (AA) and Narcotics Anonymous (NA). Teams should discuss these types of encounters and how to honor confidentiality, be respectful, and maintain professionalism.

CURRENT ISSUES AND FUTURE TRENDS

Most ACT teams are now incorporating and utilizing the principles of recovery and psychosocial rehabilitation into their clinical work.[26] In 2007, Salyers and Tsemberis[27] questioned whether the prescriptive nature of the program—for example, the requirements that the client be treated by multiple members of the team and have multiple contacts per week—can be compatible with patient choice. Person-centered care, choice, empowerment, and the belief that recovery is possible are now embraced by many ACT teams. It is now widely accepted that people with SMI can lead rich and full lives in the community of their choice.

At the heart of the work of ACT teams are questions about the ethics of providing treatment to those who refuse it.[28] Questions of autonomy versus paternalism abound, yet situations where coercion is considered life-saving are common. Williamson's review[28] discusses the difficulty of applying traditional principles of ethical treatment to persons denying the experience of illness. Frequent staff meetings, input from all concerned stakeholders, and consultations from ethics committees facilitate exploration of the complex ethical considerations inherent in community treatment. Although ACT programs have become mainstream, they continue to change in response to changing clinical populations and mental health policies. In addition to incorporating recovery principles, ACT programs have been developed for forensic populations, the homeless, adolescents, and geriatric populations.[29] Standards have been modified in some programs to address the issue of graduation from the program, and peer specialists have become an important part of many ACT teams.

WORKING WITH INDIVIDUALS WITH DUAL DIAGNOSES IN RESIDENTIAL TREATMENT SETTINGS

Individuals presenting with SMI and co-occurring SUDs have historically been treated in either mental health or substance abuse treatment settings, respectively. However, there is consistent evidence supporting the integration of mental health and substance abuse treatments within such settings.[30,31] Additionally, the high comorbidity rates associated with substance use and other disorders often makes it difficult to effectively parse out individuals into separate treatment programs. As discussed in detail in Chapter 6, effective residential treatment programs have been noted to provide empirically supported psychosocial interventions designed to address the complex clinical presentations that often accompany individuals who are dually diagnosed. Such treatment programs require components of a therapeutic milieu, engagement of a multidisciplinary treatment team, direct supervision of clientele, training and supervision of staff, and clinical and administrative oversight.[32]

One of the greatest challenges facing individuals diagnosed with SMI and SUDs is identifying a safe environment that will engage them in a range of treatment services to aid in the recovery process. Many of these individuals present with symptoms that suggest they lack the motivation to change problematic behaviors; they are unable to actively engage with providers, and, once engaged, the progress made is often at a slow pace. Additionally, these individuals tend to prematurely leave longer term programs at higher rates than do non–dually diagnosed individuals.³³ These and other factors contribute to the likelihood that dually diagnosed individuals, when compared with those without similar difficulties, will face severe psychosocial obstacles and that they will lack the necessary mental and physical resources to be able to manage living independently in the community.

Although the residential setting is quite different from outpatient care, in fact, this higher level of care allows both clinicians and individuals engaged in residential treatment to cultivate and experiment with new skill sets in various treatment domains. To do this, a well-designed residential program takes advantage of the setting as a type of therapeutic community (or a milieu): an environment in which much of the mechanism of change may be found in the opportunities for members of the community to participate in living-learning experiences.³⁴

COMPETENCIES FOR RESIDENTIAL PROGRAM STAFF

Mental health professionals must integrate into the therapeutic milieu by spending time with individuals in the residence in activities such as eating meals together, watching a sporting event, or working on an art project. The involvement of the public service mental health professional in the day-to-day therapeutic milieu is an equally vital part of this educational process. Engagement at this level provides a greater familiarity with the psychosocial struggles of those with SMI and substance use problems. Clinical staff need to develop practical skills in engagement strategies, motivational counseling, integrated mental illness and substance abuse treatments, and relapse prevention/coping skills treatments.³⁵ Residential programming should include peer support and family education and interventions, and it must focus on developing healthy life skills and community support networks. Also important is addressing criminal justice system involvement, housing challenges and resources, and vocational rehabilitation needs. Exposure to comprehensive psychosocial rehabilitative services often begins while in a residential program and is increasingly the standard purview of residential treatment.

Finally, consistent participation in supervisory meetings focused on this work is an integral component of professional development. The focus of such meetings can range from a review of a specific treatment intervention or how a crisis was managed, to education regarding recovery principles and psychosocial rehabilitation. Due to the nature of working for longer periods in a less formal residential setting, one of the major areas of supervision should be the understanding and maintaining of professional boundaries. Other important topics for supervision should include successful engagement with the interdisciplinary treatment team, establishing and improving communication with providers outside of the program, and opportunities for advocacy, as well as other professional development issues.

WORKING WITH INDIVIDUALS WITH TRAUMATIC BRAIN INJURY (TBI)

TBI describes the intracranial injury resulting from the external application of force to the head. TBI is most often an acute event, and it can either be penetrative (where the dura mater is breached) or nonpenetrative.³⁶ In contrast to many other acute traumatic injuries, TBI often causes abrupt and profound life changes. It is thought that more than 5 million US citizens are living with a TBI-related disability.³⁷ Confusion exists about what is considered an acquired brain injury (ABI) versus a TBI. By definition, any TBI (e.g., from a motor vehicle accident or assault) could be considered an ABI. In the field of brain injury, ABIs are typically considered any injury that is nontraumatic. Examples of ABI include stroke, near drowning, hypoxic or anoxic brain injury, tumor, neurotoxins, electric shock, or lightning strike.

An interdisciplinary treatment team is needed to evaluate the various layers of symptoms and disability, provide evidence-based interventions, and educate the person with the TBI and family members, as well as other professionals on the medical and rehabilitation treatment team. A comprehensive rehabilitation plan is tailored to each individual's clinical and social needs and includes the services provided by many key professionals; these often include a physiatrist (a doctor of physical medicine rehabilitation), physical therapists, occupational therapists, speech/language pathologists, rehabilitation nurses, social workers/case managers, recreational therapists, neuropsychologists, and a mental health expert.

Research exists on a wide range of psychotherapeutic treatment models for survivors of TBI. Studies on effective treatments for the emotional and cognitive sequelae of TBI have shown mixed results across a range of interventions from antidepressant therapy (ECT), transcranial magnetic stimulation (TMS), and biofeedback, to various psychotherapies including individual and group cognitive behavioral therapy (CBT), coping skills training, and behavior management to other adjunct therapies such as cognitive processing therapy (for trauma symptoms).³⁸ Psychoeducation is paramount to any treatment modality and should occur at the onset of therapy; subjects should include TBI epidemiology, symptoms/sequelae, social support and caregiving, treatment, and prevention of further injury.[38]

COMPETENCIES FOR STAFF WORKING WITH INDIVIDUALS WITH TBI

Providing treatment to survivors of TBI requires a broad understanding of the complex range of symptoms and disabilities associated with TBI. Most TBIs are mild and cause temporary loss or disruption of neurological function; however, some mild TBIs and most severe injuries can cause permanent impairment.[37] TBI is a common injury and may be missed initially when the medical team is focused on saving the individual's life. In mild TBI, physical symptoms may resolve quickly or never develop despite cognitive and behavioral problems existing—thus the need for comprehensive evaluation including clinical history, neurologic and mental status exam, and neuropsychological testing. However, TBI assessment tools are rarely utilized in the emergency or acute care setting, and the person with mild TBI is often not diagnosed and sent home. Even in the scenario of severe TBI, the life-threatening medical issues (such as hemorrhaging or increased pressure on the brain mentioned) and/or trauma to other areas of the body may minimize or obscure the diagnosis and treatment of nonphysical aspects of TBI.

The continuum of care and rehabilitation for persons with TBI is broadly segmented into three stages that follow the initial acute medical intervention (see Figure 13.1). These three stages are inpatient, community-based care, and long-term care and management and reflect a general progression in recovery. A person with a TBI does not necessarily advance through these stages in exact order. Each person's rehabilitation process is unique to his or her circumstances. Program goals focus on maximizing the patient's functional status, independence, psychosocial adjustment, and vocational/leisure skills including community reintegration.

Following acute evaluation and management of a brain injury, the survivor may need intensive, specialized inpatient rehabilitation. Family and caregiver education, as well as involvement in the rehabilitation plan, is essential if the person is to ultimately reintegrate successfully back into the community. During an inpatient rehabilitative admission, typically, a patient is assigned a case manager who acts as a liaison among the patient, family, clinical team, payer, and community.

A neurobehavioral program (NBP) is a long-term rehabilitation program that specializes in the treatment of individuals who have sustained a TBI and have been unsuccessful living in the community or in other facilities. The purpose of the NBP is to assist these individuals in managing their behaviors appropriately and in learning skills to maximize their independence and improve their overall quality of life. A behavioral approach to treatment based on initial and ongoing assessments is offered. The IDT identifies and prioritizes behaviors that present obstacles to successful community reintegration. The team also works with each person's cultural and spiritual beliefs when developing his or her individualized treatment plan. Goals should have predicted

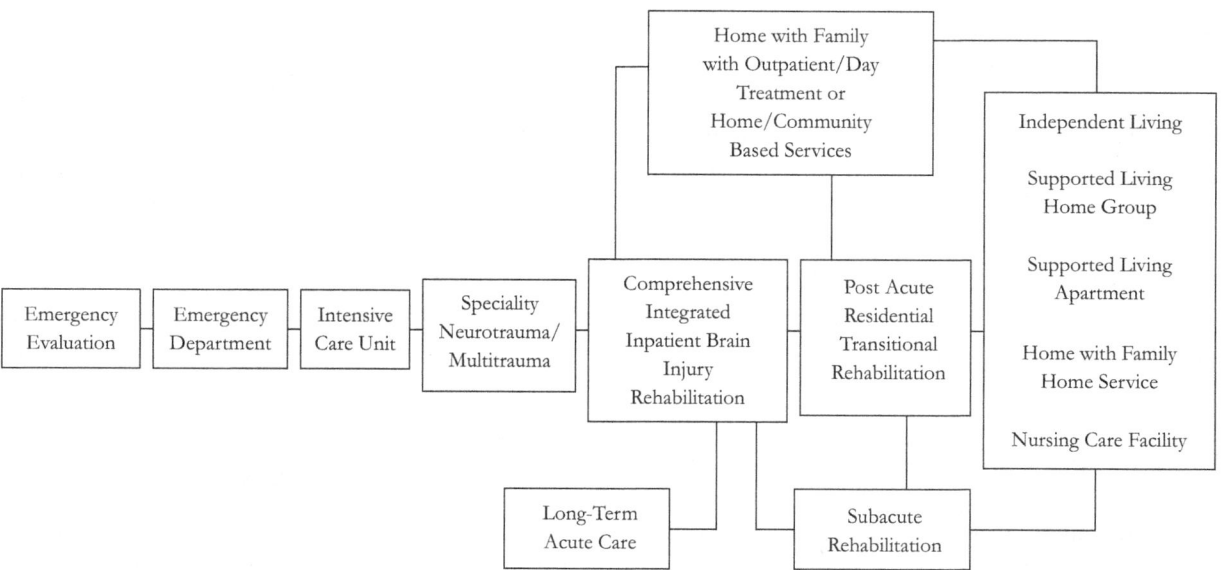

Figure 13.1 Traumatic brain injury continuum of care SOURCE: Adapted from the Rocky Mountain Regional Brain Injury System to depict the continuum of care for individuals with moderate and severe TBI.

outcomes and address the physical, cognitive, educational, and behavioral needs of each person. These may include activities of daily living (ADL), medication, mobility, nutrition, leisure and recreational needs, communication and coping skills, substance abuse, and family/caregiver training.

Longer term community care and support is also based on the specific needs of the TBI survivor. Individually developed plans often include transition to home and community services including vocational and ongoing education and support related to recovery and wellness. Cases involving higher levels of disability require comprehensive services and the need for both home- and community-based case management. It is important to know that most states fund and administer a TBI or ABI "waiver" program the waiver provides a variety of services to support an individual in the community that typically would require the individual to exhaust his or her assets and income. These individuals and their families often require case management services to navigate these critically needed resources for long-term support. Securing community resources and long-term entitlements (payment) for ongoing services can be challenging, if not impossible for this population. State ABI services often include specialized services such as care management and coordination, housing and living subsidies, vocational services, and assistive technologies.

Mental health practitioners have important roles to play in identifying and addressing the neurobehavioral burdens that caregivers face. These caregiver burdens correlate more strongly with community adaptation than with severity of injury or even cognitive impairments.[38] Behavioral symptoms, including irritability, aggression, and various forms of regressed social functioning, typically increase over time as other indicators of functional disability decrease. Increased social withdrawal over time associated with TBI often produces additional strain on the primary caregiver system to absorb and manage maladaptive behavior. As a result, caregivers of persons with TBI are often faced with significant unmet needs for professional assistance and advice, particularly in the late post-acute setting, when access to supportive services may be limited or unavailable. Additionally, there are a number of caregiver burnout issues specific to the challenging disabilities resulting from TBI.

WORKING WITH OLDER ADULTS

The US population of older adults, those age 65 and older, has been growing steadily since the turn of the last century. In 1900, 4.1% of the population was age 65 or older; by 2012, that number had grown to more than 13.7%,[39] with an anticipated growth within the next 15 years to more than 20%, representing almost 70 million people.[40] This growth is attributed to reduced death rates in those between the ages of 65 and 84, particularly for older men, who have seen a reduction of 41.6% in the period between 1990 and 2007.[39] Within the elderly population, the Census Bureau also predicts an increase in racial and ethnic minorities from 21% in 2012 to 28% in 2030—with the Hispanic population showing the greatest percentage increase (155%).[39] One other important change in the aging population is the sex ratio. Typically, women have lived longer than men, resulting in a much larger number of women, 66% as of 2012 in the oldest (85+) age group. This ratio is expected to decrease in all older age groups, with the most dramatic decrease from 66.6% to a predicted 61.9% in the 85+ age group.[40] What is less clear in our prediction of the future is how older adults will be able to function as their numbers grow during the next 35 years. A 2010 survey of noninstitutionalized elders found that, in those age 65 and older, 36% reported having a physical (e.g., hearing, vision, etc.) or mental (e.g., cognition) disability, and 28% of Medicare beneficiaries reported some difficulty performing one or more ADLs (e.g., bathing, dressing, eating, etc.). Within instrumental ADLs (IADLs) (e.g., managing money, preparing meals, managing medication, etc.), 12% of noninstitutionalized elders reported difficulty with one or more of these tasks.[39] The picture is worse for institutionalized elders, such as those in nursing homes where an estimated 1.3 million older adults are housed. Despite the fact that a growing number of older adults are in nursing homes for shorter stays, such as post-acute care, an examination of institutionalized Medicare beneficiaries showed that 76% reported difficulties with one or more ADLs.[39]

With respect to psychological difficulties, older adults are subject to the same struggles as younger adults, including anxiety disorders, mood disorders, substance abuse disorders, and psychotic disorders.[41,42] Researchers have found that, in the United States, older adults with mental health needs are less likely than their younger counterparts to receive services.[43] Studies of preferences for treatment in older adults indicate that when they seek treatment, they are more likely to do so in primary care settings rather than through specialty mental health care[44] and typically do not want pharmacotherapy.

COMPETENCIES FOR STAFF WORKING WITH OLDER ADULTS

Particular competencies are needed in working with older adults, and a number of competency models have been developed to assist in training mental health care providers.[45,46] Training models themselves tend to be discipline-specific but contain many commonalities when outlining competencies. Based on these models, competencies can be considered within three broad areas: professionalism (e.g., practitioner self-awareness and strengths-based approach), knowledge (e.g., legal/ethical issues, age-related changes), and skills (e.g., assessment and differential diagnoses, care coordination for complex needs).

Professionalism

Awareness of one's own age-related biases is foundational in working with older adults, given the impact of biases on practice. For example, it is not an uncommon assumption that a certain level of depression is expected in older adults, that a lower level of physical or mental functioning is less of a concern for older adults than for younger adults, that older adults can't or don't want to change thoughts or behaviors, or that sexual functioning is less important. Similarly, due to the age of a patient, practitioners could feel discomfort in discussing certain topics with an older person (e.g., substance abuse, sexuality, cultural or generational norms, or trauma histories). Assumptions, biases, and discomfort can result in important gaps in assessment and/or care. One of the ways to balance this is to take a strengths-based approach in working with older adults. Beginning by understanding and exploring strengths can help shape the practitioner's thought process and post-assessment interventions in a way that maximizes the likelihood of success, thus encouraging optimism and hopefulness.

Knowledge

Developmental and age-specific knowledge are critical in working with older adults. Understanding age-related physiological changes, pharmacologic knowledge (e.g., polypharmacy, risks related to psychotropic and benzodiazepine usage), interaction of common social and functional factors on psychological health (e.g., death of a spouse, hip fracture), and individual variability in possible outcomes from treatment is key, given the compounding impact of multiple, complex needs. In addition, providing treatment to older adults requires knowledge of nuanced ethical and legal issues. These include issues of confidentiality, informed consent, cognitive capacity and competency, abuse or neglect including self-neglect, and end-of-life decisions.

Skills

Assessment and differential diagnoses skills are critical when working with any population, but these are particularly challenging when working with older adults, given the common confounds of complex problems or needs in multiple areas of life and health. Relatedly, the complexity of needs of older adults requires close and continuous attention to care coordination and appropriate consultation with other treatment providers, caregivers, and family members—which often requires significant advocacy work. For example, a 75-year-old Hispanic woman, recently diagnosed with diabetes and who has a history of heart disease and who presents complaining of forgetfulness and feelings of sadness and lethargy may also report that she has a very limited income, insecure housing, and is the primary caregiver for three young grandchildren. Assessment and treatment for this woman would require teasing apart potential mood, cognitive, physical, stress (social and physical), and pharmacologic factors as well as care coordination—or referral or advocacy in the absence of adequate care provision—with primary care and specialty physical health providers, other mental health providers, a case manager, or others who could assist with social needs. Other family members may also need to be considered and consulted, and the court system could also potentially be involved should she be assessed as having significantly impaired cognitive capacity.

The growing numbers of older adults indicate a continuing demand for health care providers who can address the unique needs of this fast-growing population and who are sensitive to the disparity in mental health treatment as well as the specific needs and treatment preferences of older adults.

WORKING WITH LESBIAN, GAY, BISEXUAL, AND TRANSGENDER (LGBT) INDIVIDUALS

Individuals who identify as LGBT may present in public health settings with mental health challenges that are typical of the general population. However, it is important to have a basic understanding of several key terms associated with LGBT identities in order to offer appropriate, individualized services. Sexual orientation relates to one's attraction (e.g., physical, emotional) to another person. One can be attracted to another of the same sex, opposite sex, or both/multiple sexes. *Sex* is assigned at birth and is largely based on genetics, hormones, and other physical characteristics. *Gender*, on the other hand, is a concept that is based on the social construction of identity, and it can be thought of as one's sense of being a man or woman, boy or girl. Gender identity is one's sense of one's own gender, whereas *gender expression* is how one's gender identity is expressed. *Transgender* is difficult to define precisely but usually refers to an individual whose assigned sex at birth does not match the gender identity or expression of the person, according to societal expectations. For a more complex understanding and critical review on the background of these terms, see *The Fenway Guide to Lesbian, Gay, Bisexual, and Transgender Health*.[47]

COMPETENCIES FOR STAFF WORKING WITH LGBT INDIVIDUALS

Lyons et al.[48] recommend several strategies for developing one's multicultural competence for working with individuals who identify as lesbian, gay, or bisexual. They suggest utilizing supervision or consultation with an expert, continuing education and trainings, personal self-reflection, and self-directed training. Additionally, having an awareness of the mental health disparities that exist in the population is helpful for understanding psychosocial stressors experienced by LGBT-identified individuals. For example, Ruble and Forstein[49] reviewed the research on lesbian, gay, and bisexual populations, and they identified that these individuals were at higher risk for mood disorders, anxiety disorders, and suicidal behavior. Societal factors, such as having a stigmatized identity, experiencing discrimination or inequality, or having barriers to social support, may contribute to this increased risk.

When working with individuals who identify as transgender, additional training and knowledge is needed. For example, some individuals who identify as transgender may wish to receive cross-sex hormone treatment or complete a sex-reassignment surgery (also referred to as a gender-confirming surgery). Prior to engaging in either course of treatment, the World Professional Association for Transgender Health[50] recommends that the individual first undergo a mental health evaluation to determine eligibility, readiness for treatment, and capacity for informed consent. Mental health professionals in the public sector may be called on to complete these evaluations. It is recommended that mental health professionals be prepared, at a minimum, to diagnose mental health conditions and differentiate them from gender identity disorder/dysphoria, have some knowledge about gender nonconforming identity and expression, and receive continuing education in the assessment and treatment of gender dysphoria.[50] Additionally, the collaboration of a multidisciplinary team is essential for the treatment of transgender individuals; a comprehensive health care team often includes mental health professionals, primary care, and specialty services such as endocrinology or surgery.

WORKING WITH VETERANS

It is essential that anyone working with veterans understand the meaning of what it is to serve our country and take the time to learn about military culture and military experience. Each war brings its own unique characteristics and leads to different readjustment issues. For example, those veterans who served in World War II came home as heroes. Veterans who served in Vietnam came home to a country divided by the war. Many Vietnam veterans struggled with senses of loss and shame and entered an underfunded mental health system that was yet to understand the possible long-term impacts of combat and trauma. This led many veterans to feel misunderstood, rejected, and distrustful of the government as well as society in general. Many veterans who served in Iraq and Afghanistan faced multiple deployments and fought in battles seen in living rooms all over the world. Media and technology now play huge roles in access to information and public perception. Service members may be thousands of miles away from their loved ones yet in frequent contact through computers and smartphones. This contact can be both healthy and distracting (e.g., if a service member has a fight with his overburdened wife back home parenting their three children but must go out on patrol and remain focused).

However, unlike Vietnam veterans, current service members feel the support of the country. They have a health care system that better understands PTSD and TBI, as well as the necessity of offering mental health services both on the battlefield and as quickly as possible at home. These service members are seen as heroes. In addition, many financial, educational, and vocational supports are available to them. Despite these positive developments and lessons learned since Vietnam, these returning service members still face challenges and obstacles. Issues of substance abuse, impulsivity, suicidality, and violence seem to be the hallmarks of these new veterans.

COMPETENCIES FOR STAFF WORKING WITH VETERANS

In working with veterans, genuine listening, authenticity, and willingness to ask questions when one may not understand the meaning of what a veteran is saying are extremely important. Practitioners who do not know military jargon such as MOS (military occupational specialty) or job assignment should let the veteran educate them. The VA hires many veterans—and specifically peer specialists (veterans with lived experiences)—to help veterans in treatment feel more comfortable, safer, and provide hope, but also to help nonveteran staff understand the military and veteran experience.

Despite the fact that impact war and combat may have on an individual and/or her family, most service members are now able to live productive lives with PTSD and/or TBIs. Several evidence-based practices such as cognitive processing therapy, CBT, and computer applications help service members deal with readjustment issues. Southwick and Charney (2012) identified 10 coping mechanisms that are effective in dealing with stress and life-threatening trauma. These resiliency factors include confronting fears; maintaining an optimistic, but realistic outlook; the presence of social support; the presence of resilient role models; having an inner moral compass; a sense of religion or spirituality; finding a way to accept that which could not be changed (cognitive flexibility); being physically fit and having sense of well-being; keeping one's brain mentally sharp by being an active problem solver; and having meaning and purpose in one's life.[51] Many traumatized individuals will not possess all 10 resiliency factors, but many are skills and supports that can be developed through behavioral and psychotherapeutic interventions with their practitioners.

Women veterans represent a unique subset of the overall veteran population and are the fastest growing group of veterans presenting for services at the VA. Since 2000, the population of women veterans utilizing care through VA has doubled, and it is projected that, by 2015, there will be an estimated 2 million women veterans in the United States.[52] Among individuals presenting to the VA for mental health services, a higher proportion of women present for mental health treatment compared to men.[53] Additionally, many women veterans present with psychosocial concerns such as unemployment, homelessness, or stressors relating to acting in the caregiver role (e.g., for children, aging parents, or spouses).

Military sexual trauma (MST) is the term used by the VA to describe sexual assault or harassment experienced by a veteran while in the military. The term can be broadly used to describe experiences ranging from offensive remarks about sexual activities to forced and unwanted

---

Box 13.2 SPECIAL OUTREACH SERVICES IN A COMMUNITY SETTING

Mr. Gibbs is a well-educated 39-year-old biracial divorced combat veteran who carries the diagnosis of schizoaffective disorder, depressed. Mr. Gibbs experienced a psychotic break while in the military. Discharged with no follow-up mental health care, he quickly relapsed and was brought by his father to the local VA hospital. He spent the next 2 years in and out of psychiatric hospitals and experiencing bouts of homelessness. He was noncompliant with medications largely because of the significant weight gain he experienced secondary to the neuroleptic medications. Even when taking his medications, he continued to experience significant residual symptoms including paranoia and obsessive and ruminative thoughts that made him guarded. As he gained weight, he developed multiple medical problems including high blood pressure and diabetes.

At a very young age, Mr. Gibbs' mother died in prison of a drug overdose. He was raised by his maternal grandmother until his father was able to provide a stable home for him. Ethnic identity issues have always been a part of his life because his father, stepmother, and brother are white, and he both appears and identifies himself as black. His strengths include being intelligent, articulate, likeable, and a talented musician. His father and extended family live nearby and are positive sources of support.

After a series of psychiatric hospitalizations, Mr. Gibbs agreed to participate in a VA intensive assertive community treatment program. Initially, he was hesitant to engage with or be around people, let alone VA staff. For months, clinicians met with Mr. Gibbs where he was comfortable: at a picnic table outside the treatment center. A team approach was utilized in which the team psychiatrist focused on medication-related issues and other clinicians focused on helping him develop coping mechanisms and improve his life and social skills. As he became medication adherent, he learned to compartmentalize his obsessive ruminative thinking, which he continued to struggle with, and to share with his primary clinician. Meeting with his family helped the team to see Mr. Gibbs as an important member of that family and to learn how his illness impacted them. His wish to lose weight led to therapy often occurring over long walks where he spoke of his dreams to return to work. A supportive employment specialist helped him obtain a job as a bookkeeper at a local company. He kept this job for more than 3 years until he went back to school to become a certified peer specialist. Although his mental illness is a significant part of his life, he now uses it in a positive manner to instill hope in others. He is a living example that recovery is possible.

sexual activities. According to Kimerling, Gima, Smith, Street, and Frayne,[54] of the veterans screened for MST in the VA, 22% of the female veteran population screened positive for MST, compared to 1% of the male veteran population. Because of these rates of MST, it is suggested that psychosocial assessments for all veterans include a screening for history of MST. Competencies for working with individuals with MST should include specific training on trauma and military culture. Many, if not all, the issues illustrated in the case study in Box 13.2 are relevant regardless of the system providing the care (i.e., VA or state).

The case example in Box 13.2 highlights important community-based interventions that helped the individual move from a life of repeated hospitalizations to a rich, full life lived in the community. Engagement occurred over time in settings where the person was most comfortable and included his family and friends. The approach was person-centered and included a balance of traditional and nontraditional interventions. Most importantly, it involved setting and achieving small manageable goals that gave him a sense of accomplishment and positive self-worth. Because of the IDT approach, clinician specialties were well-utilized, and the individual's wishes and goals could be addressed. Although he had seen much trauma during his military experience, this was not a major focus of the work that he needed to address to live optimally in the community. Listening to and understanding his needs and preferences guided the treatment process. Being aware of the cultural and familial values so central to him was integral to partnering with him in each step of this therapeutic process.

SUMMARY

In meeting the needs of special populations, practitioners must obtain new sets of competencies through continuing education and seek appropriate consultation from experts in the respective areas. It is also critical to be aware of one's own biases and to develop one's multicultural competence through supervision and personal reflection. Understanding the culture and specific needs of these special populations is necessary for practitioners to develop comprehensive programs to engage these individuals in welcoming and recovery-oriented care. As acute inpatient psychiatric beds have decreased, the need to develop community structures and person-centered models of care have become essential in meeting the needs of individuals living with SMI, homelessness, TBI, and other significant psychosocial issues. These programs should be easily accessible and individualized, and the focus should be on improving functioning. Utilizing an IDT approach provides team members with both the necessary expertise and critical support on a daily basis. It is important for practitioners to understand each unique individual's perspectives, needs, beliefs, values, and preferences; this is particularly important with special populations. In addition to assuming both strengths-based and person-centered approaches, practitioners must obtain the knowledge and requisite skills to optimally serve each individual.

REFERENCES

1. US Department of Housing and Urban Development, Office of Community Planning and Development. *The 2013 Annual Homeless Assessment Report (AHAR) to Congress.* https://www.onecpd.info/resources/documents/ahar-2013-part1.pdf. Published 2013. Accessed April 20, 2014.
2. US Department of Veterans Affairs, Office of Public and Intergovernmental Affairs. News Releases—Office of Public and Intergovernmental Affairs. http://www.va.gov/opa/pressrel/pressrelease.cfm?id=1807. Accessed April 20, 2014.
3. US Interagency Council on Homelessness. *Opening Doors: Homelessness among Veterans.* http://usich.gov/usich_resources/fact_sheets/opening_doors_homelessness_among_veterans. Accessed April 20, 2014.
4. Fargo J, Metraux S, Byrne T, et al. Prevalence and risk of homelessness among US veterans. *Prev Chronic Dis.* 2012;9: E45.
5. US Department of Housing and Urban Development. *Defining Chronic Homelessness: A Technical Guide for HUD Programs.* 2007. https://www.hudexchange.info/resources/documents/DefiningChronicHomeless.pdf. Accessed April 20, 2014.
6. Levine IS, Rog DJ. Mental health services for homeless mentally ill persons. Federal initiatives and current service trends. *Am Psychol.* 1990;45(8):963–968.
7. Substance Abuse and Mental Health Service Administration, Homelessness Resource Center. *Individuals Experiencing Chronic/Long-Term Homelessness.* 2010. http://homeless.samhsa.gov/resource/individuals-experiencing-chronic-long-term-homelessness-48804.aspx. Accessed April 20, 2014.
8. Sullivan G, Burnam A, Koegel P, Hollenberg J. Quality of life of homeless persons with mental illness: results from the course-of-homelessness study. *Psychiatr Serv.* 2000;51(9):1135–1141.
9. Edens EL, Kasprow W, Tsai J, Rosenheck RA. Association of substance use and VA service-connected disability benefits with risk of homelessness among veterans. *Am J Addict.* 2011;20(5):412–419.
10. Greenberg GA, Rosenheck RA. Correlates of past homelessness in the National Epidemiological Survey on Alcohol and Related Conditions. *Adm Policy Ment Health.* 2010;37(4):357–366.
11. US Department of Veterans Affairs. *Secretary Shinseki Details Plan to End Homelessness for Veterans.* http://www.va.gov/opa/pressrel/pressrelease.cfm?id=1807. Accessed April 20, 2014.
12. Marx AJ, Test MA, Stein LI. Extrohospital management of severe mental illness. Feasibility and effects of social functioning. *Arch Gen Psychiatry.* 1973;29(4):505–511.
13. Deci PA, Santos AB, Hiott DW, Schoenwald S, Dias JK. Dissemination of assertive community treatment programs. *Psychiatr Serv.* 1995;46(7):676–678.
14. Stein LIS, AB. *Assertive Community Treatment of Persons with Severe Mental Illness.* New York: Norton; 1998.

15. Bond GR, Drake R, Mueser KT, Latimer E. Assertive community treatment for people with severe mental illness. *Dis Management Health Outcomes.* 2001;9(3):141–159.
16. Mueser KT, Bond GR, Drake RE, Resnick SG. Models of community care for severe mental illness: a review of research on case management. *Schizophr Bull.* 1998;24(1):37–74.
17. Marshall ML, Lockwood A. Assertive community treatment for people with severe mental diseases. 1998. *Cochrane Database of Systematic Reviews.*1998, Issue 2. Art.No.:CD001089. DOI:10.1002/14651858. CD001089.
18. Allness D, Knoedler W. *National Program Standards for ACT Teams.* Arlington, VA: National Alliance for the Mentally Ill; 2003.
19. Teague GB, Bond GR, Drake RE. Program fidelity in assertive community treatment: development and use of a measure. *Am J Orthopsychiatry.* 1998;68(2):216–232.
20. Bond GR, Salyers MP. Prediction of outcome from the Dartmouth assertive community treatment fidelity scale. *CNS Spectrums.* 2004;9(12):937–942.
21. Latimer EA. Economic impacts of assertive community treatment: a review of the literature. *Can J Psychiatry. Revue canadienne de psychiatrie.* 1999;44(5):443–454.
22. Gillespie M, Meaden, A. Psychological processes in engagement. In: Cupitt C, ed. *Reaching Out: The Psychology of Assertive Outreach.* New York: Routledge; 2010:15–42.
23. Rosenberg S, Mueser K, Jankowski M, Hamblin J. Trauma exposure and PTSD in people with severe mental illness. *PTSD Research Quarterly.* 2002;13(3):1–7.
24. Muskett C. Trauma-informed care in inpatient mental health settings: a review of the literature. *Int J Ment Health Nursing.* 2014;23(1):51–59.
25. Gray AJ, Johanson P. Ethics and professional issues: the universal and the particular. In: Cupitt C, ed. *Reaching Out: The Psychology of Assertive Outreach.* New York: Routledge; 2010:229–247.
26. Salyers MP, Stull LG, Rollins AL, et al. Measuring the recovery orientation of assertive community treatment. *J Am Psychiatr Nurses Assoc.* 2013;19(3):117–128.
27. Salyers M, Tsemberis T. ACT and recovery: Integrating evidence-based practice and recovery orientation on Assertive Community Treatment teams. *Community Ment Health J.* 2007;43(6):619–641.
28. Williamson T. Ethics of assertive outreach (assertive community treatment teams). *Curr Opin Psychiatry.* 2002;15(5):543–547.
29. Phillips SD, Burns BJ, Edgar ER, et al. Moving assertive community treatment into standard practice. *Psychiatr Serv.* 2001;52(6):771–779.
30. Drake RE, O'Neal EL, Wallach MA. A systematic review of psychosocial research on psychosocial interventions for people with co-occurring severe mental and substance use disorders. *J Subst Abuse Treat.* 2008;34(1):123–138.
31. Mueser KT, Drake RE, Sigmon SC, Brunette MF. Psychosocial interventions for adults with severe mental illnesses and co-occurring substance use disorders: a review of specific interventions. *J Dual Diagn.* 2005;1:57–82.
32. Butler LS, McPherson PM. Is residential treatment misunderstood? *J Child Fam Stud.* 2006;16:465–472.
33. Horsfall J, Cleary M, Hunt GE, Walter G. Psychosocial treatments for people with co-occurring severe mental illnesses and substance use disorders (dual diagnosis): a review of empirical evidence. *Harvard Rev Psychiatry.* 2009;17(1):24–34.
34. Kennard D. The therapeutic community as an adaptable treatment modality across different settings. *Psychiatr Q.* 2004;75(3):295–307.
35. Drake RE, Mueser KT, Brunette MF, McHugo GJ. A review of treatments for people with severe mental illnesses and co-occurring substance use disorders. *Psychiatr Rehabil J.* 2004;27(4):360–374.
36. Bhalerao SU, Geurtjens C, Thomas GR, Kitamura CR, Zhou C, Marlborough M. Understanding the neuropsychiatric consequences associated with significant traumatic brain injury. *Brain Inj.* 2013;27(7–8):767–774.
37. Block CK, West SE. Psychotherapeutic treatment of survivors of traumatic brain injury: review of the literature and special considerations. *Brain Inj.* 2013;27(7–8):775–788.
38. Marsh NV, Kersel DA, Havill JA, Sleigh JW. Caregiver burden during the year following severe traumatic brain injury. *J Clin Exp Neuropsychol.* 2002;24(4):434–447.
39. US Department of Health and Human Services, Administration for Community Living. *Administration on Aging.* http://www.aoa.acl.gov/Aging_Statistics/Profile/2013/4.aspx. Accessed 1/29/2015.
40. Ortman JM, Velkoff VA, Hogan H. *An Aging Nation: The Older Population in the United States.* https://www.census.gov/prod/2014pubs/p25-1140.pdf. Published May 2014. Accessed 1/29/2015.
41. Kessler RC, Berglund P, Demler O, Jin R, Merikangas KR, Walters EE. Lifetime prevalence and age-of-onset distributions of DSM-IV disorders in the National Comorbidity Survey Replication. *Arch Gen Psychiatry.* 2005;62(6):593–602.
42. Narrow WE, Rae DS, Robins LN, Regier DA. Revised prevalence estimates of mental disorders in the United States: using a clinical significance criterion to reconcile 2 surveys' estimates. *Arch Gen Psychiatry.* 2002;59(2):115–123.
43. Karel MJ, Gatz M, Smyer MA. Aging and mental health in the decade ahead: what psychologists need to know. *Am Psychol.* 2012;67(3):184–198.
44. Institute of Medicine. *The Mental Health and Substance Use Workforce for Older Adults: In Whose Hands?* Washington DC: The National Academies Press; 2012.
45. Karel MJ, Knight BG, Duffy M, Hinrichsen GA, Zeiss AM. Attitude, knowledge, and skill competencies for practice in professional geropsychology: Implications for training and building a geropsychology workforce. *Train Educ Prof Psychol.* 2010;4(2):75–84.
46. Lieff SJ, Kirwin P, Colenda CC. Proposed geriatric psychiatry core competencies for subspecialty training. *Am J Geriatr Psychiatry.* 2005;13(9):815–821.
47. Makadon HJ, Mayer KH, Potter J, Goldhammer H, American College of Physicians. *The Fenway Guide to lesbian, gay, bisexual, and Transgender Health.* Philadelphia: American College of Physicians; 2008.
48. Lyons HZ, Worthington RL, Bieschke KJ, Dendy, AK, Georgemiller R. Psychologists' competence to treat lesbian, gay, and bisexual clients: state of the field and strategies for improvement. *Prof Psychol: Res Pract.* 2010;41(5):424–434.
49. Ruble MW, Forstein M. Mental health: epidemiology, assessment, and treatment. In: Makadon HJ, Mayer KH, Potter J, Goldhammer H, eds. *The Fenway Guide to Lesbian, Gay, Bisexual, and Transgender Health.* Philadelphia: American College of Physicians; 2008:187–208.
50. Coleman E, Bockting W, Botzer M, et al. Standards of care for the health of transsexual, transgender, and gender-nonconforming people, version 7. *Int J Transgenderism.* 2012;13(4):165–232.
51. Southwick SM, Charney DS. *Resilience: The Science of Mastering Life's Greatest Challenges.* New York: Cambridge University Press; 2012.
52. Frayne SM, Phibbs, CS, Friedman SA, et al. *Sourcebook: Women Veterans in the Veterans Health Administration. Volume 1: Sociodemographic Characteristics and Use of VHA Care. Women's Health Evaluation Initiative.* Washington DC: Women Veterans Health Strategic Health Care Group, Veterans Health Administration, Department of Veterans Affairs; 2010.
53. Frayne SM, Mattocks KM. *Sourcebook: Women Veterans in the Veterans Health Administration. Volume 2: Sociodemographics and Use of VHA and Non-VA Care (Fee).* Washington, DC: Women Veterans Health Strategic Health Care Group, Veterans Health Administration, Department of Veterans Affairs; 2012.
54. Kimmerling R, Gima K, Smith, MW, Street AE, Frayne S. The Veterans Health Administration and military sexual trauma. *Am J Pub Health.* 2007;97:2160–2166.

14.

CULTURAL COMPETENCE AND PUBLIC PSYCHIATRY

Esperanza Díaz, Michelle Silva, Elena F. Garcia-Aracena, Luis Añez, Manuel Paris, Andres Barkil-Oteo, Aniyizhai Annamalai, Miriam Delphin-Rittmon, and Selby Jacobs

---

EDUCATIONAL HIGHLIGHTS

- Culture influences health outcomes.
- Public psychiatry providers need to develop culturally competent services to address disparities.
- Person-centered care is the best approach to cultural sensitivity.
- Policies influence the social determinants of mental health.
- Cultural competence trainings are essential to address health disparities.

INTRODUCTION

What does a specialist in public psychiatry need to know about mental health and cultural competence? This chapter provides a response to this question. The goal of cultural competence is to improve the quality of health care outcomes through research, education, and interventions addressing the health and mental health disparities among racial and ethnic minorities.[1] Public psychiatry has common goals with cultural competence: these are to serve the needs of the population of people with serious mental illnesses and addictions by supporting and improving appropriate mental health systems.

HEALTH DISPARITIES

We start by looking at health disparities. Health disparities are defined as measurable differences in the quality of health care when access-related factors are controlled for in certain segments of the population.[2] Health status and health outcomes are measured when studying disparities. All health professionals should be concerned with the prevalence and incidence of diseases that are often segmented by race and ethnicity, thus revealing vast differences between minorities and nonminorities.[3] Health disparities are evident in respiratory, cardiovascular and infectious diseases, child mortality, cancers, obesity, and diabetes. For example, the prevalence of high blood pressure—a major risk factor for coronary heart disease, stroke, kidney disease, and more—is 40% greater in African Americans than in whites. Consequently, African Americans have a higher rate of stroke and are twice as likely to die from it than are white Americans. Mexican American and African American mothers are more than 2.5 times as likely as non-Hispanic white mothers to begin prenatal care in the third trimester or not at all.[4]

SOCIAL DETERMINANTS OF HEALTH AND MENTAL HEALTH

Observing how society influences health is a useful starting point to understand health disparities. Researchers have identified certain main factors that are summarized as the social determinants of health (Table 14.1).[5,6]

The impact on health from a full range of social conditions, such as housing quality, neighborhood safety, fair

Table 14.1 SOCIAL DETERMINANTS OF HEALTH

Income-Affordability	Housing
Education-Literacy	Insurance
Language access	Food access
Race and ethnicity	Complex health needs
Transportation	

Table 14.2 THE SOCIAL DETERMINANTS OF MENTAL HEALTH

Poverty	Abandoned housing
Homelessness	Access to quality food
Violence	Public safety
Social exclusion	Access to health care
Racism and discrimination	Green space
Sanitation/pollution	Clean air and water
Overcrowding	Justice
	Sustainable resources

employment, distribution of political, civil and economic rights, transportation, land use planning, and economic development, highlights areas for intervention. The social determinants of health are universal processes taking a unique form in each society based on its culture, politics, and economy.[7] Some might argue that social determinants of health are separate from cultural factors. We argue they are not, essentially because we see a 100% correlation between the two. They go hand in hand in shaping the social picture of every person.

Public health and epidemiological studies frequently separate the social determinants of health from culture for the purpose of determining if they make independent contributions. Many studies focus on race and ethnicity when, in fact, they need to focus on other variables such as poverty, acculturation, language, and treatment preferences, with all these dependent on the individual's environment and the ability to access education and jobs. In order to compare groups, the sample has to be homogeneous. Ethnic group stereotypes often creep into studies and might engender false beliefs of uniformity within members of an ethnic group, thus obscuring individual differences because of other factors that might be excluded. Social determinants complicate this matter but illuminate deep understandings of cause and consequence. Statistical discrimination is a theory of gender and racial inequality based on stereotypes. Some examples of tolerated statistical discrimination are that older people are charged more for life insurance or that a college diploma assumes that better education leads to better performance. A public psychiatry specialist needs to know how to integrate appropriate variables to arrive at a fair assessment. For example, to be equitable and to address disparities in all groups, the expansion of insurance coverage would cover different services for racial and ethnic groups that require specific interventions.[8]

What about mental health? Mental health disparities are evident across racial and ethnic groups as measured by access to services, accuracy of diagnosis, type of treatment, comparative effectiveness, location of services, cultural competence, proficiency, and recovery.[5]

Minorities report psychological problems often. African American females are 20% more likely to report serious psychological problems than are non-Hispanic white females. Suicide attempts among Hispanic girls in grades 9–12 are 70% higher than for white girls in the same age group. Death rates for adolescent American Indian/Alaskan Native females are four times the rate for white females in the same age group.[4,9] And, across the United States, access to care is a major problem for these high-risk groups. A recent survey conducted by Harris Interactive and the American Psychological Association determined that 25% of the US population lacks adequate access to mental health care. One in four Americans has a mental disorder, but two-thirds of these individuals do not receive treatment.[10] Where you live and work can impact your mental health (see Table 14.2).

Living in poverty has the strongest effect on the rates of mental illness. By understanding what it means to live under constraining circumstances, clinicians can tailor treatment recommendations to address the needs of those living in these conditions.[6] Services should be organized to allow other supports, such as case management and supportive interventions, as required to address these needs within the provision of care.[11] Here, we discuss barriers to services and further develop the theme of access.

CULTURAL COMPETENCE

Cultural competence presumably improves health outcomes. But what is it? First, we need to define "culture," which is no simple task. The term "culture" is most often used to describe a "learned system of knowledge, behaviors, attitudes, beliefs, values, and norms that are shared by a group."[12] Beyond a unifying principle of group membership, however, culture entails understanding the unique social context and individual life history of each person. It assumes a fluid and dynamic process by which individuals, communities, and social systems interface with one another and are mutually influenced. Culture "influences the experience, expression, course and outcome of mental health problems, health seeking and the response to health promotion, prevention or treatment interventions."[7] Therefore, in mental health, cultural competence becomes a natural and integral component of effective care and ethical practices. To effectively support change in an individual's way of thinking, to understand his or her motivations, and to appreciate his or her emotional experience, the systems of care must take into account the individual's cultural context. The experience of psychiatric distress, help-seeking patterns, reception to prevention and intervention, and the ultimate course and outcome of treatment are undoubtedly influenced by culture.[13] When providing health care, we need to talk about culture because it differs among various people, is omnipresent, and is frequently ignored.

Having defined culture, how is cultural competence defined? Among many, a standard definition is that "cultural competence is having the capacity to function effectively as an individual and an organization within the context of the cultural beliefs, behaviors and needs presented by consumers and their communities."[11] In considering the health care systems, the following definition expands the concept in a way that is useful for truly effective services: "Cultural competence in health care entails: understanding the importance of social and cultural influences on patients' health beliefs and behaviors; considering how these factors interact at multiple levels of the health care delivery system (e.g., at the level of structural processes of care or clinical decision-making); and, finally, devising interventions that take these issues into account to assure quality health care delivery to diverse patient populations."[14] The shared goal in creating culturally competent systems is to promote services that are accessible to all communities regardless of diversity across age, race, ethnicity, gender, language, physical and mental ability, sexual orientation, religious and spiritual beliefs

---

Box 14.1 HOMELESSNESS AND MEDICATION ADHERENCE

A homeless African American male revealed his main concerns about medication: "It is not that I do not want to take it. It is more about keeping alert to defend my belongings and defend myself. Streets are tough and more if you are from a color group."

Box 14.2 TREATMENT EXPERIENCE BY A MONOLINGUAL SPANISH-SPEAKING PATIENT

"I like the groups in the clinic. In other places they do not speak Spanish. There, they speak my language. I can talk about my problems without so much embarrassment.

They understand my perspective; I can share my feelings"

---

and affiliations, socioeconomic status, educational background, structural issues, marital status, and other dimensions. Structural issues refer here to influences derived from normal operations of social institutions such residential segregation, healthcare access, neighborhood safety, etc. Structural competency is an approach to train health workers about how the environment affects health.

In health care settings, this means understanding the importance of social and cultural influences on an individual's health beliefs and behaviors, paying attention to organizational and structural processes, and integrating both in treatment to ensure quality care.[7,14,15] Addressing system-wide factors requires the development of culturally and linguistically competent systems. It also involves establishing both person-centered and recovery-oriented systems of care.[16,17] It requires clinicians and public health providers to work together to address disparities.

TERMS USED TO REFER TO CULTURAL COMPETENCE

Over the years a variety of terms have been used when referring to cultural competence. In the late 1960s, the term "patient-centered" encompassed both cultural sensitivity and cultural competence.[18] When the US Surgeon General began reporting on unequal treatment and began to document compelling scientific evidence of racial and ethnic health and mental health disparities,[2] the term "cultural competence" rose to prominence. It remains the most common term used, but to some it implies reducing this concept to a technical skill and equating culture with race and ethnicity, which may lead to stereotyping. The term "person-centered care," although referring to a model of care based on recovery principles (see Chapter 3), is also used more specifically to refer to cultural competence education in clinical interactions.[19] The concept of *cultural humility* is used to emphasize that cultural competence is a lifelong learning process.[20] *Cultural sensitivity* refers to a provider's attitudes and his or her ability to understand the person's needs and culture and to adapt treatment recommendations accordingly, taking into account how implicit bias and stereotypes may influence ways of thinking in clinical encounters. We expand on this concept in the training and education section.

The term "cross-cultural" applies in clinical practice when there are marked cultural differences between the provider and patient. In this circumstance, there is the need to learn details about a specific region or country. Language is one of those differences, and poor language competency is a major stumbling block to excellent care because it creates a need for interpreters. (For instance, in English the word "once" means one time, but in Spanish, it means the number "eleven." There are anecdotal reports of this major confusion when reading medication directions. We discuss this in greater detail in the "Language Barriers" and "Immigrants and Refugees" sections.)

BARRIERS TO SERVICE

It is important to understand the factors that get in the way of culturally sensitive services. Negative views of mental illness influence the development of mental health services, and stigma and discrimination toward the mentally ill influence access and remain the most important barriers to overcome in the community.[21] In this section, we focus on barriers for racial and ethnic minorities. We group them into four large categories: language, culture, workforce diversity, and lack of minority-specific evidence-based treatments.

LANGUAGE BARRIERS

Language not only creates a barrier to service access, but it also results in more diagnostic errors, a lower perception of quality of services, and fewer follow-ups. According to the Robert Wood Johnson Foundation survey, 20% of Spanish-speaking patients delayed or refused treatment because of language problems. Because there are an estimated 13 million Spanish-speaking people in the United States, this refusal of treatment is an urgent public health problem. The crisis-oriented nature of Hispanics reinforces their tendency to not seek help, and their lack of English proficiency is another reason to avoid a consultation. But when services are delivered in Spanish in a culturally sensitive setting, the engagement and treatment outcomes take a completely different turn, and the clinic becomes a more hospitable place for minority patients.[23]

Language barriers are not only a product of discrepancies in the language spoken between patients and providers. A commonwealth survey showed that a significant percentage of minorities who spoke English had problems communicating with their doctors because they the doctors did not understand the conversation and their questions went unanswered.

Language barriers and limited understanding of the patient's culture are major challenges in providing health care to refugees. Qualified interpreters who can translate and objectively interpret cultural nuances are critical. Even if the refugee has some English-language proficiency, it may not be sufficient to express concerns, describe symptoms, and discuss treatment. Even with qualified interpreters, subtle differences in meaning can be lost in translation. Interpreting services can take place either in-person or via telephone. The advantages of in-person services are the ability to use nonverbal communication with the patient, the ability to provide a written translations of the treatment plan, and a decreased dependence on the technological quality of telephonic communication. The advantages of telephone interpreter services are patient comfort in discussing sensitive information in the absence of a third person (especially if there are gender differences between the patient and the interpreter) and less potential for a triadic relationship involving the interpreter, in which the interpreter might impose his or her own values. A family member should not be used as an interpreter to respect privacy and allow professionals to hear the problem without interference. Table 14.3 provides some tips for working with interpreters.

CULTURAL BARRIERS

Illnesses are shaped by cultural beliefs. Culture determines how symptoms manifest, how they are described, and how they are treated. Clinicians should strive to elicit and understand patient identity, explanatory models, and the social determinants of mental health. They should be aware of their own biases and stereotyping. If not trained properly, health care providers could fail to understand sociocultural differences between themselves and their patients that could affect their ability to properly diagnose and treat, and this ultimately leads to poorer health outcomes. For

Table 14.3 WORKING WITH INTERPRETERS

- Word for word translation is needed in areas that are delicate and significant
- Summary translation in areas that require abstract interpretation
- Meaning interpretation in areas that need elaboration and explanation in addition to translation
- Coaching the interpreter in this way is useful.[22]

example, gender or family roles can be perceived very differently across different cultures. These differences can be important in conceptualizing and implementing certain therapies, such as interpersonal psychotherapy for treatment of major depression.

LACK OF DIVERSITY IN THE HEALTH CARE WORKFORCE

Minorities represent 28% of the population, but they are underrepresented in medical school, public health schools, and government agencies where decisions about health and structural influences are made. In addition, they are underrepresented in the health care workforce. This is important because many studies reveal how racial and ethnic diversity could positively impact the quality of the health care delivered. Patients tend to be more satisfied and rate the quality of their treatment higher when it is delivered by a provider of the same race who speaks their language.[24]

In the behavioral health field, minority health care professionals comprise 21.3% of psychiatrists, 6.2% of psychologists, 5.6% of advanced practice psychiatric nurses, 12.6% of social workers, and 10.7% of counselors [25] which is far below their representation in the American population.[35] Furthermore, in the addictions treatment field, 70–90% of the workforce is made up of non-Hispanic whites, whereas only 56% of all clients are white.[25]

The scarcity of behavioral health professionals with adequate training creates an unfortunate effect in that the existing pool of mental health and addiction professionals are overburdened with excessive caseloads, which can contribute to burnout.[26] It is for these reasons that attracting qualified personnel to serve in culturally specific clinics continues to be an ongoing challenge. The use of culturally appropriate patient navigators or case managers, as well as peer support, is useful in addressing structural issues.

LACK OF MINORITY-SPECIFIC EVIDENCE-BASED DIAGNOSIS AND TREATMENT

We need to be aware that research into the disparities experienced by racial and ethnic minorities poses its own methodological challenges. For example, there are intragroup differences among Hispanics. When researchers lump together statistics for a certain race, ignoring intragroup differences, the results produce an "ethnic gloss" that can be deceptive.[27] Cultural diagnostic limitations are recognized by the *Diagnostic and Statistical Manual of Mental Disorders* (DSM 5): for example, the manic phase of mood disorders in Hispanics may not be elation; irritability and aggressiveness are described as prominent presentations and are modulated by the ability to speak English.[28]

How can we best implement evidence-based treatment practices when research validating best evidence for minorities is scarce? To this end, providing effective and ongoing training and education, support for foreign language proficiency, and performance-based supervision around the integration of cultural determinants and treatment modalities is critical to the provision of appropriate client care.[29]

Cultural treatment adaptation is defined as changes to an evidence-based treatment modality to accommodate the behavior, beliefs, or attitudes of a certain group, and it provides one way of linking cultural competence to evidence-based practice.[30] These adaptations can be implemented through change in the components of the treatment or in the way the interventions are delivered. For example, translating treatment material into the native language of the target group is one example of cultural adaptation. More research is required to determine if treatment interventions affect the outcomes that matter: a patient's satisfaction with care, effective care, improved health, and reduced disparities.

IMMIGRANTS AND REFUGEES

Immigrants and refugees are special groups with unique needs that are important to understand. Immigrants and refugees are at risk for mental illness but often do not have access to quality mental health care. In this population, culturally competent care applies more specifically because the culture of the providers and the patients may differ greatly, and cross-cultural differences will be more obvious in the presence of language differences (as discussed earlier). Immigrants have added challenges: they have been left their own country and may not be able to return, they have left behind supports and family; and they must acquire a new identity and learn to understand a new culture and a new language, all while possibly grieving for substantial personal losses.[31] Undocumented immigrants usually arrive in the United States looking for a better life; many are waiting to get legal issues resolved while they send money to their countries of origin. The motivation to work and be healthy for their families is a positive influence in mental health treatments. In contrast, second-generation immigrants have a higher incidence of substance abuse, depression, and poorer mental health.[32]

Unlike immigrants, refugees have been forced to flee their homeland and have resettled in the United States or another country to avoid persecution (see Chapter 15 on

> **Box 14.3 CULTURALLY COMPETENT CARE**
>
> A Middle Eastern refugee was referred with a confused clinical picture. He had been originally evaluated by medicine and was referred with a possible diagnosis of psychosis. Interpreters were not helpful. A psychiatrist who spoke his language and understood his culture, clarified his diagnosis. Post-traumatic stress disorder and borderline intellectual functioning were the major problems. Without such expertise, the symptoms could not be assessed to arrive at this formulation.

Global Mental Health for a brief review of the global refugee burden, US resettlement, and evidence-based mental health interventions in this population). Refugees come from many different places around the world and their responses to the stressors of trauma, migration and resettlement can vary widely based on cultural background as well as on personal traits of vulnerability or resilience.

Demoralization has been defined as a syndrome that differs from depression, presenting as it does with subjective incompetence and hopelessness as its core features. Although not specifically described in refugees, it may be commonly observed in cross-cultural psychiatry.[33] Close attention should be paid to the family system and social network during a refugee's treatment. Rules of confidentiality and disclosure should be applied in a way that respects cultural context. For example, interventions for adolescents should be framed in ways that avoid alienating family members or aggravating intergenerational conflicts.[34] A similar caution is needed when state-run departments of children and family services are involved, in order to engage the families in trusting therapeutic relationships and avoiding early drop-out.

Refugee clinics are emerging in several medical centers. The Refugee Clinic of Yale New Haven Hospital, housed in the Primary Care Center, opened in 2008 and provides specialized attention to refugee populations. In addition to caring for the patients' medical needs, the staff screen for major psychiatric disorders and make referrals.[35]

CULTURAL VARIATIONS IN PSYCHIATRIC SYNDROMES

Variations in common psychiatric syndromes have also been described in refugees, recent immigrants, or cultural minorities of recent arrival. For example, multiple variations of panic attacks with significant physical components have been described in Southeast Asian refugees.[36–38] Cambodian refugees describe *khyal* attacks (or wind attacks), a variation of a panic attack, in their idiom of distress. In this syndrome, somatic symptoms trigger a catastrophic belief that "wind" and blood are rushing through blood vessels to cause bodily dysfunction or death.[39]

Culturally specific syndromes have also been seen in association with other common psychiatric diagnoses. An example is *khmaoch sangot* (literally, "the ghost pushes you down"), which is a form of sleep paralysis seen more frequently in those with post-traumatic stress disorder and is associated with visual hallucinations, panic attacks, and elaborate cultural associations.[40] *Koro* ("shrinking penis") is a culturally bound syndrome described in a case report of a refugee,[41] but it has not been reported or systematically studied in large populations of refugees or cultural minorities. Even though specific syndromes have been described, what is more commonly seen are subtle variations of commonly seen psychiatric symptoms as defined in the DSM.

Psychological distress can manifest differently from the Westernized norms of emotional crisis. Refugee patients often present with physical symptoms, and the prevalence of physical symptoms in those with mental health issues can be very high.[42] Somatization has been described,[41] and a causal association has been shown between PTSD and somatic complaints.[39,43,44] Refugees also have a high level of psychosocial problems after resettlement, but evidence is lacking to determine a direct relationship between displacement stressors and somatic symptoms.

BRIEF HISTORY OF PUBLIC PSYCHIATRY AND POLICIES ADDRESSING ETHNIC/RACIAL MINORITIES

Here, we examine how mental health systems create sustainable structures that are sensitive and responsive to individual needs and preference. This section offers a brief history of key policies that address ethnic and racial minorities.

In 1955, the government founded the National Institute of Mental Health (NIMH) to ensure that seriously mentally ill people could have a life in the community and hope for recovery. The introduction of new medications to treat mental disorders initiated the movement for deinstitutionalization. Deinstitutionalization was a great hope but did not have the expected consequences, because it soon became apparent that the mentally ill needed supports if they were to live in the community.

Starting in 1956 and continuing to the present, deinstitutionalization for mentally ill persons marked the beginning of public psychiatry.[45,46] Profound changes in mental health care took place, such as the community mental health movement subsequent to the passage of the Mental Health Center Act in 1963. This Act was crucial to the creation of the first community mental health centers, including the Connecticut Mental Health Center (CMHC). Attention to social and environmental determinants of health and the realization of the complex needs of various minorities were central to the community mental health movement and resulted in the development of policies and responsive services.[47]

Subsequently, the passing of the Civil Rights Act in 1964 reinforced the Mental Health Center Act efforts by highlighting the need to address minorities equally. The Act eliminated the Jim Crow laws that had legalized segregation in the South, and Title VI of the Act guided federal agencies' financial assistance to potential beneficiaries and program creation, with a view to promoting equality and justice. Mandated as part of Title VI, the provision of limited English proficiency (LEP) materials can improve access to services for persons who have difficulty speaking and understanding English, but most organizations have been slow to implement LEP guidelines.

In 1973, the NIMH established the Minority Fellowship Program (MFP) to support workforce diversity for mental health providers and researchers. These policies supported the development of specialized services for minorities, but did not produce the hoped-for results. In 1985, the Heckler Report published evidence of serious health and mental health disparities related to racial and ethnic minorities and supported the creation of the Office of Minority Health and Health Disparities (OMHD) as part of the Centers for Disease Control and Prevention (CDC); as well, the Agency for Healthcare Research and Quality (AHRQ) was established to reduce health care disparities.

The Culturally and Linguistically Appropriate Services (CLAS) standards were created in 1998. They are based on a national review conducted by the OMHD. The standards supported the creation of services such as minority specialty clinics (the Hispanic Clinic at CMHC, described later, is one example). In 2000, the Office of Civil Rights (OCR), empowered by the White House, published Executive Order 13166 "Improving Access to Services for Persons with Limited English Proficiency," which led to the establishment of a national framework for understanding and eliminating health disparities. The Healthy People 2010 initiative followed shortly thereafter. This initiative supported research aimed at uncovering the reasons for persistent disparities and resulted in the 2001 publication of the Surgeon General's Report on "Mental Health: Culture, Race, and Ethnicity." This report revealed that ethnic minorities do not utilize mental health services as much as the majority population and stated that "culture counts."[5,45]

Several reports followed. "Cultural Competence Standards in Managed Care Mental Health Services: Four Underserved/Underrepresented Racial/Ethnic Group" is the first report on culturally competent mental health care created by a government agency.[5] The CLAS,[11] the President's New Freedom Commission on Mental Health[5] and the IOM's "Unequal Treatment Report"[2] also confirmed that, after years of new policies and interventions, health disparities remain the same as those documented in the 1985 Heckler Report.

Follow-up with new policies continues at all levels. The Mental Health and Addiction Equity Act was passed in 2008, requiring equal coverage for mental illness and physical illness in those plans that include mental health coverage. Section 10334(b) of the Patient Protection and Affordable Care Act requires six agencies in the Department of Health and Human Services to establish offices of Minority Health. Action plans addressing reductions in health disparities (2011) and how to advance the CLAS standards were released (2013).

The Department of Mental Health and Addiction Services (DMHAS) Health Disparities Initiative (2009), a public–private partnership between DMHAS and the Yale Program for Recovery and Community Health (PRCH), was designed to identify and develop statewide systemic interventions to eliminate behavioral health disparities. In addition, this project implements transformation goals discussed in the DMHAS Commissioner's Policy on Cultural Competence and the DMHAS Office of Multicultural Affairs and Health Disparities Initiative Strategic Plans. Recovery-oriented practice follows the traditions of person-centered care, in which the individual takes charge of his or her own treatment, and it adapts principles of recovery to achieve unique treatment goals (see Chapter 3 on Recovery-Oriented Practice for more details).

MODELS OF SERVICE DELIVERY

Here we look at how mental health services respond to people from ethnic and racial minority communities struggling with high-risk factors and social determinants of illness that can contribute to overall poor health outcomes.[4]

Increasingly, with the release of the enhanced National Culturally and Linguistically Appropriate Services Standards in 2001 and further revisions,[11] health care professionals are attuned to the importance of adopting a system-wide approach to addressing culture in health care service delivery. The CLAS standards outline competencies that organizations and health care systems can implement to reduce health care disparities and ensure that their services address the cultural beliefs, values, and worldviews of those accessing care. Implementation examples are the use of interpreters to address language access to health care and the creation of state minority offices to advance cultural competency.[48]

A prototype of how these policies are implemented is the Hispanic Clinic. In 1973, the CMHC, noticing the lack of culturally sensitive services, created a clinic for Hispanics who did not speak English. The clinic began to operate one afternoon a week and was staffed by one Spanish-speaking psychiatrist and a clinical social worker. Eventually, it was named *La Clinica Hispana* (the Hispanic Clinic). The Hispanic Clinic is a model of collaboration between a state government and an academic institution. The clinic's name purposely does not include the word "mental health" to avoid stigma, and it was opened in a location near Hispanic neighborhoods. As a collaborative endeavor between Yale University and the CDMHAS, the Hispanic Clinic was created to improve access to care for monolingual Spanish speakers. The services continue to expand in response to the population's growing needs.[23,49] It has become an important training site for multiple disciplines, including on its staff, medical students, psychiatry residents, psychologists, fellows, and social workers. It is also a site that provides research opportunities to develop specific practices for Hispanic populations. The clinic is a model of culturally sensitive services, a model for cultural competence, and a provider of structural interventions. Case management assesses and addresses needs such as homelessness, poverty, transportation, health insurance, and medications for those who cannot afford them.

Another example is the Connecticut Latino Behavioral Health System (CT LBHS), opened in 2006. It was developed in response to demands for expansion of mental health services in the state's south central region with support from the CDMHAS and the Connecticut state legislature. The goal is to support a community-based collaborative model providing mental health care for the Latino population using bilingual/bicultural capacity-building efforts. A unique feature is ongoing workforce development with cultural competence training for all personnel and systems affiliated with the program and ongoing collaboration with primary care centers.

Nationally the efforts to improve continue. An innovative model of service delivery is now being implemented through the Health Impact Assessment (HIA), an intervention to elevate the importance of health and mental health in the process of decision-making. Decisions related to economic, environmental, and social determinants of health usually are made outside of the domains of health and mental health. The HIA and the Mental Health Impact Assessment (MHIA) assess the impact of policy and planning decisions on population health (e.g., consideration of the health effects of new construction). These assessments, coupled with the new paradigm proposed by "structural competency" in teaching, are promising. Public health professionals also will benefit from learning and adapting these methods in their work.[6]

An example of MHIA implementation is a substance abuse treatment program in Wisconsin's prisons that was developed to address barriers to entering the workforce after successful substance abuse treatment.[50] African Americans represented 14% of the state's general population and 28% of its prison population. Their arrest histories affect their abilities to find jobs when released, even if they were not convicted, causing stress and promoting depressive presentations.[51,52] The MHIA supported change in the legislation to facilitate employment and increase the number of previously incarcerated African Americans entering the workforce after release. Being culturally competent translates into systems that instill hope, foster empowerment, and promote individual choice in the recovery process.

There are no simple solutions. Borrowing from global health and population health perspectives, we should consider models of innovation and paradigm shift. Creative interventions could be useful in advocating for and developing programs for effective change. The nongovernmental organizations Partners in Health and Running Upstream are examples of interventions that address minorities and their needs. Paul Farmer, who investigated the root causes of the global health crisis that led to the creation of Partners in Health, sought to promote health and social justice by practicing medicine with community outreach and enlisted other appropriate partners to improve outcomes in impoverished communities.[53] Clinical and community barriers to care are removed when medical treatment is declared a "public good" and is provided free of charge. Running Upstream uses the metaphor of swimming upstream to prevent children from being swept downstream by the currents of poor health care. Rishi Manchanda, its founder, describes the need to address prevention strategies like structural interventions.[54] Understanding more about the causes of structural inequalities in health care will make medicine better.

Joining professional associations that encourage their members to think and plan critically is an effective approach to developing better service models. Ongoing collaborations fostered by professional associations that promote teaching models are useful; these collaborations are supported by American Medical Association, the American Association of Directors of Psychiatric Residency Training, the American Psychological Association, and the National Association of Social Work.

Culturally and linguistically appropriate therapeutic interventions will emerge as the norm in an environment committed to addressing the individual, his or her social environment, and the surrounding health and political systems. But empirical studies are still needed to develop and test new treatment models based on innovative ideas.[55–58] A paradigm shift is needed, one that will examine, unify, and bolster existing services in order to bridge the gaps that so many at-risk patients fall through.

TEACHING CULTURAL COMPETENCE

Effective teaching methods to train the health care workforce are useful to address health care disparities and structural issues. There is no agreement on the best method to teach cultural competence, and there are no studies on the effect of cultural competence education on health outcomes.[59] What we do know is that, between 1985 and 2001, the rate of health disparities did not change despite efforts to address cultural competence education. Health disparities suggest the importance of cultural competence but do not prove it. In a paper comparing rates of cardiac procedures after myocardial infarction between populations with and without mental disorders, the mentally ill were less likely to undergo these procedures. Implicit bias about mental illness and stigma were considered as major influences on treatment recommendations, thereby interfering with access to treatment.[21]

Educational programs should aim to reveal and eliminate stereotypes among health care providers, using methods such as person-centered care and culturally sensitive interviewing methods to allow providers to see the person behind the illness. Learning about implicit bias should be a priority in any curriculum because it is suggested as a possible contributor to health disparities.[60] Training should uncover implicit assumptions and stereotypes to show how they could interfere in cross-cultural interactions. Experiential exercises help providers understand that implicit assumptions and prejudices are part of human nature and that they influence health recommendations.

All clinicians should be encouraged to routinely take a social history of their patients to identify the social determinants of their mental health. The Cultural Formulation Interview, CFI from DSM 5,[61] a semi-structured interview, elicits information on the cultural context of the patient. It is an important tool for exploring themes such as identity, ethnic differences, social networks, and social determinants of mental health. The CFI can be used to build skills in eliciting culturally relevant information; the instrument provides sets of questions related to cultural definition of the problem, cultural perceptions of cause, context and support, cultural factors affecting self-coping, and past and current help-seeking. Video recordings of trainees' role-playing their own clinical vignettes in practice interviews using CFI questions foster self-assessment and reflection.[62] Box 14.4 shows an example of culturally competent care using the CFI as a starting point.

Considering the ongoing change occurring in the cultural and ethnic characteristics of the population in North America and around the globe, person-centered care presents the most appropriate method to practice cultural sensitivity and competence in clinical settings. Cultural competence in the person-centered care approach assures individualized understanding and also addresses health disparities, structural inequalities, and poor health outcomes in minority populations.[63]

Taking lessons from the literature and past experiences, the approach to teach cultural competence should be based on creating learning environments in which the medium is the message.[64] The faculty's clinical wisdom, self-knowledge, cultural humility, and respect for diversity create a model for teaching that contributes to the development of clinical sites that sensitively address psychiatric needs in the community. We see the concept of cultural competence as a

---

Box 14.4 **CULTURALLY COMPETENT CARE**

A challenging monolingual Hispanic patient followed at the Hispanic Clinic had been diagnosed with depression and interpersonal problems. The woman was fixated on the loss of her mother, making all interventions ineffective. Applying ethnography to understand her symptoms—the explanatory model from the CFI—we clarified that her mother practiced as a "Witch" in her country. She was sought out to read the future and to counsel people about their difficulties. The patient felt important because of her mother's special status. When her mother died and the patient moved to United States, she lost her mother, her country, her language, and her special status as the daughter of a respected person in her community. Her treatment focused on helping her resolve the mourning of these multiple losses and learn positive aspects of her new culture.

lifelong learning process of cultural humility, rather than a static one.[20]

Our institutional culture encourages diverse faculty and students to promote specialty programs that address minorities and recovery from mental illness. An example of this approach is the Hispanic Clinic, described earlier, a specialized clinic serving monolingual Spanish speakers with mental illnesses and substance abuse disorders. The trainees in these programs are exposed to culturally sensitive methods with instruction on health disparities, skills for evaluations, a system for addressing social determinants, and Latino values as they relate to engagement and retention.[65,66] The site provides the opportunity for culturally competent evaluation and treatment recommendations. Dually diagnosed treatments and mental health and substance abuse prevention are at the core of the programs and respond to the specific needs of the person and the population.

The social determinants of health and mental health discussed previously are part of "structural competency," a new approach aiming to train health workers about how the environment affects health. This approach attends to structure as an organizing principle. Trainees learn about "markers of exclusion" that cause stigma, institutionalized racism, and how city environments may promote health, among many other factors.[67] All these are crucial factors for a public psychiatry professional to master.

More research is needed to develop ways to address routinely the social determinants of health, including those that are not limited to health care providers. Effective teaching methods need to evolve to train the health care workforce to address health care disparities and structural issues. Cultural training should not be an isolated course but instead part of the main curriculum, one that teaches students how to address patient care, conduct clinical interviews, and embrace person-centered care.

ESSENTIAL QUALITY METRICS

The implementation of programs that will expand services to minorities based on research findings about disparities is key to assessment of quality. Outcome measures, like those from annual reports that evaluate a program's progress, should be used regularly: these may include workforce development and access to services assessed by number of admissions, discharges, retention, successful completions, and dropouts. Furthermore, there is a need for ongoing evaluation of health outcomes as they relate to the cultural competence training of the mental health care workforce.

SUMMARY

After defining health care disparities and cultural competence, this chapter covered a wide range of topics related to both. These include social determinants of mental health, system and structural issues, cultural competence, barriers to care, culture-bound syndromes, models of care, and the teaching of cultural competence. A central point is that cultural competence has the potential to reduce disparities in outcomes of mental health treatment for minority populations. Also, by paying attention not only to individuals but also to the system of care, there is the potential to improve the mental health of the entire population. Essential to long-term improvements in health disparities are education and development of a diverse workforce prepared to address social determinants of health and structural issues affecting mental health.

REFERENCES

1. Institute of Medicine. *How far have we come in reducing health disparities?* Washington, DC: The National Academies Press; 2012.
2. Smedley B, Stith A, Nelson A. *Unequal Treatment: Confronting Racial and Ethnic Disparities in Health Care.* Washington, DC: National Academies Press; 2002.
3. LaVeist T. *Minority Populations and Health: An Introduction to Health Disparities in the United States.* San Francisco, CA: Jossey-Bass; 2005.
4. Office of Minority Health. *A Strategic Framework for Improving Racial/Ethnic Minority Health and Eliminating Racial/Ethnic Health Disparities.* US Department of Health and Human Services; 2011.
5. US Department of Health and Human Services. *Mental Health: Culture, Race, and Ethnicity—A Suppl to Mental Health: A Report of the Surgeon General.* Rockville, MD: US Department of Health and Human Service; 2001.
6. Institute on Social Exclusion MSC. *Mental Health Impact Assessment.* Chicago, IL: Adler School Institute on Social Exclusion: Mental Health Impact Assessment; 2013.
7. Kirmayer LJ. Rethinking cultural competence. *Transcultural Psychiatry.* 2012; 49(2): 149–164.
8. Alegria M, Lin J, Chen C, Duan N, Cook B, Meng X. The impact of Insurance Coverage in Diminishing Racial and Ethnic Disparities in Behavioral Health Services. *HSR.* 2012; 47(3): 1322–1344.
9. Lopez SR, Barrio C, Kopelowicz A, Vega WA. From documenting to eliminating disparities in mental health care for Latinos. *American Psychologist.* 2012; 67(7): 511–523.
10. US Department of Health and Human Services. *Mental Health: A Report of the Surgeon General* Rockville, MD: US Dept of Health and Human Services, Substance Abuse and Mental Health Services Administration, Center for Mental Health Services, National Institutes of Health, National Institute of Mental Health; 1999.
11. National Standards for Culturally and Linguistically Appropriate Services (CLAS) in Health and Health Care. A Blueprint for Advancing and Sustaining CLAS Policy and Practice. https://http://www.thinkculturalhealth.hhs.gov/pdfs/EnhancedCLASStandardsBlueprint.pdf. Updated 2013. Accessed January 5, 2014.
12. Smith G. *Communication and Culture.* New York, NY: Holt, Rinehart and Winston; 1966.

13. Kirmayer LJ. Cultural competence and evidence-based practice in mental health: Epistemic communities and the politics of pluralism. *Social Science & Medicine.* 2012; 75(2): 249–256.
14. Betancourt JR, Green AR, Carrillo JE, Ananeh-Firempong O. Defining cultural competence: a practical framework for addressing racial/ethnic disparities in health and health care. *Public Health Rep.* 2003; 118(4): 293–302.
15. Sue S, Zane N, Nagayama Hall GC, Berger LK. The case for cultural competency in psychotherapeutic interventions. *Annual Review of Psychology.* 2009; 60: 525–548.
16. Davidson L, White W. The concept of recovery as an organizing principle for integrating mental health and addiction services. *Journal of Behavioral Health Services and Research.* 2007; 34: 109–120.
17. Delphin-Rittmon ME, Andres-Hyman R, Flanagan EH, Davidson L. Seven essential strategies for promoting and sustaining systemic cultural competence. *Psychiatric Quarterly.* 2013; 84(1): 53–64.
18. Balint E. The possibilities of patient-centered medicine. *J R Coll Gen Pract.* 1969; 17: 269–276.
19. Saha S, Beach MC, Cooper LA. Patient Centeredness, Cultural Competence and Healthcare Quality. *J Natl Med Assoc.* 2008; 100(11): 1275–1285.
20. Tervalon M, Murray-Garcia J. Cultural Humility versus cultural competence: A critical distinction in defining physician training outcomes in multicultural education. *Journal of Health Care for the poor and underserved.* 1998; 9(2): 117–125.
21. Druss BG, Bradford DW, Rosenheck RA, Radford MJ, Krumholz HM. Mental Disorders and Use of Cardiovascular Procedures After Myocardial Infarction. *JAMA.* 2000; 283(4): 506–511.
22. Westermeyer J. Working with an interpreter in psychiatric assessment and treatment. *J Nerv Ment Dis.* 1990; 178(12): 745–749.
23. Diaz E, Prigerson H, Desai R, Rosenheck R. Perceived needs and service use of Spanish speaking monolingual patients followed at a Hispanic clinic. *Community Mental Health Journal.* 2001; 37(4): 335–346.
24. Sue S. In search of cultural competence in psychotherapy and counseling. *Am Psychol.* 1998; 53(4): 440–448.
25. Hoge MA, Stuart GW, Morris J, Flaherty MT, Paris M, Jr. Goplerud E. Mental Health And Addiction Workforce Development: Federal Leadership Is Needed to Address The Growing Crisis. *Health Affairs.* 2013; 32(11): 2005–2012.
26. Paris M, Hoge M. Burnout in the mental health workforce: A review. *Journal of Behavioral Health Services & Research.* 2010; 37(4): 519–528.
27. Safran MA, Mays RA, Trachtenberg A. Mental Health Disparities. *A J Public Health* 2009; 99(11): 1962–1966.
28. Díaz E, Miskemen T, Vega WA, et al. Inconsistencies in Diagnosis and Symptoms Among Bilingual and English-Speaking Latinos and Euro-Americans. *Psychiatric Services.* 2009; 60(10): 1379–1382.
29. Miller RM, Rollnick S. The effectiveness and ineffectiveness of complex behavioral interventions: Impact of treatment fidelity. *Contemporary Clinical Trials.* 2014; 37: 234–231.
30. Whitley R, Rousseau C, Carpenter-Song E, Kirmayer LJ. Evidence-based medicine: Opportunities and challenges in a diverse society. *The Canadian Journal of Psychiatry / La Revue canadienne de psychiatrie.* 2011; 56(9): 514–522.
31. Akhtar S. A third individuation: Immigration, identity, and the psychoanalytic process. *Journal of the American Psychoanalytic Association.* 1995; 43(4): 1051–1084.
32. Vega WA, Kolody B, Aguilar-Gaxiola S, Alderete E, Catalano R, Caraveo-Anduaga J. Lifetime prevalence of DSM III R psychiatric disorders among urban and rural Mexican Americans in California. *Arch Gen Psychiatry.* 1998; 55(9): 771–778.
33. de Figueiredo JM, Gostoli S. Culture and demoralization in psychotherapy. *Adv Psychosom Med.* 2013; 33: 75–87.
34. Kirmayer LJ, Narasiah L, Munoz M, et al. Common mental health problems in immigrants and refugees: General approach in primary care. *CMAJ Canadian Medical Association* 2011; 183(12): E959–967.
35. Shaddox C. Refugee clinic fills needs for both patients and physicians in training. *Yale Medicine.* Autumn 2011; 48(1): 7.
36. Hinton D, Um K, Ba P. A unique panic-disorder presentation among Khmer refugees: The sore-neck syndrome. *Culture, Medicine and Psychiatry.* 2001; 25(3): 297–316.
37. Hinton DE, Chhean D, Fama JM, et al. Gastrointestinal-focused panic attacks among Cambodian refugees: associated psychopathology, flashbacks, and catastrophic cognitions. *J Anxiety Disord.* 2007; 21(1): 42–58.
38. Hinton DE, Hinton L, Tran M, et al. Orthostatic panic attacks among Vietnamese refugees. *Transcult Psychiatry.* 2007; 44(4): 515–544.
39. Hinton DE, Kredlow MA, Bui E, Pollack MH, Hofmann SG. Treatment change of somatic symptoms and cultural syndromes among Cambodian refugees with PTSD. *Depress Anxiety.* 2012; 29(2): 147–154.
40. Hinton DE, Pich V, Chhean D, Pollack MH. 'The ghost pushes you down': sleep paralysis-type panic attacks in a Khmer refugee population. *Transcultural Psychiatry.* 2005; 42(1): 46–77.
41. Westermeyer J, Bouafuely M, Neider J, Callies A. Somatization among refugees: an epidemiologic study. *Psychosomatics.* 1989; 30(1): 34–43.
42. Jamil H, Hakim-Larson J, Farrag M, et al. Medical complaints among Iraqi American refugees with mental health. *J Immigr Health.* 2005; 7(3): 145–152.
43. Van Ommeren VM, Sharma B, Sharma GK, et al. The relationship between somatic and PTSD symptoms among Bhutanese refugee torture survivors: examination of comorbidity with anxiety and depression. *J Trauma Stress.* 2002; 15(5): 415–421.
44. Moore LJ, Boehnlein JK. Posttraumatic stress disorder, depression, and somatic symptoms in U.S. Mien patients. *J Nerv Ment Dis.* 1991; 179(12): 728–733.
45. Jacobs S. *Inside Public Psychiatry.* New Haven, CT: Springer; 2011.
46. Manderschied RW, Atay J, Hernandez-Cartagena MR, et al. Highlights of Organized Mental Health Services in 1998 and major national and state trends. In: Manderschied RW, Henderson MJ, eds. *Mental Health, United States 2000.* Rockville, MD: US Health and Human Services, Center for Mental Health Services; 2000.
47. Foley HA, Sharfstein SS. *Madness and Government: Who Cares for the Mentally Ill.* Washington, DC: American Psychiatric Press; 1983.
48. NY State Office of Minority Health. Statewide Comprehensive Plan 2011-2015. http://nyculturalcompetence.org. Updated 2012.
49. Diaz E, Woods SW, Rosenheck RA. Effects of Ethnicity on Psychotropic Medication Adherence. *Community Mental Health Journal.* 2005; 41(5): 521–537.
50. Liners D. Healthier lives, stronger families, and safer communities: A health impact assessment of alternatives to incarceration in Wisconsin. Presented at: 141st APHA Annual Meeting and Exposition; November 4, 2013; Boston, MA.
51. Solomon AL. In Search of a Job: Criminal Records as Barriers to Employment. *NIJ Journal.* 2012; 270: 42–51. http://www.crime-scene-investigator.net/NIJ-JobCriminalRecords.pdf. Accessed August 11, 2014.
52. Safran MA, Mays RA, Huang LN, et al. Mental Health Disparities. *Am J Public Health.* 2009; 99(11): 1962–1966.
53. Famer PE, Nizeye B, Stulac S, Keshavjee S. Structural Violence and Clinical Medicine. PLoS Medicine. 2006; 3(10): 1686–1691.
54. Manchanda R. *The Upstream Doctors: Medical Innovators Track Sickness to Its Source.* Ted Books; 2013.
55. Andres-Hyman R, Ortiz J, Añez L, Paris M, Davidson L. Culture and clinical practice: Recommendations for working with Puerto Ricans and other Latinas(os) in the United States. *Professional Psychology Research and Practice.* 2006; 37: 694–701.
56. Añez L, Paris M, Bedregal L, Davidson L, Grilo C. Application of cultural constructs in the care of first generation Latina/o clients in

a community mental health setting. *Journal of Psychiatric Practice.* 2005; 11(4): 221–230.
57. Castro FG, Barrera M, Jr., Pantin H, et al. Substance abuse prevention intervention research with Hispanic populations. *Drug and Alcohol Dependence.* 2006; 84(suppl.): S29–S42.
58. Carroll KM, Martino S, Ball SA, et al. A multisite randomized effectiveness trial of motivational enhancement therapy for Spanish-Speaking substance users. *Journal of Consulting and Clinical Psychology.* 2009; 77(5): 993–999.
59. Renzaho A, Romios P, Crock C, Sonderlund A. The effectiveness of cultural competence programs in ethnic minority patient centered health care-A systematic review of the literature. *International Journal for Quality in Health Care.* 2013; 25(3): 261–269.
60. Qureshi A, Eiroa-Orosa FJ. Training for overcoming health disparities in mental health care: Interpretative-relational cultural competence. In: Barnow S, Balkir, N. *Cultural variations in psychopathology: From research to practice.* Cambridge, MA: Hogrefe Publishing; 2013: 248–269.
61. American Psychiatric Association. *Diagnostic and statistical manual of mental disorders: DSM-5.* 5th ed. Arlington, VA: American Psychiatric Publishing, Inc; 2013.
62. Diaz E, Armah T, Linse CT, Jordan A, Fiskin A, Hafler J. An Innovative Cultural Psychiatry Curriculum *Academic Psychiatry.* Accepted with final edits.
63. Horvat L, Horey D, Romios P, Kis-Rigo J. *Cultural competence education for health professionals. The Cochrane Library 2011, Issue 10.* 2011. http://www.thecochranelibrary.com.
64. Guzder J, Rousseau C. A diversity of voices: The McGill 'Working with Culture' seminars. *Cult Med Psychiatry.* 2013; 37(2): 347–364.
65. Anez LM, Paris M, Jr., Bedregal LE, Davidson L, Grilo CM. Application of cultural constructs in the care of first generation Latino clients in a community mental health setting.[see comment]. *J Psychiatr Pract.* 2005; 11(4): 221–230.
66. Delphin ME, Rowe M. Continuing education in cultural competence for community mental health practitioners. *Professional Psychology: Research and Practice.* 2008; 39(2):182–191.
67. Metzl JM, Hansen H. Structural competency: Theorizing a new medical engagement with stigma and inequality. *Social Science & Medicine.* 2014;103: 126–133.

15.

GLOBAL MENTAL HEALTH

Carla Marienfeld, Andres Barkil-Oteo, Aniyizhai Annamalai, and Hussam Jefee–Bahloul

> ## EDUCATIONAL HIGHLIGHTS
>
> - Global mental health (GMH) incorporates many fields of study, is practiced in many settings (low-income/high-income, rural/urban, public/private, etc.), incorporates many types of treatments by providers with different levels of health care training, and emphasizes the development of local research capacity and mental health infrastructure.
>
> - Ethical GMH involves access to care, the provision of high-quality care, and the incorporation of research to determine the impact or outcomes of the care provided in the specific setting so that care delivered is appropriate for the population being treated.
>
> - Mental illness comprises a significant portion of the global burden of disease, but mental health care lags in human resources to provide care and in prioritization in health budgets.
>
> - Modern phenomena of the exportation of medications and diagnoses warrant close consideration to prevent unintentional consequences but should not be an excuse to ignore the well-documented disorders and suffering of those with mental illness.
>
> - Collaborative models for the education of trainees in high- and low-income countries allow for capacity building in low- and middle-income countries (LAMICs) in terms of research expertise and human resources, often best delivered through academic partnerships.
>
> - In the absence of psychiatric care providers, training health care workers for specific interventions and the use of new technology (such as telemedicine) can help increase access to interventions and care providers.
>
> - Several populations merit additional awareness due to the increased level of vulnerability they share within an already marginalized population of mentally ill, including refugees. Refugees struggle with both pre-existing psychiatric diagnoses and often from post-traumatic stress disorder (PTSD) and an increased risk for new or worsening mental illness associated with resettlement and new psychosocial stressors.
>
> - Public psychiatry and psychiatrists are essential players in the scale-up of mental health services in the provision of expertise, capacity building (training and supervision), and research.

INTRODUCTION TO GLOBAL MENTAL HEALTH: GLOBAL MENTAL HEALTH AND ITS RELATION TO PUBLIC PSYCHIATRY

Global mental health (GMH) incorporates many fields of study including psychiatry, psychology, social work, and public health. In very simple terms, it is the provision of mental health care, predominantly in public settings, in low- and middle-income countries (LAMICs) and in high-income countries, often in collaboration with the providers and practices of care in higher income countries. This situation is changing under pressure from a movement to do more primary research in LAMICs and develop local research capacity and local mental health infrastructure and expertise.[1] The type of care provided can be psychotherapy (individual or group-based), medications, or psychosocial interventions. The delivery of this care requires knowledge and a consideration of health economics, systems of care, and health care infrastructure. GMH often requires acceptability and support from the local or national government, as well as the population in need. GMH considers the ethical challenges in both providing and not providing care, considering the cultural context and setting. In order to provide ethical care, it is essential that GMH also reflect upon and measure both intended and unintended outcomes of the interventions provided through outcome studies and health services research. Finally, GMH is also the people who provide the care, from lay health care workers, nurses, trained psychologists, social workers, and therapists to medical doctors with specialized mental health training.

Much GMH care, like most health care around the world, is provided in public settings. LAMICs comprise about 80% of the world's population but have less than 20% of the world's mental health resources.[2] Identified barriers to the provision of public psychiatry in LAMICs include public health care priorities that often omit mental health care and a lack of public health perspectives in mental health leadership.[3] There is also a devastating lack of trained health care workers (social workers, nurses, psychologists, and psychiatrists) in the public health care system in the developing world.[4] Yet the growing body of literature, evidenced by the Global Burden of Disease studies showing that mental and substance use disorders were the leading cause of years lived with a disability (YLD), demonstrates the burden that these disorders pose and the need to prioritize the prevention and treatment of these disorders through public health systems.[5]

BRIEF HISTORY

Psychiatry's exportation to other countries initially was largely through and during the colonization of countries in South Asia, the Caribbean, Africa, and elsewhere. Initially, many asylums had self-governing regimes that were then coopted and regulated by the British Empire in its colonies, and this regulation may have ultimately led to the development of a professional psychiatric workforce.[6] British colonial rule in India led to the development of more hegemony in institutional care; however, it has been argued that even within the exportation of a largely asylum-based psychiatric care model, there were active international scientific networks and benefits occurred with the introduction of concepts such as a right to health care and the state's obligation to provide treatment facilities.[7] Interestingly, much like the GMH movement today, which incorporates a diversity of academic disciplines (health economics, public health, psychiatry, etc.), psychiatric historians also acknowledge the "multilateral and multivalent interaction with various other disciplines and organizations."[8]

The power that psychiatry came to wield and the complex interplay of gender, race, and ethnicity in this history should not be minimized,[9] nor should its complexity. Histories of colonial psychiatry show that there was some encouragement to return to traditional healing practices in some colonies.[10] Deinstitutionalization movements in the West in the 1970s and '80s occurred in some former colonies as well and also supported some local practices. For example, the former Dutch East Indies country of Indonesia developed an approach toward prevention, treatment, and rehabilitation (although with increasing numbers of mental hospitals being built) during this period, and attention was given to care provided by indigenous healers.[11]

In the past several decades, psychiatry expanded its emphasis on the importance of considering the appropriateness of our diagnoses and of understanding other cultures. This led to the fields of cross-cultural or transcultural psychiatry (see Chapter 14 for further details), which were influenced by anthropological work. An example specific to GMH is the work of Arthur Kleinman, a psychiatrist and anthropologist, and his research into the concept of neurasthenia in China. He examined and characterized the local diagnosis of neurasthenia, but those carrying the diagnosis were also evaluated for criteria of major depressive disorder, somatization, pain, and other so-called "culture-bound syndromes," and the social role of the diagnosis in the lives of the patients was also explored. The concept of neurasthenia was used broadly to explore ideas of cross-cultural psychiatry, the experience of illness, culturally sanctioned idioms of distress, and coping.[12]

Revisiting lessons learned from psychiatric history, new concern has arisen about the introduction of psychiatric concepts through exportation of modern medications or pop-cultural phenomena. The large global pharmaceutical industry is rapidly expanding the introduction and sale of psychiatric medications internationally, and the diagnosis and treatment of conditions associated with these medications has subsequently also increased, thus leading to discourse on the ethics of these occurrences.[13] Furthermore, the exposure of populations to Western culture has been criticized for introducing disorders such as anorexia and bulimia (although there are several methodological challenges limiting a simple conclusion that these disorders did not exist prior to exposure to Western culture).[14] Examples such as these warrant further consideration to prevent the introduction of new disorders or unnecessary medication. However, cross-cultural research and published narratives of patients suffering with mental illness and providers trying to care for these patients overwhelmingly discourage the idea that this is the imposition of "Western" ideas or simply a form of neocolonialism.[15]

More recent concepts incorporate the idea of "historical trauma" and its legacy on the current mental health of populations in seeking a resurgence in suppressed indigenous methods for resilience, community support, and mental health combined with locally adapted and culturally appropriate medical and psychological services. This is seen, for example, in the aboriginal healing movement in Canada.[16] The combination of local models with appropriate modern medical practice, along with an understanding of the historical context of psychiatry in international settings, lends itself well to influence by and delivery from public psychiatry. With a focus on culturally appropriate care models, the recovery movement, and serving the populations most in need, public psychiatry is an ideal delivery model for modern GMH.

REVIEW OF TOPICS

THE RIGHTS OF PEOPLE WITH MENTAL DISORDERS

GMH seeks to use the principles of scientific evidence in the context of human rights. The 1948 United Nations Declaration of Human Rights affirmed health care as a right. And, as has been well-documented and declared repeatedly during the "movement for global mental health," mental health is a part of health, such that there is "no health without mental health."[17,18] In addition to the right to mental health care, many patients with mental illness hold a vulnerable place in society, in that they suffer repeated violations of their basic human rights.[19] More specifically for mental health, Mario Maj shares a more expanded conception of health care rights informed by the World Psychiatric Association. In this view, mental health rights include the right to access professionals who understand and can treat a specific disorder (given non-psychiatric physicians' limited training and expertise in accurately diagnosing mental illness), which often means the right to access a psychiatrist in the public system.[20] Furthermore, people have a right to treatment that is based in and informed by current scientific evidence, and they have a right to procure the appropriate evidence for the context if it is lacking, which is particularly relevant to mental illness in LAMICs.[20,21] Mental illness should be treated in a setting that is appropriate and humane.[20,22] Further rights are more consistent with the movement for the right to health in LAMICs, including the right for consumers of health care to be participants in decision-making about care, the right to access quality care, and the right of health promotion leading to a full life.[20]

THE EPIDEMIOLOGICAL AND ETHICAL CASE FOR INTERNATIONAL PUBLIC PSYCHIATRY

The prevalence and severity of mental illness varies from country to country, but the degree of unmet treatment needs and burden of illness is high throughout the developed and developing world. Using World Health Organization (WHO) data, one study showed that whereas severity of a disorder did correlate with the probability of receiving treatment in most countries, 35–50% of serious mental illness in developed countries and 76–85% in less developed countries received no treatment in the past year.[23] The WHO also looked at the treatment gap (the difference between those who need care and those who receive care globally) and discovered a gap for schizophrenia/psychosis of 32%, for depression and dysthymia 56%, bipolar disorder 50%, panic disorder 56%, generalized anxiety disorder 58%, obsessive compulsive disorder 57%, and alcohol abuse and dependence 78%.[24] The unmet need evidenced by treatment gaps results in substantial burden of illness and disability, and the Global Burden of Disease study shows an increasing burden of noncommunicable disease in general and mental and behavioral disorders specifically. Major depressive disorder is the second leading cause of YLD, with anxiety seventh, alcohol use disorders fifteenth, schizophrenia sixteenth, bipolar disorder eighteenth, dysthymia nineteenth, and Alzheimer's disease twenty-fourth.[25]

The prevalence of mental illness combined with the absence of quality public psychiatry for many patients and families internationally has resulted in sometimes substandard methods of coping with mental illness such as deception, coercion, and physical restraint. These methods lead to human rights violations and demands for the "ethical imperative" and "the moral case" to scale up public psychiatric services.[26,27] Building on the principle of "no health without mental health," the "moral case" for addressing treatable illnesses with cost-effective evidence-based interventions through international public psychiatry is made as our world faces increasing challenges including the cost of psychiatric medications, the loss of trained physicians from LAMICs, and the social and economic changes facing many LAMICs that are known to impact mental health.[17,27] It is also important, in the midst of large-scale data and public policy imperatives, not to lose sight of the experience of those suffering with mental illness, experiencing stigma, and not being "treated with dignity, respect, or protection by medical personnel."[28] Indeed, some of our work at Yale has revealed stigma about mental illness even among medical and nursing students in several international contexts.[29,30]

THE NEED FOR INTERNATIONAL PUBLIC PSYCHIATRY, BEYOND POVERTY AND MENTAL HEALTH

Targeting a disease while ignoring the context virtually eliminates the ability to treat the determinants of the disease,[31] although income alone poorly reflects the complex social determinants of mental illness. Reviews show weak evidence to support an association between mental illness and income level, identifying instead low education, rapid social change, physical health, the risk of exposure to violence, and harder to define experiences of insecurity and hopelessness as contributing to mental illness; these make up the social, economic, and environmental determinants of disease.[32] Another study looking across continents found that older widowed females had worse mental health outcomes and concluded that adverse events or changes in life circumstance may have a greater influence on mental health than poverty.[33] Interestingly, interventions to reduce poverty had inconclusive benefits for mental illness, but interventions to promote mental health were associated with improved economic outcomes, thus suggesting that the scale-up of mental health care services may be an economic as well as a public health intervention.[34] Combining public health approaches with clinical approaches to mental health treatment may have a more robust bidirectional benefit.

GMH WORK IS RESPONSIBLE AND BIDIRECTIONAL

In doing GMH work, be it research, education, public policy work, advocacy, or direct clinical care, the goal should always be to do the work responsibly. Good intentions can hide unintended harms. The objective of GMH work should always incorporate efficiency, effectiveness, quality, and sustainability while trying to minimize barriers such as language, cultural differences, the appropriateness or utility of the work, and competing agendas and goals. It is essential that workers be well-trained in terms of the work being done, as well as knowing about the local population, culture, and situation.

Many examples of GMH work focus on models of public psychiatry and mental health care being adapted for use in developing countries. Yet there is much to learn from other settings that may apply to public psychiatry in developing countries. For example, Yale provides a free mental health care clinic, staffed with medical students and volunteer faculty, that uses several treatment models developed in resource-poor settings in other countries and adapted for this setting. Collaborative models that truly integrate sustained contributions and models of public psychiatry from the developed world with sustained commitment from partners in the developing world are also excellent opportunities to do responsible work and learn from the experience and contributions of each collaborator. For example, Yale participates in an ongoing mental health clinic in collaboration with independent practitioners, nongovernmental groups, and academic institutions to support a recovery-oriented public psychiatry clinic in Peru.

EDUCATION AND TRAINING IN GMH

"Capacity building" is a term commonly used in global health work, and it can mean several things, including developing infrastructure to support and house treatment programs, training to increase research skills, and training to increase the number of mental health care providers. Approaches to building capacity are enhanced by academic partnerships between high- and low-income countries to develop research capabilities and educational interventions that can also inform policy.[35] An example of this is the development of a psychiatry residency training program in Addis Ababa University in Ethiopia, undertaken jointly with the University of Toronto.[36] Even in GMH education in the United States, it has been argued that psychiatry residency trainees should avoid short-term clinical experiences and instead focus on multi-year projects featuring collaborative relationships with partners in LAMICs, thus resulting in capacity building in research or other scholarly work on the part of both the resident supervised in the United States and the international collaborator.[37]

DELIVERING MENTAL HEALTH CARE WITH NO LOCAL PSYCHIATRIC STAFF

Approaches that provide specialized mental health training for primary care physicians or health care workers, or those that provide innovative use of technology, have been suggested to fill the gap in mental health care services in developing countries. The lack of psychiatrists in developing countries or rural areas has necessitated other care providers to assume a mental health care role with little or no mental health background. However, when trained, these practitioners have the potential to provide mental health services in integrated programs (also called *collaborative care models*). Systematic psychiatric assessments can be done via nonphysician providers who perform longitudinal patient monitoring, treatment interventions, and care coordination based on specialist-provided stepped-care recommendations.[38] Similar programs are being conducted in developing countries; however, most programs do not use outcome measures to test the effectiveness of such interventions.[39] A randomized controlled trial of a collaborative care intervention led by lay health counselors in primary care settings to improve the outcomes of people with common mental disorders showed a good response to the intervention and demonstrated cost effectiveness.[40] Other interventions can focus on improving primary care physicians' (PCPs) capacities to diagnose and treat mental health conditions. Medical education sessions, group teaching classes, or "telepsychiatry" can supervise, support, and other providers of mental health, PCPs, and other practitioners.[41]

Telepsychiatry is the use of telemedicine to provide psychiatric assessments and treatments or supervision to on-site care providers either via videoconferencing (synchronous telepsychiatry) or via store-and-forward approaches (asynchronous telepsychiatry) that involve saving and transmitting to experts clinical information via encrypted email or secure websites.[42] Telepsychiatry has been shown to be as effective as face-to-face care delivery in providing assessments and psychiatric treatment.[43] The use of this technology requires a functional infrastructure if it is to be effective and sustainable. Measurement of the effectiveness telepsychiatry in developing countries using standardized assessment instruments is needed.[44]

There are three settings in which telepsychiatry has been proposed to fill a mental health gap:

1. *Within the borders in developed countries.* Telepsychiatry has been widely utilized in developed countries to increase access to mental health services in rural areas[45,46] and for ethnic minorities.[47] An increasingly popular way to use telepsychiatry is in consultation–liaison services for primary care settings.[48]
2. *Within the borders in developing countries.* Telepsychiatry is used in India and Uganda to provide mental health services from urban to rural and underserved settings.[49,50] These services suffer from many shortcomings in the presence of poor-quality Internet service, unreliable electrical service and equipment, and the high costs of basic communication services in developing countries, but with infrastructure improvements, this delivery option could be valuable.
3. *Cross-border from developed to developing countries.* Cross-border use of telepsychiatry from resource-rich to resource-poor settings has been suggested, but with very few reports and no effectiveness studies.[44] One example is the utility of telepsychiatry to provide psychodynamic psychotherapy training and treatments from the United States to China, where there are no available psychoanalysts.[51] Another example is the use of telepsychiatry to provide culturally sensitive mental health assessments and treatment to multinationality refugees in Denmark by culturally matched providers available in Sweden.[52]

MENTAL HEALTH OF VULNERABLE POPULATIONS: REFUGEE MENTAL HEALTH

Several populations within the mentally ill globally merit additional awareness due to the increased level of vulnerability they share within an already marginalized population. Special attention should be paid to certain age groups, such as children and the elderly; females who are at risk of gender-based violence and often have less social standing; lesbian, gay, bisexual, and transgender (LGBT) persons at risk for sexuality-based discrimination; immigrants at risk of losing many social supports and social integration; and people being displaced due to social forces or conflict such as refugees, asylum seekers, and internally displaced persons.

Refugees and immigrants represent a special group within the public mental health system. Many of these populations face inequities such as low household incomes and levels of education, poor health morbidity status, and high mortality.[53] Immigrants may experience a higher rate of mental illness as a result of immigration. As a group, refugees are especially vulnerable to adverse psychiatric effects due to trauma exposure, direct torture, loss or separation from family, and forced migration.

According to the UN, the global burden of displaced people in the world numbered 43 million at the end of 2010. Of these, more than 15.3 million are outside the country of their nationality and are legally defined as refugees. Only a small percentage is permanently resettled in a country willing to accept them. As of 2013, the major countries from which refugees originate are Iraq, Myanmar, Bhutan, Somalia, and Democratic Republic of the Congo.

There is no single model of health care delivery that serves refugees coming into the United States. Initial health assessments are performed by public health departments, community health clinics, academic centers, or private facilities. Mental health assessments are recommended, although not always performed, during the initial health screening.

Refugees face pre-migration, migration, and post-migration stressors that place them at high risk for psychological distress. Torture, witnessed trauma, detention in camps, and death of family members are all risk factors for the development of psychiatric illness. The prevalence of psychiatric diagnoses is up to 10 times higher compared to the local population, with post-traumatic stress disorder (PTSD) and depression being the most common.[54] Somatization and pain disorders are also commonly seen in patients with a history of trauma and torture.[55] In addition, language barriers and socioeconomic factors such as unemployment, restricted economic growth, and housing problems contribute to continued distress after resettlement.[56]

Mental health services are scarce in many regions that refugees originate from or transit through. After arrival in the United States, with its relatively greater resources, refugees still do not receive adequate services due to communication barriers and the poor capacity of agencies to address the social and mental needs of displaced refugees. Refugees are insured under Medicaid, the federal government health insurance program, for a period limited to 8 months after arrival. Many are then subsequently uninsured. If care is received, it is likely through public psychiatry.

Research on mental health treatment of refugees has been mostly centered on symptoms of PTSD. Psychological treatments using culturally appropriate variations of cognitive behavioral therapy and other multimodal strategies have been successfully applied to treat PTSD and depression in refugees.[57,58] Community-based psychosocial interventions (e.g., school based programs) targeting mental health symptoms, as well as quality of life and social functioning, have also been described as being used with refugees with moderate success.[59,60]

Miller and Rasco outline the following ecological principles to guide the development and implementation of community interventions for refugees: (1) When access to resources is a problem, alternative settings should be created or capacity enhanced to adapt to existing settings. (2) Interventions should address the priorities of the community rather than those of the system and be preventive whenever possible. (3) Culturally appropriate beliefs regarding psychological well-being should be incorporated into community-based interventions and integrated into existing community settings. (4) Capacity building to foster empowerment should be the priority, rather than the direct provision of services.[61] Chapter 14, on cultural competency,

---

Box 15.1 REFUGEE MENTAL HEALTH: LINKING INTERNATIONAL AND LOCAL PUBLIC MENTAL HEALTH

Refugee mental health is an area in which western providers who might be trained in GMH or have practiced in international settings can utilize these skills for populations in their local setting.

Mr. B. is a 29-year-old male Iraqi refugee who was tortured and imprisoned for 1 month while in Iraq. He initially fled to Syria as a refugee and then was resettled in the United States. On initial mental health screening, it was noted that he had one prior suicide attempt and was treated in Syria, presumably for PTSD, with unknown medications that were discontinued prior to his coming to the United States. Upon evaluation in the Yale Refugee Clinic, he was diagnosed with PTSD with psychosis and major depressive disorder (MDD). He made a suicidal statement within 2 weeks of his arrival in the United States that resulted in his first psychiatric hospitalization. He had five total hospitalizations in a period of about 15 months, all for suicidal intent. He struggled with feeling isolated, poor English language proficiency, unemployment, and the transition to the cold New England weather. His roommates also belonged to a religious sect that persecuted people with his beliefs. He had few social supports and little contact with his family in Iraq. He was initially seen every other week in the refugee clinic, and he often reported nonspecific somatic complaints such as flank pain, headaches, and cough. He is now seeing an Arabic-speaking psychiatrist every other week and has not had any psychiatric hospitalizations in the past 5 months. The combination of refugee-specific services, seeing a provider who shared his language, and the support and stability of regular contact and visits may have allowed for this outcome.

---

can further elucidate how to provide culturally appropriate care in community settings. GMH experiences in providers may also improve their effectiveness as clinicians when dealing with different populations in their local settings as well.

FUTURE CHALLENGES

Barriers have been identified in the scale-up of GMH priorities and agendas so that they can be addressed. One important barrier is the time it takes to implement evidence-based interventions (when they exist), although other identified barriers contribute to the slow pace of change. These include the lack of mental health as a priority area for development, which leads to disproportionately low funding compared to the burden of disease; the difficulty in changing to community-based systems and interventions from centralized care delivery in institutions; the challenges of integrating mental health care into routine health care settings; the dearth of trained counselors, social workers, nurses, psychologists, and psychiatrists to provide mental health care; and the lack of public health perspectives in the design and implementation of both mental health interventions and mental health public policy.[62] In particular, given the availability of cost-effective interventions, governmental funding for mental health care is much lower than indicated based on the prevalence of mental health disorders, and this is particularly true in the poorest countries, which spend the lowest percentages of their health budgets on mental health.[4] Further compounding the issue of lack of human resources is that the shortfall is projected to grow if steps are not taken to reverse the trend (although, fortunately, there is a growing body of literature that suggests many mental health interventions can be delivered by trained nonspecialists in the public sector).[63] Some LAMICs have developed public mental health systems, and lessons can be learned from them, but many lack any national mental health policy to direct their efforts.[64] Hopefully, increased awareness of the unmet health care need of the mentally ill and the often inhumane treatment currently available in some developing countries, will engender the political will to promote changes deemed vital for success. These changes include the integration of psychiatry with primary health care settings, concurrent with development of public psychiatry infrastructure in community-based settings; the creation of training and supervision for community-based mental health care workers; and the mobilization of patients and families struggling with mental illness to advocate for humane treatment and to help decrease stigmatization.[62]

Although many barriers exist, there are many treatment interventions that are inexpensive (medications and psychotherapy) and can be delivered through public psychiatry by workers with brief, specific training and ongoing supervision.[21] Many treatments—such as those for depression, drug and alcohol use disorders, and schizophrenia—and some trials for prevention have been proved effective, although evidence is still needed in some areas (such as treating developmental disabilities or mental health in conflict and disaster settings).[21] Well-designed training programs for care providers, such that they receive supervision and auditing with feedback, can improve treatment outcomes.[65] The WHO has tried to codify cost-effective and generally available treatments through the international mental health Gap Action Programme (mhGAP) initiative in 2010, an intervention guide for mental, neurological, and substance use disorders in nonspecialized health settings.

It can be argued that GMH has a core agenda to scale-up services for people with mental disorders and to promote human rights for this population, and this has been done largely through four initiatives: the WHO's mhGAP for treatment algorithms, training for nonspecialists workers in the public psychiatry systems, the Movement for Global Mental Health as a locus for advocates to share ideas and work toward a common goal, and through the Grand Challenges in Mental Health, which has obtained input from many relevant stakeholders to set a research agenda to improve the lives of those living with mental illness.[66] A call to action has been made, one that targets mental health stakeholders, including providers, consumers, governments, multilateral agencies, and professional and consumer groups, and this call uses core and secondary indicators to track progress.[67] The number of programs and initiatives can be seen as a sign of success, although the goal of seeing programs taken to scale remains to be seen.[68]

Success has been seen with training and supervision of health care workers to deliver treatment interventions, yet psychiatrists are still too few. Psychiatrists represent a critical component in understanding, diagnosing, and treating mental illness, in addition to their vital role in training and supervising other mental health care providers. LAMICs remain lacking in psychiatrists, a key reason for their treatment gap in psychiatry, and psychiatrists are also essential in mental health leadership; in advocating for public policy, resources, and training in mental health; as well as in helping to build clinical capacity, providing referral pathways, and conducting research.[69]

ESSENTIAL QUALITY METRICS

An ethical imperative exists to know the true impact of the GMH work being done, despite the solid theory behind it or the good intentions of the intervention. As such, valid metrics must be used so that intended and unintended outcomes are noted, measured, and reported. Metrics used must be relevant to the topic and situation, and they must be independent of the interest of those conducting the work.

Several initiatives have been started to identify research priorities and measures to ensure that the most relevant and feasible work is done and that appropriate outcome measures are used to determine the impact of the research.[70] Large projects have sought input from a wide variety of mental health stakeholders to determine which research to prioritize, and good consensus has been reached in aligning research goals with the burden of mental illness.[1,71] The Grand Challenges in Mental Health project, the largest by far in terms of setting the research agenda in GMH, identified the following research goals (in very simplified terms): (1) identify root causes and risk and protective factors; (2) advance prevention and implementation of early interventions; (3) improve treatments and expand access to care; (4) raise awareness of the global burden of disease; (5) build human resource capacity; and (6) transform health system and policy responses. They also suggested a summary of principles for research, including using a life-course approach to studies, using system-wide approaches to address suffering, using evidence-based interventions, and understanding environmental influences.[1] There is some concern that research is often not utilized as it should be to guide policy-makers and the decisions of funders, and so although quality metrics are essential from an ethical and scientific standpoint, they should not be isolated from public policy, advocacy, and treatment initiatives.[72]

SUMMARY

Compared to the general population, there is a significant disparity in the provision of care and respect for human rights of persons living with mental disorders. Beyond the substantive global burden of mental diseases, the lack of expenditure on mental health treatment, and the lack of mental health professional staff in many countries, there exists the condition of local people living with mental illness in terrible conditions and experiencing pain, suffering, and discrimination. Arthur Kleinman equates the experience of living in these conditions as primarily a failure of humanity, not just a result of technical problems regarding diagnosis and treatment.[28]

The International Covenant on Economic, Social, and Cultural Rights asserts "the right of everyone to the enjoyment of the highest attainable standard of physical and mental health."[73] This standard is not limited to the right to health care, but to "a wide range of socio-economic factors that promote conditions in which people can lead a healthy life."[73] It has been shown that mental health problems are experienced to a greater degree in situations of disadvantage and that social injustice has psychological consequences.[74] Addressing GMH issues and their determinants is key to promoting human rights and social justice. This can be accomplished by creating diagnosis and treatment programs, but also by advocating for autonomy, respect, and empowerment of all people in general and of stigmatized and marginalized people in particular.[75]

Initiatives and efforts to address health must include mental health as a key part of their strategy. However, this inclusion remains incomplete. Mental health was recently excluded from a global effort to prioritize four major noncommunicable diseases (NCDs) on the global health agenda.[76] Yet, like many NCDs, mental health has a high burden of disease and disability, it results in economic loss and contributes to poverty, and there are cost-effective evidence-based interventions to address them.[77]

Ethical considerations extend beyond the lives of people with mental illness to the research done to address their disorders. In many countries, the ethical standards for research and treatment are not adequate. Addressing this issue will require the adoption of ethical standards on how to best conduct research to benefit society as a whole and the larger scientific inquiry, as well as the direct population affected and being studied. Given the lack of resources, there must be a balance between relevance and excellence.[78] Special attention should be paid to practitioners and researchers who are working with vulnerable populations, and efforts should be made to equip them with appropriate ethical education.[79] Ethical mental health research is essential in building trust, and it is the cornerstone for successful research projects.[75]

GMH challenges are not only the problem of the world's poorest communities. These collective challenges surpass the capacity of any one community to address and require coordinated efforts from governments and nongovernmental stakeholders. The interconnectedness and interdependence of the globalized world has made it more difficult to address any one global health problem, such as depression, HIV, or NCDs, without the use of knowledge, expertise, and support from many diverse stakeholders. Ethical coordination needs to occur among players ranging from financial support and financing systems to system-level evaluations, technological solutions, and even environmental experts.

The term "global health" is often construed as referring to illnesses that are endemic in developing countries and that can be addressed with solutions provided by the technologically more advanced developed countries. Some critics argue against the predominant paradigm's emphasis on technological solutions as ignoring the strong behavioral, cultural, social, political, and economic determinants that underlie most GMH problems that require comprehensive—not merely technical—approaches.[80] Julio Frenk frames the problem as "It is again the idea of the poor, ignorant, passive, and traditional societies in need of the charity and technology of the rich."[80] The problem, he continues, is that this notion of global work fails to capture the essence of the current interconnected global world. Global health and mental health need to move from an "aid mentality," which implies dependent relationships and a donor–recipient frame, to "global solidarity" that relies on interdependent relationships and equal membership. The term "solidarity" not only promotes mutual respect between equal members but also captures the nature of GMH challenges in our connected, interdependent world.[80] Knowledge of GMH informs practice in public psychiatry in developed countries, and, reciprocally, work in public psychiatry informs and benefits GMH.

REFERENCES

1. Collins PY, Patel V, Joestl, et al. Grand challenges in global mental health. *Nature*. 2011; 475(7354): 27–30.
2. Saxena S, Thornicroft G, Knapp M, Whiteford H. Resources for mental health: scarcity, inequity, and inefficiency. *Lancet*. 2007; 370(9590): 878–889.
3. Saraceno B, van Ommeren M, Batniji R, et al. Barriers to improvement of mental health services in low-income and middle-income countries. *Lancet*. 2007; 370(9593): 1164–1174.
4. Saxena S, Thornicroft G, Knapp M, Whiteford H. Resources for mental health: scarcity, inequity, and inefficiency. *Lancet*. 2007; 370(9590): 878–889.
5. Whiteford HA, Degenhardt L, Rehm J, et al. Global burden of disease attributable to mental and substance use disorders: findings from the Global Burden of Disease Study 2010. *Lancet*. 2013; 382(9904): 1575–1586.
6. Swartz S. The regulation of British colonial lunatic asylums and the origins of colonial psychiatry, 1860-1864. *Hist Psychol*. 2010; 13(2): 160–177.
7. Ernst W. Crossing the boundaries of 'colonial psychiatry'. Reflections on the development of psychiatry in British India, C. 1870-1940. *Cult Med Psychiatry*. 2011; 35(4): 536–545.
8. Engstrom EJ. Cultural and social history of psychiatry. *Curr Opin Psychiatry*. 2008; 21(6): 585–592.
9. Oyebode F. History of psychiatry in West Africa. *Int Rev Psychiatry*. 2006; 18(4): 319–325.
10. Keller R. Madness and colonization: psychiatry in the British and French Empires, 1800-1962. *J Soc Hist*. 2001; 35(2): 295–326.
11. Pols H. The development of psychiatry in Indonesia: from colonial to modern times. *Int Rev Psychiatry*. 2006; 18(4): 363–370.
12. Kleinman A. Neurasthenia and depression: a study of somatization and culture in China. *Cult Med Psychiatry*. 1982; 6(2): 117–190.
13. Schulz K. Did antidepressants depress Japan? *The New York Times*. Aug 22, 2004.
14. Cummins LH, Simmons AM, Zane NW. Eating disorders in Asian populations: a critique of current approaches to the study of culture, ethnicity, and eating disorders. *Am J Orthopsychiatry*. 2005; 75(4): 553–574.
15. Patel V, Prince M. Global mental health: a new global health field comes of age. *JAMA*. 2010; 303(19): 1976–1977.
16. Waldram JB. Healing history? Aboriginal healing, historical trauma, and personal responsibility. *Transcult Psychiatry*. 2013; 51(3): 370–386.
17. Prince M, Patel V, Saxena S, et al. No health without mental health. *Lancet*. 2007; 370(9590): 859–877.
18. Prince M. Introducing the movement for global mental health. *Indian J Med Res*. 2008; 128(5): 570–573.
19. Drew N, Funk M, Tang S, et al. Human rights violations of people with mental and psychosocial disabilities: an unresolved global crisis. *Lancet*. 2011; 378(9803): 1664–1675.
20. Maj M. The rights of people with mental disorders: WPA perspective. *Lancet*. 2011; 378(9802): 1534–1535.
21. Patel V, Araya R, Chatterjee S, et al. Treatment and prevention of mental disorders in low-income and middle-income countries. *Lancet*. 2007; 370(9591): 991–1005.
22. Dhanda A, Narayan T. Mental health and human rights. *Lancet*. 2007; 370(9594): 1197–1198.
23. Demyttenaere K, Bruffaerts R, Posada-Villa J, et al. Prevalence, severity, and unmet need for treatment of mental disorders in the World Health Organization World Mental Health Surveys. *JAMA*. 2004; 291(21): 2581–2590.
24. Kohn R, Saxena S, Levav I, Saraceno B. The treatment gap in mental health care. *Bull World Health Organ*. 2004; 82(11): 858–866.
25. Vos T, Flaxman AD, Naghavi M, et al. Years lived with disability (YLDs) for 1160 sequelae of 289 diseases and injuries 1990-2010: a systematic analysis for the Global Burden of Disease Study 2010. *Lancet*. 2012; 380(9859): 2163–2196.
26. Patel V, Bloch S. The ethical imperative to scale up health care services for people with severe mental disorders in low and middle income countries. *Postgrad Med J*. 2009; 85(1008): 509–513.
27. Patel V, Saraceno B, Kleinman A. Beyond evidence: the moral case for international mental health. *Am J Psychiatry*. 2006; 163(8): 1312–1315.
28. Kleinman A. Global mental health: a failure of humanity. *Lancet*. 2009; 374(9690): 603–604.
29. Iheanacho T, Stefanovics E, Makanjoula V, Marienfeld C, Rosenheck R. Medical and nursing students' attitudes towards people with mental illness in Nigeria: A tale of two teaching hospitals. *International Psychiatry*. 2014; 11(2).
30. Sun B, Fan N, Nie S, et al. Attitudes towards people with mental illness among psychiatrists, psychiatric nurses, involved family members and the general population in a large city in Guangzhou, China. *Int J Ment Health Syst*. 2014; 8: 26.
31. De Vos P, Stefanini A, De Ceukelaire W, Schuftan C, Movement PsH. A human right to health approach for non-communicable diseases. *Lancet*. 2013; 381(9866): 533. doi:10.1016/S0140-6736(13)60274-3
32. Patel V, Kleinman A. Poverty and common mental disorders in developing countries. *Bull World Health Organ*. 2003; 81(8): 609–615.
33. Das J, Do QT, Friedman J, McKenzie D, Scott K. Mental health and poverty in developing countries: revisiting the relationship. *Soc Sci Med*. 2007; 65(3): 467–480.
34. Lund C, De Silva M, Plagerson S, et al. Poverty and mental disorders: breaking the cycle in low-income and middle-income countries. *Lancet*. 2011; 378(9801): 1502–1514.
35. Fricchione GL, Borba CP, Alem A, Shibre T, Carney JR, Henderson DC. Capacity building in global mental health: professional training. *Harv Rev Psychiatry*. 2012; 20(1): 47–57.
36. Alem A, Pain C, Araya M, Hodges BD. Co-creating a psychiatric resident program with Ethiopians, for Ethiopians, in Ethiopia: the Toronto Addis Ababa Psychiatry Project (TAAPP). *Acad Psychiatry*. 2010; 34(6): 424–432.
37. Marienfeld C, Rohrbaugh RM. Impact of a global mental health program on a residency training program. *Acad Psychiatry*. 2013; 37(4): 276–280.
38. Huffman JC, Niazi SK, Rundell JR, Sharpe M, Katon WJ. Essential Articles on Collaborative Care Models for the Treatment of Psychiatric Disorders in Medical Settings: A Publication by the Academy of Psychosomatic Medicine Research and Evidence-Based Practice Committee. *Psychosomatics*. 2014; 55(2): 109–122.
39. Ssebunnya J, Kigozi F, Kizza D, Ndyanabangi S, Consortium MRP. Integration of Mental Health into Primary Health Care in a rural district in Uganda. *African journal of psychiatry*. 2010; 13(2): 128–131.
40. Patel V, Weiss HA, Chowdhary N, et al. Effectiveness of an intervention led by lay health counsellors for depressive and anxiety disorders in primary care in Goa, India (MANAS): a cluster randomised controlled trial. *The Lancet*. 2010; 376(9758): 2086–2095.
41. Chipps J, Ramlall S, Mars M. Practice guidelines for videoconference-based telepsychiatry in South Africa. *African journal of psychiatry*. 2012; 15(4): 264–270.

42. Butler TN, Yellowlees P. Cost analysis of store-and-forward telepsychiatry as a consultation model for primary care. *Telemedicine and e-Health*. 2012; 18(1): 74–77.
43. Garcia-Lizana F, Munoz-Mayorga I. What about telepsychiatry? A systematic review. *Prim Care Companion J Clin Psychiatry*. 2010; 12(2).
44. Jefee-Bahloul H, Mani N. International telepsychiatry: a review of what has been published. *Journal of telemedicine and telecare*. 2013; 19(5): 293–294.
45. Rabinowitz T, Murphy KM, Amour JL, Ricci MA, Caputo MP, Newhouse PA. Benefits of a telepsychiatry consultation service for rural nursing home residents. *Telemedicine journal and e-health: the official journal of the American Telemedicine Association*. 2010; 16(1): 34–40.
46. Rohland BM, Saleh SS, Rohrer JE, Romitti PA. Acceptability of telepsychiatry to a rural population. *Psychiatric services*. 2000; 51(5): 672–674.
47. Yeung A, Johnson DP, Trinh N-H, Weng W-CC, Kvedar J, Fava M. Feasibility and effectiveness of telepsychiatry services for Chinese immigrants in a nursing home. *Telemedicine and e-Health*. 2009; 15(4): 336–341.
48. Hilty DM, Yellowlees PM, Cobb HC, Bourgeois JA, Neufeld JD, Nesbitt TS. Models of telepsychiatric consultation–Liaison service to rural primary care. *Psychosomatics*. 2006; 47(2): 152–157.
49. Mars M. Telepsychiatry in Africa—a way forward? *African journal of psychiatry*. 2012; 15(4): 215–217.
50. Thara R. Using mobile telepsychiatry to close the mental health gap. *Current psychiatry reports*. 2012; 14(3): 167–168.
51. Fishkin R, Fishkin L, Leli U, Katz B, Snyder E. Psychodynamic treatment, training, and supervision using internet-based technologies. *The journal of the American Academy of Psychoanalysis and Dynamic Psychiatry*. 2011; 39(1): 155–168.
52. Mucic D. International telepsychiatry: a study of patient acceptability. *Journal of telemedicine and telecare*. 2008; 14(5): 241–243.
53. Pumariega AJ, Rothe E, Pumariega JB. Mental health of immigrants and refugees. *Community Ment Health J*. 2005; 41(5): 581–597.
54. Fazel M, Wheeler J, Danesh J. Prevalence of serious mental disorder in 7000 refugees resettled in western countries: a systematic review. *Lancet*. 2005; 365(9467): 1309–1314.
55. Van Ommeren M, Sharma B, Sharma GK, Komproe I, Cardeña E, de Jong JT. The relationship between somatic and PTSD symptoms among Bhutanese refugee torture survivors: examination of comorbidity with anxiety and depression. *J Trauma Stress*. 2002; 15(5): 415–421.
56. Carswell K, Blackburn P, Barker C. The relationship between trauma, post-migration problems and the psychological well-being of refugees and asylum seekers. *Int J Soc Psychiatry*. 2011; 57(2): 107–119.
57. Nickerson A, Bryant RA, Silove D, Steel Z. A critical review of psychological treatments of posttraumatic stress disorder in refugees. *Clin Psychol Rev*. 2011; 31(3): 399–417.
58. Palic S, Elklit A. Psychosocial treatment of posttraumatic stress disorder in adult refugees: a systematic review of prospective treatment outcome studies and a critique. *J Affect Disord*. 2011; 131(1-3): 8–23.
59. Murray KE, Davidson GR, Schweitzer RD. Review of refugee mental health interventions following resettlement: best practices and recommendations. *Am J Orthopsychiatry*. 2010; 80(4): 576–585.
60. Williams ME, Thompson SC. The use of community-based interventions in reducing morbidity from the psychological impact of conflict-related trauma among refugee populations: a systematic review of the literature. *J Immigr Minor Health*. 2011; 13(4): 780–794.
61. Miller KE, Rasco LM. *The mental health of refugees : ecological approaches to healing and adaptation*. Mahwah, NJ: Lawrence Erlbaum; 2004.
62. Saraceno B, van Ommeren M, Batniji R, et al. Barriers to improvement of mental health services in low-income and middle-income countries. *Lancet*. 2007; 370(9593): 1164–1174.
63. Kakuma R, Minas H, van Ginneken N, et al. Human resources for mental health care: current situation and strategies for action. *Lancet*. 2011; 378(9803): 1654–1663.
64. Jacob KS, Sharan P, Mirza I, et al. Mental health systems in countries: where are we now? *Lancet*. 2007; 370(9592): 1061–1077.
65. Rowe AK, de Savigny D, Lanata CF, Victora CG. How can we achieve and maintain high-quality performance of health workers in low-resource settings? *Lancet*. 2005; 366(9490): 1026–1035.
66. Patel V. Global mental health: from science to action. *Harv Rev Psychiatry*. 2012; 20(1): 6–12.
67. Chisholm D, Flisher AJ, Lund C, et al. Scale up services for mental disorders: a call for action. *Lancet*. 2007; 370(9594): 1241–1252.
68. Eaton J, McCay L, Semrau M, et al. Scale up of services for mental health in low-income and middle-income countries. *Lancet*. 2011; 378(9802): 1592–1603.
69. Patel V. The future of psychiatry in low- and middle-income countries. *Psychol Med*. 2009; 39(11): 1759–1762.
70. Saraceno B. Mental health systems research is urgently needed. *Int J Ment Health Syst*. 2007; 1(1): 2.
71. Sharan P, Gallo C, Gureje O, et al. Mental health research priorities in low- and middle-income countries of Africa, Asia, Latin America and the Caribbean. *Br J Psychiatry*. 2009; 195(4): 354–363.
72. Araya R. Invited commentary on ... Mental health research priorities in low- and middle-income countries. *Br J Psychiatry*. 2009; 195(4): 364–365.
73. Substantive Issues Arising In The Implementation Of The International Covenant On Economic, Social And Cultural Rights. Committee on Economic, Social and Cultural rights 2000; http://daccess-dds-ny.un.org/doc/UNDOC/GEN/G00/439/34/PDF/G0043934.pdf. Accessed March 15, 2014.
74. Sheppard M. Mental health and social justice: Gender, race, and psychological consequences of unfairness. *British Journal of Social Work*. 2002; 32(6): 779–797.
75. Ngui EM, Khasakhala L, Ndetei D, Roberts LW. Mental disorders, health inequalities and ethics: A global perspective. *Int Rev Psychiatry*. 2010; 22(3): 235–244.
76. Becker AE, Kleinman A. Mental health and the global agenda. *N Engl J Med*. 2013; 369(14): 1380–1381.
77. Patel V, Simon G, Chowdhary N, Kaaya S, Araya R. Packages of care for depression in low- and middle-income countries. *PLoS Med*. 2009; 6(10): e1000159.
78. Tol WA, Patel V, Tomlinson M, et al. Relevance or excellence? Setting research priorities for mental health and psychosocial support in humanitarian settings. *Harv Rev Psychiatry*. 2012; 20(1): 25–36.
79. Roberts LW, Hammond KA, Warner TD, Lewis R. Influence of ethical safeguards on research participation: comparison of perspectives of people with schizophrenia and psychiatrists. *Am J Psychiatry*. 2004; 161(12): 2309–2311.
80. Frenk J, Gómez-Dantés O, Moon S. From sovereignty to solidarity: a renewed concept of global health for an era of complex interdependence. *Lancet*. 2014; 383(9911): 94–97.

PART IV

SYSTEM DEVELOPMENT IN PUBLIC PSYCHIATRY

16.

EDUCATION AND WORKFORCE DEVELOPMENT IN PUBLIC PSYCHIATRY

Jeanne L. Steiner, Chyrell Bellamy, Michael A. Hoge, Joanne DeSanto Iennaco, Anne Klee, Allison N. Ponce, Robert M. Rohrbaugh, David A. Ross, Thomas H. Styron, and Selby C. Jacobs

---

EDUCATIONAL HIGHLIGHTS

Public mental health education and training emphasizes the value of:

- Understanding systems of care, including fiscal, political, and organizational principles
- Working within interdisciplinary teams
- Participating in joint educational ventures in which trainees from different disciplines can learn together and develop collaborative working relationships
- Expanding the public mental health workforce by including peers, families, community groups, and medical providers in the network of resources available to the individuals we serve.

INTRODUCTION AND BRIEF HISTORY

The educational philosophy, structure, and content of Yale's educational programs in public psychiatry mirror the national trends in community mental health. The Yale Department of Psychiatry has a long history of teaching public psychiatry and mental health, starting shortly after the Community Mental Health Centers Act of 1963 enabled the construction of these institutions across America. The Connecticut Mental Health Center (CMHC) itself opened in 1966,[1] and, from its inception, has been an academic community mental health center. Now, after nearly 50 years, its academic programs have been sustained within the institution and the community it serves.[2]

In the late 1960's, for example, an interdisciplinary Masters of Public Health program for psychiatrists, psychologists, social workers and nurses provided clinical experience as well as courses in research methods and program development and evaluation. As of 1978, CMHC was able to support the core residency of the Department of Psychiatry at a time when federal funding for training positions in psychiatry was diminishing, and residents began to rotate through its Clinical Community Psychiatry module and other clinical/educational programs. Psychology trainees and psychiatric nursing students came to CMHC in connection with educational programs associated with the Department of Psychiatry, for psychology, and the Yale School of Nursing. Although there is no school of social work at Yale, graduate students in social work affiliated with other universities had regular clinical placements at CMHC. Thus, from the earliest years of CMHC's development as a center of excellence for research, clinical care, and community engagement, its educational components included each of the major mental health disciplines. The value of interdisciplinary teamwork was highlighted and strengthened by experiences in which students and trainees from several professional disciplines worked and learned together in their clinical placements.

The inpatient units of the West Haven Veterans Administration (VA) hospital served as training sites for Yale residents in psychiatry starting in the early 1960s. In the 1980s an inpatient unit focusing on rehabilitation was developed, and, in the 1990s, as the VA shifted to a capitated model of care, inpatient services were drastically reduced and staff resources were shifted to outpatient services. These outpatient services, organized into diagnoses-related "firms," included the development of comprehensive community-based outpatient psychosocial rehabilitation (PSR) programs including an Assertive Community Treatment (ACT) team and work and housing programs, many of which originated at VA-Connecticut (VA-CT) before being disseminated nationally in the VA system.

As the Department of Psychiatry at Yale and other academic medical centers throughout the United States turned the spotlight in the 1980s and 1990s on research programs aimed at the neurobiology of mental disorders, clinical programs for persons with serious and persistent mental illness evolved and adapted significantly to the needs of the individuals they served. The paradigm shifts toward recovery-oriented care and an emphasis on enhancing the quality of life in the community brought necessary changes to the training programs as well.

In the late 1990s, the boundaries between Yale-New Haven Hospital (YNNH), a large general hospital, and its public neighbor, CMHC, became more permeable. Up to that point, YNNH's payer mix included primarily privately insured and some publicly funded individuals on its inpatient psychiatry service, and uninsured patients were admitted primarily to CMHC's inpatient programs. In the late 1990s, due to a number of factors related to the shift of publicly funded care to general hospitals (see Chapter 11 on Inpatient Services), YNNH's psychiatric service opened admissions more widely to the uninsured. The considerable effect of this shift was a large increase in the utilization of YNNH's inpatient services by persons who received outpatient treatment at CMHC. The implications for the service system and for the residency training programs were profound in that this nonprofit teaching hospital became a "public-sector" setting by virtue of its patient population, comprising a large proportion of individuals with serious and persistent mental illness who were poor.

By the 2000s, it became increasingly clear to residency training directors that specific knowledge and skills were required to prepare trainees to meet the needs of the patients they would encounter in inpatient and ambulatory settings.[3] Educational venues, such as CMHC, the VA, and the inpatient psychiatric service of YNNH, offered rich environments in which learning could take place. The complex needs of patients with comorbid conditions, legal entanglements, cross-cultural challenges, and increasingly powerful self-advocacy efforts are addressed through encounters with patients, clinical supervision, seminars, and mentorship in these settings. Several formal and informal interdisciplinary training endeavors within inpatient and ambulatory services took place at CMHC since its earliest days. One example that was evaluated was a seminar held at CMHC from 2004 to 2006. Its participants included students and trainees from nursing, social work, psychology, and psychiatry, and its "dual aims" were "to provide a knowledge base for treating individuals with serious mental illness (SMI) and to teach how to work collaboratively with other disciplines."[4]

By the mid-2000s, when the basic tenets of community psychiatry from the 1960s regained prominence—both nationally and within the Yale Department of Psychiatry—postgraduate fellowship programs were developed at CMHC and the VA. They were launched in order to provide advanced training in leadership and management skills to psychiatrists and psychologists who want to apply that expertise to the needs of those served within the public sector. In 2003, the VA Interprofessional Fellowship in Psychosocial Rehabilitation and Recovery-Oriented Services began accepting fellows from multiple disciplines to complete a 1-year period of postgraduate training. This fellowship has graduated 38 fellows to date. Most recently, VA-CT has become a national leader in employing consumers of mental health care to provide care to individuals who are earlier in their recovery process.

An academic division of public psychiatry, launched at Yale in 2015, will serve as a vehicle to enhance collaboration across sites and professional disciplines within the department. In addition to providing an infrastructure for research development and dissemination, the division will enable educators to communicate, coordinate, and evaluate training initiatives. Junior faculty can be connected with academic mentors, and efforts to recruit promising trainees into public-sector–based positions can be strengthened.

The long tradition of population-based service management and evaluation in the public sector has become the predominant mode for much of health care development in 2014. In almost any setting, mental health professionals need to learn the fundamentals of care that have been promulgated within the public sector, primarily how to (1) understand systems of care, (2) work collaboratively within interdisciplinary teams and with providers of community support services, and (3) translate evidence-based practices into person-centered care. This chapter provides an overview of several educational programs that can serve as models for educational initiatives in other settings.

Education of a workforce prepared to work in public psychiatry and sufficient in number is essential for the continuing development of the field. For this reason, the ultimate significance of education in public psychiatry is workforce development. As this chapter illustrates and a section on workforce development herein discusses, this is a complex task.

The authors recognize that development of a professional workforce includes discipline-specific, foundational education and training activities as well joint learning experiences. In that vein, they present models for discipline-based efforts and emphasize how interdisciplinary collaboration can be woven into these programs.

DISCIPLINE-BASED EDUCATION AND TRAINING

PSYCHOLOGY

Clinical psychology is considered to have originated in 1896, when Lightner Witmer established the first psychological clinic at the University of Pennsylvania. The American Psychological Association (APA), now the largest association for psychologists in the United States, was founded just 4 years earlier, in 1892. For the next 50 years, many psychologists focused on the development and application of methods of assessing intelligence and personality. However, formal education and training programs in clinical psychology were not established until the late 1940s, when World War II saw large numbers of soldiers in need of mental health services returning from the battlefields. The VA created hospital and clinic positions for psychologists to provide assessment and treatment and also established the first paid internships for training clinical psychology graduate students. Concurrently, the National Institute of Mental Health began providing support to departments with clinical psychology programs, and the APA formalized a required curriculum for becoming a clinical psychologist. In the 1950s, the newly formalized clinical psychology profession began to be recognized by state licensure, and psychology has since been a licensed profession in every state in the United States. There are currently approximately 105,000 licensed psychologists in the United States.[5]

A doctoral degree in psychology is typically considered the standard for entry into the profession as designated by licensing jurisdictions across the United States and Canada. Although there is some range in terms of focus on populations, types of treatments, and theoretical orientations, clinical and counseling psychologists emerge from training programs that offer the Doctor of Philosophy degree (PhD) or Doctor of Psychology degree (PsyD). The APA accredits training programs, thereby designating them as having met defined standards and objectives that are accepted as indicating quality training meant to protect the public. APA-accredited doctoral programs require the completion of a 1-year doctoral internship, and most licensing jurisdictions also require the completion of a postdoctoral training experience. The Yale Department of Psychiatry offers an accredited doctoral internship, as does the VA, and both settings offer many opportunities for postdoctoral training. This chapter includes a discussion of the elements of these programs that focus on psychology training in the public sector.

The practice of psychology in the public sector pertains to work with marginalized and disenfranchised groups, often with SMI as the focus.[6] Psychologists are underrepresented in settings that serve adults with SMI in comparison to other disciplines, including social workers, nurses, and psychiatrists,[7] with relatively few psychologists engaged in this work.[8] As the recovery movement has gained momentum, many opportunities to reinvigorate psychology as a discipline using recovery-oriented evidence-based practices in public mental health have emerged.[9,10]

Psychology doctoral internship training programs in public mental health embrace the scientist-practitioner or practitioner-scholar framework. Although there is variation across training programs, doctoral interns are generally engaged in training experiences that encourage the development of professional and scientific skills and competencies and the conduct of ethical practice and research. Interns work with a range of patients under close supervision in an apprenticeship model that features increasing clinical responsibility over the course of the training year. The goal is to prepare those doctoral psychology intern with entry-level skills in health service psychology with generalist skills and competencies. Core competencies that are consonant with the guidelines and principles of the APA's accreditation model include assessment, evaluation, and case conceptualization skills; intervention and consultation skills; supervision, teaching, and presentation skills; scholarly inquiry, knowledge, and research skills; and professionalism. Diverse clinical and theoretical perspectives are represented in treatment and supervision, including cognitive behavioral, psychodynamic/interpersonal, evidence-based, and integrative approaches. Generally, this public-sector–based work is grounded in the recovery model and its principles and philosophy.

Psychology postdoctoral training enhances many components of the fellows' previous basic training and equips them with a specialized set of skills. Intervention, assessment, consultation, program evaluation, and advocacy are essential competencies identified in the psychology competency benchmarks model[11] and are integrated into the training year.

Consultation, both individual- and program-based, is often another central component of the experience, as are contributions to systems-based performance evaluation and improvement projects. Consistent with other models of mental health professionals as trainers,[12,13] fellows may also participate in the training and education of front-line staff. In addition to other professionals, such as their psychiatry and social work colleagues, fellows often work with a range of nonpsychologist mental health providers who offer PSR and homeless services including supportive and supported housing, employment supports, and community integration programs. Although there are some predefined elements of a fellowship year, the trainees are generally encouraged to explore their interests as they engage with concepts of recovery and social justice and propose projects that build on their current skills and prepare them for advanced work in public-sector mental health care. In public mental health settings, psychologists and postdoctoral psychology fellows can provide leadership on interdisciplinary teams; consultation to providers and systems of care; program design, implementation and evaluation; and policy analysis and advocacy.

Clinical practice is often a central component of the psychology training experience in public mental health settings and involves multiple elements including individual and group therapy and assessment and evaluation activities. The traditional model of psychotherapy is expanded upon, and fellows work with people in recovery in a variety of natural settings and across systems of care.

Working in public mental health settings with individuals with SMI and substance use disorders (SUDs), trainees learn that mental illness has an impact upon individuals in ways that extend far beyond the experience of psychiatric symptoms. Poverty, unemployment, homelessness, and stigma are disproportionately experienced by many people who have SMI,[14-16] with far-reaching social justice implications. Psychology trainees and those with whom they work stand to benefit from supervision that helps them understand their class privilege and relationship with power in a framework that promotes social justice.[17]

NURSING

Currently, there are several pathways to enter the nursing profession; all are academically based educational programs including associate- and baccalaureate-level diplomas leading to eligibility for licensure as a Registered Nurse (RN). The RN is considered an entry level into professional nursing; the role of the RN in psychiatric settings involves assessment and planning care, medication administration, patient and family education, and individual or group counseling.[18]

Graduate programs for RNs at the master and doctoral levels lead to eligibility for licensure as an advanced practice nurse (APRN) and board certification as a psychiatric mental health nurse practitioner (PMH-NP). For many years certification as a psychiatric-mental health clinical nurse specialist was the recognized advanced practice role, although the certification in this area has been phased out, leaving only one path to certification in the psychiatric advanced practice specialty. The PMH-NP role includes preparation as a nurse therapist able to assess, diagnose, and treat individuals, groups, and families. Psychiatric nurses pioneered the development of graduate education in the 1940s, when the National Mental Health Act was passed.[19] This eventually led to development of the advanced practice role and certification through the American Nurses Association.

Historically, nursing education was based within hospital settings, where nurses were educated in apprenticeship programs with an emphasis on hands-on clinical training combined with some didactic classroom-based education. The focus of the training was often to perform procedures, as opposed to providing comprehensive holistic care. Often, student nurses were used as a source of labor for the hospital, actually staffing whole units or floors and working more than 40 hours a week. This was common in both medical-surgical hospital settings as well as in psychiatric settings. The first psychiatric nursing program was opened in 1913 at the Johns Hopkins Hospital.[19] Early clinical experiences for nurses in psychiatric settings required that the nurses lived in a residence or dormitory on the grounds of psychiatric hospitals during their training experience.

Reforms in nursing education occurred after reviews of nursing preparation and a landmark report by the Rockefeller Foundation, now known as the Goldmark Report,[20] identified problems associated with training programs that were more focused on staffing hospitals than providing an education to students. This focus provided momentum to efforts to base nursing education programs within educational settings. It was during this time period, in 1923, that Yale School of Nursing was founded, thus providing the first independent university-based educational program for nurses.[21] The school has offered a master's degree program in psychiatric nursing since 1949, and many students have gained clinical experience in psychiatric nursing in public psychiatric settings that include the CMHC, state psychiatric hospitals, and community-based clinics. These settings offer students opportunities to meet educational competencies, and they provide rich experiences with individuals with complex mental and physical health needs. Yale School of Nursing and its faculty serving in joint appointments played a role in the partnership between the state of Connecticut and the Yale School of Medicine in developing CMHC and its programs focused on community-based psychiatric care. Some of the first directors of nursing at CMHC were faculty members at Yale School of Nursing. With these appointments came a strong presence of nursing education at CMHC.

Many nursing education degree programs use public psychiatric settings to provide their students with hands-on clinical experiences with psychiatric patients. Associate and baccalaureate degree programs in nursing typically have a clinical rotation in a psychiatric setting, with most placements in inpatient psychiatric units or day treatment or partial hospital programs. Outcomes of baccalaureate nursing programs include expectations that graduates would assume the role of provider of care, evaluating patient change and progress over time, and designing, managing, and coordinating care as well as participating with the interdisciplinary team.[22:35] In these experiences, students have opportunities for assessment and care planning activities, individual supportive counseling, co-leading patient groups, and administration of medications to psychiatric patients. Patient education is also an important competency of the inpatient psychiatric experience.

Graduate degree programs in nursing require clinical work in psychiatric settings. Students have academic coursework in advanced physical health assessment, pathophysiology, and pharmacology. In addition, they have specialty-focused education in mental health assessment, psychopathology, and neurobiology, as well as in psychopharmacology. During clinical experiences, students are mentored by experienced clinicians in assessment and differential diagnosis; individual, group, and family psychotherapy; and prescribing psychopharmacologic agents. Students are often placed in public psychiatric outpatient clinics, psychiatric emergency departments, intensive outpatient programs, and inpatient hospital units. They are mentored by psychiatric nurse practitioners and psychiatric clinical nurse specialists, as well as by experienced therapists (including social workers and psychologists) and psychiatrists. Recently, doctoral programs in nursing leading to the Doctor of Nursing Practice (DNP) have been developed to provide advanced education for those seeking further clinically focused education. This program is contrasted with the PhD in nursing, which is considered a research-focused terminal degree that is often required for individuals interested in working as an academic faculty member.

Once students graduate and are certified and licensed, they are prepared to provide care to those with psychiatric problems, including psychotherapy and psychopharmacologic management. Depending on the state they live in, they may pursue independent practice, or they may be required to collaborate with a physician to provide care to patients. It is expected that, in the future, most advanced practice nursing will be done by graduates of doctoral-level DNP programs. A current trend is to offer advanced practice residency programs or fellowships to newly graduated APRNs so that they can further build their knowledge and skills in a program designed to provide real work experience in the clinician role with strong supervision and academic support in the process.

SOCIAL WORK

Although Yale University does not have its own academic department of social work or graduate training program, the Department of Psychiatry has worked closely with its social work faculty and professional staff in each of its academic and clinical missions.

Brief History of Social Work and Developing a Discipline-Specific Knowledge Base

Psychiatric social work began in the early 1900s and was primarily developed in communities to assist people with psychiatric illnesses. At that time, social workers played an important role acting as liaison among the psychiatrist, patient, and the patient's family. They were responsible for assessing the patient's social history, which psychiatrists used to provide more accurate diagnoses. These social histories also provided the social worker with first-hand information to develop interventions to help integrate persons back into their community. With attention to personality factors gaining ground in the field of psychology in the 1920s, some in the social work profession began to raise criticisms regarding the "social" approach, arguing that caseworkers should focus only on the individual rather than the family, which would "enable the social worker to deal with the personality of the patient in his social setting as intelligently and constructively as the psychiatrist deals with it in the hospital."[23:34] Thus, social integration soon afterward took a back seat to the more psychologized practices.

The question about whether social work could lay claim to discipline-specific knowledge was first raised by Abraham Flexner, in his 1915 speech entitled "Is Social Work a Profession?" presented to the National Conference of Charities and Corrections.[24] His assertion that it was not a profession had a negative impact on the social work profession. Social work was seen as woman's work, low-paid work, the purview of do-gooders. For years since Flexner's comment, some social work scholars have searched to define social work discipline-specific knowledge, however, this is a challenge for a field of work that has "borrowed or assimilated knowledge from the behavioral and social sciences."[25] According to Thyer: "knowledge does not know discipline-specific boundaries ... the concept of overlapping knowledge makes sense because we share the same subject matter—human behavior." Some would argue that Flexner was saying that social work should have a definite purpose and not confine itself to a single aim.[24] Social work is unique because of its array of professional services: person-in-environment perspective, strengths-based approach, social justice component, and community organizing (a comprehensive scope of professional services). Others might say that if we look closely, other fields are also preparing professionals (psychologists, psychiatrists, occupational therapists) to perform similar roles and duties.[25] The difference, however, might be social work's values and ethical principles that reinforce practice that is based on empowerment and self-determination of the individuals and families served.

Social work has made strides as a profession because of the shared knowledge from various schools of thought from the social sciences; they offer an interdisciplinary framework that lends itself to working with others within the field of psychiatry. Social workers comprise 60% of the mental health profession, compared to 10% psychiatrists, 23% psychologists, and 5% nurses.[26] According to the National Association of Social Workers (NASW), social workers have been charged, based on their professional ethics, to promote human well-being with an emphasis on the needs and "empowerment of people who are vulnerable and oppressed, and living in poverty." This is done by focusing on not only the individual, but also on the individual within the context of his or her environment.

Social work is guided by a set of ethical principles and values, all of which can be used to better define the role of social workers on interdisciplinary teams:

1. Social workers' primary goal is to help people in need and to address social problems.
2. Social workers challenge social injustice.
3. Social workers respect the inherent dignity and worth of the person.
4. Social workers recognize the central importance of human relationships.
5. Social workers exhibit integrity; they behave in a trustworthy manner.
6. Social workers are competent; they practice within their areas of competence and develop and enhance their professional expertise.[27]

Although all of these are important to the field of social work, the value "dignity and worth of the person" specifically calls for social workers' practice to be person-centered and recovery-oriented. Social workers treat each person in a caring and respectful fashion, mindful of individual differences and cultural and ethnic diversity. Social workers promote patients' socially responsible self-determination and seek to enhance patients' capacity and opportunity to change and to address their own needs. Social workers are cognizant of their dual responsibility to patients and to the broader society and seek to resolve such conflicts in a socially responsible manner consistent with the values, ethical principles, and ethical standards of the profession.[27]

Person-centered care approaches are inherent in the values and ethical principles of social work. Social work training emphasizes a strengths-based approach to working with individuals, family, and systems with a focus on patients having an active versus passive role in decisions about their care. The Council on Social Work Education (CSWE), which is the accrediting body for schools of social work, has recently joined in with the Substance Abuse and Mental Health Services Administration (SAMHSA)'s Recovery to Practice (RTP) initiative and has expressed its commitment to integrating the mental health recovery model within social work education and practice.[28] This joint resolution was also signed by other professional organizations, including the American Psychiatric Association, American Psychiatric Nurses Association, and the National Association of Peer Specialists.

Social workers enjoy a long and solid tradition of working within teams.[29] Use of interdisciplinary teams in psychiatric settings seems to be the preferred approach. Rarely are professionals working solely with individuals and making decisions that do not involve other professionals or other systems. The social work values and ethical principles regarding human relationships provide a foundation for the importance of establishing partnerships with others. Social workers understand that relationships between and among people are an important vehicle for change. They engage people as partners in the helping process and seek to strengthen relationships among people in a purposeful effort to promote, restore, maintain, and enhance the well-being of individuals, families, social groups, organizations, and communities.[27]

To move toward improving interdisciplinary teams in psychiatry, much work needs to be done from the start in developing "good teams," where all team members feel a part of rather than peripheral to the process. According to Hackman,[30] the place to start is for groups to be "set up right in the first place." The following elements of good teamwork should be considered:

1. Clear structure and accountability
2. Good leadership
3. Delegation of tasks
4. Shared goals
5. Role delineation—having a reciprocal respect of roles
6. Maintenance of strong professional support linkages
7. Mechanisms to resolve conflict[31]

Learning and development of professionals is more likely to occur when those elements are addressed. As stated by Rosen and Callaly, "rather than focusing on within-team rivalries and ideological differences over treatment philosophies, these should be put aside in favour of the principle 'the service user comes first,' and focusing on the combined tasks of the team to meet the needs of that individual and their family."[31:235]

Because of shared discipline knowledge among all the team's members, role blurring and flexibility need to be acknowledged and perhaps welcomed by participants in order to provide the best service to the client.

PSYCHIATRY RESIDENTS

Requirements for postgraduate medical education or residency training in the United States are set by a national organization, the Accreditation Council for Graduate Medical Education (ACGME). Traditionally ACGME has set standards for residency training based on a set of didactic (coursework) and clinical (experiential) requirements. Those clinical requirements deemed most important to the formation of a competent psychiatrist have been awarded required time during the 48 months of psychiatry residency. For example, according to current regulations, residents must have 6 months of inpatient psychiatric clinical experience, 2 months of experience in consultation-liaison psychiatry, 2 months of experience with child and adolescent psychiatry, 12 months of outpatient experience, etc. There is no timed requirement in public or community psychiatry, only this statement regarding community psychiatry:

> This experience must expose residents to persistently and chronically-ill patients in the public sector (e.g., community mental health centers, public hospitals and agencies, and other community-based settings). The program should provide residents the opportunity to consult with, learn about, and use community resources and services in planning patient care, as well as to consult and work collaboratively with case managers, crisis teams, and other mental health professionals.[32]

Although the first sentence of this statement mandates involvement with chronically ill patients in the public sector, the use of the word "should" in the second sentence means that programs do not have to provide an experience using community resources or consulting and working collaboratively with programs usually associated with public-sector settings. This is in stark contrast with requirements mandating experiences with, for example, psychodynamic, cognitive behavioral, and supportive psychotherapy.

There are 37 pages of other ACGME requirements for residency training in psychiatry. Of the hundreds of requirements contained in these regulations, there are very few (perhaps seven) other statements that mandate training in tenets important to education in public psychiatry, including the following from Section IV.A:

- Residents must be comfortable managing and treating the chronically mentally ill with appropriate psychopharmacologic, psychotherapeutic, and social rehabilitative interventions.

- Residents must understand American culture and subcultures, particularly those found in the patient community associated with the educational program, with specific focus for residents with cultural backgrounds different from those of their patients.

- Residents must be trained in the use of case formulation that includes neurobiological, phenomenological, psychological, and sociocultural issues involved in the diagnosis and management of cases.

- Residents must communicate effectively with patients, families, and the public, as appropriate, across a broad range of socioeconomic and cultural backgrounds.

- Residents must display sensitivity and responsiveness to a diverse patient population, including but not limited to diversity in gender, age, culture, race, religion, disabilities, and sexual orientation.

- Residents must learn to practice cost-effective health care and resource allocation that does not compromise quality of care, including an understanding of the financing and regulation of psychiatric practice, as well as information about the structure of public and private organizations that influence mental health care.

- During their outpatient year, residents must have opportunities to apply psychosocial rehabilitation techniques and to evaluate and treat differing disorders in a chronically ill patient population.

There are no ACGME requirements that mandate a recovery-oriented approach to care or specify the types of psychosocial rehabilitative treatments that residents must be exposed to, even though these treatments may have a better established evidence base than some other treatments (such as psychodynamic psychotherapy) that are specifically ACGME mandated. The ACGME has recently instituted another set of requirements, The Milestone Project, which seeks to improve assessment of outcomes of residency training. Here again, tenets important to education in public psychiatry are not emphasized. For example, in a milestone related to treatment planning, residents are encouraged to utilize "an array of modalities and providers [that] may include consideration of complementary and alternative medicine, occupational therapy, and physical therapy." Housing programs, work rehabilitation, cognitive remediation, and other therapies often employed in public psychiatry settings are not mentioned.

Although the ACGME requirements do not promote education in public psychiatry, they also do not prohibit residency programs from utilizing public psychiatry settings to meet the ACGME timed clinical training requirements. Programs that are based in institutions with a strong public psychiatry mission can craft a didactic and clinical curriculum that provides residents with a strong foundation in public psychiatry, which is what Yale has tried to do in its own residency program.

A focus on public psychiatry in the Yale residency begins during recruitment, when departmental leaders highlight the importance of public psychiatry in the history of the department and the ways in which that historical mission continues to animate the work of the modern department of psychiatry. They review the special Yale University-state of Connecticut partnership that underlies the CMHC and the pioneering work done at VA-CT in providing PSR to veterans returning from our nation's wars with the signature wounds of post-traumatic stress disorder and traumatic brain injury. They emphasize the importance of the patient narrative and an evidence-based bio-psychosocial approach to care as the philosophical underpinning of the residency and discuss the expectation that Yale residents will understand how to function in a multidisciplinary team that provides a recovery-oriented approach to caring for underserved populations. By explicitly discussing these values during recruitment, the department has been fortunate to recruit residents who are primed to want to learn about public psychiatry.

Resident education in public psychiatry begins in the very first year, when residents do a rotation on the inpatient service of VA-CT. A foundation of this 3-month rotation is a weekly class on *bio-psychosocial formulation*. Consistent with the focus on patient narrative, residents present a patient that they are working with on the inpatient unit. The small group (usually four to six residents) work together to identify data pertinent to a formulation from the patient's story and begin to develop hypotheses about the patient's presentation and, when time permits, about potential treatment options. In the *social formulation*, the participants consider a cultural and spiritual formulation as well as thinking through more specific social factors that may be contributing to the patient's presentation. In addition to this clinical and didactic experience in their postgraduate year 1 (PGY1), residents will soon also have clinical experiences with patients engaged in PSR. This will include making home visits with an ACT team and working in variety of other settings, such as a recovery-oriented day program, an integrated medical and psychiatric team treating homeless veterans, and a wellness center providing medical and recovery-oriented services to indigent patients with severe mental illness.

In the PGY2, residents have the option of immersing themselves in a public psychiatry setting by selecting a 3-month rotation on an inpatient unit at the CMHC where care is provided for severely ill patients who have intense psychosocial challenges and difficulty managing outside the hospital. In addition to usual inpatient learning goals of medical management, residents also learn about the challenges of developing outpatient treatment plans in a resource-limited system. The PGY2 didactics begin with residents introducing themselves through affiliation groups that they belong to through their family (such as ethnicity and spiritual groups), as well as affiliation groups they may have joined (such as sexual orientation) and the ways in which these affiliation groups might influence their assumptions about the world and especially toward the mentally ill. In this way, educational leaders begin to train residents to think about affiliation groups, their own implicit assumptions, and possible stigma toward the mentally ill. Rather than passively learn about homelessness, residents tour homeless shelters and permanent housing with a homeless outreach team. Residents learn the robust evidence base for PSR interventions in a series the organizers have named "Social Psychiatry Boot Camp."

PGY2 residents also participate in a year-long weekly case conference series using patient narrative and a bio-psychosocial perspective. Cases are selected to span the range of psychopathology typically encountered at their level of training. One resident writes a protocol that is posted on an internal website prior to the session, and all members of the class are expected to complete a full bio-psychosocial formulation of the material. The session begins with the author sharing his or her own formulation, following which time is reserved for peer supervision and discussion. Three faculty members of diverse clinical perspectives are then invited to share their thoughts on the material. Throughout the year, a diverse group of individuals represent the "social" perspective, including nurses, social workers, peer support specialists, family members, National Alliance on Mental Illness (NAMI) representatives, and psychiatrists from a wide range of clinical settings (e.g., ACT teams, state hospitals, community clinics).

This paradigm accomplishes several important goals. Foremost, the leaders model for residents, early in their training, the value of a robust social psychiatry perspective as a core component of patient-centered care. By directly linking these teachings to the patients whom residents are treating, faculty demonstrate the relevance of complex concepts that may otherwise seem less pertinent or less tangible (e.g., PSR and the recovery movement). Finally, this method allows faculty to explore complex systems of care and demonstrates the role of interdisciplinary collaboration. Having faculty representing a public psychiatry perspective participate in these weekly case conferences ensures that residents learn material relevant to public psychiatry and emphasizes the value the department places on resident education in public psychiatry (Figure 16.1).

In the PGY3 outpatient-oriented year, resident placements include CMHC and the VA-CT, where residents work largely with severely mentally ill patients in public psychiatry settings. Residents have the opportunity to work with individual patients and to experience how outpatient teams operate. Each setting has developed didactics that have been tailored to the specific populations treated at each site. For example, CMHC also has a seminar in which residents and faculty meet together to discuss literature pertinent to the population treated at the institution and to discuss ways in which this literature might be translated to improve patient care in this public psychiatry setting.

These public psychiatry settings present several challenges to meeting the ACMGE-mandated learning objectives for outpatient treatment, including developing resident competence in pharmacology and psychotherapy because many of the patients have failed multiple medication trials and have complicated psychosocial presentations that are challenging for inexperienced residents to manage.

The PGY4 year is largely an elective year in which residents choose a major placement and have additional time to choose among many elective opportunities. Residents can learn in several public psychiatry settings, including (1) walk-in and initial assessment service at CMHC, (2) La Clinica Hispana, an outpatient clinic for Latino patients at CMHC; (3) a young adult service at CMHC; and (4) a comprehensive PSR program at VA-CT. In the 2014–15 academic year, the department piloted a program in which a PGY4 resident worked in a large state hospital and participated in the didactic learning relevant to the public psychiatry fellowship.

ADVANCED EDUCATION EXPERIENCES

In addition to subspecialty fellowships in addictions, geriatrics, psychosomatic medicine and law and psychiatry, three postgraduate fellowship programs were launched within the Yale Department to provide advanced training and expertise to young professionals with an interest in the public sector. Each of the fellowships was built on the existing rich clinical and academic environments of CMHC and the West Haven Campus of VA Connecticut Healthcare System, where the integration of evidence-based treatment and rehabilitation programs for individuals with SMI and SUDs were well-established sites for education. They are examples of public–academic partnerships, in which the support of stipends and faculty effort is provided through federal or state funding mechanisms.

In 2003, the VA Interprofessional Fellowship in Psychosocial Rehabilitation and Recovery Services was created at the West Haven VA. The purpose of the program is "to develop future mental health leaders with vision,

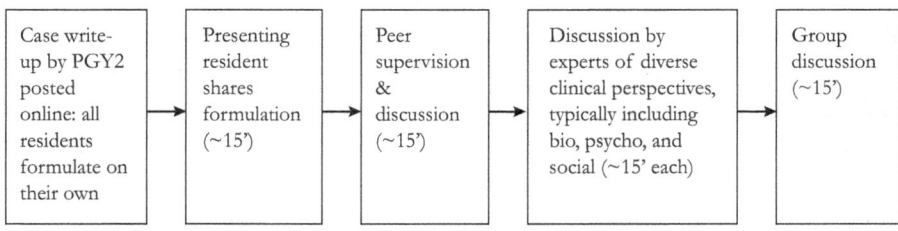

Figure 16.1 PG 2 Case Conferences

knowledge, and commitment to transform mental health care systems in the 21st century by emphasizing functional capability, rehabilitation, and recovery."[33] Although the majority of fellows are postgraduate psychologists and social workers, the program also trains individuals from nursing, psychiatry, occupational therapy, and rehabilitation counseling. Trainees learn through clinical work on interdisciplinary teams, in seminars, and through close mentorship by faculty who are engaged in the development and evaluation of community-based initiatives. An associated goal for fellows when working with individuals, groups, and families is to learn and then apply evidence-based psychotherapeutic and psychoeducational techniques. Using their knowledge and acquired skills, residents engage in an educational dissemination project or a scholarly pursuit with faculty mentorship that culminates in a presentation that each resident makes at a national conference.

A core seminar, on Leadership in Public Mental Health Systems, was started at the VA for the PSR fellows but is now open to the fellows in the two other programs listed here and is offered as an elective through the Department of Psychiatry. It is based on the premise that most professional graduate programs focus on clinical work and research but that there is little education and training on program management and leadership development. The monthly seminar brings together leaders from the Yale Medical School and community to discuss career trajectories, management styles, negotiation skills, decision-making, politics in organizations, and other pertinent topics. Participants also engage in their own leadership exploration and development over the course of the year through mentored exercises.

A separate fellowship in public mental health and administration was developed in 2009 for postdoctoral psychology fellows. Each year, one to two fellows in this program are funded by various federal grants to deliver clinical services to adults at CMHC and to concurrently serve as consultants and evaluators within the large network of community providers affiliated with CMHC. These psychology fellows attend the leadership seminar based at the VA and a second core seminar on public mental health and administration, based at CMHC, whose participants also include the public psychiatry fellows (described later) and junior faculty. Presenters include the commissioner and other senior staff from the Connecticut Department of Mental Health and Addiction Services (DMHAS) and other faculty with expertise in this arena. Specific topics include financing of public mental health systems, recovery and transformation in public mental sector mental health systems, creating and implementing change, developing culturally sensitive programs, and becoming an effective consultant. The curriculum also includes interactive visits to the state's legislative office building, homeless shelters, a forensic inpatient hospital, and other sites where experts in those fields provide informal talks.

Public psychiatry fellowships (PPFs)—for physicians who have completed residencies in psychiatry—have existed for several decades, the most prominent of which is the Columbia PPF established in 1980.[34] Although many of these fellowships were phased out in the 1970s as federal funding cuts occurred, a renaissance of sorts began to take place in the 2000s when several academic centers across the country launched new programs by developing alternative funding strategies.[35] They differ somewhat in their structures and funding mechanisms, yet many are based on public–academic partnerships, in which the local or state government provides financial support in return for clinical service and an opportunity to recruit trainees into permanent positions.[36] Dr. Jules Ranz from Columbia University created a network of PPF directors that provides a mechanism to exchange ideas and data about program development and strategies for success. PPFs have based their curricula on established guidelines, and these core competencies were published by the Columbia group[37] and the American Association of Community Psychiatrists.[38] A certification process for public psychiatry and recognition as a subspecialty is in development for a 2015 launch.

In addition to the Columbia program, CMHC is another example of a successful and long-standing academic–public partnership. When the Yale PPF was developed in 2007, funding for fellowship positions was built into an existing relationship between DMHAS and Yale to provide professional services to CMHC through a staffing contract, originally established in 1966. DMHAS added funds to covers the fellows' stipends as well as program support. The fellows' commitment for 50% clinical time is spent within ambulatory services at CMHC or on inpatient services at Connecticut Valley Hospital, a 900-bed state facility.[39] The fellows' other 50% effort is devoted to academic activities such as seminars, Department of Psychiatry grand rounds, and scholarship. This PPF attracts psychiatrists who are interested in improving the care of individuals served within public-sector settings by increasing their level of expertise in clinical care, administration, performance improvement, and evaluation of services. The vast majority of the Yale PPF graduates accept jobs within the public sector, some of which are combined with academic roles, and many have assumed medical director positions within those institutions.

TEACHING PSYCHOSOCIAL REHABILITATION

As discussed in Chapter 4, PSR is a process or approach that utilizes a wide variety of techniques, many of them evidence-based, to help an individual with SMI and addictions reach his or her highest potential in the community. This expertise and practice can be considered a subspecialty within public psychiatry. PSR training programs provide opportunities for community psychiatrists and other mental health professionals to develop their core skill set in the treatment of individuals with SMI, including how to integrate clinical treatment with rehabilitation in a person-centered, recovery-oriented plan of care. A comprehensive PSR training approach utilizes formal training complemented by "on the job" in vivo experience.

Trainees are taught the theories and principles of evidence-based practices identified through the updated Schizophrenia Patient Outcomes Research Team (PORT) project, which systematically reviews all schizophrenia interventions studies for empirical support. These evidence-based psychosocial treatment interventions include ACT, supported employment, skills training, cognitive behavioral therapy, token economy interventions, and family-based services. Trainees working with individuals with schizophrenia and comorbid SUDs learn psychosocial interventions for alcohol and substance use disorders. Likewise, when working with persons with schizophrenia, they incorporate structured psychosocial intervention for weight loss into treatment planning.[40]

The Psychiatric Rehabilitation Association, a national trade organization, along with the Boston University Center for Psychiatric Rehabilitation and the Center for Psychiatric Rehabilitation at the University of Chicago, offer ongoing leadership and training in PSR. Over the past three decades, the Boston University Center for Psychiatric Rehabilitation has taken the lead in developing detail-oriented training curricula to guide students and practitioners through the rehabilitation process.[41:106] This approach focuses on helping individuals understand their values and preferences and then systematically working with them to set and achieve goals in desired residential, educational, vocational, and social environments. It includes an evaluation of their skill functioning and resources needed for each person to be successful and satisfied in his or her particular environment. This is followed by teaching the person the requisite skills and helping him or her obtain the necessary resources and supports.[41:106–107]

With regard to "on the job" or in vivo experience, trainees learn first-hand how to provide wrap-around case management, supported employment, money management, and other technical skills directly in the community through an apprenticeship model. ACT teams, for example, can provide a rich training ground for psychiatry residents, social work postmaster residents, and psychology postdoctoral residents. Psychiatry residents can be integrated into the team for full-year placements or longer. For many psychiatry residents, this may be their first time seeing patients in the community. The psychiatry resident is responsible for providing mental health care, case management, and PSR services for the client. Their work is supervised by the team psychiatrist and, to a lesser extent, by the program manager, usually a social worker, who receives and provides feedback from and to the entire interdisciplinary team at daily rounds. The vignette in Box 16.1 is an example of what a psychiatry resident might expect and learn with regard to PSR.

INTEGRATION OF EDUCATION IN PUBLIC PSYCHIATRY

Having reviewed discipline-based education programs, it is important to emphasize the value of interdisciplinary education in public psychiatry. Advanced fellowships provide this experience as an essential feature. The authors believe that learning together fosters working together. In the process, students learn how to build strong teams that function optimally in serving people with SMIs and addictions. It is important that an interdisciplinary approach be carried out at the level of academic departments as well, for the reasons discussed earlier and in Chapter 19. Interdisciplinary academic teams within divisions of public psychiatry create a model that can be replicated in the sphere of practice learned in advanced fellowships.

IMPLICATIONS FOR WORKFORCE DEVELOPMENT

The ultimate goal of teaching public-sector psychiatry and mental health is to create a workforce that is sufficient in size and skill to meet the needs of individuals with behavioral health conditions. As the content of this chapter reveals, that challenge is exceptionally complex and goes far beyond the simple act of teaching. The lessons from these Yale-based efforts to train practitioners illustrate the major challenges nationally within the public sector in addressing workforce development needs.

The SAMHSA commissioned a national workforce strategic plan that was authored by the Annapolis Coalition on the Behavioral Health Workforce, with a Yale faculty

> **BOX 16.1**
>
> *Immersion in Community Practice to Acquire Advanced Professional Skills*
>
> The first time Dr. Zack Smith, a PGY4 psychiatry resident met his newly assigned client Adam, a 28-year-old white man, Adam was living in his older sister's home in a town 10 miles away from the clinic. Adam had a history of psychiatric inpatient treatment stays for hallucinations, paranoid thinking, and suicidality. While in the hospital, he would agree to take his medications again, but he routinely discontinued taking them upon leaving the hospital. After Adam's eighth stay in 2 years, the ACT team started working with him in hopes of avoiding additional inpatient hospitalizations and helping him live stably in the community. The ACT team had seen Adam for a year when he began to work with Dr. Zack. When they met Adam, he was starting to focus on setting and achieving various life goals.
>
> The first few times Dr. Zack went to see Adam in the community, he was joined by a team member until both he and the team felt he could comfortably handle community visits on his own. As Dr. Zack shadowed his team members, he learned from them, including observing environmental and behavioral cues and adopting a relaxed demeanor, which included taking off his tie, tucking his ID badge in his shirt, and refraining from asking personal or probing questions in public about symptoms and relationships. At first, Adam would barely look at him, mumbled many of his words, and seemed shy and quiet. Dr. Zack asked Adam many questions about his goals and dreams and received mostly one-word answers. After about a month or so, Adam invited Dr. Zack into his home, where he discovered that Adam loved cats and was a devout Yankees baseball fan. He saw that his medication bottles looked full and untouched. Later, while accompanying Adam to the supermarket, he noted that Adam barely made eye contact with the cashiers and yet comfortably conversed with the same teller at his local bank about her dogs and cats.
>
> Over time, Dr. Zack disclosed to Adam that he was a Chicago Cubs fan and had a Golden Retriever, which opened up more discussions about baseball and animals. By their seventh or eighth visit, Adam began to talk about himself. Over the course of the 30-minute car ride to a medical appointment, Adam shared that he one day wanted to live in his own apartment, get a car, have a girlfriend, and go back to school to become a veterinary assistant. Dr. Zack shared this important information in a treatment team meeting, which triggered a supported employment referral to support Adam's vocational goal and included arranging a volunteer position at an animal shelter. As Adam became more confident, the supported employment specialist on the team started to work with him on his resume, identified part-time jobs in the community, and took him out to job sites. The peer specialist also offered to join Dr. Zack on some upcoming visits to offer his support around social opportunities in the community and later to help Adam build social skills. Dr. Zack also worked with Adam to map out his rehabilitation plan, including his goals and skills and the resources he would need to achieve them. Together, they created a budget for Adam to live on and reviewed his spending and savings each week. Over time, Adam was able to ask questions and share concerns about medication side effects, and Dr. Zack talked openly about various medications and about good nutrition and exercise. Adam agreed to start on a low dose of antipsychotic medication.
>
> Helping an individual with SMI and frequent psychiatric inpatient stays live successfully in the community can take significant collaboration between the individual and his provider team. Residents like Dr. Zack learn to "meet the person where they are," despite his or her wishes for the individual to take medications, engage in psychotherapy, and work on particular goals. Residents first learn to focus on building rapport and trust and then help the individual set and achieve life goals. Accomplishing goals typically involves a combination of resource attainment and skill development with the support of the clinician. Psychotherapy happens naturally in the community during conversations in the car or a person's home. Working on an ACT team, residents learn to apply and adapt the tools they learned earlier in their training to community settings with patients who are less comfortable with office-based psychotherapy.

member as lead author.[42] The resulting blueprint for action, which is known as the Annapolis Framework,[43] identifies a set of goals, six of which are illustrated in this chapter and described here:

Strengthening the Traditional Workforce

1. The initial goal is to systematically recruit and retain individuals to work with the populations served in the public sector. This chapter describes, for example, how difficult it has been for professions such as psychology to interest students in learning about and pursuing careers in public-sector work and for all professions to recruit persons of color. Successful recruitment seems to involve early exposure during training to persons with SMI, to effective treatments for this population, and to mentors who are skilled and strongly committed to this

work. Stipends and loan repayment strategies have also been used successfully.

2. The second goal is to effectively train individuals once recruited. It has been a constant challenge for academic training programs to keep pace with changes in health care practice and with constantly evolving evidence-based interventions. For the public sector, innovation has involved shifting training into community-based settings, such as PSR programs and ACT teams, and immersing students in models of care focused on recovery and resilience.

3. An effective workforce requires not only training skilled practitioners, but also developing supervisors and leaders who can train students, supervise staff, lead teams, and manage programs. This has been accomplished at Yale and in other systems through the development of fellowships and other forms of advanced training that teach the administrative, financial, human resource, and change management skills that are key to managing groups and organizations.

Broadening the Concept of Workforce

4. The shift to recovery-oriented care in the public sector has had major implications for the field's concept of "workforce." It has become clear that expanded workforce roles for persons in recovery and their family members are essential, whether as paid peer specialists, volunteer mentors, or as supportive members of a consumer's family and social network. Peer and family support is a powerful and effective complement to the services offered by traditional providers.

5. Similarly, expanded caregiving roles for community groups and organizations are necessary to meet the housing, financial, vocational, and social needs of persons with behavioral health conditions. Citizen-based coalitions have also been effective in preventing and addressing co-occurring substance abuse problems within local communities.

6. Last, there is a compelling rationale for expanded roles for medical health care providers in meeting behavioral health needs because individuals and families seeking help more frequently turn to these providers than to behavioral health professionals.

The cross-cutting theme for the public sector that echoes throughout these goals is the imperative to teach students to work well with others: in multidisciplinary teams, in interprofessional collaborations with primary and specialty medical care, and in partnerships with persons in recovery, their family members, and community service organizations. Working well with others in such complex relationships requires strong interpersonal and communication skills, self-confidence, respect for the contributions of others, and the abilities to both lead and follow. Developing such competencies within the public-sector workforce is perhaps the greatest ongoing challenge.

SUMMARY

In summary, this chapter describes the development and implementation of both discipline-based and interdisciplinary training and education programs for public psychiatry. The value of these specialized programs is not only to develop the workforce necessary to perform clinical and administrative tasks, but also to reinforce the commitment of professionals to work with an historically underserved segment of our population and to do so by collaborating closely with other members of a team. Advanced programs provide a cadre of mentors who encourage their trainees to engage in life-long education and continued affiliation with professional networks. These elements can promote recruitment and retention into systems of care that may be lacking in financial or other tangible resources. System development and recovery-oriented services can flourish when the professionals within their ranks are inspired and gratified by the work they accomplish and the professional relationships they form.

REFERENCES

1. Jacobs SC. *Inside Public Psychiatry*. Shelton, CT: People's Medical Publishing House-USA; 2011.
2. Steiner JL, Anderson N, Belitsky R, et al. Public psychiatry training and education at the Connecticut Mental Health Center. In: Jacobs SC, Griffith EEH, eds. *40 Years of Academic Public Psychiatry*. West Sussex, England: Wiley and Sons; 2007: 160–173.
3. Yedida MJ, Gillespie CC, Bernstein CA. A survey of psychiatric residency directors on current priorities and preparation for public-sector care. *Psychiatric Services*. 2006; 57: 238–43.
4. Steiner JL, Ponce AN, Styron T, Aklin EA, Wexler BE. Teaching an Interdisciplinary Approach to the Treatment of Chronic Mental Illness: Challenges and Rewards. *Academic Psychiatry*. 2008; 32(3): 255–258.
5. Freedheim DK, Weiner IB, eds. *Handbook of Psychology, History of Psychology* (Vol. 1). Hoboken, NJ: John Wiley & Sons; 2003.
6. Chu JP, Emmons L, Wong J, et al. Public psychology: A competency model for professional psychologists in community mental health. *Professional Psychology: Research and Practice*. 2012; 43(1): 39–49. doi: 10.1037/a0026319.
7. Roe D, Yanos PT, Lysaker PH. Overcoming barriers to increase the contribution of clinical psychologists to work with persons with severe mental illness. *Clinical Psychology: Science and Practice*. 2006; 13: 376–383. doi: 10.1111/j.1468-2850.2006.00051.

8. Duffy FF, West JC, Wilk J, et al. Mental health practitioners and trainees. In: Manderscheid RW, Henderson M, eds. *Mental Health, United States*. Rockville, MD: U.S. Department of Health and Human Services; 2002.
9. President's New Freedom Commission Report. *Achieving the promise: Transforming mental health care in America. Final Report*. Rockville, MD: President's New Freedom Commission on Mental Health; 2003.
10. Reddy F, Spaulding WD, Jansen MA, Menditto AA, Pickett, S. Psychologists' roles and opportunities in rehabilitation and recovery for serious mental illness: A survey of Council of University Directors of Clinical Psychology (CUDCP) clinical psychology training and doctoral education. *Training and Education in Professional Psychology*. 2010; 4(4): 254–263. doi: 10.1037/a0021457.
11. Fouad NA, Grus CL, Hatcher RL, et al. Competency benchmarks: A model for understanding and measuring competence in professional psychology across training levels. *Training and Education in Professional Psychology*. 2009; 3: S5–S26. doi: 10.1037/a0015832.
12. Maguire, N. Training for front-line homeless workers: Practicalities and ethics of teaching cognitive behavioural and dialectical behavioural psychological therapeutic techniques. *Housing, Care and Support*. 2012; 15: 177–85. doi: 10.1108/14608791211288589.
13. Substance Abuse and Mental Health Services Administration. *Integrated treatment for co-occurring disorders: Training frontline staff*. Rockville, MD: Center for Mental Health Services, Substance Abuse and Mental Health Services Administration, U.S. Department of Health and Human Services. http://store.samhsa.gov/shin/content/SMA08-4367/TrainingFrontlineStaff-ITC.pdf. Published 2009. Accessed January 27, 2015.
14. Corrigan PW, Kerr A, Knudsen, L. The stigma of mental illness: Explanatory models and methods for change. *Applied and Preventive Psychology*. 2005; 11(3): 179–190. doi: 10.1016/j.appsy.2005.07.001.
15. Folsom DP, Hawthorne W, Lindamer L, et al. Prevalence and risk factors for homelessness and utilization of mental health services among 10,340 patients with serious mental illness in a large public mental health system. *American Journal of Psychiatry*. 2005; 162(2): 370–376. doi: 10.1176/appi.ajp.162.2.370.
16. Stuart H. Mental illness and employment discrimination. *Current Opinion in Psychiatry*. 2006; 19: 522–526. doi: 10.1097/01.yco.0000238482.27270.5d.
17. Goodman LA, Liang B, Helms JE, Latta RE. Training counseling psychologists as social justice agents: Feminist and multicultural principles in action. *The Counseling Psychologist*. 2004; 32: 793–837. doi: 10.1177/0011000004268802.
18. American Nurses Association. *Nursing: Scope and Standards of Practice*. Silver Spring, MD: American Nurses Association; 2010.
19. American Psychiatric Nurses Association (APNA), International Society of Psychiatric-Mental Health Nurses (ISPN). *Psychiatric-Mental Health Nursing: Scope and Standards of Practice*. Silver Spring, MD: American Nurses Association; 2007.
20. Goldmark J. *Nursing and Nursing Education in the United States: Report of the Committee and Report of a Survey*. New York, NY: The Macmillan Company; 1923.
21. Varney H. *Yale University School of Nursing: A Brief History*. New Haven, CT: Yale School of Nursing; 1998.
22. American Association of Colleges of Nursing. *The Essentials of Baccalaureate Education for Professional Nursing Practice*. 2008
23. Stuart PH. Community care and the origins of psychiatric social work. *Social Work in Health Care*. 1997; 25(3): 25–36.
24. Morris P. Reinterpreting Abraham Flexner's Speech, 'Is Social Work a Profession?' Its Meaning and Influence on the Field's Early Professional Development. *Social Service Review*. 2008; 82(1): 29–60.
25. Thyer BA. Developing discipline-specific knowledge for social work: Is it possible? *Journal of Social Work Education*. 2002: 38(1): 101–114.
26. Mental Health. National Association of Social Workers (NASW) Website. http://www.naswdc.org/pressroom/features/issue/mental.asp. Published 2014. Accessed January 27, 2015.
27. Code of Ethics of the National Association of Social Workers. National Association of Social Workers Website. http://www.naswdc.org/pubs/code/code.asp. Approved 1996. Published 2008. Accessed January 27, 2015.
28. Recovery to Practice Pledge. Council on Social Work Education (CSWE) Website. http://www.cswe.org/CentersInitiatives/DataStatistics/42850.aspx. Published 2014. Accessed January 27, 2015.
29. Bronstein LR. A model for interdisciplinary collaboration. *Social Work*. 2003; 48(3): 297–306.
30. Hackman JR. *Groups that work (and those that don't)*. San Francisco, CA: Jossey-Bass; 1990.
31. Rosen A, Callaly T. Interdisciplinary teamwork and leadership: issues for psychiatrists. *Australasian Psychiatry*. 2005; 13(3): 234–240.
32. ACGME Program Requirements for Graduate Medical Education in Psychiatry. Accreditation Council for Graduate Medical Education Website. http://www.acgme.org/acgmeweb/Portals/0/PFAssets/ProgramRequirements/400_psychiatry_07012014.pdf. Published 2014. Accessed January 27, 2015.
33. Klee A. Interprofessional Fellowship in Psychosocial Rehabilitation and Recovery Oriented Services, program description. US Department of Veteran Affair's Website. http://www.va.gov/oaa/fellowships/psychosocial-rehab.asp. Accessed March, 2014.
34. Ranz JM, Rosenheck S, Deakins S. Columbia University's Fellowship in Public Psychiatry. *Psychiatric Services*. 1996; 47: 512–516.
35. Le Melle SL, Mangurian C, Ali OM, et al. Public Psychiatry Fellowships: A developing Network of Public-Academic Collaborations. *Psychiatric Services*. 2012; 63(9): 851–854.
36. Steiner JL, Giggie M, Koh S, Ranz J. The Evolution of Public Psychiatry Fellowships. *Academic Psychiatry*. 2014; 38(6): 685–9.
37. Ranz JM, Deakins SM, Le Melle SM, Rosenheck SD, Kellermann SL. Core Elements of a Public Psychiatry Fellowship. *Psychiatric Services*. 2008; 59: 718–720.
38. American Association of Community Psychiatrists: Guidelines for Developing and Evaluating Public and Community Psychiatry Training Fellowships. http://www.communitypsychiatry.org/pages.aspx?PageName=Guidelines_for_Developing_and_Evaluating_Public_and_Community_Psychiatry_Training_Fellowships. Published 2008. Accessed January 27, 2015.
39. Steiner JL. Yale Fellowship in Public Psychiatry program description. Yale School of Medicine Website. http://medicine.yale.edu/psychiatry/education/clinfell/public.aspx. Revised January 2014. Published January 2014. Accessed March 1, 2014.
40. Kreyenbuhl J, Buchanan R, Dickerson FB, Dixon LB. The Schizophrenia Patient Outcomes Research Team (PORT): Updated Treatment Recommendations 2009. *Schizophrenia Bulletin*. 2010; 36(1): 94–103.
41. Anthony WA. *Psychiatric rehabilitation*. 2nd ed. Boston, MA: Center for Psychiatric Rehabilitation, Sargent College of Health and Rehabilitation Sciences, Boston University; 2002.
42. Hoge MA, Morris JA, Daniels AS, Stuart GW, Huey LY, Adams N. *An action plan for behavioral health workforce development: A framework for discussion*. Rockville, MD: Substance Abuse and Mental Health Services Administration, U.S. Department of Health and Human Services; 2007.
43. Hoge MA, Stuart GW, Morris J, Flaherty MT, Paris M, Goplerud E. Mental health and addiction workforce development: Federal leadership is needed to address the growing crisis. *Health Affairs*. 2013; 32(11): 2005–2012.

17.

EVIDENCE-BASED PUBLIC PSYCHIATRY

Jack Tsai, Joanne DeSanto Iennaco, Julienne Giard, and Rani A. Hoff

---

EDUCATIONAL HIGHLIGHTS

- Evidence-based psychiatry is necessary for advancement of the field.
- Requirements for evidence and definitions of evidence-based practices vary.
- Well-conducted randomized controlled trials represent the most rigorous research designs.
- Implementation of evidence-based psychiatry involves training and fidelity.
- Patients' values, preferences, needs, and choices must be considered in practice.
- Integrating new technologies into psychiatry can help the field be evidence-based.

BRIEF HISTORY

Public psychiatry and the mental health system began somewhat inauspiciously. The treatment and care of individuals with mental illness and addictions as we know it today has evolved through various paradigm shifts, including decades of different practices and methods. Admittedly, some of these practices have been inhumane, ineffective, and inadequate. Thus, it is important to recognize this history to appreciate the invaluable need for the field of psychiatry to be evidence-based, self-critical, and constantly evolving.

Organized, institutional public psychiatry was predated by the creation of privately funded or public, charitably funded "lunatic asylums." These lunatic asylums for the "insane" proliferated in Europe during the 19th to early 20th century.[1,2] For example, by the 1900s, there were thousands of lunatic asylums in England alone. Inhabitants of these asylums lived in dirty, crowded conditions; were subject to beatings, starvation, and imprisonment; and received inadequate treatments for their mental conditions.[3,4] More humane and moral treatment was promoted during that time through the work of Phillip Pinel in France, William Tuke in England, Dorothea Dix in the United States, and many other reformers. Eventually, the lunatic asylums were transformed into modern state psychiatric hospitals in the United States, which ultimately led to deinstitutionalization and the creation of community mental health centers. Of course, these changes occurred over decades of other embarrassing, esoteric, and ineffective practices, such as bloodletting, phrenology, hydrotherapy, lobotomies and other psychosurgeries, insulin shock therapy, and various other drug treatments.[5,6] These dark moments in psychiatry's history illustrate the necessity to systematically evaluate outcomes, develop treatments based on data, and move toward patient-centered care.

Despite inauspicious beginnings, psychiatry has risen to become an indispensable part of the public health system and a well-respected specialty within the medical community. Today, public psychiatry can be broadly defined as mental health services primarily financed by local, state, federal, or other public funds with mandates to serve the poor, needy, and disabled. Institutions that provide these services include community mental health centers, state hospitals, Department of Veterans Affairs (VA) medical centers, and various other public sector programs. Because public dollars are being used to fund these institutions and services, there is particular scrutiny and attention on their practices being evidence-based and cost-effective.

IMPORTANCE OF EVIDENCE-BASED PUBLIC PSYCHIATRY

Several federal and legislative actions have occurred in recent years that have made evidence-based psychiatry a priority for the nation's public health. In 1999, the first ever Surgeon General's Report on Mental Health alerted the public, mental health advocates, and policy-makers that mental illness was the second leading cause of disability and premature mortality in the country. The report reported the "urgent need for research evidence that supports strategies for mental health promotion and illness prevention"[7:454] and "delivery of state-of-the art treatments."[7:455] A few years later, in 2002, President George W. Bush announced the President's New Freedom Commission on Mental Health, which was charged to examine the state of mental health care delivery. The Commission's final report recommended a "fundamental transformation of the nation's approach to mental health care" (p. 1), including advancing evidence-based practices through dissemination and demonstration projects and changing reimbursement policies to more fully support evidence-based practices.[8,9] More recently, in 2008, Congress passed the Paul Wellstone and Pete Domenici Mental Health Parity and Addiction Equity Act, which essentially required group health insurance plans to cover mental and physical health equally. This act ensured that benefits for mental health or substance use disorders were on par with medical/surgical benefits.[10] The 2010 landmark passage of the Patient Protection and Affordable Care Act (ACA) under President Obama's administration extended this equity in coverage to also apply to individual health insurance coverage, and so coverage of mental health conditions and substance use disorders will become mandatory for most insurance providers by 2014.[11–13]

Together, these developments have elevated the importance of evidence-based mental health care. Moreover, many private and public payers, including Medicare and Medicaid, are moving toward "pay-for-performance" systems in which providers are compensated by payers for meeting certain established measures for quality and efficiency, which often rely on evidence-based guidelines for care.[14,15] This represents a fundamental change from the fee-for-service system, in which, inherently, there is less emphasis placed on evidence-based care.[16,17] Thus, it is important to recognize that there is an increasing demand for medical care that meets standards of safety and efficacy in order to be reimbursable both in the private and public sectors.

This chapter provides an introduction to evidence-based care in public psychiatry. The era of evidence-based medicine is described; certain evidence-based practices in psychiatry are reviewed; challenges with training, fidelity, and implementation are discussed; and future directions of evidence-based psychiatry are considered.

EVIDENCE-BASED MEDICINE

Evidence-based medicine can be defined as the "conscientious, explicit and judicious use of the current best evidence in making decisions about the care of individual patients."[18:71] This definition means that individual clinical expertise should be integrated with empirical evidence from systematic research to make clinical decisions. The role of the patient must also not be overlooked because a patient's values, preferences, needs, and choices should be considered with the evidence. Empirical evidence can consist of studies using a wide range of methodologies and research designs, differing in the precision by which variables of interest are measured and the scientific rigor by which inferences and conclusions can be reliably and accurately drawn. In other words, the evidence can range from expert opinion to meta-analyses of randomized controlled trials (RCTs).

Systems have been developed to classify evidence in a body of literature by using a hierarchy of scientific rigor and quality. In the United States, a recognized authority in assessing scientific clinical research is the Agency for Healthcare Research and Quality (AHRQ), which evaluates evidence in four key domains: risk of bias (low, medium, or high), consistency (consistent, inconsistent, or unknown/not applicable), directness (direct or indirect), and precision (precise or imprecise). Additionally, when appropriate, studies are evaluated for coherence, dose–response association, residual confounding, strength of association, publication bias, and applicability. The strength of evidence is then assigned an overall grade of High, Moderate, Low, or Insufficient.[19] There are various other systems in use in the United States and internationally, such the system used by the US Preventive Services Task Force;[20] the Oxford Centre for Evidence-Based Medicine (CEBM);[21] the Grading of Recommendations Assessment, Development, and Evaluation (GRADE) system;[22] the Strength of Recommendation Taxonomy (SORT);[23] and others.[24–26]

There is currently no universal system to rate the scientific evidence available for a medical test, treatment, or recommendation. The requirements for evidence used by different groups vary, but, in general, the highest standard is RCTs. In RCTs, an intervention is compared to an alternative treatment or no intervention among study participants who are randomly assigned to one group. A meta-analysis of RCTs aggregates the results over a series of studies and provides the strongest evidence for a treatment effect. Slightly lower standards of evidence are *quasi-experimental studies*, which include comparison groups that are not assigned by randomization. Often ranked below that standard are *open clinical trials*, which lack independent comparison groups. And usually at the lowest levels of evidence are *clinical observations* and *case studies*.

Using the available evidence to make sound clinical decisions is essential to good practice. It is important to note though, that evidence-based medicine is not "cookbook" medicine.[18] Evidence-based medicine ideally requires a bottom-up approach that takes into account individual clinical expertise and patient choice, as well as evidence from systematically conducted research. The field of psychiatry has made great efforts in establishing itself as a medical specialty by adopting the methods of evidence-based medicine, and the field needs to continue to do so to advance science and improve clinical care.

EVIDENCE-BASED PRACTICES IN PSYCHIATRY

The practice of evidence-based medicine has been formalized in various forms, including the development of evidence-based guidelines, treatment algorithms, and work group recommendations. In psychiatry, certain treatment packages, service models, and manualized interventions have been developed, collectively referred to as *evidence-based practices*. Different lists of evidence-based practices have been disseminated by different private, nonprofit, state, and federal organizations, including the Substance Abuse and Mental Health Administration (SAMHSA), the Robert Wood Johnson Foundation, and the National Alliance on Mental Illness (NAMI).

There is variability in how an evidence-based practice is defined, and there is no universal definition. There has, however, been consensus developed within various groups. For example, Chambless and Hollon[27] established criteria that a psychotherapy can be considered evidence-based (or what they termed an empirically supported therapy) if (1) the therapy is shown to be statistically significantly superior to a comparison group in at least two independent RCTs, controlled single case experiments, or equivalent time-sample designs; (2) a treatment manual or its logical equivalent was used; (3) and the target population had a specified problem with valid, reliable inclusion criteria used. Therapies can be designated as "possibly efficacious" if only one rigorous study exists showing the therapy is statistically significantly superior to a comparison group. This set of criteria has been used by Division 12 of the American Psychological Association (APA) to develop a list of more than 50 evidence-based psychotherapies for conditions ranging from depression to sexual dysfunction[28] (refer to the resource list at the end of this section).

To give readers an example of another set of evidence-based practices that is broader in scope and used beyond psychotherapies, in 1998, the Robert Wood Johnson Foundation convened a consensus panel of researchers, clinicians, administrators, consumers, and family advocates to determine which practices currently demonstrate a strong evidence base. They initially identified six evidence-based practices for adults with severe mental illness, which has since been expanded to 11 evidence-based practices for a wider range of patient populations. The SAMHSA has created a Knowledge Informing Transformation (KIT) series for these 11 evidence-based practices, which are briefly described in Table 17.1. These evidence-based practices extend beyond symptom relief from mental illness and addictions to psychosocial rehabilitation and community supports for other domains of life, such as housing, employment, and education. This is in line with the current movement toward recovery-oriented care as opposed to the medical model of care.[29,30] For each of the 11 evidence-based practices, SAMHSA offers toolkits and resources to guide design and implementation.

In addition to these 11 evidence-based practices, SAMHSA also maintains a national registry of more than 320 evidence-based programs and practices (refer to the resource list at the end of this section). Individuals or organizations can submit their practices for review by SAMHSA, which determines whether they meet minimum requirements; these include (1) the intervention has produced one or more statistically significant positive behavioral outcomes over a comparison group over time, (2) evidence of the positive behavioral outcomes has been demonstrated in at least one experimental or quasi-experimental study, (3) results have been published in a peer-reviewed publication or documented in a comprehensive evaluation report with sound methodology, and (4) training and implementation resources have been developed and are available to the public.

Unfortunately, clinical practice is not always evidence-based. The term "evidence-based practice" is not always used in such a rigorous fashion, and many clinicians claim to follow evidence-based approaches when the methods they use are unsubstantiated by systematic research,[31] or they overestimate their ability to deliver evidence-based practices.[32] In reality, there is often a large gap between what research has shown to be effective and actual practice. Many clinicians

Table 17.1 EVIDENCE-BASED PRACTICES FROM THE SUBSTANCE ABUSE AND MENTAL HEALTH SERVICES ADMINISTRATION (SAMHSA) KNOWLEDGE INFORMING TRANSFORMATION (KIT) SERIES

EVIDENCE-BASED PRACTICE	TARGET POPULATION	DESCRIPTION
Assertive Community Treatment (ACT)	Adults with severe mental illness	Service delivery model (treatment, rehabilitation, and case management) provided by interdisciplinary teams offering weekly visits, 24-hour support, and individualized services
Illness Management and Recovery (IMR)	Adults with severe mental illness	Step-by-step approach to educate individuals about their mental illness, set meaningful personal goals, and acquire skills to make progress in their goals
Permanent supported housing	Homeless adults	Subsidized housing (i.e., rental subsidy) with case management services (usually ACT-like services)
Supported employment	Adults with severe mental illness	Model that focuses on consumer choice, rapid job search, competitive employment, on-site job support, and time-unlimited support
Supported education	Adults with mental illness	Various program models that prepare, assist, and support individuals to pursue postsecondary education or training
Integrated Dual Disorders Treatment (IDDT)	Adults with mental illness and comorbid substance use disorders	An interdisciplinary team approach that offers mental health and substance abuse services at the same time, tailors interventions to the individual's stage of change, and emphasizes motivational interviewing and harm reduction
Family psychoeducation	Families of adults with severe mental illness	Interventions that elicit the collaboration and support of family members to foster an individual's recovery
Medication Treatment, Evaluation, and Management (MedTEAM)	Adults with severe mental illness	Principles of medication management that include appropriate use and dosing of psychotropics, documented rationale for medication selections, measurement of medication-related outcomes, and patient involvement in medication decisions.
Consumer-operated services		Programs operated by mental health consumers that emphasize peer support, self-help, and social inclusion
Treatment of depression in older adults	Older adults with depression, including dysthymia	An array of practices, including geriatric outreach services, psychogeriatric assessment, antidepressant medication, reminiscence therapy, cognitive-behavioral therapy, problem-solving treatment, and interpersonal psychotherapy
Interventions for disruptive behavior disorders	Children with disruptive behavior disorders	Various tools to prevent or reduce severe aggressive behavioral, emotional, and development problems by enhancing knowledge of parents, caregivers, and providers

lack training in evidence-based approaches, and members of the public are often unaware that evidence-based practices exist. Consequently, patients do not always receive the most effective, safe, and cost effective treatments available.

As mentioned, there are a number of resources of evidence-based practices for various psychiatric conditions. Lists of evidence-based and best practices have been maintained by different organizations with different criteria of what constitutes an evidence-based practice. Interested readers are referred to these resources:

- SAMHSA has a searchable online registry called the National Registry of Evidence-based Programs and Practices (NREPP) that contains more than 320 substance abuse and mental health interventions that have been determined to be evidence-based (http://www.nrepp.samhsa.gov/)
- Chambless and APA Division 12 provide a list of empirically supported therapies (http://www.div12.org/empirically-supported-treatments/)
- APA Task Force on Serious Mental Illness and Severe Emotional Disturbance have catalogued best practices for people with serious mental illness (http://www.apa.org/practice/resources/grid/catalog.pdf)
- Many state mental health departments have their own lists of evidence-based practices. For example, the Connecticut Department of Mental Health and

Addiction Services (DMHAS) currently has a list of 20 evidence-based practices with information and resources available for each evidence-based practice (http://www.ct.gov/dmhas/cwp/view.asp?q=472912)

In considering evidence-based practices in psychiatry, it would be remiss to not discuss the important role of patients in treatment and the fundamental shifts made toward person-centered care in mental health care and health care in general. Originating in the psychiatric rehabilitation field in the 1990s, there has been a national movement emphasizing the empowerment of patients in their own care and expanding the notion of recovery beyond symptom relief to quality of life and other life domains.[29] As stated in the 1999 US Surgeon General's report, mental health services are being called upon to be "consumer oriented and focused on promoting recovery,"[7:455] and the President's New Freedom Commission stated that mental health services should help patients to be "able to live, work, learn and participate fully in their communities."[8:44] Of course, the role of patients and the extent to which recovery-oriented practices may differ are influenced by treatment setting and circumstances.[30] But patients should be seen as active participants in their treatment and should be informed of their treatment options and the evidence for these options. The practice of psychiatry needs to offer evidence-based treatments that incorporate the individual needs and preferences of patients.

There may also be clinical conditions or situations in which there are no established evidenced-based practices, their use is inappropriate, or there are inadequate resources. In these situations, a less structured approach may have to be taken in which the best evidence available is used with clinical judgment to make informed clinical decisions about a specific population or setting where a clinical problem has been identified. This approach balances the clinical realities in practice with implementing an established evidence-based intervention. Some clinical settings are limited in their ability to pay for costs to train clinicians or change clinical practice. In these settings, a clinical team may assess the resources and barriers to implementing change and decide on a course of intervention as close to the evidence-based practice as feasible for them. For example, in a setting where a specific intervention like dialectical behavioral therapy may be recommended by the current "best evidence," it might impose cost on a setting to train an entire team in interventions; thus, approaches might involve training only a single clinician who uses this approach with the specified population, clinical consultation on implementation in the specific setting, or introduction of specific techniques targeting the problem or issue for that setting. However, clinicians using these approaches should be cautioned that these approaches may be divergent from the actual evidence-based practice and may not result in the same outcomes as found in the research.

TRAINING AND FIDELITY

Implementing principles of evidence-based medicine and evidence-based practices requires time and costs for training. Two main barriers to staff implementation of evidence-based practices are that clinicians often lack the necessary knowledge and skills to use these practices and certain organizational dynamics undermine the treatment teams' ability to implement and maintain innovative approaches.[33] Proper training can help overcome these barriers and is quintessential to encouraging and teaching staff how to use evidence-based practices. Training that is contextual and incorporates active learning can improve staff knowledge and attitudes.[34] Adequate training and staff adherence also ensures that evidence-based practices will be delivered as intended (i.e., fidelity), an issue that will be described later. Training can take a variety of forms, from in-service on-site trainings to intensive training retreats or workshops. Usually, a variety of materials are provided to trainees, such as treatment manuals, demonstration videos, worksheets, and other resources. Well-conducted trainings typically include an initial intensive training period followed by regular supervision and follow-up periods to ensure the training has been integrated into practice appropriately.

Expert consultants who have had experience with evidence-based practices often serve as the trainers. Clinicians can also be trained to be trainers by expert consultants, known as the *train-the-trainers* approach. Train-the-trainer models have also become widely used across various disciplines,[35–37] including for practices in the mental health field.[38,39] Technical assistance centers exist for some evidence-based practices to help and support organizations in training and implementation.[40,41]

Fidelity is an important indicator of training and implementation, and one that is necessary for quality assurance.[42] *Fidelity* refers to the degree to which a particular program follows a prescribed model of care or, in this case, an evidence-based practice. In other words, fidelity monitors the accuracy and consistency with which an intervention is implemented as planned. Fidelity measures are tools developed to assess a program's fidelity to an evidence-based practice model and increasingly are becoming standard requirements in monitoring implementation and for research.[43] Fidelity measures typically contain various domains that are rated on scales with anchor points indicating the degree to which a program's actual practice adheres to the evidence-based practice model. These scales are usually rated by independent consultants outside of the agency, such as from a technical assistance center, and information is gleaned from reviews of patient charts, interviews with various staff and leadership at the agency, consultant observations, and sometimes interviews with patients.

Examining fidelity over time is a crucial component of monitoring implementation because "fidelity drift" does occur.[44] Fidelity drift occurs when an agency's practice begins to deviate from the evidence-based practice model because of various factors, including time, staff turnover, insufficient leadership, and inadequate ongoing monitoring. These issues may need to be addressed with feedback from fidelity monitors, refresher trainings, working with leadership, finding champions for the cause, and the like. Research has shown that agencies that have greater fidelity to evidence-based practices tend to have better patient outcomes[44] and less staff turnover.[45,46]

An example of a large dissemination effort is the National Implementing Evidence-Based Practices project,[42] which disseminated five of the evidence-based practices shown in Table 17.1 in routine public mental health settings. Over a 2-year period, 53 community mental health centers across eight states implemented one of those evidence-based practices with moderate to high fidelity, with the first year being a critical time period for implementation.[42] This project showed that public mental health centers can implement evidence-based practices successfully, although there are various factors to consider and a multipronged implementation strategy is most effective.[47]

In breadth and scope, the VA has had the largest evidence-based practice dissemination initiative in the United States to date.[48] The VA is working to transform its mental health care system by nationally disseminating and training staff to implement a select number of evidence-based practices for mental and behavioral health conditions (refer to Table 17.3). The VA has focused on providing competency-based training for these evidence-based psychotherapies, which include participation in an in-person, experiential workshop and ongoing telephone-based clinical consultation on actual patient cases with an expert; this training lasts approximately 6 months and includes rating of sessions. To facilitate local implementation, there is a local evidence-based coordinator at each VA medical center throughout the country who acts as liaison to facilitate and monitor the implementation of these evidence-based psychotherapies (Table 17.2).

Table 17.2 TRAINING AND DISSEMINATION OF EVIDENCE-BASED PSYCHOTHERAPIES IN THE VETERANS HEALTH ADMINISTRATION[a]

EVIDENCE-BASED PSYCHOTHERAPY	CONDITION
Cognitive processing therapy	Post-traumatic stress disorder
Prolonged exposure therapy	Post-traumatic stress disorder
Cognitive-behavioral therapy for depression	Depression
Acceptance and commitment therapy	Depression
Interpersonal psychotherapy	Depression
Behavioral family therapy	Severe mental illness
Multiple family group therapy	Severe mental illness
Social skills training	Severe mental illness
Integrated behavioral couples therapy	Relationship distress
Cognitive-behavioral therapy for insomnia	Insomnia
Cognitive-behavioral therapy for chronic pain	Chronic pain
Motivational interviewing	Motivation and adherence
Motivational enhancement therapy	Substance use disorders
Contingency management	Substance use disorders
Behavioral couples therapy for substance use	Substance use disorders
Cognitive-behavioral therapy for substance use disorders	Substance use disorders

[a]Reprinted with permission[48]

In addition to psychotherapies, the VA has been diligent in ensuring that its formal policy documents outlining mental health treatment policy are informed by evidence-based practice literature. For example, handbooks that govern the delivery of services for specific conditions such as post-traumatic stress disorder (PTSD) include treatment guidelines that promote evidence-based psychotherapies and pharmacotherapies, as well as discourage pharmacotherapies found in the literature to be ineffective (e.g., the prescribing of benzodiazepines for patients with PTSD). The primary policy document for VA mental health services, the Uniform Mental Health Services Package, details what every VA facility is either required or strongly encouraged to provide for patients with mental health diagnoses. This document, which is written by the senior mental health leadership in VA and informed by content matter experts in each clinical area, incorporates the most recent evidence-based data to ensure that the mental health services provided have a proven track record of effectiveness. In addition to mandating that services be evidence-based, the VA also monitors compliance with these mandates through a large and extremely comprehensive evaluation program that tracks access, quality, and outcomes of mental health services.

The national VA initiative to implement evidence-based psychotherapies has also been followed by two national initiatives to improve prescribing practices for mental health disorders in VA. The first, a national psychotropic prescribing initiative, employs the electronic medical records system in VA to identify (1) variance in prescribing ("possible overprescribing"), such as patients on three or more classes of medication for depression, PTSD, or psychosis; 2) poor clinical management, such as patients on antipsychotics who have not been monitored for metabolic side effects and patients with gaps in antipsychotic medication possession; (3) poor alignment of prescribing, such as people receiving an antidepressant or a benzodiazepine with no documented mental health disorder or medical indication for the drug; and (4) under-met needs ("possible under-prescribing") such as patients with opiate dependence who have not been prescribed an opiate agonist or bipolar patients who have not been prescribed a mood stabilizer or atypical antipsychotic. Measures related to these four categories are calculated at the facility level quarterly, and facilities work collaboratively with mental health leadership to create action plans to address poor practices and to monitor improvement.

In collaboration with the psychopharmacology initiative, the VA also employs a program of *academic detailing* to assist facilities in making positive changes in prescribing practices. Itself an evidence-based intervention, albeit at the clinician as opposed to the patient's level, academic detailing programs partner content matter experts in psychotropic prescribing with clinical teams at each VA facility to review areas of improvement, establish likely points of effective intervention, assist with training and education for prescribers, and assist facilities to set reasonable and meaningful targets for change.

OTHER CHALLENGES WITH IMPLEMENTING EVIDENCE-BASED PRACTICES

The field of public psychiatry, like other fields, conducts research to identify evidence-based practices that yield the best outcomes for individuals in need, and it also needs to identify the best practices to implement those evidence-based practices. The field is further along in identifying evidence-based practices than it is in identifying how to fully implement the practices in real-world settings. The Schizophrenia Patient Outcomes Research Team (PORT) recommendations are an example of evidence-based practices being identified, but implementation lagging.[49] The average time for research-based interventions to be translated and implemented, even to modest degrees, is 17 years.[50] Identifying more evidence-based practices and evidence-based implementation strategies and shortening the time from discovery to delivery are the challenges.

Implementation challenges vary across settings. In public-sector programs, they commonly include workforce issues (e.g., high staff turnover), lack of agency resources to use a comprehensive implementation strategy, and clinicians' perceptions of evidence-based practices.[51] In particular, the workforce development issues are daunting, including low compensation, lack of cultural diversity, and limited competence in evidence-based treatments.[52]

IMPLEMENTATION STRATEGIES

Progress has been made in the emerging field of implementation science.[53,54] Fixsen's landmark monograph in 2005 provided an important articulation of stages of "implementation" and "core implementation components" or "implementation drivers" across diverse fields of inquiry. The stages are listed and defined in Table 17.3.

Core implementation components include recruitment and selection of staff, training, supervision and coaching, performance assessment, decision support data systems, facilitative administrative supports, systems interventions, and leadership. All these components may be necessary for full implementation and sustainability. For example, an implementation plan including only training, which is, unfortunately, common, is most likely to yield a small sustainable degree of implementation, if any, in comparison to an implementation plan that encompasses all eight implementation drivers. Research is beginning to tie degrees of fidelity improvement with specific implementation strategies.[55]

The Institute for Healthcare Improvement's Collaborative Model for achieving breakthrough improvement is another example of promising work done from an implementation perspective.[56,57] In this model, experts and participating organizations or teams are identified. Teams identify specific measurable aims that they want to achieve

Table 17.3 STAGES OF IMPLEMENTATION

STAGE OF IMPLEMENTATION	DESCRIPTION
Exploration and adoption	Organization explores which innovation to implement.
Program installation	Active preparation to do activities in accordance with the EBP (e.g., funding obtained, human resource activities, policy development).
Initial implementation	Changes begin for the implementation to take place. Challenges include people's fear of change, inertia, and investment in the status quo.
Full operation	New learning becomes integrated into practitioner and organizational practices, policies and procedures.
Innovation	Based on skillful performance of the EBP, it may be discovered that the practice needs to refined or expanded in one or more ways. Important to distinguish this from fidelity drift.
Sustainability	Despite internal and external changes and factors, long-term survival or implementation of the EBP is achieved.

(e.g., implementation of an evidence-based practice). Learning lessons are held, and teams go through action periods between learning sessions, including a series of Plan, Do, Study, Act cycles.

The SAMSHA offers models to guide change or process improvement in behavioral health settings that can be useful in practice or process innovation. They have a series of Technical Assistance Publications that offer information and resources on implementing change in practices (http://store.samhsa.gov/list/series?name=Technical-Assistance-Publications-TAPs-). For example, the "Implementing Change in Substance Abuse Treatment Programs"[58] publication provides guidance about ways to conceptualize the change process and steps to implement best practices. There are other sources of information and links to models that can be used in process improvement, such as the Network for the Improvement of Addiction Treatment or NIATx (http://www.niatx.net/Home/Home.aspx). NIATx offers information on how to plan focused changes in organizations that consider feasibility to promote outcomes and sustainability of results. These materials offer ways to implement evidence-based interventions in the reality of clinical practice settings, thoughtfully bringing together the two described approaches of research-based and practice-based implementation.

USING TECHNOLOGY IN EVIDENCE-BASED PSYCHIATRY

COMPUTERIZED SEARCHES FOR EVIDENCE

A multitude of electronically available resources can be used to assist the practice of using evidence in clinical settings. They include web-based resources on clinical problems and interventions, organization-specific health information about patient care, online databases and search engines that offer efficient ways to find evidence about clinical practice, and web-based information from organizations and governmental agencies that catalog completed research.

There are various electronic databases to find research evidence to answer particular clinical questions that arise in practice. These databases include peer-reviewed articles, official reports, dissertations, monographs, and various other sources of information. Some of these databases are available to the general public (e.g., Google Scholar, PubMed), whereas others are available through academic institutions and health care systems (e.g., Web of Science, Scopus). Specific databases of the medical and psychiatric literature (e.g., MEDLINE), psychology (e.g., PsycINFO), sociology (e.g., Sociological Abstracts), nursing (e.g., CINAHL), and many other health-related fields should also be utilized when searching for evidence to guide practice. A few additional databases are worth noting, such as the Health and Psychosocial Instruments (HAPI) database, which is a resource for various instruments, measures, rating scales, and studies using these measures or reporting on their development and validity; and Embase, a multipurpose database suited for studies related to pharmacology, drugs, and the biomedical literature.

Secondary sources also exist that provide summarized reports of the evidence available. For example, the British Medical Journal (BMJ) Group has a series of journals: *Evidence-Based Medicine* (http://ebm.bmj.com/), *Evidence-Based Mental Health* (http://ebmh.bmj.com/), and *Evidence-Based Nursing* (http://ebn.bmj.com/). The American College of Physicians (ACP) Journal Club, UpToDate, and the Turning Research into Practice (TRIP) database are also good secondary sources for review of studies, practice guidelines, and critically appraised topics and articles. A well-known organization that synthesizes research literature by conducting systematic reviews and meta-analyses on a range of topics is the Cochrane Collaboration, which operates the Cochrane Library (http://www.thecochranelibrary.com/view/0/index.html). The Cochrane Library includes the Cochrane Database of Systematic Reviews, the Database of Abstracts of Reviews of Effectiveness, and the National Health

Service Economic Evaluation Database. Many government agencies also offer reviews of studies and health-related topics on their websites, including the National Institutes of Health, the National Institute of Mental Health, and the SAMSHA.

There are now even phone-based applications for some of these aforementioned databases that provide access to the medical literature as well as drug references, medical calculators, and diagnostic aids.[59] However, further research is needed on their use and the best ways to incorporate these applications into regular clinical practice.

USE OF ELECTRONIC MEDICAL RECORD SYSTEMS

With increasing adoption of electronic medical records and health policy initiatives supporting their adoption,[60,61] electronic medical record systems represent great potential in improving health care not only through improving documentation methods,[62,63] but also because they can provide recommended treatment approaches to clinicians in real-time and provide feedback on outcomes and benchmarks in clinical practice on the back-end. Aggregated information from medical records may also be useful for administrators and for program evaluation purposes, as well as for monitoring implementation of evidence-based practices.

There are many tiers or levels of electronic information available that can contribute to a better understanding of clinical problems identified in practice, ranging from availability of basic electronic data to implementation of fully integrated electronic medical records. Basic administrative data available in many settings provide information to inform clinicians about patient characteristics and relevant outcomes including length of stay, admission and discharge information, work and housing information, and clinical diagnoses. As systems evolve to include fully integrated electronic medical records, specific information about clinical status, medications, health service use, interventions, and outcomes can be used to inform clinical decisions and provide follow-up information to evaluate outcomes of the use of evidence-based practices. Various advanced features are being developed for electronic medical records to support real-time evidence-based guidelines, clinical reminders, communication with patients and between health care providers, and other computerized clinical decision support systems in addition to medical charting.[64-66]

The electronic information available within psychiatric settings can also be useful sources of information about the quality of mental health services provided. Mining information available in the organization provides an efficient way to answer clinical questions and examine ways to improve the quality of services. Challenges in the future will be in developing user-friendly management systems that allow clinicians to input data and measures to track the implementation of interventions and receive feedback on their effects. In addition, designing measures to monitor fidelity to evidence-based practices is critical to attaining successful outcomes. Making these advances in psychiatry will improve the process by which clinical questions are answered, evidence-based practices are implemented, outcomes are evaluated, and progress is made in improving systems of care in public psychiatry.

FUTURE OF EVIDENCE-BASED PSYCHIATRY

The future of psychiatry holds great promise, especially as the field continues to emphasize and focus on using systematic evidence to guide its development. Although great strides have been made to increase our understanding of effective treatments in psychiatry and to disseminate those treatments to clinicians who can effectively employ them, much remains to be done. Efforts at every level of the system can be brought to bear in order to continue to improve mental health services nationally. These include the incorporation of empirical data into legislation and policy for agencies delivering mental health services; funding rigorous research to identify and disseminate existing and novel interventions, along with defined standards for what constitutes an acceptable evidence base; having informed research agendas that guide scientists toward expanding the evidence base and away from further testing of interventions that do not meet standards; and increasing academic partnerships with public laboratories, such as community mental health centers and national mental health care systems like as the VA, so that research can be conducted in real-world settings and so that scientific findings can be more quickly translated into practice.

Legislative and policy bodies continue to improve in the incorporation of evidence-based research in their deliberations. However, it can be a struggle to define what constitutes evidence[67] and to overcome political agendas that may contradict the evidence base. For example, pharmaceutical companies, who are large campaign contributors, have effectively blocked legislative and policy decisions that would damage sales of their particular drugs even when research shows them to be ineffective. Similarly, powerful lobby groups such as clinician associations (e.g., American Medical Association, American Psychiatric Association, etc.) and advocacy groups (e.g., NAMI) can use political and financial arguments to preserve treatment practices that have been shown to be ineffective. The future of evidence-based psychiatry must continue to have champions who challenge these positions and continue to be the voice for implementing evidence-based practices. For public agencies with mental health policies, such as the VA and state mental health programs, leadership should be vigilant in ensuring that policy is informed by and supportive of evidence-based practices.

In Connecticut, the state spends hundreds of millions of dollars on mental health services and addiction treatment through at least five state agencies that vary on how much money they spend on evidence-based programs or "best practice" approaches. For example, in 2013, the Department of Mental Health and Addiction Services reportedly spent about 31% of $259 million in grants to private, nonprofit organizations for evidence-based programs.[68] The Department of Social Services reportedly spent 15% of $153 million on behavioral health programs that were evidence-based, and the Department of Children and Families reportedly spent 20% of $125 million on programs that had some evidence base.[68] Similar rates have been observed in other states as well, although many are moving toward more state-wide implementation of evidence-approaches in mental health.[70,71] For example, Oregon passed a law to ensure that 75% of state-funded mental health services are evidence-based,[69] which has led to more widespread adoption of evidence-based practices and demonstrates the power of legislation. It is reasonable for legislatures and taxpayers to demand accountability for public dollars being spent on mental health services. The question is how to best purchase, measure, and document the use of evidence-based approaches. There have been a couple of national policy initiatives working on this, such as Results-Based Accountability (RBA)[70] and Results First.[71]

Research funding is, of course, a cornerstone to improving our understanding of effective treatment in mental health. However, funding agencies effectively make policy statements through their strategic funding decisions. Calls for proposals, strategic plans, and other documents issued by funding agencies help set the tone for what is considered to be an adequate evidence base and what areas of research are most likely to be considered favorably. Requiring a sufficient level of rigor in grant proposals and funded studies helps to improve the evidence base. In addition, however, strategic decisions about funding priorities will drive researchers toward identifying more effective interventions. Funding agencies can also reduce the time between research and implementation by continuing to require realistic but effective dissemination plans. To this end, traditional mechanisms, such as conference presentations and manuscript publication, should be enhanced through the use of the great advances in digital technology seen in the past decade in order to reduce the time it takes for effective interventions to become known and disseminated.

Funding agencies can set funding priorities, but they rely on review panels of researchers to peer-review proposals. Although peer review is an essential part of a rigorous health research environment, it can also fall prey to pressure to fund "business as usual" and studies of least incremental effect. Study groups and their review officers should, of course, strive to maintain methodological rigor, but they should also allow for much more innovation and creativity. The fact is that there is unlikely to be any miracle drug that cures any psychiatric disorder, and much more research needs to be done to support the development of psychotherapeutic interventions, psychosocial interventions, skills building, and recovery-oriented services.

Finally, public psychiatry takes place in huge national "laboratories," in clinical settings where services are delivered. Academic partnerships between public agencies and faculty not only supply agencies with talented clinical staff, they also provide the opportunity for those staff to identify innovation opportunities, to test new ideas, and to monitor the effects of established interventions in real-world settings. In addition, academic partnerships allow agencies to tap the talent of faculty in order to accurately assess whether services are evidence-based, whether they are being delivered as intended, and how effective they are. For this reason, formal program evaluation strategies should continue to be implemented in these settings to continually monitor service structures, processes, and outcomes. Such data can not only serve to inform the evidence base itself, but can also shape service systems by identifying gaps, opportunities, deficiencies, positive deviance, and effective implementation strategies.

SUMMARY

If the field of psychiatry is to advance, it must rely on research, be patient-oriented, and utilize data-driven approaches. Identifying and implementing evidence-based practices can be challenging, but are necessary for care that is accountable and reimbursable. Psychiatry must rise beyond its unscientific beginnings to an era of practice based on systematic research to best serve our patients. Although the quality of mental health treatment has improved dramatically since even the mid-20th century, much remains to be done.

As so much of mental health care is delivered in this country through federal and community agencies, the role of public psychiatry is immensely important. Establishing firm values to identify and support interventions that are actually shown to be effective through rigorous testing and are receptive to patients will not only improve mental health systems nationally, but improve the mental health of the nation as a whole.

REFERENCES

1. Porter R. *Madmen: A Social History of Madhouses, Mad-Doctors & Lunatics.* Stroud, UK: Tempus; 2004.
2. Scull AT. *Madhouses, Mad-Doctors, and Madmen: The Social History of Psychiatry in the Victorian Era.* Philadelphia: University of Pennsylvania Press; 1981.
3. Foucault M. *Madness and Civilization: A History of Insanity in the Age of Reason.* New York: Random House; 1988.
4. Conolly J. *The Treatment of the Insane without Mechanical Restraints.* New York: Cambridge University Press; 2013.
5. Davison GC, Neale JM. *Abnormal Psychology.* 8th ed. New York: Wiley; 2001.
6. Overholser W. Modern trends in psychiatry. *Psychiatr Q.* 1950;24(4):645–656.
7. Department of Health and Human Services. *Mental Health: A Report of the Surgeon General.* Rockville, MD: US Department of Health and Human Services, Substance Abuse and Mental Health Services Administration, Center for Mental Health Services, National Institutes of Health, National Institute of Mental Health; 1999.
8. President's New Freedom Commission on Mental Health. *Achieving the Promise: Transforming Mental Health Care in America.* Rockville, MD: President's New Freedom Commission on Mental Health; 2003.
9. Hogan MF. New Freedom Commission report: the president's New Freedom Commission: recommendations to transform mental health care in America. *Psychiatr Serv.* 2003;54:1467–1474.
10. Barry CL, Huskamp HA, Goldman HH. A political history of federal mental health and addiction insurance parity. *Milbank Q.* 2010;88:404–433.
11. Barry CL, Huskamp HA. Moving beyond parity: mental health and addiction care under the ACA. *N Engl J Med.* 2011;365:973–975.
12. Busch SH. Implications of the Mental Health Parity and Addiction Equity Act. *Am J Psychiatry.* 2012;169:1–3.
13. Consolidated Appropriations Act., §Section 8(o)(19) (2008).
14. Petersen LA, Woodard LD, Urech T, Daw C, Sookanan S. Does pay-for-performance improve the quality of health care? *Ann Intern Med.* 2006;145:265–272.
15. Epstein AM. Will pay for performance improve quality of care? The answer is in the details. *N Engl J Med.* 2012;367:1852–1853.
16. Dudley RA, Miller RH, Korenbrot TY, Luft HS. The impact of financial incentives on quality of health care. *Milbank Q.* 1998;76:649–686.
17. Schroeder SA, Frist W. Phasing out fee-for-service payment. *N Engl J Med.* 2013;368:2029–2032.
18. Sackett DL, Rosenberg WM, Gray JA, Haynes RB, Richardson WS. Evidence based medicine: what it is and what it isn't. *Br Med J.* 1996;312:71.
19. Agency for Healthcare Research and Quality. *Methods Guide for Effectiveness and Comparative Effectiveness Reviews.* AHRQ Publication No. 10(14)-EHC063-EF. Rockville, MD: Agency for Healthcare Research and Quality; 2014.
20. Harris RP, Helfand M, Woolf SH, et al. Current methods of the US Preventive Services Task Force: a review of the process. *Am J Prev Med.* 2001;20:21–35.
21. Centre for Evidence-based Medicine. Oxford Centre for evidence-based medicine- levels of evidence. http://www.cebm.net/?o=1025. Published March 2009. Accessed March 3, 2014.
22. Guyatt G, Oxman AD, Akl EA, et al. GRADE guidelines: 1. Introduction- GRADE evidence profiles and summary of findings tables. *J Clin Epidemiol.* 2011;64:383–394.
23. Ebell MH, Siwek J, Weiss BD, et al. Strength of recommendation taxonomy (SORT): a patient-centered approach to grading evidence in the medical literature. *J Am Board Fam Pract.* 2004;17:59–67.
24. Lohr KN. Rating the strength of scientific evidence: relevance for quality improvement programs. *Int J Qual Health Care.* 2004;16:9–18.
25. West S, King V, Carey TS, et al. *Systems to Rate the Strength of Scientific Evidence: Summary.* AHRQ Publication No. 02-E015. Rockville, MD: Agency for Healthcare Research and Quality; 2002.
26. Atkins D, Eccles M, Flottorp S, et al. Systems for grading the quality of evidence and the strength of recommendations. I: critical appraisal of existing approaches. The GRADE Working Group. *BMC Health Serv Res.* 2004;4:38.
27. Chambless DL, Hollon SD. Defining empirically supported therapies. *J Consult Clin Psychol.* 1998;66:7.
28. Chambless DL, Baker MJ, Baucom DH, et al. Update on empirically validated therapies, II. *Clin Psychol* 1998;51:3–16.
29. Anthony WA. Recovery from mental illness: the guiding vision of the mental health service system in the 1990s. *Psychosoc Rehabil J.* 1993;16:11–23.
30. Tsai J, Salyers MP. Recovery orientation in hospital and community settings. *J Behav Health Serv Res* 2010;37:385–399.
31. Berke DM, Rozell CA, Hogan TP, Norcross JC, Karpiak CP. What clinical psychologists know about evidence-based practice: familiarity with online resources and research methods. *J Clin Psychol.* 2011;67:329–339.
32. Brosan L, Reynolds S, Moore RG. Self-evaluation of cognitive therapy performance: do therapists know how competent they are? *Behav Cogn Psychother.* 2008;36:581–587.
33. Corrigan PW, Steiner L, McCracken SG, Blaser B, Barr M. Strategies for disseminating evidence-based practices to staff who treat people with serious mental illness. *Psychiatr Serv.* 2001;52:1598–1606.
34. Beidas RS, Kendall PC. Training therapists in evidence-based practice: a critical review of studies from a systems-contextual perspective. *Clin Psychol Sci Pract.* 2010;17:1–30.
35. Orfaly RA, Frances JC, Campbell P, Whittemore B, Joly B, Koh H. Train-the-trainer as an educational model in public health preparedness. *J Pub Health Manag. Pract.* 2005;11: S123–S127.
36. Green ML. A train-the-trainer model for integrating evidence-based medicine training into podiatric medical education. *J Am Podiatr Med Assoc.* 2005;95:497–504.
37. Corelli RL, Fenlon CM, Kroon LA, Prokhorov AV, Hudmon KS. Evaluation of a train-the-trainer program for tobacco cessation. *Am J Pharm Educ.* 2007;71:109.
38. McHugh RK, Barlow DH. The dissemination and implementation of evidence-based psychological treatments: a review of current efforts. *Am Psychol.* 2010;65:73.
39. Fitzgerald MA, Chromy B, Philbrick CA, Sanders GF, Muske KL, Bratteli M. The North Dakota Mental Health and Aging Education Project: curriculum design and training outcomes for a train-the-trainer model. *Gerontol Geriatr Educ.* 2009;30:114–129.
40. Salyers MP, McKasson M, Bond GR, McGrew JH, Rollins AL, Boyle C. The role of technical assistance centers in implementing evidence-based practices: lessons learned. *Am J Psychiatr Rehabil.* 2007;10:85–101.
41. National Association of State Mental Health Program Directors. *Technical Assistance for State Mental Health Agencies.* http://www.

nasmhpd.org/TA/NTAC.aspx. Published 2013. Accessed May 3, 2014.
42. McHugo G, Drake RE, Whitley R, et al. Fidelity outcomes in the national implementing evidence-based practices project. *Psychiatr Serv.* 2007;58:1279–1284.
43. Bond GR, Evans L, Salyers MP, Williams J, Kim HW. Measurement of fidelity in psychiatric rehabilitation. *Ment Health Serv Res.* 2000;2:75–87.
44. McGrew JH, Bond GR, Dietzen L, Salyers MP. Measuring the fidelity of implementation of a mental health program model. *J Consult Clin Psychol.* 1994;62:670.
45. Aarons GA, Sommerfeld DH, Hecht DB, Silovsky JF, Chaffin MJ. The impact of evidence-based practice implementation and fidelity monitoring on staff turnover: evidence for a protective effect. *J Consult Clin Psychol.* 2009;77:270.
46. Rollins AL, Salyers MP, Tsai J, Lydick JM. Staff turnover in statewide implementation of ACT: relationship with ACT fidelity and other team characteristics. *Adm Policy Ment Health Ment Health Serv Res.* 2010;37:417–426.
47. Bond GR, Drake RE, McHugo GJ, Rapp CA, Whitley R. Strategies for improving fidelity in the national evidence-based practices project. *Res Social Work Pract.* 2009;19:569–581.
48. Karlin BE, Cross G. From the laboratory to the therapy room: national dissemination and implementation of evidence-based psychotherapies in the US Department of Veterans Affairs Health Care System. *Am Psychol.* 2014;69:19.
49. Aarons GA, Hurlburt M, Horwitz SM. Advancing a conceptual model of evidence-based practice implementation in public service sectors. *Adm Policy Ment Health Ment Health Serv Res.* 2011;38:4–23.
50. Aarons GA, Wells RS, Zagursky K, Fettes DL, Palinkas LA. Implementing evidence-based practice in community mental health agencies: a multiple stakeholder analysis. *Am J Public Health.* 2009;99:2087–2095.
51. Dixon LB, Dickerson F, Bellack AS, et al. The 2009 schizophrenia PORT psychosocial treatment recommendations and summary statements. *Schizophr Bull.* 2010;36:48–70.
52. Hoge MA, Stuart GW, Morris J, Flaherty MT, Paris M, Goplerud E. Mental health and addiction workforce development: federal leadership is needed to address the growing crisis. *Health Aff (Millwood).* 2013;32:2005–2012.
53. Fixsen DL, Naoom SF, Blase KA, Friedman RM, Wallace F. *Implementation Research: A Synthesis of the Literature.* Tampa: University of South Florida, Louis de la Parte Florida Mental Health Institute, The National Implementation Research Network; 2005.
54. Institute for Healthcare Improvement. *The Breakthrough Series: IHI's Collaborative Model for Achieving Breakthrough Improvement.* Boston, MA: Institute for Healthcare Improvement; 2003.
55. Institute of Medicine. *Crossing the Quality Chasm: A New Health System for the 21st Century.* Washington, DC: National Academy Press; 2001.
56. Kilo CM. A framework for collaborative improvement: lessons from the Institute for Healthcare Improvement's Breakthrough Series. *Qual Manag Health Care.* 1998;6:1–14.
57. McGovern MP, Lambert-Harris C, McHugo GJ, Giard J, Mangrum L. Improving the dual diagnosis capability of addiction and mental health treatment services: implementation factors associated with program level changes. *J Dual Diagn.* 2010;6:237–250.
58. Substance Abuse and Mental Health Services Administration. *Implementing Change in Substance Abuse Treatment Programs, TAP 31.* Rockville, MD: Substance Abuse and Mental Health Services Administration; 2009.
59. Mosa ASM, Yoo I, Sheets L. A systematic review of healthcare applications for smartphones. *BMC Med Inform Decis Mak.* 2012;12:67.
60. Berner ES, Detmer DE, Simborg D. Will the wave finally break? A brief view of the adoption of electronic medical records in the United States. *J Am Med Inform. Assoc.* 2005;12:3–7.
61. Palacio C, Harrison JP, Garets D. Benchmarking electronic medical records initiatives in the US: a conceptual model. *J Med Syst.* 2010;34:273–279.
62. Tsai J, Bond G. A comparison of electronic records to paper records in mental health centers. *Int J Qual Health Care.* 2008;20:136–143.
63. Hillestad R, Bigelow J, Bower A, et al. Can electronic medical record systems transform health care? Potential health benefits, savings, and costs. *Health Aff (Millwood).* 2005;24:1103–1117.
64. Bates DW, Kuperman GJ, Wang S, et al. Ten commandments for effective clinical decision support: making the practice of evidence-based medicine a reality. *J Am Med Inform Assoc.* 2003;10:523–530.
65. Garg AX, Adhikari NKJ, McDonald H, et al. Effects of computerized clinical decision support systems on practitioner performance and patient outcomes: a systematic review. *JAMA.* 2005;293:1223–1238.
66. Tsai J, Rosenheck RA. Use of the internet and an online personal health record system by US veterans: comparison of Veterans Affairs mental health service users and other veterans nationally. *J Am Med Inform Assoc.* 2012;19:1089–1094.
67. Tanenbaum SJ. Evidence-based practice as mental health policy: Three controversies and a caveat. *Health Aff (Millwood).* 2005;24:163–173.
68. State must benchmark human services programs. *Hartford Courant.* http://www.courant.com. Published April 26, 2013.
69. Oregon Addiction and Mental Health Services. *Evidence-based Practices.* http://www.oregon.gov/oha/amh/pages/ebp/main.aspx. Accessed April 1, 2014.
70. Fiscal Policy Studies Institute. *Results-Based Accountability (RBA) & Outcomes-Based Accountability (OBA).* http://www.resultsaccountability.com/. Accessed April 1, 2014.
71. The Pew Charitable Trusts. *Pew-MacArthur Results First Initiative.* http://www.pewstates.org/projects/pew-macarthur-results-first-initiative-328069. Accessed April 1, 2014.

18.

ADMINISTRATIVE BEST PRACTICES IN PUBLIC PSYCHIATRY

Andres Barkil-Oteo, Margaret Bailey, Robert Cole, Miriam Delphin-Rittmon, Susan Devine, Selby C. Jacobs, Jeanne L Steiner, Louis Trevisan, and Michael J. Sernyak

> ### EDUCATIONAL HIGHLIGHTS
>
> - The field of public psychiatry must develop knowledge on the current best practices in administration and leadership in public psychiatry.
>
> - Arguments to whether psychiatrists make good administrators are as old as the field itself.
>
> - Psychiatrists are afforded multiple opportunities for meaningful involvement within public-sector settings in the role of a medical director.
>
> - A Population health perspective is becoming increasingly important for leaders and managers of health systems.
>
> - Although there are many effective treatments for mental health disorders, there is a discrepancy between what's known to be effective and the care delivered to patients. Quality improvement practices efforts could help mitigate this gap.
>
> - Meaningful Productivity measures should focus on outcomes measures along process measures.
>
> - Program development and innovation in public psychiatry often occurs through informal trial-and-error strategies. However systematic program planning can lead to a more nuanced and effective programs.
>
> - Psychiatry trainees should be actively encouraged to pursue careers in leadership and administration in public psychiatry through specialized tracks in residency.

BRIEF HISTORY

As early as the expansion of community mental health centers in the 1960s, a debate ensued as to whether mental health professionals would make suitable administrators. The reason clinicians were employed originally was due to a lack of qualified mental health administrators—business administrators with no mental health experience were seen as unfit for the role—and because clinicians were deemed qualified by virtue of their experience working with patients. Furthermore, it was suggested that the knowledge clinicians would use in dealing with patients could also be used for dealing with employees.[1] While admitting the difficulties in having clinicians with nonmanagerial experience running program centers, there was general agreement that the model of clinician-executive was the best fit for mental health systems, despite some notable dissent from people arguing that clinicians should be true to their training and leave administrative activities to administrators.[2]

Proponents of the clinician as administrator based their arguments on the clinicians' knowledge and awareness of the purposes and needs of mental health care clinics. One of the earliest studies on the position of psychiatric administrator found that because the clinician executive could navigate the fiscal and the clinical aspects of patient care, he or she was especially effective in advocating for patients' well-being.[3] A second benefit was that the clinician's highly developed interpersonal skills could be helpful in managing conflicts within the organization. Many authors conceded that, despite any shortcomings in the clinician-executive managerial idea, clinicians were more equipped to lead mental health systems, and they would be more successful overall, than administrators with no clinical background. Levinson and Klerman agreed that clinicians may be particularly suited to become administrators because their "appropriate concern for the feelings and personal needs of the organization's members will facilitate, not hinder, their efforts to build the organization."[4] O'Neill emphasized that "only a good practicing psychiatrist can really be a good administrative psychiatrist."[1]

Dissenters found these arguments overly optimistic. Watchel found the presumption of administrative expertise in clinicians to be somewhat dubious and warned about specialty bias: that is, whether one's clinical training would lead him or her to favor one therapeutic modality over another, regardless of its appropriateness for the center's needs, or whether one's focus on individual pathologies could lead to neglect of systemic problems.[5] There have been many calls to fill knowledge gaps common among clinician administrators in such diverse areas as politics, finance, labor management, and negotiation with outside agencies.[6]

INTRODUCTION: THE STRUCTURE OF LEADERSHIP

The topic of adopting administrative best practices in the changing public psychiatry system begs the question of whether the current administrative structures of public psychiatric programs are optimal. The constellation of senior leadership usually includes a chief executive officer (CEO), a chief operating officer (COO), a medical director, and a director of clinical services (CD), often with the support of a chief financial officer (CFO) and/or a chief information officer (CIO). Many community mental health centers also have a director of community-based services (CSD). For the purpose of this discussion, the "structure of administration" will refer exclusively to the structure of senior leadership in community behavioral health centers, even though this structure is replicated down throughout the organization's administration of clinical divisions and units.

The senior leadership group in community behavioral health centers is responsible for articulating the vision, defining the mission, upholding the values, deploying the strategies, and implementing all the functions described as "best practices." One example of the latter is the employment of an interdisciplinary team (IDT) approach, which provides a model for administrative interaction within the entire organization. The IDT approach is reflected at the service level by the clinical team, where we have collaboration between a CD who is responsible for clinical services (implementing new evidence-based treatments and new electronic medical record-keeping, dealing with human resources issues, and coordinating services among inpatient, outpatient, community, and emergency units), and a medical director, who heads the medical programs. The CD relates not only to the COO, but also to all the other officers in senior leadership. Communication and cooperation permeate the administration of community behavioral health centers.

ROLE OF MEDICAL DIRECTOR

Psychiatrists are afforded multiple opportunities for meaningful involvement within public-sector settings and among them is the position of medical director. A medical director can be situated at various levels within an organization or system of care: from a team, program, or agency to a hospital, service system, or state. The specific duties and job descriptions will be adapted to the needs of the entity and the expertise of the individual psychiatrist. Because the actual title of medical director can denote a diverse array of responsibilities and levels of authority based on the breadth and hierarchy of a particular organization, it is useful to consider several roles and tasks that are relevant to the position in many public psychiatry venues.

The leadership of clinical teams or programs is a role for psychiatrists that has been examined closely for several decades.[7-10] Such leadership positions generally combine varying proportions of administrative oversight and direct service, and there is evidence that the overall job satisfaction for many program medical directors is associated with higher degrees of administrative responsibility.[11] There are five key responsibilities of these positions: (1) to provide medical and psychiatric assessments of individual patients and to synthesize these data with other perspectives within an interdisciplinary team, (2) to evaluate and oversee a risk management plan, (3) to promote collaboration among team members by recognizing and addressing group dynamics that might reflect patient characteristics or organizational conditions, (4) to recommend appropriate levels of care for patients within the program, and (5) to ensure adherence to regulatory guidelines and standards of care. Other tasks or responsibilities may include the supervision of other physicians and clinical staff, leading initiatives to improve unit performance, and monitoring staff development.

Medical directors at the agency level perform the same basic tasks as just outlined, with an expanded scope and level of authority. A detailed list of guidelines, principles, and a "model job description for the system medical director" can be found on the American Academy of Community Psychiatry (AACP) website.[12] Physician leaders are responsible, along with senior colleagues from other disciplines, for assuring the overall quality of clinical care provided within an institution, which requires them to oversee many aspects of the delivery of care. Risk management, which is described in more detail in Chapter 8, comprises a complex set of medical-legal considerations that can be particularly challenging in settings designed for individuals with serious mental illness and substance use disorders. The medical director must be knowledgeable about the clinical, ethical, and legal aspects of risk management and be able to access appropriate expert consultation when indicated.

Medical directors can and should assume leadership roles for program development and innovation in order to participate in the quality of the care provided by their organizations. With their background in scientific method and critical examination of evidence, these physician leaders should facilitate the application of new findings into clinical practice, along with the measurement of the outcomes of these interventions. In addition to assuring compliance with the requirements of relevant regulatory agencies, such as the Joint Commission, Centers for Medicare and Medicaid Services (CMS), and the Commission on Accreditation of Rehabilitation Facilities (CARF), psychiatrists in administrative positions ought to establish meaningful performance improvement initiatives based on the needs of the individuals served in that setting.

Advocacy within the system of care is another critical role for medical directors at any level of authority. This includes advocating for patients under care who are vulnerable by virtue of their symptoms, stigma toward those with mental illness, poverty, and other social factors. Physicians must collaborate with the CEO, other administrators, staff, and consumers to ensure that the service system is recovery-oriented and that the policies and procedures set forth by the medical staff and administrators promote patient-centered care in a healing environment. Advocacy for staff and patients includes the assurance of adequate staffing, appropriate physician caseloads, and professional work conditions.

Perhaps the most critical and meaningful duty of medical directors within public-sector settings is to promote the training, recruitment, and retention of other medical staff. The medical director serves as a role model in each day of her or his work, providing expertise and direction in the six areas of competency delineated by the Accreditation Council for Graduate Medical Education (ACGME): patient care, medical knowledge, practiced-based learning and improvement, interpersonal and communication skills, professionalism, and system-based practice.[13] Leadership can be demonstrated in numerous venues, including formal and informal teaching, case discussions, consultation, individual supervision, and facilitation of communication between clinical staff and administration.

As described in Chapter 16, the skills and knowledge necessary for modern-day medical leadership are taught within psychiatric residency programs and public psychiatry fellowships, but all medical directors have the opportunity to promote the development of their successors by inspiring others to assume leadership roles and improve care for the individuals served. The mentoring of other psychiatrists and providing them with the resources and support they require to work effectively within IDTs and to provide the highest quality of patient-centered care benefits the profession and its institutions.[14]

ROLE OF CLINICAL DIRECTOR

The role of a CD within a public psychiatric service setting is generally held by a professional who is licensed, certified, or registered to practice in one of several core disciplines: psychiatry, nursing, psychology, or social work. The CD is generally responsible to the CEO for the direction of the clinical staff, often in collaboration with the heads of specific disciplines and other clinical leaders. The CD typically possesses significant clinical skill and experience, which is brought to bear on the range of administrative and supervisory responsibilities attendant to the position.

In a large organization, the CD typically works as a member of a larger management team, with duties that vary and may be carried out in collaboration with other team members. In a public psychiatry service setting with academic affiliations, the CD must also support and contribute to both the education of trainees from a variety of disciplines and the implementation of research protocols within the organization's clinical teams and programs.

As part of the management team, the CD contributes to the development of the organization's infrastructure by participating in decisions about service design. These may include helping to clearly define the portals of entry to services and the criteria for admission to various clinical programs, as well as the selection, implementation, and evaluation of evidence-based treatments and other service initiatives. In addition, the CD plays a major role in the establishment and maintenance of collaborative relationships with referral sources and with other members of the community provider network, including area hospitals; providers of housing, social rehabilitation, and vocational programming; the Probate Court; and the criminal justice system.

Perhaps the most satisfying but complex responsibility of the CD in a public psychiatric setting involves accountability for the quality of patient care and for workforce development. The CD is often charged with the development of policies and procedures to guide patient care, as well as with the adherence to regulatory guidelines for clinical programs. In addition, the CD is responsible for addressing difficult clinical problems, often in collaboration with the organization's risk manager and other clinical leaders: providing or accessing consultation; facilitating communication and collaboration between clinical staff and community providers in order to obtain a higher level of care; or advocating for additional clinical and/or fiscal resources to better address a client's treatment or community support needs. Workforce development responsibilities include accountability for the selection of clinical staff and maintenance of the staffing schedule: the crafting of job descriptions, orientation requirements, and performance measures, as well as the assignment of staff, comprise a significant part of the CD's work in this regard. The CD must be accountable for the adequacy of staffing within the budget constraints that frequently impact the public service system, thus necessitating an ability to assess service needs, reallocate resources, and support clinicians who may become overwhelmed when clinical demands exceed staffing resources. Often, the CD must be able to negotiate service and staffing changes made necessary by budgetary limitations in the context of union influence and oversight. Accountable for the overall supervision of staff performance—much of which is delivered by team- or program-level clinical supervisors—the CD must collaborate with other organization leaders to assess staff development needs and facilitate access to appropriate consultation, clinical supervision, training, and education. Opportunities to support the professional development of staff are extremely important to the culture of the public service system, contributing to workforce satisfaction and retention, as well as to the delivery of high-quality, recovery-oriented care.

ROLE OF THE ADMINISTRATIVE LEADER: OPERATING AND FINANCING PUBLIC PSYCHIATRY

It is a commonly held misconception that the role of the administrative leader in public psychiatry begins and ends with budgeting and accounting. Although the critical nature of fiscal/budgetary management cannot be overemphasized, there are any number of equally vital roles and responsibilities typically under the direction of the administrative leader. These range from taking a leadership role in high-level strategic planning to the provision of adequate parking. They also include the direction and oversight of information management (including medical records, clinical information systems, and network/LAN management); internal and external communications; community and legislative relations; fundraising and donor relations; clinical support services; care management (including admission/registration, utilization management, billing interface, and liaison with entitlement agencies); security and safety programs; collaboration with risk management; liaison and/or oversight over legal affairs; housekeeping and plant operations; food and nutritional services; monitoring the pharmacy and clinical laboratory; HIPAA and CMS compliance; regulatory affairs, including Joint Commission accreditation and licensure if applicable; staff training; and patient advocacy. Understanding the breadth and depth of the administrative leader's role will help clinical leaders to appreciate the importance of their close coordination with administrative leaders.

As is the case in any organization, it is simply not possible to plan, manage, or evaluate in a reasonable way without paying close attention to financial (revenue and expenses), human, and capital resources. Without strategic and operational attention to resources, the organization will neither thrive nor survive, so all individuals with leadership responsibilities must recognize the critical roles that resource planning and management play. Key aspects of resource management include the generation of revenue from clinical encounters and allocations or grants (from government or other sources); the covering of operating expenses, including the costs of labor and contractors, utilities, and supplies; human resource management, including staff recruitment, retention, performance evaluation, credentialing and privileging, and labor relations (especially when organized labor is involved); and capital planning, budgeting, and project management.

The role of the administrative leader in public psychiatry is broad and multifaceted but focused on finances and resources. A close, collaborative working relationship between the individual occupying this role (usually titled chief administrative officer, COO, deputy director for administration, or executive director) and clinical leaders is of key strategic and operational importance to the organization. Although it is essential that clinical leaders possess a certain level of knowledge and degree of comfort with financial and human resource management and other administrative/operational functions, it is of equal or greater significance that they appreciate the importance of a symbiotic relationship with those in the organization charged with administrative leadership roles.

WHY POPULATION HEALTH?

A population health perspective is becoming increasingly important for leaders and managers of health systems. Population health emerged recently as a conceptual term that transcends existing notions of public health, going beyond collective actions to assure general health (e.g., water and sewer systems, public sanitation agencies, pollution guidelines, mandatory vaccinations) by incorporating analysis and research into the widest possible number of determinants that influence the health of populations (for a more detailed discussion, see Chapter 7). Population health defines and measures the personal, social, and environmental conditions, and systematic variations among these variables, that ought to be considered in the development of policies to improve a population's health and well-being. The ultimate purpose of population health policy is "to improve the health of individuals and populations by investments in the determinants of health through policies and interventions that influence these determinants."[15]

The term requires us to define two essential concepts: health and population. Over the years, the term "health" meant strictly physical health, but this is changing as mental health is being increasingly recognized as an essential part of health: there is "no health without mental health," according to the World Health Organization (WHO). Populations, on the other hand, used to be defined according to geographical location but now include any group of people who share common attributes, like the population served by one clinic or having one condition like diabetes or depression.

To make an impact on the determinants of mental health, services must be organized accordingly. Services must affect determinants on the individual and societal level. Studies shows that while some people seem to be overtreated, others have problems accessing services: such problems could be an artifact of the way services are organized, where limited capacity in clinics in terms of physical space and trained personnel result in many barriers to accessing services. This in turn leads to specialty mental health services dealing exclusively with severe mental illness. As a result, mental health programs are often criticized for their lack of access to the general population.

A population health approach offers a different paradigm. By providing interventions to mitigate risks across the total population (vaccination and anti-smoking campaigns, exercise promotion) and identifying social factors that contribute to poor health (e.g., the socially disadvantaged have poorer health outcomes in every domain, including higher rates of morbidity, disability, and mortality),[16] a population health approach looks beyond the treatment of specific conditions found in one segment of the population; instead it concerns itself with the health concerns of the whole population and provides interventions to mitigate risk across the total population.

A health system that aims to provide for both the general population and vulnerable groups must provide a spectrum of interventions, from universal interventions to after-care. As described in an Institute of Medicine (IOM) report[17] these interventions should be evidence-based whenever possible.

Prevention of conditions may be achieved through universal, selective, or indicated interventions. *Universal interventions* aim to improve mental health at the population level through psychoeducation and outreach over mass media in order to promote awareness, enhance resilience, and mitigate risk factors, including suicide and violence among people with mental illness. *Selective interventions* focus on special populations who are at higher risk of developing disorders, seeking to work by providing specific interventions to mitigate risk. Examples of this approach are found in school-based programs (e.g., preschool programs for children from poor neighborhoods), maternal health programs, group therapy (e.g., support groups for people in bereavement), and the debriefing of those suffering from trauma. *Indicated interventions* are aimed at individuals who are at very high risk of developing a disorder, such as programs that target prodromal teenagers.

Early intervention, diagnosis, and treatment of well-known short-term conditions are carried out through *case identification* and *standard treatment*. Effective case identification targets individuals who are identified in clinical settings or through outreach programs, and it is essential to providing effective treatment, especially for conditions that are underrecognized and exhibit access problems, like depression in primary care and people with first-break psychosis. *Standard treatment of known disorders* refers to the provision of evidence-based treatment for patients who have been assessed, diagnosed, and followed-up, with the goal of restoring well-being and achieving recovery.

Longer term treatment interventions are *rehabilitation* (sometimes called *tertiary prevention*) and *after-care*. The former targets people with chronic conditions, aiming to provide treatment, rehabilitation, and support to prevent recurrence. This category includes rehabilitation services, such as educational, vocational, and social programs that aim to introduce people with mental illness to the workforce and enhance their cognitive functioning. After-care provides long-term maintenance and care for people with severe mental illness. Its goals are to maintain quality of life and functioning and to provide continuous support. Such treatment should commence as early as possible after diagnosis.

From a public health perspective, there is always tension in the way services are organized, between focusing on the general population (*improving the average* approach) and the vulnerable population (*high-risk* approach). The high-risk approach focuses on individuals with the highest possibility of developing the disease, either to bring their risk down to that of the general population or to help them recover quickly. Improving the average approach focuses on the entire population and aims to mitigate the risk for everyone. Both approaches are important, and a preference for one or the other depends on the specific situation. Mental health care has traditionally preferred the high-risk approach, giving greater focus to the vulnerable population sometimes at the expense of the general population. This reflects too great an emphasis placed on the concept of mental illness (alterations in thinking, mood, or behavior associated with distress or impaired functioning) and not enough emphasis placed on mental health (the successful performance of mental function resulting in productive activities, fulfilling relationships, and the ability to adapt to change and adversity).

RISK MANAGEMENT

Another important issue for systems is risk and managing risk. Risk management programs in public psychiatry are an integral, essential component in ensuring that the system fulfills its mission and meets its commitments to patients, staff, and the community. The goals of risk management policies are to identify areas of current or anticipated risk and maintain a preventative strategy to limit injuries to patients, staff, guests, and the community at large. It is essential to create highly specific and comprehensive work rules aimed at minimizing injury. Risk management activities, to be effective, must be broad-based and multidisciplinary, highly sensitive to patient and staff needs, and understood as a responsibility of every employee. Regular educational programs (for current clinical and administrative staff) and thorough orientation (for new employees) in service education, along with special meetings in response to high-risk clinical events (e.g., peer-reviewed critical incident reviews), are specific examples of activities targeted to mitigate risk among staff members.

From the patients' perspective, risk management begins from the commencement of the staff–patient relationship: the most significant factor contributing to patient dissatisfaction and potential litigation is the breakdown of communication between a staff person and a patient.

Effective oral and written communication diminishes potential risks and contributes to positive outcomes. Because the patient's medical record captures all aspects of the patient's care and provides an ongoing source of information regarding all aspects of the patient's treatment in written form, skill and attention to detail in completing this record are paramount. Direct, authentic oral communication and a clinical staff who maintain a respectful, recovery-oriented approach, listen carefully to their patient's concerns, and share with their patients specific insights regarding their condition make positive steps in supporting patient satisfaction and mitigating risk. Staff who communicate poorly and disrespectfully incite patient dissatisfaction and escalate the risk of litigation. Sensitivity and respect for patients and their vulnerabilities and rights are key components in decreasing dissatisfaction and enhancing positive patient outcomes. Overall risk is decreased by professional, sensitive awareness of patient vulnerabilities: family, social, and community pressures; poverty and homelessness; lack of social support and stigma; and medical and legal problems. A sound risk management approach (as well as good clinical practice) includes sensitivity to each patient's unique vulnerabilities.

Actively *involving patients in all aspects of their care* enhances the care provided. Inherent in active patient involvement and recovery-oriented care is protection of patients' rights. Public psychiatry practices should be committed to ensuring that all patients' rights are respected and that all persons understand the rights that they are entitled to, particularly the right to be treated in a humane and dignified manner, free from coercion, abuse, or harm at all times. One key right is that all persons must be afforded the greatest possible degree of freedom. Adult patients must not be detained if they want to leave, except as prescribed by statute. The use of involuntary seclusion or restraint should be limited to cases when the patient presents an imminent physical risk. Privacy is another crucial patient right: patients expect that all information about themselves, including their medical record, will be kept confidential.

All patients must be informed of the identity and role of all persons involved in their care. Competent adults have the right to refuse care from their care providers without consequences. They also have the right to participate and be present and involved in all aspects of their treatment. Adequate, understandable information must be provided to patients in order for them to give informed consent for any treatment. Finally, when unexpected and/or negative outcomes occur, patients and/or appropriate family/significant others should be informed as soon as possible.

The recovery process from serious and persistent mental illness always involves some exposure to risk because it is inherently part of this process. Although risk can never be eliminated, it can surely be minimized by maintaining an awareness of the principles just described, including attention to effective oral and written communication, providing ample opportunity for staff education and development, and maintaining scrupulous respect for the rights and dignity of all patients.

PRODUCTIVITY IN THE WORKFORCE

Although the US health system spends twice as much as other developed nations, health outcomes in the United States are comparably poor. Improving the productivity of health care systems is often cited as one of the most difficult tasks for administrators and policy-makers. In economics, *productivity* is defined as the measure of output that can be produced given a combination of inputs. Productivity can be measured at the unit level or globally as a system. At the unit level, for example, the productivity of a hospital might be measured by examining the health outcomes (output) resulting from the resources (input) invested by the hospital. It is also important to distinguish between the average and marginal productivity of systems. The average productivity of a system measures total output relative to total input, whereas marginal productivity is the change of the output resulting from a change in input. Average productivity is useful for the purpose of comparing existing systems, whereas marginal productivity is better suited for a consideration of whether more money should be spent on health care. For example, if we were interested in comparing the productivity of US hospitals, we would look at their average productivities in order to decide which one has the greatest output per input unit. However, if we wish to measure how many more visits per physician would result after investing in a new health system, then we would need to look marginal productivity.[18]

Some authors argue that our current measures of productivity tend to reflect an interest of the health care system—that is, to provide more services—rather than the interests of the population, which are to stay healthy and avoid the need for hospitalization. Current health productivity indicators largely measure the utilization of health services quantitatively: number of visits, missed appointments, discharge rates, bed occupancies, and average length of stays.[19] Such "throughput" measures reflect a metric common in service industries—productivity as number of units delivered. However, in health care, the ultimate goal is not to deliver surgeries, computerized tomography (CT) scans, or outpatient visits, but to utilize these services in order to produce a qualitative output, which is the health of the people utilizing these services.

Useful measures of health care productivity must include those that consider whether treatments are evidence-based, of high quality, and inclusive of patients' values. Measuring providers' productivity by number of visits won't account for either the quality of the visits or whether clients are benefiting, because a highly productive provider could be one providing low-quality service and vice versa. The Patient-Centered Outcomes Research Institute (PCORI) (created under the Affordable Care Act), will encourage research on identifying interventions that have meaningful impacts on health outcomes.

QUALITY IMPROVEMENT IN PUBLIC MENTAL HEALTH SERVICES

More than 34.6 million adults (14.6% of the adult population) received mental health treatment in an inpatient or outpatient setting in 2012.[20] Millions more stated that they want mental health or substance use treatment but didn't receive it.[20] According to the Substance Abuse and Mental Health Services Administration (SAMHSA), only 44.7% of adults with any mental illness and 68.5% of adults with serious mental illness received mental health services.[20]

Although there are many effective treatments for mental health disorders, there is a discrepancy—similar to that found in medical care—between what's known to be effective and the care delivered to patients. A major review of studies assessing the quality of care for many mental illnesses and substance use disorders concluded that only 27% of the studies reported satisfactory rates of adherence to recognized clinical practice guidelines.[21] This difference between the quality of care delivered and established clinical guidelines is defined as the *quality gap*. Later studies documented the same quality gap in the treatment of many specific mental health disorders, including attention deficit hyperactivity disorder, anxiety disorders, depression in both adults and children, and schizophrenia.[22] One notable study highlighted that the quality gap for alcohol dependence treatment is as great as 90%.[23] Such poor-quality treatment has many consequences. Failure to accurately diagnose and treat mental illness can lead to fatalities in some cases. Approximately 9.3 million American adults (3.9%) had serious thoughts of suicide in the past year; of these, 2.7 million (1.1%) made suicide plans and 1.3 million (0.6%) attempted suicide. In addition, the use of seclusion and restraints in inpatient mental health facilities is estimated to cause 150 deaths in the United States each year.[24]

These qualitative shortcomings in the delivery of mental health care are another manifestation of the inconsistencies in quality of care being delivered throughout our entire health care system. The issues of the quality gap and inadequate treatments received wide attention after two IOM reports: *To Err Is Human: Building a Safer Health System*,[25] and *Crossing the Quality Chasm: A New Health System for the 21st Century*,[26] The Quality Chasm report proposed a six-point framework for achieving improved quality in health care. Following the same paradigm, the IOM published another report devoted entirely to mental health and substance use delivery systems.[27] The report highlighted some of the attributes of the mental health sector that distinguish it from the general health sector, including the higher stigma faced by people with mental health and substance use disorders, the need for better coordination between clinicians and agencies treating the wide range of mental health and substance use problems, and the incomplete development of a system to capture data on the quality of care and ways to improve it.

The report highlighted the issues of providing patient-centered care and avoiding coercion. Clinicians and systems of care should aim to incorporate patient-centered decision-making tools in their practices. To ensure informed decisions, different options for treatment should be explained. Patient values are denied by default whenever a patient's choice of treatments is restricted to a limited number of similar options. A meaningful choice experience should include options that are significantly different but complementary. The treatment process should be based on a collaborative approach that is balanced with the provision of informed choices and an offer of all evidence-based alternatives. People with mental illness, like all other members of our society, have the right to self-determination, which means that the patient will decide the direction and nature of the intervention, with the provider occupying a consultative and supportive role.[28] This process could be made more transparent by sharing with patients and family members the policies that guide the evaluation and determination of endangerment and of impairment of one's decision-making capacity. The use of psychiatric advance directives should be explained and encouraged, and wider adoption of screening instruments and evidence-based treatments should be implemented.

Among the screening instruments feasible for daily use are patient questionnaires and other patient assessment tools such as the Audit C and CAGE questionnaire, for alcohol abuse; the Patient Health Questionnaire-2 (PHQ2) or PHQ9, for depression; and the Post-traumatic Stress Disorder Checklist (PCL) for PTSD. These tools are designed to capture patient progress and outcomes over the course of treatment. To encourage the delivery of evidence-based treatments, the report suggested implementing coordinated efforts to disseminate evidence-based treatment among clinicians in order to build a system capable of measuring the quality of care it delivers and encouraging quality improvement projects in clinical sites to diagnose problems in delivery and to devise local solutions to any issues that are discovered.

PROGRAM DEVELOPMENT, INNOVATION, AND EVALUATION IN PUBLIC PSYCHIATRY

Program development, innovation, and evaluation are vital to carrying out a public mental health center's vision and mission. Program development involves a process of planning, implementing, and evaluating a program or intervention in response to an identified need at the service delivery, community, organization, or health care system level, and it is aimed at improving outcomes related to the identified need. Innovation can be defined as the "introduction of a new concept, idea, service or product aimed at improving treatment, diagnosis, education, outreach, prevention, and research, with the long-term goal of improving quality, safety, outcomes, efficiency and costs."[29] Program development and innovation are related processes in that program development typically involves the implementation of an innovation; however, not all innovations are carried out through the development of a program (e.g., a policy requiring clinicians to provide clients with a signed copy of their treatment plan is an innovation that can be implemented without a specific program being developed).

Leadership within a public mental health setting is continually faced with the challenge of needing to prioritize which service delivery, workforce, or other need to address and in what manner and timeframe. An important initial step in this process is the gathering of information about areas where change or innovation is needed. Formal measures such as needs assessments, consumer satisfaction or staff cultural climate surveys, and reviews of client and agency performance and outcome data can all inform prioritization of needed programming. In addition, the use of informal approaches, such as observation and discussions with community members and other relevant stakeholders, can inform decisions about how to prioritize program development and innovation.

Once needs have been identified, several strategies can be used by leadership to inform decision-making about where to intervene. First, alignment of possible interventions with the mental health center's current vision, mission, and strategic priorities should be considered. Although needs that are particularly aligned may be important to prioritize, those that are not well-aligned should also be considered because they may highlight new areas of needed innovation not previously considered that could significantly improve health or other organizational outcomes.

Second, leadership will need to consider both fiscal resources and existing staffing capacity when deciding when and how to address identified needs. Planning programs in a staggered manner based on short, intermediate, and long-term timelines may help to offset budgetary or staff constraints. In addition, planning more costly innovations in combination with less costly programs, rather than implementing high-cost interventions simultaneously, may help to reduce overall point-in-time costs.

Finally, because innovation can emerge from brainstorming and discussions among members of complex teams, convening interdisciplinary committees can be beneficial. These should include people in recovery from mental health and substance use disorders, front-line staff, and community members to assist with program prioritization and planning. Adopting such a participatory action approach, in which collaboration, equity, and diversity in ideas are valued, can lead to increased credibility, trust, and cultural responsiveness to a service or program. In addition, including community members and recovering individuals in the program planning and implementation processes can help to reduce stigma and improve access and engagement in care.

STEPS TO REALIZING A PROGRAM OR INNOVATION

Program development and innovation in public psychiatry often occurs through informal trial-and-error strategies, as well as through the use of more systematic and established program development approaches. Although trial-and-error program development can lead to the development of impactful innovations, such approaches are usually less efficient and more costly if multiple "tweaks" and iterations of the program are put in place before a preferred or successful model is identified.

Systematic program planning can lead to the development of more nuanced and effective programs. Key steps in the program development process are these:

- *Identify the problem.* The problem is the need to be addressed through the program. Problem identification can occur through the needs assessment strategies described earlier.

- *Establish the program development team.* As in problem prioritization, convening an IDT that includes diverse staff and relevant stakeholders, including people in recovery, will help to ensure that important program details are considered in the innovation planning process.

- *Develop a program description and model.* A program description presents the issue to be addressed through the program along with its intended outcomes and may be used to inform the development of a program model. A program model, in turn, outlines the broader theory of change for a program and presents the relationship between major program components. A logic model is a commonly used framework for presenting how a program will create specific changes over time. Figure 18.1 presents an example of a logic model for an outreach training program. As illustrated, a logic models displays the relationship between program activities and includes specific detail regarding short-, intermediate-, and long-term outcomes, which can be particularly useful for evaluation planning.

- *Plan the evaluation.* An evaluation of a program should be planned as part of the program development process. The evaluation directly relates to the program model in that the evaluation plan addresses the manner in which components of the program model will be assessed.

INPUTS	ACTIVITIES	OUTPUTS	SHORT-TERM OUTCOMES	INTERMEDIATE OUTCOMES	LONG-TERM OUTCOMES
• Training team which includes peer trainers • Budget • Community Partners • Evaluation team • Training space • Time	• Focus groups • Design curriculum • Advertise workshop • Conduct workshop series • Conduct follow-up technical assistance	• Case managers attend training • Supervisors attend training • Outreach workers attend training • Peer providers attend training	• Increased knowledge of cultural issues in help-seeking • Increased knowledge of outreach strategies and community resources • increased knowledge of one's own cultural beliefs and values	• Providers network with churches, shelters, and other community supports • Providers ask about cultural preferences • Increased client access • Increased client engagement	• Increase in days housed • Reduced criminal justice involvement • Reduced substance use • Increased employment • Improved quality of life

Figure 18.1 Institute of Medicine Report[17]

In planning an evaluation, both process and outcome evaluations should be considered because each provides important information about the overall program. Process evaluations assess the outcomes related to the program activities and outputs, whereas outcome evaluations assess the extent to which the proposed short-, intermediate-, and long-term outcomes are achieved. An evaluation plan also includes the data analytic strategy to be used to synthesize information collected during the evaluation process.

- *Implement and evaluate the program.* Development of a project plan or workflow that outlines tasks, timelines, persons responsible, and benchmarks for specific implementation and evaluation activities can be a useful tool for carrying out and keeping a project on track. A project workflow can serve as a blueprint for project staff and can be used by the project director to guide oversight and supervision.

- *Use evaluation findings for program improvement.* Program evaluation findings can be used by program staff to improve and strengthen an innovation over time. Components of the program found to work can be continued, whereas those that do not produce the intended outcomes can be modified or discontinued. Creating such continuous quality improvement feedback loops contributes to the sustainability of a program and helps to ensure alignment of the innovation with the mental health center's vision and mission.

TRAINING LEADERS FOR TOMORROW'S HEALTH CARE SYSTEM

People enter health care from different professional disciplines and have a wide variety of career goals, including research, teaching, and providing direct clinical care. Acknowledging the lack of administrative training, some programs are moving toward specialized tracks for trainees who want more exposure to leadership roles. These tracks largely focus on three components: specialized curriculum, experiential learning in the form of a project, and mentorship by a clinician leader.[30] Although, currently, mental health professionals are often identified and promoted to leadership positions based on their career achievement, there is a need to move toward the idea "cultivated leadership," in which trainees are exposed early on to leadership training and opportunities.

The goal here would not be to prepare every clinician to be a CEO, but to cultivate leadership skills as an important component within the training of students. Front-line clinician leaders, those delivering the day-to-day services, are as important as the CEO to the success of health delivery system because they are the catalysts for effective clinical teams.[31] There is strong evidence that good leadership skills lead to good clinical outcomes. Once we understand that leadership traits are essential to the delivery of effective clinical services in our increasingly complex health care system, we are compelled to make leadership one focus of our training.

Leadership requires not only business experience but also elements of self-control. The leader's mood and behavior drive the mood and behavior of everyone else in the organization, which ultimately affects the bottom line.[32] Emotional Intelligence Research showed that managing for financial results begins with the leader managing his or her inner life, so that the right emotional and behavioral elements appear. A leader's mood has the greatest impact on performance when it's upbeat, but it must also be attuned with the people around him, which is called "resonance." Goleman's article[32] argued that the process of self-awareness and mood management can be taught. As part of their training, mental health professionals tend to be very familiar with these skills. Is it possible that this ability makes them better leaders not just for mental health services, but also for health care in general? Obviously, not all trainees will have this ability, and many of them may not be good leaders or want to have anything to do with administration; but, if we emphasize the importance of these skills for students both for the success of their clinical duties as well as for potential leadership roles in the future, more trainees will be disposed to take managerial roles. One particular educational activity, *quality and patient safety rounds,* is being adopted in several training programs in an effort to involve trainees not simply in providing clinical services, but also in reviewing system performance and brainstorming different solutions. These rounds provide a mechanism for reviewing cases in any venue of the system that has become problematic. Cases are brought to the attention of staff members because of poor outcomes of treatment, missed handoffs, suicide attempts, medication overdoses or mistakes, patient complaints, and complaints from ancillary or other medical/consulting services. This meeting primarily emphasizes systems improvement and does not allow accusations, blaming, or complaining about other staff behavior. It is meant to look at the sentinel event, the facts of the case, and then trace the actions back to see how the system of care operated. One effective tool to use in these discussions is the *fishbone (Ishikawa) diagram*.[33] These meetings help to delineate factors in poor outcomes or near misses and organize finding appropriate solutions. Staff and trainees, along with quality management and interested administrative personnel, are invited to learn from the case and to share their expertise in this attempt to reduce the probability of a recurrence of similar incidents.

SUMMARY

In this chapter, we discussed some of the administrative issues that individuals leading public mental health systems today will face. It is evident that this is an increasingly complex system that requires proficiency in many aspects of leadership. Understanding these different leadership modalities, how they interact with each other, how to think about the mission of the system as a whole, and how to evaluate and improve the system are crucial elements of leadership in public mental health systems. Many of these skills are not formally taught in training programs and are only acquired on the job. Thus, there is a need for clinicians to become competent in a variety of management skills if they are to lead and change our current system into one featuring high-performing, high-quality services that adopt patient-centered care and evidence-based practices.

REFERENCES

1. O'Neill FJ. On administrative psychiatry. *Psychiatr Q.* 1970;44:359–365.
2. Kal EF. Are we losing psychiatrists to administrative positions? *Am J Psychiatry.* 1971;128:365–366.
3. Hawkes RW. The role of the psychiatric administrator. *Adm Sci Q.* 1961;6:89–106.
4. Levinson DJ, Klerman GL. The clinician-executive: some problematic issues for the psychiatrist in mental health organizations. *Psychiatry.* 1967;30:3–15.
5. Wachtel AS. Therapeutic orientation: a handicap in mental health administration. *American Journal of Psychiatry.* 1966;8:916–919.
6. Hinkle A, Burns M. The clinician-executive: a review. *Adm Ment Health.* 1978;6:3–21.
7. Langsley DG, Barter JT. Psychiatric roles in the community mental health center. *Hosp Community Psychiatry.* 1983;34:729–733.
8. Clark GH Jr, Vaccaro JV. Burnout among CMHC psychiatrists and the struggle to survive. *Hosp Community Psychiatry.* 1987;38:843–847.
9. Ranz J, McQuistion HL, Stueve A. The role of the community psychiatrist as medical director: a delineation of job types. *Psychiatr Serv.* 2000;51:930–932.
10. Pollack D, Minkoff K. The medical director's role in organized care delivery systems. In: Talbot J, Hales R, eds. *The Textbook of Administrative Psychiatry.* 2nd ed. Arlington, VA: APPI; 2001:83–92.
11. Ranz J, Stueve A. The role of the psychiatrist as program medical director. *Psychiatr Serv.* 1998;49:1203–1207.
12. American Association of Community Psychiatrists. AACP guidelines for psychiatric leadership in organized delivery systems for treatment of psychiatric and substance disorders. *Comm Psychiatrist.* 1995;9:6–7. http://www.communitypsychiatry.org/publications/clinical_and_administrative_tools_guidelines/leadership.aspx. Accessed March 2014.
13. Accreditation Council for Graduate Medical Education. *ACGME Common Program Requirements.* http://www.acgme.org/acgmeweb/Portals/0/PFAssets/ProgramRequirements/CPRs2013.pdf. Published 2013. Accessed March 2014.
14. Sowers W, Pollack D, Everett A, Thompson KS, Ranz J, Primm A. Progress in workforce development since 2000: advanced training opportunities in public and community psychiatry. *Psychiatr Serv.* 2011;62:782–788.
15. Kindig DA, Stoddart G. What is population health? *Am J Public Health.* 2003;93:380–383.
16. Marmot M. Social determinants of health inequalities. *Lancet.* 2005;365:1099–1104.
17. Institute of Medicine. *Reducing Risks for Mental Disorders: Frontiers for Preventive Intervention Research.* Washington, DC: National Academy Press; 1994.
18. McKellar R, Chernew M, Colucci J. *Productivity Measurement in the United States Health System.* The New America Foundation. http://www.newamerica.org/downloads/McKellar_Chernew_Colucci_NAF_10_2013.pdf. Published 2013. Accessed January 2015.
19. Hussey PS, De Vries H, Romley J, et al. A systematic review of health care efficiency measures: health care efficiency. *Health Serv Res.* 2009;44:784–805.
20. Substance Abuse and Mental Health Services Administration. *2013 National Survey on Drug Use and Health: Mental Health Findings.* Rockville, MD: Substance Abuse and Mental Health Services Administration; 2014.
21. Bauer MS. A review of quantitative studies of adherence to mental health clinical practice guidelines. *Harv Rev Psychiatry.* 2002;10:138–153.
22. Pincus HA, Page AEK, Druss B, Appelbaum PS, Gottlieb G, England MJ. Can psychiatry cross the quality chasm? Improving the quality of health care for mental and substance use conditions. *Am J Psychiatry.* 2007;164:712–719.

23. McGlynn EA, Asch SM, Adams J, et al. The quality of health care delivered to adults in the United States. *N Engl J Med*. 2003;348:2635–2645.
24. Substance Abuse and Mental Health Services Administration. *Roadmap to Seclusion and Restraint Free Mental Health Services*. Rockville, MD: Substance Abuse and Mental Health Services Administration; 2014.
25. Institute of Medicine. *To Err Is Human: Building a Safer Health System*. Washington, DC: National Academy Press; 2000.
26. Institute of Medicine. *Crossing the Quality Chasm: A New Health System for the 21st Century*. Washington, DC: National Academy Press; 2001.
27. Institute of Medicine. *Improving the Quality of Health Care for Mental and Substance-Use Conditions*. Washington, DC: National Academy Press; 2006.
28. Corrigan PW, Angell B, Davidson L, et al. From adherence to self-determination: evolution of a treatment paradigm for people with serious mental illnesses. *Psychiatr Serv*. 2012;63:169–173.
29. Omachonu VK, Einspruch NG. Innovation in healthcare delivery systems: a conceptual framework. *Innovation J*. 2010;15:1–20.
30. Ackerly DC, Parekh A, Stein D. Perspective: a framework for career paths in health systems improvement. *Acad Med*. 2013;88:56–60.
31. Blumenthal DM, Bernard K, Bohnen J, Bohmer R. Addressing the leadership gap in medicine: residents' need for systematic leadership development training. *Acad Med*. 2012;87:513–522.
32. Goleman D. What makes a leader? *Harv Bus Rev*. 2004;8:91–114.
33. QAPI. *How to Use the Fishbone Tool for Root Cause Analysis*. Centers for Medicare and Medicaid Services. http://www.cms.gov/Medicare/Provider-Enrollment-and-certification/QAPI/downloads/FishboneRevised.pdf. Accessed February 10, 2015.

19.

CONCLUSION AND FUTURE CHALLENGES

Selby C. Jacobs, Samuel A. Ball, Larry Davidson, Esperanza Díaz, Joanne DeSanto Iennaco, Thomas J. McMahon, Robert M. Rohrbaugh, Jeanne L. Steiner, Thomas H. Styron, Michael J. Sernyak, and Howard Zonana

---

EDUCATIONAL HIGHLIGHTS

- Public psychiatry concerns itself with the pragmatics of caring for people with serious mental illnesses and addictions.
- The field of public psychiatry is in the midst of a major transition. Change and evolution of public psychiatry is the norm during the modern era.
- Multiple new policies and factors are contributing currently to change. They include policies on reform of insurance, service delivery, and practice; expansion of access; accountability; quality control; prevention; person-centered care; recovery; protection of society; social challenges; and scientific discovery.
- Analysis of the variables currently changing the system and practice of public psychiatry provides a framework for thinking about institutional and professional development.
- Public–academic partnerships can play important roles in supporting and advancing the field of public psychiatry.
- Divisions of public psychiatry in academic departments of psychiatry are instrumental in supporting careers in the public sector.
- In light of its scope and significance, public psychiatry is a true subspecialty of psychiatry with an essential mission of serving people with serious mental illnesses and/or substance use disorders.

INTRODUCTION

This textbook was planned and written to describe public psychiatry as we know it at present. Yet public psychiatry is hardly a field in a steady state. New policies are molding the system, and public practice will change significantly over the next several years. What are the forces of change? What are the implications of these developments for the practice of public psychiatry? How might academic centers support public authorities and professionals who pursue careers in public psychiatry? How might public authorities and academic centers partner to manage change? How might academic departments better organize to prepare professionals for public psychiatry? This final chapter addresses these questions.

The first chapter introduced the textbook, providing definitions, an overview of the content, and editorial comments on the significance of public psychiatry as well as the need for a textbook at this point in time. In addressing the questions posed in the Introduction, here, we continue in the vein of editorial comment, pulling together the broad and disparate topics covered throughout the textbook. Through this editorial voice, the first and last chapters serve as bookends for the textbook.

INTELLECTUAL DIALECTICS AND PRAGMATISM

A recent vision for community mental health, offered on the 50th anniversary of landmark 1963 legislation and published in a leading professional journal, called for "a new vision of community mental health for the next 50 years, exploring the inner space of the brain."[1] Appealing and desirable as this scientific agenda is, unfortunately, it is not enough for public psychiatry. It ignores the immediate needs of people with serious mental illnesses (SMIs) and co-occurring or independent substance use disorders (SUDs). It neglects the system of services and the developmental, integrative tasks it faces.

Public psychiatry needs a bigger vision. The profession of psychiatry as a whole needs to pay attention not only to an intellectual, scientific, and research agenda but also, based on evaluation, to the pragmatic development, improvement, and stewardship of its system of care, especially for the most vulnerable people it serves. Public psychiatry, as a subspecialty of general psychiatry, plays an essential role in this broader agenda and needs a broader vision for it.

A historical perspective of modern psychiatry suggests that it periodically averts its attention from immediate, pragmatic tasks. Prior to World War II, Kraepelinian, organic, and diagnostic theory dominated practice. Practice took place largely in state hospitals. In the post-World War II era, military psychiatrists returned from service overseas with great optimism for psychiatric services in the United States and a "can do" attitude. Psychoanalysis eventually prevailed as the dominant intellectual discipline, creating not only distance between psychiatry and the rest of medicine but also diversion from the task of treating large numbers of people with chronic illnesses in state psychiatric hospitals. The community mental health movement of the 1960s, infused with ideas from public health and a commitment to community-based services, emerged out of these postwar circumstances as an alternative. The first phases of community psychiatry focused on the construction of community mental health centers, but the early movement failed to adequately care for chronically ill people coming out of state hospitals and struggling in the community. Gathering steam in the 1980s, neuroscience became the preeminent scientific and intellectual discipline, promising that biological psychiatry would soon solve the etiologic and pathogenetic puzzles of severe and persistent psychiatric diseases. Although each of these movements offered incremental change through insights, new treatments, and new community-based services, none of them relieved psychiatry from the task of caring for people with persistent and disabling SMIs and/or SUDs.

Through these intellectual currents, public psychiatry has had to appropriate discoveries to the extent they were useful and steer a course for the here and now that was always more pragmatic than the hoped-for developments and discoveries. In doing so, public psychiatry has taken charge of the vulnerable, core population of people with SMIs and/or SUDs. Public psychiatry must continue to shoulder these responsibilities until new breakthroughs in understanding etiology and treatment arrive. For the professional in public psychiatry, just as important as discoveries from the inner space of the brain are discoveries and evidence from clinical research, clinical trials, services research, evaluations of rehabilitation and community supports, and psychiatric epidemiology.

In short, invoking a Pascalian notion of the infinitely small and infinitely large, professionals in public psychiatry must attend not only to the molecular function of the brain, but also to the environment, society, and a system of services, and everything in between, needed to serve people with SMIs and SUDs. The building block of public psychiatry is the encounter between a person seeking help and an interdisciplinary team of professionals who, in a person-centered recovery context, mobilize a system of care in service of the person who is ill. Person-centered care has become a vehicle for achieving a more pragmatic clinical process that is optimal for meeting the variable and complex needs of people with severe and persistent behavioral disorders. Through person-centered care, professionals in public psychiatry bring their skills to an individual encounter in order to make the system work as effectively as possible. This textbook aims to support the public psychiatry enterprise through contributing to the education of professionals who pursue careers in this vibrant, challenging subspecialty of psychiatry.

A SERVICE SYSTEM OF PUBLIC PSYCHIATRY IN TRANSITION

The system of modern public psychiatry for people with SMIs and SUDs began to develop in the 1960s as community services were added to existing public hospitals. The system was consolidated in the 1980s, with the development of a wide range of community-based support services for people living in the community. Subsequent to that, the system began to fray as economic recessions starting in the early 1990s led to cutbacks. By 2003, the Presidential New Freedom Commission concluded that the system was "a shambles." Subsequently, the service system was cut severely during the economic recession of 2008 and ensuing years, as states strived to balance their budgets. Psychiatric hospital beds, as one index of services, were severely cut in number. As a result, people with SMIs and SUDs have difficulty accessing hospital treatment and have been transinstitutionalized to nursing homes, emergency rooms, jails, and homeless shelters. Forty percent of people with SMIs and co-occurring addictions do not access treatment, 60% of all people with any psychiatric disorders do not, and close to 90% with addictions do not. These cuts in services have occurred in circumstances in which psychiatric disorders account for a substantial burden of disease in American society, and mortality rates from psychiatric disorders are high from suicide and untreated, co-occurring chronic medical conditions. In short, contemporary public psychiatry faces many challenges. Although it is possible to assess the current status of the service system—and this assessment is important for efforts to improve it—it is also important to appreciate that the system is perpetually evolving. This is an essential point.

The system is not static and never has been. Chapter 2 reviewed the historical development of the service system in order to help describe it. At the same time, the history illustrates that the system is practically in constant development, sometimes retrenching and sometimes evolving with new services. The present is no exception. The following sections of this chapter discuss some of the major policy, scientific, professional, political, and economic factors that are currently shaping the service system of public psychiatry. Given that the pace of change is very rapid, resulting in an evolving picture of the system from year to year, the fundamental purpose of this discussion is to develop a way of thinking about a dynamic system so that the professional in public psychiatry will be able to monitor and adapt to the change.

CONTEMPORARY DEVELOPMENTS IN THE SERVICE SYSTEM

THE 2010 AFFORDABLE CARE ACT

The 1999 Surgeon General's report describing the de facto system of public psychiatry at that point and the 2003 New Freedom Commission report laid a foundation that led to legislative initiatives in 2008 establishing parity of insurance coverage for psychiatric disorders. The enactment of the 2010 Affordable Care Act (ACA) built on these previous policy landmarks and opened the 21st century era of health care reform. Health care reform has profound implications for public psychiatry.

Although the momentum of development under the ACA has swung from local and state innovation to federally stimulated initiatives, it is important to remember that the public system has always evolved collaboratively between the federal and state governments. Before the ACA, as noted in Chapter 2, the 2003 New Freedom Commission encouraged local experimentation and development. Now, under the ACA, states using Medicaid waivers are scrambling to respond to new programs spelled out in federal legislation that is shaping the service system. Taking Connecticut as an example of this turning tide, while responding to new federal programs such as behavioral health homes, most initiatives of the state authority itself are now limited in scope and directed at special populations, such as transitioning youth, people with first episodes of psychosis, or high-risk populations. On the state level, under a state "partnership," local initiatives since the ACA are driven as much by the state budget office and the state Medicaid agency as by the behavioral authority. It is as if state authorities, in responding to federal policy initiatives, are waiting to see how insurance and service delivery reform play out under the ACA. A key consideration for the states is the residual population of people with SMIs and/or SUDs who will be left with no insurance benefits under Medicaid or subsidized private insurance. Estimated at 5–8% of the population needing behavioral services, they will need services funded directly by state general fund dollars through state-owned and -operated facilities or through grants and contracts with private, nonprofit community mental health centers.

The 2010 ACA is a large, complex piece of legislation that will reform all of health care. In particular, it has the potential to transform behavioral health care and the service system of public psychiatry[2] over the course of its 9-year implementation period. Three major areas of reform emerged from the legislation: reform in insurance, reform in service delivery models, and reform in practice. Reforms in each domain mutually support the others.

HEALTH INSURANCE REFORM

Health insurance reform occurs through individual mandates, insurance subsidies for disadvantaged people, elimination of exclusions for preexisting conditions, and community ratings for risk of morbidity. Health insurance exchanges, a central mechanism of reform that began to operate in 2014, provide a place to sign up for health insurance coverage. This mechanism increases access for previously uninsured people to all medical services, including behavioral services. About half of the increase in access comes through Medicaid. As a result of insurance reform and the increased number of people with health insurance, meeting the demand for behavioral services is a current challenge in public practice.

As part of insurance reform, the legislation offers new reimbursement strategies that are alternatives to fee-for-service. These include bundled or episode financing and adjusted capitation for populations. Also, insurance reform includes new reimbursement for preventive care, such as depression detection. Furthermore, it emphasizes care coordination, under Medicaid's Home and Community Based Services option, such as targeted case management, which is of particular importance for high-risk, high-service–utilizing populations. These insurance reforms dovetail into new service delivery models.

Expanded Medicaid eligibility and other program elements of the ACA enhance and protect access for disadvantaged people with SMIs and/or SUDs. Single people are now eligible for Medicaid, which opens access for many with behavioral disorders. Ambulatory services for SUDs are now reimbursed as part of insurance reform, thus setting the stage for equity with mental illnesses in access to services for treatment and addressing long-standing constraints for addiction services. In addition, along with the expansion of Medicaid coverage, block grant funds to states, if not cut in response to the expanded Medicaid revenue stream under the ACA, can be redirected to fund recovery supports for those who are not considered Medicaid eligible.

SERVICE DELIVERY REFORM

Service delivery reform is another thrust of the ACA. Reform occurs by providing incentives to reorganize the structure of practice. New service delivery models provide alternatives to traditional fee-for-service reimbursement, which created a pernicious incentive to generate as many services as possible to maximize income, with limited attention to longitudinal care. Service delivery reform involves promotion of accountable care organizations (ACOs). These incorporate integrated primary and behavioral health care, attend to comprehensive or long-term care, and place a value on prevention (see Chapter 6). The new financing mechanisms under insurance reform and incentives for the reorganization of care are designed to bend the cost curve of services while improving models of care for people with long-term illness, disabilities, and comorbidities. Obviously, this has implications for people with serious behavioral disorders, which are discussed in more detail later in the sections on reform of service delivery models and practice.

As an aside, the ACA does not propose a national health service or a comprehensive structure, as did the Mental Health Systems Act of 1980. Rather, the ACA contains incentives, such as prospective payment mechanisms, to accomplish this change.

PRACTICE REFORM

The ACA also contains elements that lead to reform of practice. Two conceptual cornerstones of practice reform serving as building blocks for accountability are integrated health care (see Chapter 3) and population health, including prevention (see Chapter 8). In the realm of practice, public psychiatry is out in front of the change in some respects. For example, the ACA encourages person-centered, recovery-oriented practice (see Chapter 3) and interdisciplinary team practice (see Chapters 2 and 16). Much less well-developed in public psychiatry at present are the ideas of practice-based population health, integrated health care, and integrated mental health and substance use services, the latter a long-term but elusive goal for public psychiatry.

Under the ACA, public psychiatry must renew a community and population perspective of practice, a goal of community-based practice in the 1960s that has been lost over time. The triple-aim policy of the Centers for Medicare and Medicaid (CMS) and its accompanying metrics shapes practice not only by supporting improved clinical care, but also improved population health, such as reducing rates of depression and suicide and reducing unnecessary costs (such as repeated, avoidable hospitalizations), thereby conserving finite resources for the comprehensive care of an entire population.

Furthermore, under the ACA, public psychiatry must commit to the goal of integrated primary and behavioral health practice. Thus, the new service delivery models rely on collaborative practice among psychiatry and primary care medicine.

AN ALTERNATE PERSPECTIVE ON SERVICE AND PRACTICE REFORM

Integrated health care models might serve as the central theme for conceptualizing the unfolding transformation of service delivery in public psychiatry (see Chapter 5). A number of demonstration projects are under way funded by Substance Abuse and Mental Health Services Administration (SAMHSA)'s Primary and Behavioral Health Care Integration (PBHCI) program.[3] The effectiveness of these integrations is still not well demonstrated. Nevertheless, the integration of primary care and behavioral health, as a fundamental, underlying process, is driving much of the transformation of the system of public psychiatry.

Yet the perspective of integrated health care in not enough to capture the full scope of the integrative and organizational challenges faced at present by public psychiatry. First, integrated health care does not take into consideration insurance reform and accountable care, which have already been discussed. Also, integrated health care, by concentrating on psychiatry and primary care, does not fully consider the spectrum of integrative tasks facing public psychiatry. For example, the addiction treatment system, at least up until this point and despite many policy initiatives over the past 20 years, has been largely segregated from the mental health and physical health care systems. Unless this integration is done correctly, with great vigilance to parity and equity issues for addiction medicine, the substance abuse treatment needs of patients could actually get worse. This might occur if addiction medicine becomes lost in the competing physical and mental health priorities within a capitated system of care. It may well fall primarily on the shoulders of the professional leaders of public psychiatry (particularly those with addiction training) to make sure this does not happen.

Furthermore, the integrative tasks for public psychiatry are even more complex, including public health and forensic psychiatry, and demand attention. Chapter 7 on psychiatric public health demonstrates the cogency of public health for attaining a population perspective and implementing prevention as part of reform of current practice. Chapter 8 on forensic psychiatry presents the essential and growing interplay between public psychiatry and forensic psychiatry, manifest in collaborations with officers of the criminal justice system and in risk management. The discussion in the "Reform of Practice" section picks up these themes.

In summary, the integration agenda for public psychiatry with respect to primary care, addiction medicine, public health, and forensic psychiatry must be comprehensive. Also, the agenda for reorganization of service structures under the ACA is complex. For these reasons, the editors have chosen a broad framework within which to discuss service delivery and practice development.

NEW SERVICE DELIVERY MODELS

On a local level, the "hodgepodge" system of public psychiatry (see Chapter 2) is about to become even more Byzantine, at least during a period of transformative transition under current policies. The CMS, the SAMHSA, and the Health Resources and Services Administration (HRSA), in collaboration with state Medicaid authorities and legislatures using Medicaid waivers, are implementing and evaluating new service delivery models. For Medicaid populations, several new federal Medicaid policies serve as incentives at a local level, as states strive to increase the federal share of Medicaid expenses while relieving their own budgets and also reducing overall costs by efficient management of the system. These service delivery initiatives include higher than customary federal Medicaid assistance percentage (FMAP) reimbursement to states, new Medicaid reimbursement for community services related to comprehensive coordination and management of care, and cost-based reimbursement opportunities for community behavioral health centers.

At this point (2015), it looks like three models for the organization of service delivery hold promise for people with SMIs and/or SUDs: (1) safety net ACOs for Medicaid and dually eligible populations, including those with behavioral disorders; (2) certified, community behavioral health clinics (CCBHC) under the 2014 Excellence in Mental Health Act (EMHA); and (3) behavioral health homes, a service delivery model enabled by section 2703 of the ACA, implemented by state authorities under Medicaid, and designed to expand person-centered medical homes to people with SMIs and addictions. The current pace of development of these new models is high. Although it is possible to describe them, evaluations have not been done.

There are both similarities and distinctions among the three service delivery models under discussion. The shared features, in addition to the health home concept and integrated health care, include fiscal and quality accountability, high-cost case management, and practice-based population health with adherence to CMS's triple-aim policy. All three models are designed to coordinate services for people with chronic illnesses and physical, mental, and substance use comorbidities. As a person traverses an episode of illness, these models foster the comprehensive coordination of services from the hospital to the clinic and the community, including community supports and rehabilitation.

Also, the new models are distinct and different in origin, governance, mission, resources (especially behavioral personnel), and function. The distinctions among them may play a role in how existing service delivery models in public psychiatry adapt and evolve toward these new models.

THE SAFETY NET ACO

Under CMS, the Medicare Shared Savings Program (MSSP) is promulgating regulations for ACOs that share three basic components: a beneficiary population, annual financial benchmarks, and responsibility to measure and report 33 quality metrics.[4,5] Two basic types are possible: the MSSP model, in which the health care provider is not at financial risk, and the Pioneer model, in which larger health care organizations accept risk. This new, safety net ACO, a more recent addition to ACO service delivery models, is directed at populations under Medicare. It is particularly interesting in its implications for serving people with SMIs and SUDs. Medicaid recipients, including dual-eligibles, and uninsured are included as target beneficiaries. The integration of primary care with psychiatric services in a health home is an explicit goal with accompanying quality metrics. Finally, the safety net ACOs address social determinants of health through population-based prevention programs and the coordination of services across medical and social service agencies. For behavioral health, they include only one quality metric, which is depression screening; however, the features just described offer potential for helping the core target population of people with SMIs and SUDs.

THE CERTIFIED COMMUNITY BEHAVIORAL HEALTH CLINIC

In 2014, Congress enacted the EMHA. It offers existing community mental health centers the opportunity to become CCBHCs provided they meet certain criteria. Although historic in the parochial sphere of public psychiatry as the single, most important piece of behavioral health legislation per se since 1963, the EMHA is best understood in the context of general health care reform, in which it plays a special and specific part.

The EMHA set new standards for community behavioral health clinics. It appropriated $900 million to expand access to community mental health centers and improve the quality of mental health care for all Americans. The enactment of the legislation created an enormous incentive for community behavioral health centers in the form of cost-based reimbursement of Medicaid behavioral services. For fiscally hard-pressed, private, nonprofit behavioral agencies, this incentive is essential because the PR costs of expanding service to newly enrolled people in Medicaid under the ACA often exceed any new revenue from Medicaid under preexisting reimbursement rates.

The EMHA provides for 2-year demonstrations in eight states. It sets new standards for provider organizations, which are certified by individual states according to federal criteria. The legislation requires the CCBHCs to provide a broad range of mental health and substance abuse services.

These include 24-hour psychiatric crisis services, child mental health programs, psychosocial rehabilitation programs, mental health peer-support programs, outpatient addiction treatment programs, acute detoxification services, and consumer-directed programs. Additionally, the CCBHCs are required to provide all the services required by the state plan for all the people covered by their particular plan. And, the CCBHCs must offer on-site primary care or have contracts with federally qualified health centers (FQHCs). Part of the budget appropriated under the EMHA is devoted to infrastructure development, including the construction and modernization of facilities. The EBHA requires that states develop prospective payment systems for services offered at CCBHCs under Medicaid. Having done so, the FMAP rises to 90% for the state. This rise in FMAP, along with cost-based reimbursement to the CCBHCs, puts behavior health centers, depending on the states where they are located and successful revenue generation, on a stronger fiscal footing. This can lead to expansion of services. Finally, CCBHCs are eligible to serve as medical homes for people with SMIs and/or addictions. As a result of this legislation, CCBHCs may develop into a cornerstone of integrated health care for the traditional target population of public psychiatry.

Implementation of the EMHA, including demonstration projects by 2017, plays out over 7 years, with Health and Human Services responsible for evaluating the new clinics and reporting back to Congress by 2021. Although it offers another pathway for the development of service delivery, the long implementation schedule raises questions of whether it will be in time, given the current rapid pace of development of other service delivery models.

BEHAVIORAL HEALTH HOMES

Behavioral health homes, enabled by Section 2703 of the ACA, which permits states to modify their state Medicaid plans, are a third service delivery model in development and of interest. The behavioral health home derives from the model of person-centered medical homes in primary care, which, among its other features, intends for FQHCs to serve as the medical home for people with SMIs on Medicaid.[6-8] The SAMHSA-HRSA Center for Integrated Health Solutions (SAMHSA-HRSA) and an AHRQ publication regarding the integration of mental health care into patient-centered medical homes (HRSA) guide the development of the behavioral health home. Behavioral health homes may have the most steam for serving the most disadvantaged people with SMIs and addictions who are left without health insurance benefits under the ACA. This is true because they are driven both by state Medicaid agencies and mental health authorities.

Behavioral health homes have considerable state-by-state variation, given local histories and the status of local systems. To take Connecticut as an example, the state has formed a Connecticut Behavioral Health Partnership made up of the departments of (1) Mental Health and Addiction Services, (2) Children and Families, and (3) Social Services (the Medicaid agency). The Connecticut plan uses an administrative services organization (ASO) to manage services under a noncapitated contract with performance incentives related to access, economy, and quality. It offers a variety of Medicaid-covered clinical and community support services to a Medicaid population estimated to number about 115,000 people. Local behavioral agencies are responsible for service delivery in their respective communities.

THE ROAD AHEAD IS UNCLEAR AT PRESENT

It is too early at this point to know how these innovative service delivery models will play out in the service system of public psychiatry. In states where political opposition to the ACA and Medicaid expansion exists, the picture is particularly murky. Still, it is useful to speculate and monitor the evolution of models.

It helps to start with an understanding of existing service delivery models. Three models of service delivery currently exist in public psychiatry for ambulatory care: (1) state-owned community mental health centers, (2) private nonprofit community mental health centers, and (3) mental health services in (FQHCs; see Chapter 2). The distinctions among the three existing models position them differently in how they respond to the new incentives for service delivery reform. Indeed, largely as a function of their governance and fiscal structures, it appears that they may emerge in different niches of a new system of public psychiatry.

As solo entities, private nonprofit agencies may gravitate to CCBHCs, given the potential that cost-based reimbursement provides for expanding services and access under the ACA. Some may also contract with state authorities as behavioral health homes. FQHCs may have large enough budgets and reserves to go at risk as safety net ACOs. State-owned agencies, given their tie into community-based supports and psychosocial rehabilitation financed by state authorities, will be linked to state initiatives for behavioral health homes as the ultimate safety net service delivery model for the most disadvantaged and disabled people with no insurance or benefits (the 5–8%).

The fundamental question for public psychiatry, one that runs through these service delivery permutations, is how well these developments serve the most disadvantaged and disabled people with serious and persistent mental illnesses and/or SUDs, especially those who do not enroll in Medicaid. Of interest to public psychiatry in this regard are current demonstration programs under the ACA for dually eligible people (eligible for both Medicare and Medicaid) to address the needs of poor, disabled people with mental illnesses and addictions who are high utilizers of service. Also, demonstration projects for people who are high risk for hospitalization, aimed at limiting the number of days spent in the hospital and controlling costs, may help to ensure that people with serious behavioral disorders have lower cost and better quality alternatives to hospital care. Serving the most vulnerable is the ultimate test of the public system and the criterion that public psychiatry must keep its eyes on.

In the end, at this point in time, the conceptual framework of the scenarios discussed herein is more important than the conclusions. The concepts provide a context for professionals in public psychiatry on the local level to develop strategic options to lead their agencies forward.

REFORM OF PRACTICE

Given the major transition occurring in public psychiatry at present, what are the consequences for professional practice in order to maintain clinical and management competency? Previous chapters have foreshadowed much of this discussion, which is drawn together here in the light of health care reform. Also, this discussion recapitulates some of the issues introduced earlier but now with an emphasis on practice. The following considerations create a complex, multivariate equation of change for professional practice in public psychiatry.

Integrated health care, the latest phase of mainstreaming behavioral care with general medical care, challenges behavioral health agencies to consider partnering or merging with primary care centers and clinics. As people enroll in medical homes, primary care may become a gateway to behavioral services. CCBHCs and behavioral health homes may become medical homes for people with SMIs and/or SUDs, provided they have demonstrated a capacity for primary care. As a result, behavioral professionals need to hone their consultative skills for collaboration with colleagues in primary care. Also, they need to understand essential aspects of primary care such as metabolic syndrome, common chronic diseases, basic medical treatments, and drug interactions. Many already work principally in FQHCs and have adapted to this new practice.

Another important integrative task for public psychiatry is a continuing effort to bring together psychiatry and addiction medicine. This agenda, which figured in the report of the New Freedom Commission and stems from earlier initiatives in the 1990s, is far from complete. The integration of the two, encouraged under integrated health care but important in its own right, is an important criterion for behavioral health centers as they establish their credentials and credibility under the EMHA. Expertise in treating co-occurring disorders is a cornerstone. New procedures for evaluation, brief treatment, and quick referral of people with SUDs may help to increase access to care. The integration of mental health and addiction medicine into comprehensive behavioral health programs calls for professionals in public psychiatry to attend to bridging, collaborating, maintaining basic competencies, and, in some cases, subspecializing in addiction medicine. Indeed, given the demands made on primary care and the limited number of addiction specialists by comparison to professionals in public psychiatry, the latter may play a critical role in accomplishing this integrative task.

Practice-based population health establishes quality standards for practice that focus not only on the health of the individual but also on a whole panel of people served by the practice. A population perspective, in conjunction with new, capitated financing mechanisms, engenders a concern for finite resources. In addition, preventive interventions, such as depression screening, emerge as an essential part of clinical service in the public arena. Suicide prevention becomes an essential, routine clinical function. Prevention of substance abuse is another low-cost example of a powerful early intervention. Outreach to transitioning youth, veterans with behavioral conditions returning from war, and early intervention for first episodes of psychosis offer hope of avoiding frank and prolonged illnesses. Professionals in public psychiatry need to understand, contribute to, and implement these initiatives as part of an overall program of population health in psychiatry.

Contemporary interest in social determinants of heath focuses attention on social problems, such as poverty, homelessness, and access to services, that intersect with health status. For example, homelessness will continue to demand attention until adequate residential resources are easily accessible and behavioral services are available for all people with SMIs and/or SUDs in the community. Elections and political changes at the local, state, and federal level, as well as economic cycles, will sharpen or attenuate attention to social determinants of health and shape behavioral policy accordingly. Professionals in public psychiatry, as they did at the dawn of the modern era of community psychiatry, need to renew and incorporate a broad social and community perspective into their viewpoint of disorders and services. They need the skills for successful, clinical outreach and involvement in community life.

Forensic issues now loom large in public practice. Recently, the Vera Institute of Justice, focusing on social determinants of health, characterized the health effects of mass incarceration as a major public health crisis facing American society.[9] In public psychiatry, the large number of people applying for treatment, especially young men from disadvantaged neighborhoods who are exiting prisons and seeking community services, and who have a history of SUDs, mental illnesses, or comorbidity, are a reflection of this problem. In addition, an emphasis on protection of society is an inevitable consequence and outgrowth of the recent American social and community disasters at Sandy Hook, Connecticut; the Washington Naval Yard; and others. As a result, collaborations with the criminal justice system are essential and require special knowledge and skills of the professional in public psychiatry. Court, parole, and probation officers become part of the team, and compliance with treatment and risk management are explicit parts of the clinical process. Professionals in public psychiatry need to know how to work with forensic populations and incorporate risk management into routine practice.

Accountability in health care also has fundamental implications for practice. The need to control health care costs, which is politically necessary to protect the viability of expanded access, requires that the new access to care go hand in hand with efficient use of resources. Utilization management (similar to that proposed in the 1990s), internal to an organization or imposed from outside, is an inevitable result. Professionals in public psychiatry need to contribute to these procedures in their practice. Public authorities also need to move in this direction to efficiently manage state-funded services for high-risk, vulnerable parts of their target populations as part of contemporary demands for accountability.

Quality improvement is a counterpoint to accountability and cost control in a value proposition for clinical services, expressed in the equation $v = q/c$ (value equals quality over cost). A focus on quality, along with cost consciousness, aims at improving the value of clinical services. In 2014, the CMS launched a Transforming Clinical Practice Initiative to help clinicians and hospitals to replace volume-based practice with value-based practice. To implement the equation, health care providers have to measure, monitor, and report the process and outcomes of their services. Under the CMS's triple-aim policy, public psychiatry has to develop the information technology to measure and report quality metrics not only for individuals but also for the populations served. There are also related incentives to implement evidence-based interventions. Professionals in public psychiatry cannot leave these concerns to "management" and need to understand and master the quality improvement strategies for success in contemporary practice.

As part of quality initiatives, it is essential to address disparities in health care outcomes for people from cultural and ethnic minorities. A byproduct of insurance reform may be greater numbers of previously uninsured people from these groups entering the system of care. This increase in access reinforces the need to correct disparities in health care outcomes. Doing so requires cultural competence and quality measures for these special populations. Many professionals entering public psychiatry already speak a second language, have cultural competence in two spheres, and can expand from there. Other professionals, in order to become culturally competent, must cultivate a career-long, cultural curiosity. Learning second-language skills is a building block for this and facilitates the engagement and retention of people from minority groups in a plan of care. Finally, cultural competence is a fundamental strategy for the professional in public psychiatry who wishes to succeed in a clinical process that is person-centered and recovery-oriented.

A vast expansion of access to mental health services for previously uninsured people under the ACA, enhanced by parity of insurance benefits for behavioral services, challenges agencies and providers to accommodate the demand. Many single and many homeless people now have access to services financed by Medicaid. Many people with primary SUDs also have greater access. Professionals in public psychiatry must expand practice and manage access to efficient evaluation and treatment through walk-in and urgent care services under expanded hours of operation. At the same time, they need to monitor the risk of diffusing focus on the core, most vulnerable target population of people with SMIs and/or SUDs, a perennial unintended consequence.

Recovery principles empower recipients of service as consumers and engage them as never before. The SAMHSA and state authorities have identified recovery as a key initiative and are linking policies, grants, and demonstrations to its achievement. New metrics for personal outcomes to supplement clinical outcomes are in development. As a result, white-coated behavioral professionals no longer exclusively encounter the people they serve in the consultation room. Recipients of service and their families, defined as partners in care, are playing larger and more essential roles in the stewardship of the system of public psychiatry. They exercise their influence through participation in governance, completion of patient satisfaction reports, collection of other quality assessments, focus groups, and, ultimately, through their personal choice of where to seek services. Professionals in public psychiatry need to master the skills of meeting recipients of service in all these venues and incorporating them into the process of care. Also, they need to expand their clinical vision to integrate clinical care, community supports, rehabilitation, recovery, and social inclusion in responding to personally defined goals of care.

There is the perennial promise of discovery from basic neurobiological, clinical, and services research on etiology, treatments, and programs. Precision medicine and the Research Domain Criteria, alternative to descriptive diagnosis based on the *Diagnostic and Statistical Manual of Mental Disorders* (DSM), may lead to breakthroughs. A multitude of treatments, practices, and programs are being systematically tested. The accumulation of this evidence over time fundamentally shapes professional practice in public psychiatry. Health care reform boosts this process by emphasizing the use of evidence-based practices in service delivery. The challenge for professionals in public psychiatry is to remain abreast of the latest scientific and clinical literature, to become experts in evaluation of evidence, and to strive to make the translation from discovery to practice as efficient as possible.

As a footnote to this discussion of practice reform, some may believe that the list of variables contributing to the evolution of practice in public psychiatry gives short shrift to the role of science and the evidence it engenders. In that regard, it is important to remember that it is the reform of practice as a function of health care reform that is under discussion. While respecting the role of science and evidence in revealing the road ahead, the point of view here is pragmatically anchored in the politics and economics of policy making.

Policy-making in relation to health care reform is an essential companion process to science. Interestingly, the processes of science and policy-making are different. Science continuously generates evidence, which behavioral health care professionals follow in real time. Academic centers, utilizing the scientific method, generate most of the evidence and debate it step by step on a micro level. Policy-making is a larger, messy, complex, often opportunistic social process at the federal, state, and local levels. It is more deadline-driven, leap-frogging rather than evolving continuously, and it advances, then sometimes retreats. It is more macro, political, consensus-building, economic, cost-conscious, and pragmatic.

SOME IMPLICATIONS OF SYSTEM TRANSITION AND PRACTICE REFORM

Evolution of the service system of public psychiatry has been practically constant since the early stages of community psychiatry in the late 1960s. As the discussion so far illustrates, the service system and public practice continue to evolve rapidly. It is important to monitor this evolution and embrace change in order to help shape it, improve it, and ultimately apply it, along with evidence-based practice, in service of people seeking help. The service system is an essential constellation of resources and a context for practice in public psychiatry. System wisdom—the accumulated, hard-earned knowledge of the system of public psychiatry—and making the service system work for people with SMIs and/or SUDs, is a defining characteristic of professionals in public psychiatry, distinguishing them from their colleagues in the rest of behavioral health and medicine.

The earlier discussion of insurance reform, transition in service delivery models, and evolving practice in public psychiatry is long and complex. Indeed, the agenda for reform of the service system and practice seems daunting. This conclusion emphasizes the need for special, advanced education for careers in this challenging and rewarding field. As a corollary, there is a need to recognize public psychiatry as a subspecialty of general psychiatry in order to support proper preparation of professionals for careers in this field and to stimulate the development of excellent, educational structures to provide it.

PUBLIC-ACADEMIC PARTNERSHIPS

What strategies are available to public psychiatry and its professionals to manage the reforms in insurance, service delivery, and practice discussed so far? We suggest that a public-academic partnership, among others, is a powerful strategy for adaptation to a rapidly evolving system. A recent article[9] summarizes the potential relationships between the two. It highlights four areas: (1) recruitment, career development, and retention; (2) structural and fiscal connections, (3) program evaluation, research, and policy; and (4) collaborations in integrated health care. The following discussion incorporates these facets of the relationships.

For public authorities, a partnership with academic institutions offers advantages in recruitment, continuing educational and career development, retention of professional staff, and the development of academic units for special purposes. The latter might include units for traumatic brain injury or patients in the criminal justice system who are not guilty by reason of insanity. For academic departments, a partnership offers the advantages of (1) support for faculty positions, with time protected for education and research; (2) educational slots for advanced fellows; and (3) underwriting research. These partnerships are mutually beneficial for innovation in services. Several examples of this over the years in the Yale Department of Psychiatry include law and psychiatry programs, recovery programs, substance abuse programs, dual-diagnosis programs, gambling programs, prevention, Latino services, and early intervention programs. Another current example of innovation is the development of collaborations with primary care for the purpose of integrated health care of people with SMIs and SUDs. In each case, the program innovation is also well-evaluated, garnering evidence for public authorities and publications for academic faculty members. The faculty members involved become valued policy advisors for the public authorities. The leadership of the state authorities, while paying much attention to federal and state policy initiatives, has this intellectual resource from which they can seek opinions about the latest evidence in the scientific and academic arena. The partnership also enriches academic departments by substantively supporting divisions of public psychiatry as an essential part of clinical services, education, and research.[10]

By first educating and then fostering and supporting careers, academic departments contribute to career development and retention of the workforce in public psychiatry. Doing so addresses a vital concern of public authorities regarding manpower development. After graduation from fellowships, academic centers for teaching public psychiatry can continue to play an important role in the continuing education of professionals pursuing careers in the field. In turn, graduating behavioral professionals need to nurture their relationship to their respective academic centers. Clinical faculty appointments are possible for those interested in teaching. Some professionals in public psychiatry may remain as full- or part-time faculty members in their departments. Many academic programs establish networks for their graduates. All these relationships reduce the isolation and grind of day-to-day work on the job.

Academic departments, or more specifically divisions in them, can be seen as "institutes" designed to preserve, develop, and improve services for people with SMIs and/or SUDs, as well as other special, target populations. Such institutes might be seen as agencies of change in public psychiatry, of interest not only to academic centers but also public authorities. The institute idea is not to suggest that academic departments become ivory towers. Rather, the academic agenda would center on the problems of and services for people with SMIs and/or SUDs. The academic departments in which these institutes would be found would still have to maintain a full spectrum of productive, clinical services for teaching purposes. An institute model would have to include an opportunity and a responsibility to preserve and demonstrate services, especially innovative interventions, for populations served by programs of the state behavioral authority. For example, growing evidence for early interventions in psychosis supports this clinical strategy, one that is potentially game changing in the practice of public psychiatry. Strategies for coping with metabolic syndrome among people with SMIs and SUDs could prove to be both lifesaving and cost-saving by preventing diabetes, hypertension, and heart disease. Also, academic departments might shoulder responsibility for consulting to state-owned institutions. If a return to an institute model were to occur, academic departments would have come full circle to concepts that were in play in the late 1950s at Yale, Columbia, Harvard, Einstein, and other places and that led to the development of the Connecticut Mental Health Center.

The partnerships between public authorities and academia can be multiple and function with mutual benefit. Given the considerations just discussed, partnerships ought to flourish and endure going forward. For example, in 2016, the partnership between the state of Connecticut Department of Mental Health and Addiction Services and the Yale Department of Psychiatry will celebrate it 50th anniversary. It helps if professionals in public psychiatry understand this relationship and build their own connections within its context. Indeed, each professional's relationship is a building block, a basic unit of the public–academic partnership.

A DEPARTMENTAL DIVISION OF PUBLIC PSYCHIATRY

In the Yale Department of Psychiatry, the number of contributors and the implications of this textbook have grown over 2 years, exceeding the original expectations envisioned during the process of writing. By its completion, 74 clinical and research faculty members of the Department contributed to the textbook. In addition, the process of writing the textbook catalyzed the development of a division of public psychiatry within the Yale Department. In short, the medium has become the message, one focused on the importance of academic divisions of public psychiatry. The emergence of a division of public psychiatry, uniting faculty from the veterans' facility, the general hospital, and the community behavioral health center, established it alongside other academic divisions of the Department of Psychiatry. These included substance abuse, forensic psychiatry, and prevention. The new departmental status facilitated essential conversations, at least for public psychiatry, among the divisions, which supported key integrative challenges for public psychiatry (see Part II of this textbook). These dialogues are an example of how the interplay between academic programs and public practice is instrumental in keeping public psychiatry comprehensive, contemporary, and vibrant, sometimes by breaking new ground (e.g., in law and psychiatry, SUDs, recovery, and early intervention) and in other cases by sustaining programs when times are hard (prevention, law and psychiatry, SUDs).[11,12] Not least, the creation of an interdisciplinary division for educational and research purposes serves as a model for an interdisciplinary team approach to practice. This local experience in a large department, amplified in the following paragraphs, may serve as a case example for other departments.

Fundamentally, the creation of a division with attention to education, research, clinical services has supported the development of careers in public psychiatry in the Yale Department of Psychiatry. Previously, the organizational structures of the Department did not map well onto the needs of faculty members specializing in public psychiatry. The new division put professionals who choose public psychiatry on a more equal footing with their departmental colleagues. In postgraduate years, the division also provided continuing education for its members. The leadership of the division also more effectively advocated for the importance of careers in public psychiatry in departmental life. The utility of a division of public psychiatry for supporting career development breaks down into four functions: teaching, investigation, fiscal management, and public–academic partnerships.

This textbook embraces the principle that the most effective advanced education in public psychiatry is interdisciplinary. As a result, interdisciplinary collaborations, already prominent in the department, have deepened. The major professional groups and three institutions (the community mental health center, the veterans' facility, and the general hospital) in the Yale Department of Psychiatry already had education programs in public psychiatry. The new departmental division served to concentrate the teaching resources, blend the professional traditions, and coordinate educational principles, thereby creating a stronger, more coherent and comprehensive teaching program. It offered a forum for faculty members to share ideas and resources, consider interrelated topics and identify the strengths and weaknesses of the content. These interest groups are now poised to more effectively apply for training grants relevant to public psychiatry.

The division also facilitated collaborations and strategic plans for comprehensive portfolios of investigation and for seeking research funding from National Institute of Mental Health, the veteran's system, and foundations. Studies ranged through clinical research, services research, and basic research. Both teaching and investigative initiatives in the division made important contributions to the academic programs of the larger Department of Psychiatry.[13] Aggregating the individual, independent initiatives of seeking research support created a critical mass of investigation that highlights this domain of research in the department.

Given recent reductions in sources of research funding, the fiscal picture in the Yale Department of Psychiatry is stringent. It is necessary to piece together salary packages that include clinical placements and research or teaching grants. As the division progressively developed teaching and research programs, it was able to put together a complete package. The diversified salary structure, while averting faculty reductions, helped to fill the demand for high-quality professionals on clinical services, not only in institutions of the department but also at the facilities of public authorities.

Last, but certainly not least, a division of public psychiatry effectively supported the relationship of the Yale Department of Psychiatry with local and state public authorities in mental health and addictions. Not many departments have well-developed and sustained relationships, and they require consistent attention and effort to maintain. As noted earlier, there is a potential for considerable mutual benefit to both sides. The partnership enhances the fundamental missions of both: to better serve, understand, adapt to change, and innovate services for people with SMIs and/or SUDs.

A FUNDAMENTAL PROFESSIONAL PROPOSITION

A fundamental professional proposition is that society, after a person completes a period of accredited study, accords that person a special status and role as a professional. In return, the social expectation is that professionals will apply their special knowledge and skills on behalf of those in society who need help and services. In the case of public psychiatry, it is important to keep an eye on and maintain a commitment to the core, target population of people with SMIs and/or SUDs, the population that the Mental Health Services Act of 1980 characterized as the most needy and vulnerable of all the people served by American psychiatry and medicine. This is the nucleus of the professional persona that characterizes all professionals in public psychiatry. Reminding ourselves periodically of this proposition renews the social contract and keeps faith with society and the people served by public psychiatry.

SUMMARY

This textbook of public psychiatry, edited and authored by faculty members of the Yale Department of Psychiatry, covers the treatment, rehabilitation, community supports, recovery, and public health of people with SMIs and co-occurring or independent SUDs served in organized, publicly funded systems of service. The book is intended as an introductory, comprehensive textbook for advanced professional students of public psychiatry. It is a text informed by unifying educational aims, an educational philosophy, and educational principles developed in the Yale Department of Psychiatry. It supports a pedagogical structure of clinical placements and teaching, clinical supervision, seminars, and development of leadership and academic skills mentored by faculty members. By virtue of being interdisciplinary, by covering both clinical practice and public health, by accepting the integrative challenges of contemporary public psychiatry, and by confronting the challenges of health care reform, the textbook strives to be comprehensive. The completion of this textbook has reinforced the already strong conviction of its editors and authors that public psychiatry is a vast, complex, vibrant, and evolving subspecialty of psychiatric practice.

For the reasons discussed in this chapter, high-quality educational programs in public psychiatry have never been more in need. Preparation of high-quality professionals in public psychiatry is a top priority to assure the future of public practice. Well-educated public psychiatry professionals are those who implement, manage, evaluate, innovate, and, in turn, teach the next generation in public psychiatry. The authors and editors of this textbook hope it will make a contribution to the educational mission.

REFERENCES

1. Kennedy PK, Greden JF, Riba M. The next 50 years: a vision of a "community of mental health." *Am J Psychiatry*. 2013;170:1097–1098.
2. Mechanic, D. Seizing opportunities under the Affordable Care Act for transforming the mental and behavioral health system. *Health Aff*. 2012;31:376–382.
3. SAMHSA-HRSA Center for Integrated Health Solutions. *Behavioral Health Homes for People with Mental Health and Substance Use Conditions: The Core Clinical Features*. http://www.integration.samhsa.gov/clinical-practice/cihs_health_homes_core_clinical_features.pdf. Published 2012, accessed 3/31/15.
4. Scharf DM, Egerhardt NK, Harkbarth NS, et al. *Evaluation of the SAMHSA Primary and Behavioral Health Care Integration (PBHCI) Grant Program: Final Report (Task 13)*. Santa Monica, CA: RAND; 2014.
5. Maxwell J, Baillett M, Toby R, Bannon C. Early observations show safety net ACOs hold promise to achieve the triple aim and promote health equity. *Health Aff*. http://healthaffairs.org/blog/2014/09/15/early-observations-show-safety-net-acos-hold-promise-to-achieve-the-triple-aim-and-promote-health-equity/. Published 2014., accessed 3/31/15.
6. Alakeson V, Frank RG, Katz RE. Specialty care medical homes for people with severe, persistent mental disorders. *Health Aff*. 2012;29:967–973.

7. Croghan TW, Brown JD. *Integrating Mental Health Treatment into the Patient Centered Medical Home.* Rockville, MD: Agency for Health Care Research and Quality; 2010. AHQR Publication No. 10-0084-EF.
8. Maust DT, Oslin DW, Marcus SC. Mental health care in the accountable care organization. *Psychiatr Serv.* 2013;64:908–910.
9. Lemelle S, Ali OM, Giggie MA, et al. Public psychiatry fellowships: a developing network of public-academic collaborations. *Psychiatr Serv.* 2012;63:851–854.
10. Steiner JL, Anderson N, Belitsky R, et al. In: Jacobs SC, Griffith EEH, eds. *40 Years of Academic Public Psychiatry.* West Sussex, UK: Wiley and Sons; 2007.
11. Jacobs SC. The community support and system development period and CMHC, 1982 to 1993. In: Mehta L, ed. *Inside Public Psychiatry.* Shelton, CT: People's Medical Publishing; 2011.
12. Jacobs SC. The period of mainstreaming and CMHC, 1993 to 2003. In: Mehta L, ed. *Inside Public Psychiatry.* Shelton, CT: People's Medical Publishing; 2011, Chapter 7, pp. 127–154.
13. Cloud C. *On life Support: Public Health in the Age of Mass Incarceration.* New York: Vera Institute of Justice; 2014.

INDEX

Acamprosate, 87
Acceptance and commitment therapy, 254t
Accountable care organizations (ACOs), 109–10, 276–78
Accreditation Council for Graduate Medical Education (ACGME), 241–42, 263
Acquired brain injury (ABI), 202
Activities of daily living (ADLs), 204
Actuarial instruments, 124–25
Addiction medicine integration, 8, 82–85. *see also* substance use disorders (SUDs)
ADHD, 144t
Administrative best practices
　administrative leader, 264–65, 270–71
　advocacy, 263
　case identification, 265–66
　clinical director, 263–64
　communication, 266
　high-risk approach, 266
　history of, 261–62
　improving the average approach, 266
　leaders, training, 270–71
　leadership structure, 262
　logic models, 269–70, 270t
　medical director, 262–63
　overview, 10, 261
　patient involvement, 266–67
　population health, 265–66, 280
　program development, innovation, evaluation, 268–70, 270t
　quality improvement, 267–68
　refusal of care, 267
　resource management, 264–65
　resources, 252
　risk management, 263, 266–67
　screening instruments, 268
　standard treatment, 265–66
　workforce productivity, 267
Administrative leader, 264–65, 270–71
Adolescents. *see* children, adolescent, young adult services
Advance directives, 268
Advanced practice nurse (APRN), 177, 238
Affordable Care Act
　accountable care organizations (ACOs), 109–10, 276–78
　behavioral health, 186
　behavioral health homes, 277–79
　CCBHCs, 277–79
　cost control initiatives, 109
　health insurance reform, 275–76, 281
　hospital clinical services, 173
　integrated health care requirements, 37, 63, 109
　mental health services access, xi, 10–11, 250, 275, 281
　minority health requirements, 217
　patient-centered medical home, 72–73

practice reform, 276, 279–81
service delivery models, 15, 18–20, 29
service delivery reform, 276
After-care, 266
Agency for Healthcare Research and Quality (AHRQ), 250
Alcohol, alcoholism, 82–83, 86t, 104, 107, 268. *see also* substance use disorders (SUDs)
Alcoholics Anonymous, 40, 41, 83
ALDH 2 gene, 84
Ambulatory behavioral health services
　cognitive behavioral therapy (CBT), 30, 66, 89, 160–61, 191, 254t
　competencies, 190–91, 194–95
　continuing care treatment, 189–92, 189t
　crisis intervention teams, 193, 194
　history of, 186–88
　homeless outreach teams, 194
　IDDT, 90, 191, 252t
　inpatient admissions, discharges, 192–93
　involuntary treatment, 190
　liaison role, benefits of, 192–93
　medication management, 189–90
　overview, 9, 185–86, 195
　psychosocial interventions, 190–91
　self-management principles, 190
　somatic treatments, 190
　specialty teams, 193–94
　system integration, 188
　walk-in services, 188–89, 188t
American Association of Community Psychiatrists, 5
American Association for the Cure of Inebriety (AACI), 82–83
American Board of Addiction Medicine (ABAM), 83–84
American Psychological Association (APA), 237, 251
Americans with Disabilities Act (ADA), 35
Amitriptyline (Elavil), 144t
Amminger, G. P., 161
Amphetamine (Adderall), 144t
Anafranil (clomipramine), 144t
Anthony, W., 34–35
Antidepressants, 104–5
Antipsychotics, 30, 65, 100, 143, 161, 166, 190, 255
Antisocial personality disorder, 104, 125–26
Aripiprazole (Abilify), 144t
Arnett, J., 146
Assertive Community Treatment (ACT) model, 17, 54, 164, 186, 193, 198–201, 200t, 252t
Atomoxetine (Strattera), 144t
Attenuated positive symptoms syndrome (APS), 157t, 159

Barefoot v. Estelle, 124
Bariatric surgery, 67
Beers, C., 16, 34
Behavioral couples therapy, 89, 254t
Behavioral family therapy, 254t
Behavioral health homes, 73–74, 277–79
Behavioral Health Primary Care Integration Model, 106
Behavioral health services (ambulatory). *see* ambulatory behavioral health services
Bellack, A. S., 42
Berwick, D. M., 109
Best Pharmaceuticals for Children Act (BPCA), 143
Bio-psychosocial formulation, 242
Bipolar disorder, 51, 104, 107, 144t
Bond, G. R., 200
Boston University Center for Psychiatric Rehabilitation, 245
Brief intermittent psychotic syndrome (BIPS), 157t, 159
British Medical Journal publications, 256
Broadhead, W., 107
Brown, S. A., 93
Buprenorphine, 87
Bupropion, 67, 87
Burden of disease, 3, 99–100, 103, 106–8
Burgess, P., 42
Bush Administration, 18

Cancer, 68
Carpenter W. T., 35
Carter Administration, 17, 34, 136, 186
Case studies, 251
Center for Psychiatric Rehabilitation, University of Chicago, 245
Centers for Medicare and Medicaid Services (CMS), 20
Certified, community behavioral health clinics (CCBHC), 20, 277–79
Chambless, D. L., 251
Charney, D. S., 207
Child and Adolescent Service System Program, 136–37
Children, adolescent, young adult services
　access to, 142
　child guidance movement, 135
　child study movement, 134–35
　community mental health centers, 136
　cultural competence, 216
　emerging adulthood, 146
　engagement in treatment by, 142
　evidence-based practice, 143–45, 145t
　forensic evaluation of, 124–25
　history, 134–37
　Medicaid, 136, 143
　overview, 8–9, 133–34, 150
　patient characteristics, 137–41, 146–47
　principles, 134, 137, 138t
　professional development, 148–50

psychiatric diagnosis, 143
psychoanalysis, 135–36
psychopathology developmental perspectives, 147
psychopharmacology, 143, 144t
publicly funded system challenges, 142–46, 144–45t
public system characteristics, 137
service delivery system gaps, 147–48
substance use disorder treatment, 90, 102
suicide risk, 105
supported education, 52–53, 90
systemic integration, 145–46
system of care concept, 136–37
terminology, 134
transitioning youth, 146–48
Children's Health Insurance Program (CHIP), 25, 26
Chinman, M., 53
Chlorpromazine (Thorazine), 144t, 171
Chronic pain, 254t
Civil Rights Act of 1964, 217
Clifford Beers Child Guidance Clinic, 16
Clinical Antipsychotic Trials of Intervention Effectiveness (CATIE), 64
Clinical director, 263–64
Clinical observations, 251
Clinic of Child Development, 134
Clinton Administration, 17–18, 99
Clomipramine (Anafranil), 144t
Clozapine, 30, 190
Clubhouse International, 55
Clubhouses, 54–55
Cognitive behavioral therapy (CBT), 30, 66, 89, 160–61, 191, 254t
Cognitive processing therapy, 254t
Cognitive remediation, computer-based, 52
Commitment laws, 116–17, 117f, 123–24
Commonwealth Fund, 135
Community-based supports. *see also* psychosocial rehabilitation
　ACT model, 17, 54, 164, 186, 193, 198–201, 200t, 252t
　clubhouses, 54–55
　cognitive impairments, 51–52
　community inclusion, 56–57
　employment, education, 50–53, 90, 252t
　history of, 17, 17t
　housing, 49–50
　identification, implementation, coordination, 55–56
　immigrants, refugees, 215–16, 227–28
　interdisciplinary case management, 54
　life skills training, 54
　NGRI patients, oversight of, 122–24
　overview, 7, 8, 49, 57
　peer support, 37, 39–42, 53–54, 66
　psychosocial rehabilitation, 54–56, 228

287

Community-based supports (Cont.)
  quality improvement, 56
  TBI/ABI, 204
  veterans, 198, 199, 206–8
Community Mental Health Act of
    1963, 173
Community mental health centers,
    136, 186–87
Community Mental Health Centers Act of
    1963, 2, 16, 98, 116
Community Mental Health Services Block
    Grants, 56
Community reinforcement approach
    (CRA), 89
Community reinforcement approach and
    family training (CRAFT), 89
Community treatment, 118–21
Competencies
  ACT staff, 200–201
  administrative leaders, 270–71
  advanced opportunities, 243–44
  advanced practice nursing, 149–50
  ambulatory services, 190–91, 194–95
  child and adolescent psychiatry, 149
  clinical child and adolescent
      psychiatry, 149
  cultural competence, 219–20
  global mental health, 226
  homelessness, 198–99
  immersion training, 246
  interdisciplinary, integration of, 245
  LGBT individuals, 206
  multicultural, 206
  nursing, 177, 238–39
  older adults, 204–5
  overview, history of, 235–37, 247
  principles of, xi, 5–7, 9–10
  psychiatry residency, 241–43, 243f
  psychology, 237–38
  psychosis early intervention, 167
  psychosocial interventions, 190–91
  psychosocial rehabilitation, 241–42, 245
  public psychiatry fellowships (PPFs), 244
  residential care, 202
  social workers, 150, 177–78, 239–41
  TBI staff, 203–4, 203f
  training goals, 245–47
  train-the-trainers model, 253
  veterans, 206–8
  walk-in services, 188–89, 188t
Comprehensive Community Mental
    Health Services for Children and
    Their Families Program, 137
Computer-based searches, 256–57
COMT, 84
Connecticut Latino Behavioral Health
    System (CT LBHS), 218
Connecticut Mental Health
    Center (CMHC)
  addiction medicine, 83
  The Consultation Center, 110–11
  educational programs, 5, 235–36,
      238–39, 242–44
  Hispanic Clinic, 218–20
  history of, ix, 16, 64, 83, 98–99
  integrated health care case study, 74–76
  psychosis early intervention, 156–58
  service system, 2, 21–23
  Wellness Center, 74–76
Connecticut Valley Hospital, 16, 171
Consolidated Appropriations Act of
    2014, 158
The Consultation Center, 110–11
Contingency management, 89, 254t
Continuing care treatment, 189–92, 189t

Coombs, T., 42
Coordinated Specialty Care guidelines,
    163–64, 164t
Crisis intervention teams, 193, 194
*Crossing the Quality Chasm: A New Health
    System for the 21st Century*, 37
Cultural competence
  children, adolescent, young adult
      services, 216
  CLAS standards, 217–18
  concepts, definitions, 212–14
  essential quality metrics, 220, 281
  health, social determinants of, 211–12,
      212t, 219–20, 280
  health disparities, 211, 219
  immigrants, refugees, 215–16, 227–28
  interpreters, 214, 214t
  minority-specific diagnosis, treatment, 215
  overview, 9, 211, 220
  professional associations, 218–19
  service barriers, 214–15
  service delivery history, 216–17
  service delivery models, 217–19
  teaching methods, 219–20
  workforce diversity, 215
Cultural Formulation Interview (CFI), 219
Culturally and Linguistically Appropriate
    Services (CLAS) standards, 217–18

DAT (dopamine transporter), 84
Deegan, P., 34
Deinstitutionalization, 8, 16, 35–36,
    49–50, 98, 115, 171–73, 192, 200,
    216, 224, 249
Demoralization, 216
Department of Mental Health and
    Addiction Services (DMHAS), 20,
    92, 157–58, 217, 244, 252–53, 258
Depression, depressive disorders, 51, 69–
    70, 104, 107, 144t, 228, 252t, 254t
Dexmethylphenidate (Focalin), 144t
*Diagnostic and Statistical Manual, Fifth
    Edition* (DSM 5), 4, 91, 125,
    143, 215
Diagnostic related groupings (DRGs), 99
Dialectical behavior therapy (DBT), 90
DIAMOND model, 70
Disability, 99, 106–8
Disability Adjusted Life Year (DALY),
    99, 107
Disaster preparation, prevention, 108–9
Disulfiram, 87
Dix, D., 16, 34, 171
Doctor of Nursing Practice (DNP), 239
Donaghue Foundation, 158
Dopamine receptor D3/D4, 84

Early Psychosis Prevention and
    Intervention Centre (EPPIC), 156
Education. *see* competencies
Eisenhower, Dwight D., 98
Elderly patients, 204–5
Electroconvulsive therapy, 190
Electronic medical records, 74, 255, 257
Emerging Adults Initiative, 147
Employee unions, 182–83
Employment, education, 50–53, 90, 252t
Enuresis, 144t
Epidemiologic Catchment Area
    (ECA), 97, 99
Epidemiology, psychiatric, 100–101, 101f
Errera Community Care Center, ix
Escitalopram (Lexapro), 144t
Eskalith (lithium), 144t
Estelle, Barefoot v., 124

Evidence-Based Medicine, 256
Evidence-Based Mental Health, 256
Evidence-Based Nursing, 256
Evidence-based practice
  ACT model, 17, 54, 164, 186, 193,
      198–201, 200t, 252t
  children, adolescent, young adult
      services, 143–45, 145t
  cognitive behavioral therapy (CBT), 30,
      66, 89, 160–61, 191, 254t
  computer-based searches, 256–57
  electronic medical records, 257
  fidelity, 253–55, 254t
  history of, 249
  IDDT, 90, 191, 252t
  implementation of, 255–58,
      256t, 280–81
  importance of, 250
  legislative policy, 257–58
  minority-specific, 215
  overview, 10, 249, 258–59
  person-centered care, 37–39, 57, 190,
      213–14, 219, 240, 253
  principles, 250–51
  psychiatry, principles of, 251–53, 252t
  psychosis early intervention, 161t,
      164, 164t
  psychosocial rehabilitation as, 251, 278
  research-enhancing treatment
      outcomes, 91–92
  research funding, 258
  research-informed clinical risk
      assessment, 126–27
  resources, 251–53, 252t, 256
  SAMHSA registry, 251
  training, 253–55, 254t
Excellence in Mental Health Act (EMHA)
    of 2014, 19, 29, 277, 278, 280
Executive Order 13166, 217

FACT programs, 118–21
Family psychoeducation, 54, 145t, 252t
Farmer, P., 218
Federally qualified health centers
    (FQHC), 70, 75, 186–88, 279
Federal Medicaid matching reimbursement
    (FMAP), 17
First-episode services (FES), 158–60,
    162–64, 165t, 169
Fishbone (Ishikawa) diagram, 271
Fluoxetine (Prozac), 144t
Fluvoxamine (Luvox), 144t
fMRI, 91
Forensic psychiatry
  actuarial instruments, 124–25
  ambulatory services, 193
  civil patients, dangerous, 122
  clinical risk assessment, 126–27
  commitment laws, 116–17,
      117f, 123–24
  community treatment, 118–21
  comorbid illnesses, 120
  competency restoration
      patients, 121–22
  conditional release, 124
  confidentiality, 121
  convicted prisoners, 122
  criminal justice collaboration, 120–21
  crisis intervention, 120
  discharge planning, 122, 128–29
  history of, 116–17, 117f
  inpatient units, 121–22
  jail diversion programs, 117–18,
      118f, 193–94
  mental health courts, 117–18, 118f

mental illness/violence
    correlation, 126
  outpatient civil commitment, 119
  overview, 8, 115–16, 129
  patients, oversight of, 122–24
  practice reform effects, 280
  psychopathy, 104, 125–26
  psychotropic medications, 120
  reasonable standard of care,
      128–29, 128t
  risk assessment, 120, 124–27
  risk management consultation,
      127–29, 128t
Forstein, M., 206
Fountain House, 54–55
Four Quadrant Model, 69, 69t
Freud, A., 135
Freud, S., 135
Friedman, R., 137
Friend's Hospital, 16, 116

GABA receptors, 84
Gender expression/identity, 205–6
Genetic risk and functional deterioration
    psychosis risk syndrome (GRD),
    157t, 159
Gesell, A., 134
Global Burden of Disease Study, 107, 225
Global mental health
  capacity building, 226
  essential quality metrics, 229–30
  funding, 228–29
  history of, 224–25
  human rights, 225
  immigrants, refugees, 215–16, 227–28
  overview, 9, 223–24, 230–31
  prevention, 229
  principles of, 226
  public psychiatry benefits, 225–26
  service delivery, 226–29
Goldmark Report, 238
Good Lives Model (GLM), 120
Gordon, R. S., 102
Grand Challenges in Mental Health, 229
Guanfacine (Intuniv), 144t

Hall, G. S., 134
Haloperidol (Haldol), 144t
Hampstead Child Therapy Course/
    Clinic, 135
Harding, C. M., 35
Hare, R., 125
Harrison Act of 1914, 83
Hartford Retreat, 116
Health, social determinants of, 211–12,
    212t, 219–20, 280
Health Care for the Homeless
    Programs, 187
Health Impact Assessment (HIA), 218
Healy, W., 135
Hispanic Clinic, 218–20
HIV/AIDS, 67–68
Hoagwood, K., 142
Hollon, S. D., 251
Home-based intervention, 145t
Homelessness
  competencies, 198–99
  legislative history, 198
  outreach, special populations services,
      198–99, 213
  outreach teams, 194
  practice reform effects, 280
  residential (housing) resources,
      22–23, 27
  in SMI/SUD patients, 198–99, 213

Hospital clinical services
    acute care, 173–74
    ancillary, 175–76
    APRNs, 177, 238
    behavioral intervention teams, 179
    community agencies, 182
    crisis intervention units (urgent care), 174
    discharge planning, 174
    emergency, 174–75
    employee unions, 182–83
    history, 171–73
    interdisciplinary team, 174–80
    long-term, 175
    mental health assistants, 179
    neuropsychological evaluation, 178
    nurses, 177
    overview, 9, 171
    partial hospitalization, 181–82
    patient autonomy, 181
    patients, patient advocates, 179–80
    positive behavioral support plans, 178
    psychiatrists, 176–77
    psychological evaluation, 178
    psychologists, 178–79
    quality metrics, 183–84
    regulatory agencies, 183
    rehabilitation therapists, 177
    social workers, 150, 177–78, 239–41
    systemic challenges in, 182–83
    treatment, recovery plan, 180–81
Housing
    community-based supports, 49–50
    congregate, 50
    custodial, 50
    permanent supportive housing, 50, 252t
    residential care, 50, 201–2
    resources, 22–23, 27
    scattered-site, 50
    supported, 198
Housing and Urban Development Supportive Housing grants, 27
Housing array model, 50
Housing Assistance Fund Program (Connecticut), 27
Housing continuum models, 50
Hypnotics, 86t

Illness Management and Recovery (IMR), 43t, 54, 252t
Imipramine (Tofranil), 144t
Immigrants, refugees, 215–16, 227–28
Improving Mood Promoting Access to Collaborative Treatment (IMPACT) model, 70
Independent Living Movement, 37
Indiana, Jackson v., 123
Indicated interventions, 265
Indicated preventive interventions, 102, 102t
Individual Placement and Support (IPS) model, 51
Inpatient units, 121–22
Insomnia, 254t
Institute of Living, 16
Institutions for mental disorders (IMDs), 16–17
Integrated behavioral couples therapy, 89, 254t
Integrated Dual Disorders Treatment (IDDT), 90, 191, 252t
Integrated health care
    access issues in, 65
    barriers to, 64–65
    challenges to, 75–76, 277

chronic conditions, 66–68
CMHC case study, 74–76
core competencies, 71
effectiveness, 276–77
funding of, 70, 73–75
history of, 64
levels of, 70–71, 71t
medication ADRs, 65
models of, 68–69, 69t
need for, 64
overview, 8, 63–64, 77
patient-centered medical home, 72–74
patient issues in, 65
peer support, 37, 39–42, 53–54, 66
practice reform, 276, 279–81
in primary care, 69–70
principles, 71
psychiatric providers in, 64–66
quality metrics, 76–77
wellness strategies counseling, 65–66
International Association of Peer Supporters, 53
Interpersonal psychotherapy, 254t
Interpreters, 214, 214t
Intuniv (guanfacine), 144t

Jackson v. Indiana, 123
Jail diversion programs, 117–18, 118f, 193–94
Jick, S. S., 105
Johns Hopkins Hospital, 238
Johnson, G., 53
Jones v. US, 123
Juvenile Psychopathic Institute, 135

Kahn, E., ix
Kazdin, A., 142
Kennedy, J. F., 16, 173
Khmaoch sangot, 216
Khyal attacks, 216
Kitchener, J./E., 108
Klein, M., 135
Kleinman, A., 224
Knitzer, J., 136
Knowledge Informing Transformation (KIT), 251, 252t
Koro, 216
Korsakoff, S., 83
Kraeplin, E., ix

L. C. by Zimring, Olmstead v., 123–24
Lambeth Early Onset (LEO) study, 162, 163
Language barriers, 214
Laura Spelman Rockefeller Memorial, 134
Leadership in Public Mental Health Systems, 244
Learning-based recovery, 51–52
Lexapro (escitalopram), 144t
LGBT individuals, 205–6
Life skills training, 54
Lisdexamfetamine (Vyvanse), 144t
Lithium (Eskalith), 144t
LOCUS tool, 28
Logic models, 269–70, 270t
Luvox (fluvoxamine), 144t
Lyons, H. Z., 206

MAOA (monoamine oxidase A), 84
McCabe, O. L., 109
McGlashan, T. H., 156, 161
Mead, S., 53
Medicaid/Medicare
    children, adolescent, young adult services, 136, 143

cost shifting, 27–28
dual eligibility, 25
eligibility expansion, 276, 279
functions of, 19–21, 24–25
history of, xi, 2, 3, 16–18, 29, 192
Home and Community Based Services option, 276
hospital clinical services, 173
low-income adult programs, 25–26, 26f
pay-for-performance systems, 250
peer-delivered services, 39
population health, practice-based, 109–10
reimbursement, 17, 277
service delivery models, 277
Medicaid Rehab Option, 53
Medicaid Supplemental Security Income (SSI), 17
Medical director, 262–63
Medicare Shared Savings Program (MSSP), 277–78
Medication management
    ADRs, 65
    continuing care services, 189–90
    overview, 54
    prescribing, over-prescribing, 255
    psychotropic medications, 120
Medication Treatment, Evaluation, and Management (MedTEAM), 252t
Medline, 42, 43t
Mental health assistants, 179
Mental Health Center Act of 1963, 217
Mental health courts, 117–18, 118f
Mental Health First Aid (MHFA), 108
Mental health Gap Action Programme (mhGAP), 229
Mental Health Impact Assessment (MHIA), 108
Mental Health Integration Program, 70
Mental health intervention spectrum, 103
Mental Health Parity and Addiction Equity Act of 2008, 92, 173, 217
Mental Health Services Act of 1980, 3
Mental Health Study Act of 1955, 173
Mental Health Systems Act of 1980, 17, 136, 186, 276
Mental Retardation Facilities and Community Health Centers Construction Act of 1963, 136, 173
Metabolic syndrome, 64, 66–67, 106, 166, 283
Metformin, 66
Methadone, 87
Methylphenidate, 144t
Migrant Health Centers, 187
Milestone Project, 242
Military sexual trauma, 207–8
Miller, K. E., 228
Miller, W. R., 93
Mindful-based relapse prevention (MBRP), 89
MindMap: A Clear Path to Mental Health, 162
Minkoff, K., 93
Minority Fellowship Program, 217
Mitchell, A., 101, 101f
Morgan, Z., 101
Moses, H., 24
Motivational enhancement therapy, 89–90, 254t
Motivational interviewing, 89–90, 254t
Movement for Global Mental Health, 229
MRI, 91
Multiple family group therapy, 254t
Multisystemic intervention, 145t

Naltrexone, 67, 87
NAPLS, NAPLS 2, 157, 161
National Comorbidity Survey (NCS), 97, 99
National Implementing Evidence-Based Practices project, 254
National Institute of Mental Health (NIMH), 17, 34, 100, 107, 156–58, 163, 216–17, 237, 257, 283
National Mental Health Act of 1946, 172
National Registry of Evidenced-based Programs and Practices (NREPP), 89
National Survey of Substance Abuse Treatment Services (N-SSATS), 92
National Technical Assistance Center for Children's Mental Health, 137
Network for the Improvement of Addiction Treatment (NIATx), 92, 256
Neurobehavioral programs, 203–4
New Freedom Commission report, 18, 28, 33, 99–100, 137, 250, 253, 274–75
New Hampshire–Dartmouth Psychiatric Research Center, 51
Nicotine replacement therapy, 67, 87
Nursing, 177, 238–39

Obama, Barack, 19
Obesity, 64, 66–67
Obsessive-compulsive disorder (OCD), 107, 144t, 164
Office of Minority Health and Health Disparities (OMHD), 217
Olanzapine, 161
Older adults, 204–5
Olmstead v. L. C. by Zimring, 123–24
Omnibus Budget Reconciliation Act (OBRA) of 1981, 186
On Your Own Without a Net (Osgood), 147
Open clinical trials, 251
Opiate addiction, 86t, 87
OPRM1, 84
OPUS study, 162, 163
Oregon, 123–24, 182, 258
Osgood, D. W., 147
Outpatient civil commitment, 119
Outreach, special populations services
    ACT model, 17, 54, 164, 186, 193, 198–201, 200t, 252t
    dual diagnoses/residential treatment programs, 201–2
    homelessness, 198–99, 213
    LGBT individuals, 205–6
    neurobehavioral programs, 203–4
    older adults, 204–5
    overview, 9, 197–98, 208
    traumatic brain injury, 202–4, 203f, 207
    veterans, 198, 199, 206–8

Paliperidone (Invega), 144t
Parent intervention, 145t
Parole, 121
Partial hospitalization, 181–82
Partners in Health, 218
Patient-centered medical homes, 72–74, 277–79
Patient Outcomes Research Team (PORT), 30
Patrick, C., 125
PCL-R, 125–26
Pediatric Research Equity Act (PREA), 143
Peer support, 37, 39–42, 53–54, 66. *see also* community-based supports
Pellens, M., 83
Permanent supportive housing, 50, 252t

Person-centered care, 37–39, 57, 190, 213–14, 219, 240, 253
PET imaging, 91
Pinals, D. A., 194
Pinel, P., 39–40
Pirkis, J., 42
Point-in-time (PIT) counts, 198
Population health, 265–66, 280
Post-traumatic stress disorder (PTSD), 51, 90, 206–7, 216, 228, 254, 254t
Prevention
   disaster preparation, prevention, 108–9
   EPPIC, 156
   global mental health, 229
   indicated preventive interventions, 102, 102t
   mindful-based relapse prevention, 89
   psychosis early intervention, 159, 160, 165–66
   rehabilitation (tertiary prevention), 266
   selective preventive interventions, 102, 102t
   service system services, 22
   US Preventive Services Task Force (USPSTF), 68
Primary and Behavioral Health Care Integration (PBHCI) grants program, 70
Primary Care Access, Referral, and Evaluation (PCARE) trial, 70
Probation, 121
Program for the Prevention of Juvenile Delinquency, 135
Prolonged exposure therapy, 254t
Prozac (fluoxetine), 144t
Psychiatric epidemiology, 100–101, 101f
Psychiatric mental health nurse practitioner (PMH-NP), 238
Psychiatric Rehabilitation Association, 245
Psychiatric security review boards (PSRBs), 123–24
Psychiatric technicians, 179
Psychiatrists, 176–77
Psychiatry residency, 241–43, 243f
Psychologists, 178–79
Psychology training, 237–38
Psychopathy, 104, 125–26
Psychosis early intervention
   benefits of, 165–66
   challenges, clinical considerations, 164–65
   classification, 166–67
   cognitive behavioral therapy (CBT), 30, 66, 89, 160–61, 191, 254t
   Coordinated Specialty Care guidelines, 163–64, 164t
   cultural context, 165
   diagnosis, 157t, 164, 165t
   disease progression mechanisms, 166–67
   duration of untreated psychosis (DUP), 155, 156, 162
   early detection, 162
   engagement in treatment, 167
   essential quality metrics, 168–69, 168t
   evidence-based practice, 161t, 164, 164t
   first break transition, 159
   first-episode services (FES), 158–60, 162–64, 165t, 169
   funding, 167–68
   goals of, 155
   history, 83, 156–58, 157t
   involuntary commitment, 165
   methods, 160–64, 161t, 166–68
   overview, 9, 108, 155–56, 169
   prevention, 159, 160, 165–66
   prodromal phase, 159
   professional development, 167
   psychosis risk syndrome, 159–61, 161t
   risk criteria, 156–57, 157t, 165t
   terminology, 158–59
   timing of, 159
   treatment-related fears, 165
Psychosis Risk Identification, Management, and Education (PRIME), 156–58, 157t, 166
Psychosocial rehabilitation. *see also* community-based supports
   clubhouses, 54–55
   community-based supports, 54–56, 228
   competencies, 241–42, 245
   disability, 99, 106–8
   as evidence-based practice, 251, 278
   history of, 99
   interdisciplinary case management, 54
   life skills training, 54
   need for, 2–4
   nursing in, 177, 238–39
   outpatient services, 236
   overview, ix–x, 49
   service delivery models, 21, 22t, 279
   special populations, 197, 201–2
   VA Interprofessional Fellowship, 236, 243–44
Psychotherapy, individual, 145t
PsycInfo, 42, 43t
Public-academic partnerships, 282–83
Public health concepts
   aggression/violence risk, 103–4
   burden of disease, 3, 99–100, 103, 106–8
   case study, 110–11
   definitions, 98
   descriptive epidemiology outcomes, 103–8, 105f
   disability, 99, 106–8
   disaster preparation, prevention, 108–9
   early intervention, 108
   history, 98–100
   intervention matrix, 102, 102t
   Mental Health First Aid (MHFA), 108
   mental health intervention spectrum, 103
   morbidity, 103–4
   mortality, 103–5, 105f
   outcomes, disparities in, 109
   overview, 8, 97–98
   population health, practice-based, 109–10
   premature death/chronic disease, 105–6
   prevention, 101–3, 102t, 111
   psychiatric epidemiology, 100–101, 101f
   suicide, 102t, 103–5, 105f
Public Housing Primary Care Programs, 187
Public policy, 2, 16–17, 257–58, 281. *see also specific legislative acts*
Public psychiatry
   accountability, 280
   clinical competence in, 4–5
   definitions, 1–2
   departmental division of, 283–84
   education (*see* competencies)
   intellectual dialectics, 274
   overview, 1, 273
   population served by, 2–3
   practice reform, 276, 279–81
   pragmatism in, 274
   quality improvement, 280–81
   readiness screening, 57
   referral procedures, 57
   significance of, 10–11
   as subspecialty, 5
Public Psychiatry Fellowships (PPFs), 244

Quality Chasm report, 268
Quasi-experimental studies, 251
Quetiapine (Seroquel), 144t

RAISE Project, 163
Randomized controlled trials (RCTs), 250–51
Ranz, J., 244
Rapid Risk Assessment for Sex Offense Recidivism (RRASOR), 125
Rasco, L. M., 228
Reagan Administration, 17, 34, 136, 186
Reasonable accommodations, 35
Reasonable standard
   of care, 128–29, 128t
Recovery, recovery-oriented practice
   acute care *vs.* recovery management model, 35–36, 41
   advocacy, 37
   approaches to, 36
   community forensic treatment, 118–21
   definitions, 34–35, 37, 194
   discrimination issues in, 40
   funding for, 34, 35
   history of, 17, 18, 34–35
   learning-based, 51–52
   outcome, quality assessment, 42–43, 43–44t
   outcomes, 39–41, 281
   overview, 8, 33–35, 43–44
   peer support, 37, 39–42, 53–54, 66 (*see also* community-based supports)
   person-centered care, 37–39, 57, 190, 213–14, 219, 240, 253
   principles, 36–37, 49, 253
   psychiatric rehabilitation, 37
   reasonable accommodations, 35
   self-determination in, 38–39
   twelve-step facilitation, 18, 36, 40–41, 54, 87, 90, 93
Recovery After an Initial Schizophrenia Episode (RAISE), 158
Recovery Assessment Scale (RAS), 43t
Recovery-Oriented Practices Index (ROPI), 44t
Recovery Oriented Systems Indicators Measure (ROSI), 44t
Recovery Process Inventory (RPI), 43t
Recovery Promotion Fidelity Scale (RPFS), 44t
Recovery Self-Assessment (RSA), 43, 44t
Recovery to Practice (RTP) initiative, 240
Redlich, F., ix
Reef, J., 101
Refugees, immigrants, 215–16, 227–28
Rehabilitation (tertiary prevention), 266
Reproductive health, 68
Research Domain Criteria, 281
Residential care, 50, 201–2
Residential (housing) resources, 22–23, 27
Results-Based Accountability (RBA), 258
Results First, 258
Risperidone (Risperdal), 144t
Robert Wood Johnson Foundation, 251
Rogers, C., 37
Rosen, A., 42
Ruble, M. W., 206
Running Upstream, 218
Rush, B., 82

Salyers, M., 201
Scale of Prodromal Symptoms (SOPS), 156
Schizophrenia. *see also* psychosis early intervention
   burden of disease, 107
   cancer rates in, 68
   continuing care treatment, 189–90
   functional recovery, 155
   obesity, metabolic syndrome in, 64
   outcomes measurement, 245
   pharmacological treatment, 144t
   psychosocial interventions, 190–91
   recovery, recovery-oriented practice, 35, 51
   risk of violence in, 103–4
Schizophrenia Patient Outcomes Research Team (PORT) project, 245, 255
Section 8 housing assistance, 27
Sedatives, 86t
Seeking Safety, 90
Selective interventions, 265
Selective preventive interventions, 102, 102t
Sequential Intercept Model, 118, 118f
Serious mental illnesses (SMIs)
   aggression/violence risk, 103–4
   ambulatory services (*see* ambulatory behavioral health services)
   burden of disease, 3, 99–100, 103, 106–8
   community supports (*see* community-based supports)
   evidence-based practice, 254t
   homelessness, 198–99, 213
   mental illness/violence correlation, 126
   natural supports, fostering, 54
   overview, 1–3, 10
   patient characteristics, 3
   premature death/chronic disease, 105–6
   recovery (*see* recovery, recovery-oriented practice)
   service system (*see* service system)
   smoking cessation, 67, 68
   work capacity recovery, 51–52
SERT (serotonin transporter), 84
Sertraline (Zoloft), 144t
Service system
   ACA (*see* Affordable Care Act)
   budget cuts in, 28–29
   catchment, 3, 186
   consumer empowerment, consumerism, 31
   cost shifting, 27–28
   delivery models, 277, 279
   features of, 1, 3–4, 8, 15–16
   federal level, 20
   financing of, 23–31, 26f
   health care reform, 17t, 18–19
   history of, 16–19, 17t
   interdisciplinary team in, 23, 31
   local level, 20–22
   mainstreaming, 17–18, 17t
   management, utilization, 28
   overview, 15–16, 31–32
   payer status, 18
   pharmacology, polypharmacy in, 29–30
   prevention services, 22
   rehabilitative programs, 7
   residential (housing) resources, 22–23, 27
   responsibility, accountability, 28
   service delivery models, 20
   skew in, 29–30
   state general funds, 25
   status of, 28–29, 82–84
   structure, components of, 19–23

structure of, 19–20
transformation of, 17t, 18, 30–31, 274–75, 281–82
Sexually transmitted diseases, 67–68
Short-cycle process improvements, 92
Sklar, M., 42
Smith, R., 83
Smoking, 67, 68, 87–89, 88t
Social determinants of health, 211–12, 212t, 219–20, 280
Social formulation, 242
Social Psychiatry Boot Camp, 242
Social Security Amendments of 1965, 136
Social Security Disability Insurance (SSDI), 26
Social skills training, 254t
Social workers, 150, 177–78, 239–41
Society for Clinical Child and Adolescent Psychology, 145
Sociopathy, 104, 125–26
Somatization, 216, 228
Southwick, S. M., 207
Specialized Treatment Early in Psychosis (STEP), 156, 158, 162–63, 166, 169
Special populations. *see* outreach, special populations services
Stages of Recovery Instrument (STORI), 43t
State Children's Health Improvement Plan, 136
State hospitals. *see* hospital clinical services
STEP Early Detection (STEP-ED) study, 162
Stewart B. McKinney Homeless Assistance Act of 1987, 198
Strauss, J. S., 35
Stroul, E., 137
Substance Abuse and Mental Health Services Administration (SAMHSA), 4, 15, 18, 20, 36, 49, 70, 137, 145, 147, 194, 251, 256
Substance use disorders (SUDs). *see also* addiction medicine integration
addiction medicine history, 82–83
ambulatory services (*see* ambulatory behavioral health services)
assessment, 85
burden of disease, 3, 99–100, 103, 106–8
children, adolescent, young adult services, 90, 102
co-existing disorders approaches, 90
cognitive behavioral therapy (CBT), 30, 66, 89, 160–61, 191, 254t
community forensic treatment, 118–21
comorbid factors, 85
definitions, 98
diagnostic interview, 85
disposition/placement, 86–87
education, 93
environmental factors, 85
evidence-based practice, 254t
expenses by payer, 26f
family-focused approaches, 90
fellowship models, 83
genetic factors, 84, 91
homelessness, 198–99, 213
integrated models of, 92–93
intoxication, withdrawal management, 86, 86t
mortality, 103–5, 105f
neurobiology, 84–85
neuroimaging, 91
overview, 1, 2, 81–82
patient characteristics, 3
peer-delivered supports, 41–42
personality traits, 84
pharmacological intervention, 86t, 87
program standards, 92
psychotherapeutic interventions, 89–90
recovery (*see* recovery, recovery-oriented practice)
research-enhancing treatment outcomes, 91–92
resources, 256
service system, 82–84 (*see also* service system)
tobacco, 67, 68, 87–89, 88t
transcriptional, epigenetic mechanisms, 84–85
treatment outcome measurement, 92
treatment selection, 90–91
twelve-step facilitation, 18, 36, 40–41, 54, 87, 90, 93
Suicide, 102t, 103–5, 105f
Sullivan, G., 198–99
Sullivan, H. S., 40
Supplemental Security Income (SSI), 17, 26–27
Supported education, 52–53, 90, 252t
Supported employment, 51, 90, 252t
Supportive Housing (Connecticut), 27
Surgeon General's report, 10–11, 18, 28, 34, 99–100, 105, 109, 173, 194, 213, 217, 250, 253, 275
Syphilis, 67–68

Targeted preventive interventions, 102, 102t
TEAMcare model, 70
Technical Assistance Publications, 256
Telepsychiatry, 227
Terry, C., 83
Thorazine (chlorpromazine), 144t, 171
TIPS study, 156, 158, 162
Tobacco dependence, 67, 68, 87–89, 88t
Tobacco Use and Dependence Clinical Practice Guidelines, 87
Tofranil (imipramine), 144t
Topiramate, 67, 87
Tourette's disorder, 144t
TPH1 (tryptophan hydroxylase 1), 84
Transgender, 205–6
Transinstitutionalization, 99, 116–17, 117f
Traumatic brain injury, 202–4, 203f, 207
Treatise on Insanity (Pinel), 39
Treatment Improvement Protocol 42, 92–93
TRIP database, 256
Tsemberis, T., 201
Twelve-step facilitation, 18, 36, 40–41, 54, 87, 90, 93

United Nations Declaration of Human Rights, 225
Universal interventions, 265
Universal prevention, 102
US, Jones v., 123
US Preventive Services Task Force (USPSTF), 68

VA Connecticut Healthcare System (VACHS), ix, 2
VA Interprofessional Fellowship in Psychosocial Rehabilitation and Recovery-Oriented Services, 236, 243–44
Van Dorn, R., 103
Varenicline, 67, 87
Veterans, 198, 199, 206–8
Veteran's Administration (VA), 2, 39, 199, 236, 237, 254–55, 254t
Violence Risk Assessment Guide (VRAG), 125
Vocational rehabilitation, 51
Vyvanse (lisdexamfetamine), 144t

Walk-in services, 188–89, 188t
Weisz, J., 103
Wellness Center, CMHC, 74–76
Wellness Recovery Action Plan, 53
Wernicke, C., 83
West Haven Veterans Administration (VA) hospital, 235–36
Williamson, T., 201
Wilson, R., 83
Witmer, L., 237
Women veterans, 207–8
Work capacity recovery, 51–52
Workforce development. *see* competencies

Yale Department of Psychiatry, ix–xi, 2, 5, 9–10, 74, 110, 235–37, 242, 244, 282–84. *see also* Connecticut Mental Health Center (CMHC)
Yale-New Haven Hospital (YNHH), ix, 2, 236
Yale School of Nursing, 238–39
Young adults. *see* children, adolescent, young adult services

Zoloft (sertraline), 144t